The Nurse Practitioner in Urology

Susanne A. Quallich • Michelle J. Lajiness
Editors

The Nurse Practitioner in Urology

A Manual for Nurse Practitioners, Physician Assistants and Allied Healthcare Providers

Second Edition

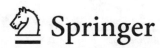

Springer

Editors
Susanne A. Quallich
Department of Urology
Michigan Medicine, University of Michigan
Ann Arbor, MI
USA

Michelle J. Lajiness
Department of Urology
University of Toledo Physicians Group
University of Toledo
Toledo, OH
USA

ISBN 978-3-030-45266-7   ISBN 978-3-030-45267-4   (eBook)
https://doi.org/10.1007/978-3-030-45267-4

This Springer imprint is published by the registered company Springer Nature Switzerland AG
The registered company address is: Gewerbestrasse 11, 6330 Cham, Switzerland

We dedicate this book to all our patients we have worked with in the past. Our patients, especially the most challenging ones, have motivated and inspired us to look to the literature and beyond to help manage their conditions. Their patience with, and perseverance through, their urologic conditions has helped us to become better clinicians.

We also thank the colleagues with whom we have worked with over the years. Many of them have encouraged us, mentored us, and supported us as we pursued explanations to those clinical questions that had unclear answers.

Finally, we would not have succeeded without our families. We offer heartfelt thanks to our families for their support and encouragement (and tech support) in allowing us to spend many hours away from them to encourage our professional growth.

SQ and SL

Introduction

We have been gratified by the response to the first edition of our book and are thankful that its success has enabled us to proceed with a second edition. We continue to be surprised and impressed by the number and skills of nurse practitioners and physician assistants that have chosen to specialize in urology and their enthusiasm for taking care of this group of patients. We have updated this book to include several additional chapters to guide providers; highlights include preoperative and postoperative management, LGBTQ matters in urology, basics of radiology, and an introduction to pain management issues. Urology continues to offer countless opportunities for NPs and PAs to blend medical and surgical care to meet the needs of their patient population.

This book continues to function as a guide giving readers direction about individual GU topics and provide other resources that will help further refine both knowledge and skills from an advanced practice perspective. This book again highlights the pathophysiology, assessment, and diagnoses specific to GU conditions and promotes advanced critical thinking. We still avoid recommending specific medications and in-depth pathophysiology but may address classes of medications as appropriate. This book is not a compendium of specific, detailed treatments for patients with a specific urologic issue—these details can be found in a variety of medical textbooks and journals.

There continues to be a lack of literature that describes or defines the role of NPs and PAs in specialty environments, and urology is no different in this regard. However, for those of us currently working with urology patients, it is clear that we are not only moving into the care of GU patients but excelling in the management of these patients, particularly those diagnoses that need chronic management and are less amenable to surgical solutions. Our colleagues working in urology realize that our roles are not restricted to providing access for general urology concerns, but many specialize in urologic oncology, sexual dysfunction, incontinence, men's health urology, or stone disease.

Nurse practitioners and physician assistants are dynamic, adaptive, and vital providers that contribute to the care and management team of GU patients by improved access, management of chronic GU conditions, and increased patient satisfaction. This is becoming more important as the well-documented shortage of urologists continues, coupled with the continued aging of the US population who will need urologic care services.

We have a combined 40 years of experience as nurse practitioners working in urology, and we have consulted several authors with a variety of specialties. We hope that this book will give the reader insight into the rapidly expanding potential for the NP and PA roles within outpatient and ambulatory care urology. It is our hope that this book will continue to serve as an introduction and guide to nurse practitioners and physician assistants to reach their potential and provide high-quality, cost-effective care for adult urology patients.

Susanne A. Quallich
Division of Andrology, General and Community Health,
Department of Urology,
Michigan Medicine, University of Michigan,
Ann Arbor, MI, USA

Shelley Lajiness
Department of Urology,
University of Toledo Physicians Group
University of Toledo,
Toledo, OH, USA

Contents

Transitioning Pediatric Urology Patients (and Their Families) to Adult Urology Care

1

MiChelle McGarry

Contents

Objectives
1. Define transition care.
2. Illustrate specific barriers to transition care.
3. Discuss specific pediatric genitourinary conditions that require consideration for transition care
4. Provide an overview of the unique care needs as patients transition to adult urology providers

M. McGarry (✉)
Pediatric Effective Elimination, Program Clinic & Consulting, PC, Littleton, CO, USA
e-mail: michelle@peepclinic.com

© Springer Nature Switzerland AG 2020
S. A. Quallich, M. J. Lajiness (eds.), *The Nurse Practitioner in Urology*,
https://doi.org/10.1007/978-3-030-45267-4_1

Introduction

The "official" definition for the age of pediatric patient care is 0–21 years. For many years, children with congenital urological issues received their urology medical care from pediatric urologists for their entire life span, which was usually in their 20s. Modern medicine has extended the life span of this population of children with congenital urologic conditions, and now this group of patients are living well into adulthood and encountering adult urology issues in addition to their congenital urology diagnoses. This ideally means that their care is transitioned to adult urology providers. The universal goals for pediatric urology providers as they care for these patients are to preserve upper and lower tract function, provide for safe urine storage and drainage, and attain and maintain continence, fertility, sexual function, and genital cosmesis, generally in this order. The last three are not necessarily on the minds of patients and parents until adolescence, but still need to be considered in all pediatric surgical and medical decisions throughout the life of the patient. The last three tend to become bigger concerns as the patient ages. The actual transition of care is complex and unique to each child, family, diagnosis, pediatric care given, developmental status, and pediatric urology team. It is the pediatric urology team that bears the responsibility of initiating transition.

Currently, this issue of transition of complex pediatric patients to adult care is being addressed at many levels. Kelleher et al. (2015) describe the issues with transitions of complex pediatric patients to adult care, citing the challenges of spina bifida patients in particular, who require management from urology, neurosurgery, orthopedics, and general medical services well into adulthood. There is guidance for this transition: "Federal Policy Supporting Improvement in Transitioning from Pediatric to Adult Surgical Services" (Kelleher et al. 2015; Box 1.1). Furthermore, the American Academy of Pediatrics (2011) states that "optimal health care is achieved when each person, at every age, receives medically and developmentally appropriate care." The process includes multiple entities, including the patient, family and/or other caregivers, the pediatric and adult providers and support staff, as well as adult and pediatric hospitals and insurance companies and the health-care system as a whole. With the passage of the Patient Protection and Affordable Care Act of 2010 (PPACA), children are able to remain on their parents' insurance until age 26, providing time to identify resources for coverage due to their disability.

Ideally this transition from pediatric to adult care should be a process that aligns with the adolescent developmental process, specifically identity versus role conflict. But there can be many practical obstacles to this actually happening. Developmental delay of the patient, difficulties with the patient taking responsibility, difficulty with the parents relinquishing responsibility, a lack of adult providers knowledgeable and/or desiring to care for these kids as adults, and the reluctance of pediatric urology providers to relinquish their patient's care to adult urology providers can all be factors. Another obstacle is the coordination of other needed medical specialties such as nephrology, PT/OT, orthopedics, neurology, neurosurgery, or endocrinology. In the pediatric hospital model, all these specialties are housed in one system, and electronic medical records facilitate seamless care transitions between specialties. Many institutions promote multidisciplinary clinics where the providers come to the patients, providing not only convenience for the patient and families but also more opportunities for provider to provider communication and continuity of care. This includes access to ancillary team members such as social work, therapeutic play specialists, and pediatric psychologists.

Because this is an emerging, and needed, area of pediatric urology care, there have been many articles, working groups, and research focused on it over the last 5 years. Zillioux et al. (2018) refers to transitional urology care as a new field that he calls "congenitalism." The authors go on to state that "despite the onset of transitional care clinics, these patients remain difficult to care for due to resource availability, insurance coverage, and multi-disciplinary needs." Their article employed a 20-question survey to members of the Society for Pediatric Urology that had a 53% response rate with 124 respondents and 32% identifying a formal transition clinic. The respondents that identified a formal transition clinic also reported higher enthusiasm for caring for this patient population and believed that they gave better care compared to respondents who did not have formal clinics. Interestingly, and likely, one of the biggest issues contributing to difficulty in caring for this population is that 64% of the providers felt that these patients were best cared for by adult specialists, (urology reconstructive or neuro-urology) the care was continuing to be provided by pediatric specialists in 54% of the clinics. The vast majority of clinics described (61%) were in tertiary care centers. These authors noted that the opinion versus the practice concerning the best model for transition clinics of this type still needs work done to establish evidence-based standards.

The Health and Human Services and National Alliance to Advance Adolescent Health Policy to Improve Transitional Care identifies six core elements needed for a transition clinic:

1. Develop practice-specific transition policy
2. Establish criteria to identify patients ready for transition
3. Assess transition readiness beginning at age 14
4. Transition Planning: Identify adult providers, insurance resources
5. Transfer of care should occur in a period of stability
6. At completion of transfer, there should be Peds-Adult feedback.

The generalized definition of transition in health care is the following: A process for ensuring that high-quality, developmentally appropriate health-care services are available in an uninterrupted manner as a patient moves from adolescence to adulthood according to Dr. Mark Rich, Chief of Pediatric Urology at Arnold Palmer Hospital for Children and USF Health, when he presented on this topic at the Advances in Urology in Key West 2017. Another well-taken point from this presentation is that adolescents need transition care in all aspects of life, not just health care. They also need help to manage medication, physicians, knowledge of their medical condition, hospitals, and medical resources. The patients also need help with resources for independent living, education, vocation, insurance coverage, community inclusion, and sexuality.

According to Martinez et al. the incidence of congenital urological diagnoses in the US in 2016 was 5252. This number includes 2765 patients living with spina bifida with an incidence of 7/10,000 live births, 118 exstrophy diagnoses indicating an incidence of 7/100,000 live births, 293 posterior urethral valves diagnoses, an incidence of 1/8000, 790 patients with an anorectal anomaly diagnosis with an incidence of 1/5000, cloaca in 197 patients, an incidence of 1/20,000, 99 patients with prune belly syndrome representing a incidence of 1/40,000, and 790 patients with diagnoses of disorders of sexual differentiation showing an incidence of 1/5000. These 5252 patients will likely represent a disproportionate use of the medical health-care system resources, especially if we are not able to successfully transition these patients to adult care in a proactive process.

Due to reconstruction of the GU tract, facilities need to have pediatric-sized instruments (such as cystoscopes) available at the adult hospital, introducing the need for planning and introducing potential financial impact. Finally, radiologists who are familiar and comfortable with the appearance of genitourinary systems that have been reconstructed are essential.

Box 1.1 The Patient Protection and Affordable Care Act of 2010 Provisions That Benefit Adolescents with Chronic GU Conditions Transitioning to Adult Care

1. Adolescents and young adults are able to remain on their parents' coverage until age 26. This means that youths with chronic medical and surgical conditions will remain insured on commercial plans.
2. Health insurance plans are prohibited from discrimination based on preexisting conditions or health status. Youths that age out of their parents' insurance or purchasing individual insurance will not have any chronic health conditions held against them through denials, higher premium rates, or complete refusal to insure.
3. Annual/lifetime limits on dollars or benefits are excluded in the PPACA.
4. The PPACA sets the minimum Medicaid eligibility for young adults at 133% of the federal poverty level (for those states expanding Medicaid).
5. The PPACA establishes rules and requirements for the availability of insurance exchanges for the purchase of insurance by individuals in each state. These exchanges provide for new coverage of preventive benefits and provide subsidies prorated based on income.

The most pediatric urology issues and diagnoses present very early in life or even prenatally, but they can also arise throughout adolescence. The conditions can be mild to life-threatening and also have a very variable effect on the child's psychosocial well-being depending on the specific disease process and how the family has coped with the disease and its effects. Their success in management depends on the support system in place to help them and the skill of knowledgeable providers.

Lambert (2015) identified the following as impeding the transition process from pediatric to adult urology care to be altering a patient and caregiver paradigm, locating adult urologists with special expertise, coordinating care with other adult specialties such as nephrology, and navigating the adult health-care environment. Another significant barrier is lack of training for urology health-care providers. There are some calling for transitional urology, or congenitalism, to become a subspecialty of pediatric urology (Peters 2016). Dr. Peters also queries an excellent question, *should these providers be primarily pediatric with additional training in adult urology or be adult urologists with additional training in pediatrics?* In either case, the needs of the population also call for the health-care providers to be savvy beyond just the medical care and to assist with resources for independent living, medication management, insurance navigation, etc. And transition needs to be addressed in health-care provider training programs, which it currently is not.

The American Urological Association 2015 Working Group on Urological Congenitalism provided recommendations for the following: management of pregnancy in young woman with bladder exstrophy and one with reflux nephropathy, as well as a young man with spina bifida with chronic kidney disease seeking undiversion. They also stated that given the lack of long-term data for patients with congenital genitourinary diseases, management of complex urological disease in these patients can be difficult. Consensus discussion with urological providers across the spectrum of the life course of these patients may help provide clinical guidance (Eswara et al. 2016).

Another resource is www.gottransition.org, a program of the the National Alliance to Advance Adolescent Health. There are separate sections for patients and families, including a quiz to assess readiness to transition, health-care providers, and researchers and policymakers. The resource page is very comprehensive.

Another very important issue is that of billing and the ability to be paid for providing transitional services. There are some codes that have been added to ICD-10 that can be used for providing transitional care management. Available on the www.gottransition.org website, there is guidance on these billing codes and the requirements to use them. The resource guide is thorough, 28 pages and includes sample vignettes. A future issue with insurance is trying to change the reimbursement to be based on value rather than volume. It is also important to continue to expand reimbursement for time spent for meaningful use activities such as generating medical and clinical summaries. Another reimbursement area that needs to be addressed is that of having both the pediatric and adult providers be able to bill for the time spent transitioning a patient.

Facilities are also essential in this process. Due to reconstruction of the GU tract, facilities need to have pediatric-sized instruments (such as cystoscopes) available at the adult hospital, introducing the need for planning and potential financial impact Finally, radiologists who are familiar and comfortable with the appearance of genitourinary systems that have been reconstructed are essential.

Transitioning

Transition to adult care obviously happens frequently in pediatrics, but one component making the urology transition different is that the conditions are uniquely pediatric and until recently have been cared for solely by pediatric providers. Both cardiology and pulmonology disciplines have led the way in pediatric to adult care transitioning with specialized fellowships. The European model as described at the European Association of Urology (EAU) 25th Annual Congress: Abstract 811 (Presented April 19, 2010) has specialized providers in pediatric to adult care, including in urology. The newness of these transitions in urology can create stress, ambivalence, and resistance among members of the team, with the patient/family feeling fear about a new system that does not know them personally. They may feel they are being abandoned by the people "who saved their child's life," while the pediatric urology team may fear that all they have "fixed" will be undone.

Depending on the child's cognitive level, issues also begin to arise regarding confidentiality, informed consent, and patient/physician decision-making versus patient/physician/family decision-making. These issues are vital in the process of ongoing care and benefit from being addressed at the same time as any physical issues are being addressed. The majority of parents/caregivers who have children with chronic disabilities that involve multiple systems have been fierce advocates for their children. While this is good, for them the process of letting go and having their children become as responsible as possible needs to start early and be directed by the care team. It can become very difficult for these families, and they can feel that they are losing control of their child's health care, which has consumed a large part of their own adult lives.

Subspecialty certification in Pediatric Urology began in 2008 for those urologists whose practice is a minimum of 75% pediatric urology. Applicants approved by the Board to enter the process of subspecialty certification must be engaged in the active practice of pediatric urology and must hold a current unrestricted general certificate in urology issued by the American Board of Urology (http://www.abu.org/subspecialtyCert_PSCOverview.aspx). With the pediatric certificate of added qualification, pediatric urologists must not have non-pediatric patients comprising more than 25% of their work in order for them to keep their specialty qualification. It is essential to note that if adult patients stay in a pediatric practice, there is reduced time to see pediatric patients, meaning that patients must be "aged out" of the pediatric urology practice.

Nurse practitioners (NPs) and physician assistants (PA) are uniquely qualified and positioned to help families with this preparation and transition process owing to their unique knowledge of child development, family systems, and disease processes. This process happens with families primarily through education within the context of the clinic visits, the strength of nurse practitioners. After training as either pediatric or family NPs, the transition to caring for patients within a specialty practice offers the opportunity for NPs to focus their training on the specific needs of pediatric GU patients.

Looking at the generalized process, it is important to start and keep a concise summary of all diagnoses, interventions, and surgical procedures. The actual surgical notes are important as there are different techniques, and which one was used originally and what any revisions were is important to future adult surgical decisions. There should be a notebook for each patient with all of this information for each child that the family/caregiver keeps and is added to with every visit and procedure so that it is complete with all surgical, procedural, and interventional information at transition. This avoids a time-consuming task to review years of care as a family presents for their last visit. A second vital issue is encouraging pediatric GU patients to enroll with a primary care provider; it is more likely for children to have a pediatrician than for adults to be able to identify a primary care provider. This is important, as pediatric providers are not trained or equipped to manage "adult" issues such as smoking prevention and cessation, obesity, type II diabetes, sexuality, birth control, or hypertension as they pertain to the adult patient.

There is a distinct need to develop transition plans for pediatric urology patients to move to adult urology providers. Some facilities have created formal plans that can be adapted to other environments. Since 2016, nearly every tertiary pediatric urology program has developed a transition clinic www.gottransition.org Toronto's Hospital for Sick Kids *Good 2 Go* is another successful program that is available on their website and has materials for transition of care for clinicians, patients, and families. This program is based on a shared management model between family, providers, and the young adult.

Several diagnoses necessitate the transition from pediatric to adult urology care: neurogenic bladder (caused by a variety of diagnoses, one being spina bifida), bladder exstrophy, hypospadias, epispadias, disorders of sex development, posterior urethral valves, cloaca, vesicoureteral reflux, ureteropelvic obstruction, nephrolithiasis, pediatric genitourinary tract cancers, undescended testes, varicoceles, and upper tract anomalies. The remainder of the chapter is a disease-by-disease review of the items for adult care providers to remember, assess, and measure for the most common pediatric genitourinary diseases that will require lifelong care.

Discussion of Specific Pediatric Genitourinary Conditions

Neurologic Conditions

Neurologic conditions include myelomeningocele, tethered spinal cord, cerebral palsy, sacral agenesis and spinal dysraphisms, and Hinman's syndrome (nonneurogenic, neurogenic bladder). Spina bifida is the most common birth defect in the USA (www.spinabifidaassociation.org), but all of these conditions have the potential to be part of a syndrome as well. Males and females with spina bifida are the largest population of persons with urogenital anomalies in the USA. There are many treatment options for them as adults, with clean intermittent catheterization (CIC) being responsible for the marked increase in life expectancy over the last 20 years. Other treatment interventions can include augmentation cystoplasties, botulinum toxin, catheterizable channel creation (Mitrofanoff), anticholinergics and other meds to increase bladder capacity, antegrade continence enema creations (ACE or MACE), and other older types of urinary diversions. The main issue for these patients is the inability to store and release urine safely and in a controlled manner.

The primary goal for the medical team is always protection of the upper tracts, but for patients and families, their goal is likely to be socially acceptable continence. These two goals can be directly opposed to each other at any time during the patient's life span. Due to the reconstructions that they undergo, both to protect upper tracts and to achieve the continence, these patients are at a lifelong risk for true infection that can cause urosepsis (not from colonization due to CIC), nephrolithiasis, stricture of their cathing channel (urethra or surgically created channel; stenosis of a surgically created channel is an expected occurrence), upper tract damage, and bladder cancer. To effectively monitor for the upper tract damage, the most important sequelae to avoid, they need serial urodynamics (with baseline communicated to the adult urology team), renal and bladder ultrasounds, and reassessment of continence, and any change in status also necessitates a spinal cord evaluation for new tethering. Awareness of the presence of a VP shunt and avoidance of infecting this are also essential.

For any child who underwent an augmentation cystoplasty, he/she needs lab work to assess for metabolic acidosis (specifically hyperchloremic acidosis), renal function, and vitamin B12 deficiency (if terminal ileum was used). The other things that the patient (and possibly caregivers) needs to be taught are signs and symptoms of bladder rupture, as well as that not catheterizing increases this risk, bowel obstruction due to adhesions, and bladder stones due to mucous from the bowel mucous settling in the bladder (46% of patients have recurrent bladder stones (Wood 2015). Bladder malignancy is also increased in the population which has had an augmentation. The risk of bladder cancer in patients with bladder augmentations is higher than the general population, but it is unclear if this is related to the augment itself or the underlying disease process (Higuchi et al. 2010). The vast majority of these patients will be on anticholinergics or antimuscarinics, and monitoring for side effects of these medications is essential.

The final considerations for patients with neurologic issues are sexuality and fertility, and these may be best and most appropriately addressed in a transitional setting as the children continue to age. It is also important to review birth control, STD prevention (remember, the risk for latex allergies is increased in pediatric urological patients due to frequent instrumentation; this has been decreasing recently due to early elimination of latex exposure), and sexual abuse prevention, especially considering the cognitive level of the patient.

Many young adult and teen spina bifida patients are sexually active, and healthcare professionals at all levels of care may be faced with issues regarding relationships and sexuality among young adults with spina bifida. Ideally these should be addressed with patients by adult specialists in these areas before sexual activity is initiated. Nevertheless, it is important to establish the information patients already have, even in the pediatric environment; some patients report they have never discussed sexuality issues with a provider and some report they would have discussed these issues if the provider had initiated the topic (Sawyer and Roberts 1999). Males with neurologic GU conditions will have possible issues with erections and retrograde ejaculation, while females will be able to conceive, but body habitus may be an issue and factor into potential delivery concerns as they become pregnant. Female spina bifida patients are less likely to use hormonal contraception and to be using no method of birth control (Cardenas et al. 2010). There is a higher incidence of precocious puberty and premature activation of hypothalamic-pituitary-gonadal axis in spina bifida girls than is seen with their healthy counterparts, and the timing of puberty may be earlier, at 10.9–11.4 years (Trollmann et al. 1998), making this a consideration in their ongoing care.

Obstructive Uropathy

Obstructive uropathy includes some degree of neurogenic bladder; these children are all born with renal disease. Posterior urethral valves are the most common diagnosis in this group and occur exclusively in males. These patients demonstrate some degree of chronic kidney disease, from either primary renal dysplasia or due to the presence of obstruction to urine flow or both of these factors. The initial damage occurs prenatally, and the timing of this directly relates to the severity of the renal involvement and damage, resulting in significant kidney disease present in 13–28% of patients with posterior urethral valves (Holmdahl and Sullen 2005). It is unclear whether timing of valve ablation (ideally done as soon as the valves are known, in the newborn period) changes the degree of renal damage. These patients are at continued risk of incomplete bladder emptying, which may be related to recurrence of or incomplete ablation of these valves, secondary bladder neck obstruction, or side effects of anticholinergic medications.

All of these patients will need routine urodynamic studies and repeat ones for any reported changes. Again, the baseline at transition of care is essential, and patients and their parents may need reminding that preservation of upper tracts is the most essential goal of care. The most common time to see renal deterioration is at and during puberty; the reason and pathophysiology for this is unclear (Ardissino et al. 2012). Blood pressure monitoring, serum creatinine, and urinalyses need to be routinely performed throughout the life span as it is not known if the natural history of end-stage renal disease lasts throughout the life span (Glassberg et al. 2013).

Infertility and retrograde ejaculation in male patient can be an issue, but erectile dysfunction usually is not an issue. Any potential infertility issues should be referred for additional evaluation.

Nephrolithiasis is an increasing pediatric urology issue with the incidence increasing by 6–10% per year and affecting 50 per 100,000 adolescents (Tasian and Copelovitch 2014). Many of these children have a syndrome or lab finding that makes them at high risk, and with adult stone specialists, this may be one of the easiest pediatric urology diseases to transition to adult providers. It becomes more complicated when stones are present in children with complex urological states (such as bladder exstrophy or myelomeningocele) or with metabolic diseases (such as growth delay due to renal issues or decreasing bone density due to reabsorption of urine through a bladder augmentation) with which adult providers may not be familiar (Lambert 2015).

Bladder Exstrophy

Bladder exstrophy and associated epispadias are very complex anomalies and are more and more often diagnosed prenatally, but if not, immediately at birth. These children undergo complex reconstructions that are usually staged; many of these patients require bladder augmentation and the creation of a catheterizable continent channel. Incontinence is a huge quality of life issue as is sexual function and cosmesis. This is due to the widened pubic symphysis creating shortened penile length and ejaculation issues and for women, sexual function, and pelvic organ prolapse. Pregnancy is possible with a higher incidence of preterm birth and a planned C-section at 37 weeks is recommended (Creighton and Wood 2013). Most of these patients are able to live a normal life span, but will continue to have the issues associated with complications of their childhood bladder surgeries such as bladder stones, UTIs, catheterization issues, and continence issues.

Disorders of Sexual Development

Disorders of sexual development and anorectal malformations are another complex group of congenital urogenital disorders. No matter what the specific disease process, these kids require endocrine, psychosocial, and urologic care throughout the life span, and a full discussion is beyond the scope of this book. Congenital adrenal hypoplasia is one of the most common genetic diseases in humans and 21-hydroxylase deficiency is the most common of these (Lambert et al. 2011). Patients with this require long-term steroid and hormone replacement, initially to achieve adult height and pubertal development, but with changing goals in adulthood. Children with congenital adrenal hypoplasia are at risk for infertility and adrenal tumors and so routine renal ultrasounds are indicated. Gonadectomy may be indicated in late adolescence or early adulthood as the incidence of gonadal malignancy in adulthood is 14% (Deans et al. 2012).

Dr. Rick Rink (2013) from Riley Hospital for Children provides the following list of concerns for transitions for patients with disorders of sexual development: sexual function, sexual identity, emotional well-being, concerns regarding intimacy, counseling patient on disclosure of their condition to others, informing the patient of their condition, gender dysphoria, vaginal stenosis, fertility, hormonal deficiencies, steroidal deficiencies, gonadal tumors, endocrine management, gynecological care, mucous-producing neovagina, tumors in neovagina, worsening virilization due to poor adherence to medical therapy, poor cosmesis, and bladder dysfunction.

Pediatric Urologic Cancer Survivors

Children who are genitourinary cancer survivors will have lifelong urologic needs. Adult survivors of genitourinary pediatric cancer (including Wilm's tumor, germ cell tumors, and rhabdomyosarcoma) are at risk for long-term complications and require serial follow-up and surveillance. Children are at risk for complications from chemotherapy and radiotherapy as well as complications and side effects from extirpative and reconstructive operations (Lambert 2015). These will depend on the tumor type and stage, treatment, and reconstructive procedures performed, but will affect multiple organ systems. With an 80% cancer survival rate, the number of childhood cancer survivors is increasing, and National Cancer Institute Surveillance Epidemiology and End Results estimates 1 in every 250 young adults will be child-hood cancer survivors (Howlader et al. 2011). Of nonprogression, nonrecurrent causes of mortality, second malignancies are the leading cause of death among long-term childhood cancer survivors (Rink 2013).

Fertility is also a likely issue for these patients and something that pediatric providers need to address in any age-appropriate child (meaning at or approaching adolescence), as egg and sperm collection and storage are widely available, but these services are dependent on the developmental age of the child. Patients and their family must be offered information regarding these services and can be directed to organizations such as the American Society for Reproductive Medicine or Resolve in addition to information regarding facility or local services.

Congenital Kidney and Urinary Tract Anomalies

Vesicoureteral reflux, ureteropelvic junction obstruction, multicystic dysplastic kidney disease, ureterovesical junction obstruction, ectopic ureteral insertion, renal ectopia, duplicated collecting systems, ureteroceles, or a solitary kidney make up a broad diagnosis group of congenital kidney and urinary tract anomalies. These can vary greatly in severity and thus have wide-ranging impacts on adult life and consideration upon transition from pediatric to adult care. Children with chronic kidney disease require lifetime follow-up to prevent progression of the disease and monitor for early signs of renal deterioration (Mertens et al. 2008). The long-term effects of these varied congenital anomalies range in severity from none to end-stage renal disease. Many patients with these diagnoses need comanagement by urology and nephrology.

Hypospadias is a common complaint and surgical case in pediatric urology practices. The incidence is approximately 1 in 200–300 live male births (Lambert 2015). This condition encompasses a wide range of severity with the most mild being a mega meatus and the most severe with a perineal urethral meatus and/or penoscrotal transposition. The goals of correction are a normal urinary stream from an ortho-topic urethral meatal position, prevention/correction of chordee, satisfactory cosmesis, and preservation of future ability to have intercourse. Unfortunately, at times, even a simple appearing repair can need grafting and multiple surgeries resulting in scarring, poor function, and poor cosmesis. All of these issues can be magnified during puberty with penile and scrotal growth. Some of the complications that can occur at any time are urethral stricture, chordee, persistent hypospadias, urethral diverticulum, cosmesis issues, voiding dysfunction, and sexual function issues (Rink 2013).

Varicoceles and cryptorchidism are two other pediatric urologic issues that require long-term education and adult follow-up; both can be repaired surgically and both have a potential to contribute to male-factor infertility in adulthood. Varicoceles in adolescent boys are repaired for indications including pain, testicular asymmetry, or abnormal semen parameters (which can be a challenge to obtain in pediatric patients).

The undescended testicle should be repaired and brought into the scrotum as soon as is reasonably safe; this is determined by discussion with pediatric anesthesia. This correction of an undescended testicle can take one or more surgeries, depending on the position of the testicle, so that the patient can more effectively perform testicular self-examination, to facilitate identification of a potential neoplasm. The incidence among men with an undescended testicle is approximately 1 in 1000 to 1 in 2500 (Misseri 2013). Although significantly higher than the risk among the general population (1:100,000), it does not warrant removal of all undescended testicles, and there are times when the neoplasm is actually on the contralateral side to the undescended testicle. As adults, these men must be reminded of their need for follow-up periodically with ultrasounds.

Summary

The goals of attaining preservation of kidneys and upper tracts, safe and effective urine storage and elimination, continence, sexual function, fertility, and genital cosmesis can only happen throughout the life span with planned and coordinated transitions from pediatric to adult urologic care. This takes time and is not simply saying "here are your records; your next appointment should be with an adult urologist." This approach is destined to fail pediatric patients for whom all on the pediatric urology team have worked diligently, usually throughout the patient's entire life to date, to achieve the abovementioned goals.

The obstacles that have been outlined include the need to shift patient/caregiver paradigms, locating and encouraging adult urologists with interest in these complex and challenging patients to take them into their practices, providing adult urologists' and other adult urology team providers' appropriate support from the pediatric team, coordinating care with other necessary specialists, and navigating the adult health-care world. These issues must be negotiated and overcome to provide exemplary care for complex pediatric urology patients as they transition to become complex adult urology patients.

Clinical Pearls
- Children should transition to adult-oriented health care between ages of 18 and 21.
- Adult specialists and subspecialists may not be prepared for the medical and social support needs of young adults with a history of multiple surgeries in the setting of chronic or uncommon GU conditions.

- Patients may need significant support, especially relative to medical decision-making, as they transition to more independence from parents.
- Patients need to be encouraged to be actively involved in their own health care as they transition.
- Development of a checklist can be helpful. Include a medical summary, a transition readiness skill assessment, plan of care, and legal documents (if needed for young adults with special health-care needs).

Resources for the Nurse Practitioner

Kelleher K, Deans KJ, Chisolm DJ (2015) Federal policy supporting improvements in transitioning from pediatric to adult surgery services. In: Seminars in pediatric surgery, vol 24(2), pp 61–64. WB Saunders.

Resources for the Families

The Urology Care Foundation, the official foundation of the American Urological Association has resources for the transition process including handouts, podcasts, and video clips. These are all directed to patients and families.

References

American Academy of Pediatrics (2011) American academy of family practice, american college of physicians, transitions clinical reporting group, Cooley WC, Sagerman PJ. Supporting the health care transition from adolescence to adulthood in the medical home. Pediatr 128: 182–199

Ardissino G et al (2012) Puberty is associated with increased deterioration of renal function in patients with CKD: data from the ItalKid project. Arch Dis Child 97(10):885–888. https://doi.org/10.1136/archdischild-2011-300685

Cardenas DD, Martinez-Barrizonte J, Castillo LC, Mendelson S (2010) Sexual function in young adults with spina bifida. Curr Bladder Dysfunct Rep 5(2):71–78

Creighton SM, Wood D (2013) Complex gynecological and urological problem in adolescents: challenges and transition. Postgrad Med J 89:34–38

Deans R, Creighton DM, Liao LM, Conway GS (2012) Timing of gonadectomy in adult women with complete androgen insensitivity CAIS: patient preferences and clinical evidence. Clin Endocrinol 76:894–899

Eswara JR, Kielb S, Koyle MA et al (2016) The recommendations of the 2015 american urological association working group on genitourinary congenitalism. Urol 88:1–7

Glassberg K, Van Batvia JP, Combs AJ (2013) Posterior urethral valves: transitional care into adulthood. Dialogues Pediatr Urol 34(4):5–20

Higuchi TT, Granberg CF, Fox JA, Husmann DA (2010) Augmentation cystoplasty and risk of neoplasia: fact, fiction and controversy. J Urol 184(6):2492–2496. https://doi.org/10.1016/j.juro.2010.08.038. Epub 2010 Oct 18

Holmdahl G, Sullen U (2005) Boys with posterior urethral valves: outcome concerning renal function, bladder function and paternity at ages 31 to 44 years. J Urol 174:1031

Howlader N, Noone AM, Wladron W et al (2011) SEER cancer statistics review 1975–2008. National Cancer Institute, Bethesda. Based on November 2011 SEER data submission, posted to the SEER website. http://www.seercancergov/csr/1975-2008

http://www.abu.org/subspecialtyCert_PSCOverview.aspx. Accessed 13 Jul 2015

Kelleher K, Deans KJ, Chisolm DJ (2015) Federal policy supporting improvements in transitioning from pediatric to adult surgery services. Semin Pediatr Surg 24(2):61–64. https://doi.org/10.1053/j.sempedsurg.2015.01.001. Epub 2015 Jan 8

Lambert SM (2015) Transitional care in pediatric urology. Semin Pediatr Surg 24(2):73–78

Lambert SM, Snyder HM, Canning DA (2011) The history of hypospadias and hypospadias repairs. Urology 77(6):1277–1283

Mertens AC, Liu Q, Neglia JP et al (2008) Cause-specific late mortality among 5-year survivors of childhood cancer: the Childhood Cancer Survivor Study. J Natl Cancer Inst 100:1368–1370

Misseri R (2013) Transition into adulthood: concerns and considerations for the pediatric urologist. Dialogues Pediatr Urol 34(4):2–3

Peters CA (2016). Tope stories in urology: the transition to transitional urology. Urol 17(10):71

Rink R (2013) DAD, transitions and my concerns. Dialogues Pediatr Urol 34(4):6–8

Sawyer SM, Roberts KV (1999) Sexual and reproductive health in young people with spina bifida. Dev Med Child Neurol 41(10):671–675

Tasian E, Copelovitch L (2014) Evaluation and medical management of kidney stones in children. J Urol 92:1329–1336

Trollmann R, Strehl E, Wenzel D, Dörr HG (1998) Arm span, serum IGF-I and IGFBP3 levels as screening parameters for the diagnosis of growth hormone deficiency in patients with myelomeningocele—preliminary data. Eur J Pediatr 157:451–455

Wood (2015). http://www.springer.com/us/book/9783319140414

Zillioux, JM, Jackson, JN, Herndon CDA et al (2018) Caring for urologic transition patients: Current practice patterns and opinions. J pediatr urol 14(3);242–e1

Testosterone Deficiency Evaluation, Management, and Treatment Considerations

2

Kenneth A. Mitchell

Contents

K. A. Mitchell (✉)
Meharry Medical College Physician Assistant Sciences Program, Nashville, TN, USA
e-mail: kmitchell@mmc.edu

© Springer Nature Switzerland AG 2020
S. A. Quallich, M. J. Lajiness (eds.), *The Nurse Practitioner in Urology*,
https://doi.org/10.1007/978-3-030-45267-4_2

Objectives
1. Define testosterone deficiency based on clinical and laboratory evaluation
2. Discuss other clinical conditions that have a relationship with low testosterone levels
3. Review treatment options and monitoring schedules for available testosterone products

Introduction

Hypogonadism is a medical term for decreased functional activity of the male gonads. In humans, the gonads (ovaries or testes) produce hormones (testosterone, estradiol, antimullerian hormone, progesterone, inhibin B, activin) and gametes (eggs or sperm) (Yialamas and Hayes 2003). In 2018, an expert panel assembled by the American Urological Association, Inc., (AUA) published a guideline for the Evaluation and Management of Testosterone Deficiency. In their deliberations, and in an effort to be more scientifically accurate, the panel agreed to cease usage of the term hypogonadism and proceed henceforth with the term testosterone deficiency (TD). The panel defined the index patient for TD as having low testosterone levels <300 ng/dL *and* associated signs or symptoms (Mulhall et al. 2018).

Signs and symptoms can vary and may include decreased libido, fatigue, erectile dysfunction, loss of body and facial hair, decreased bone mineral density, increased body fat, decreased lean muscle mass, weakness, depressed mood, sleep disturbance, and anemia. Prevalence of TD in men aged ≥45 years visiting primary care practices in the United States is estimated to be approximately 38.7%. Further evidence indicates that there is a higher prevalence of TD in men with obesity, diabetes, hypertension, rheumatoid arthritis, hyperlipidemia, and osteopenia/osteoporosis (Mulligan et al. 2006). Testosterone therapy (TTh) preparations have been available to clinicians as a medical therapy since the 1930s; however, testosterone replacement therapy was relatively uncommon until the last 15–20 years, at which point prescription rates began to increase at a rapid rate. The increase in prescribing TTh is attributed to a combination of factors, including pervasive consumer marketing increasing awareness of TD as a treatable condition, numerous published studies documenting benefits of TTh, and decreased concern regarding safety risks, particularly prostate cancer (Morgentaler et al. 2014).

Evaluation of Hypogonadism

Initial evaluation of men with hypogonadism should include a comprehensive medical history to assess the presenting symptoms and identify any associated comorbidities. Patients with one or more objective symptoms of hypogonadism (Table 2.1) should undergo a complete physical examination to identify gynecomastia and the presence of secondary sex characteristics (decreased body hair (pubic/axillary),

Table 2.1   Clinical presentation of testosterone deficiency

Physical	Psychological	Sexual
Anemia	Decreased mood	Decreased spontaneous
Decreased bone mineral density	Diminished energy, sense of	erections
Decreased muscle mass and	vitality, or well-being	Difficulty achieving
strength	Impaired cognition and	orgasm
Enlarged liver/elevated LFT's	memory	Diminished libido
Fatigue		Erectile dysfunction
Frailty		
Gynecomastia		
Increased body mass index (BMI)		
Insulin resistance		
Sleep disturbances		

decreased beard growth). Examination of the testes will the size, symmetry and consistency of the testicles (adult testes are ovoid, approximately 3 cm (Anterior/Posterior) × 2–4 cm (transverse) × 3–5 cm (length), with a volume of 12.5–19 mL); size of the testes decreases with age. A full examination also includes prostate examination and Body Mass Index (BMI) (Kim et al. 2007; Bhasin et al. 2010; Petak et al. 2002).

Laboratory testing parameters vary between the published guidelines; however, all agree that a morning total testosterone level by a reliable assay confirmed by repeat measurement should be obtained to confirm a diagnosis of testosterone deficiency. Men with total testosterone values near the lower limit of normal, or in men at risk for SHBG abnormality (e.g., older men, men with obesity, diabetes mellitus, chronic illness, liver disease, or thyroid disease) should have additional lab testing. This can include serum LH and FSH levels to distinguish between testicular failure and hypothalamic-pituitary disruption, especially in the context of a desire for ongoing fertility.

Use of the quantitative Androgen Deficiency in Aging Males (qADAM) questionnaire can help initiate a conversation about any symptoms the patient may have, help identify patients with a high probability of having testosterone deficiency, quantify the severity of testosterone deficiency in older men, and monitor symptom relief in response to treatment (Mohamed et al. 2010).

Testicular Failure (Primary Hypogonadism or Hypogonadotropic Hypogonadism)

Testicular failure, historically known as primary hypogonadism, is caused by failure of the testicles to produce testosterone or sperm due to various etiologies. Specifically, testicular failure is characterized by low serum total testosterone and elevated LH and FSH concentrations. Testicular failure is commonly attributed to testicular injury, tumor, infection (e.g., mumps orchitis), genetic defects (e.g., Klinefelter syndrome), chemotherapy, radiation therapy, and alcohol abuse (Petak et al. 2002; Seftel 2006).

Hypothalamic-Pituitary Disruption
(Secondary Hypogonadism)

Hypothalamic-pituitary disruption is characterized by low serum testosterone and low or normal LH concentrations; levels in men with hypothalamic-pituitary disruption (HPD) may be below the normal range or in low-normal range, but notable in relation to the low serum testosterone. In men when HPD is suspected, further evaluation includes measurement of serum prolactin, pituitary function testing, and often magnetic resonance imaging (MRI) of the pituitary gland.

In men with testicular failure of unknown etiology and a physical examination yielding low testicular volume or absent testes, obtaining a karyotype to exclude Klinefelter syndrome (47-XXY male) is recommended with potentially a scrotal ultrasound to confirm presence of testicular tissue. Men with Klinefelter syndrome can benefit from genetic counseling and need surveillance for certain disorders (Table 2.2) for which they are at increased risk (Dean et al. 2015; Dobs and Matsumoto 2009).

Infertility

Contemporary best practice indicates that an endocrine evaluation should be suggested when there is: (1) an abnormal semen analysis (sperm concentration less than 10 million/ml); (2) impaired sexual function (such as ED or ejaculatory issues); or (3) clinical findings suggestive of a specific endocrinopathy. In men being evaluated for infertility and/or suspected testosterone deficiency, the Endocrine Society Guidelines and the AUA publication, "The Optimal Evaluation of the Infertile Male: AUA Best Practice Statement" both recommend performing an endocrine evaluation on all infertile males. The initial hormonal evaluation consists of measurements of serum follicle-stimulating-hormone (FSH) and serum total testosterone concentrations. If the testosterone level is low, a repeat measurement of total and free testosterone (or bioavailable testosterone), serum luteinizing hormone (LH), and prolactin levels should be obtained. Two seminal fluid analyses separated by an interval of several weeks should be performed. The sample should be evaluated

Table 2.2 Klinefelter syndrome complications

Physical conditions	Psychological conditions	Sexual dysfunction
Breast cancer	Anxiety disorders	Erectile dysfunction
Cardiovascular disease	Depression	Infertility
Metabolic syndrome	Emotional and behavioral disorders	
Obesity	Impulsivity disorders	
Osteoporosis	Low self-esteem	
Peripheral vascular disease	Social phobias	
Rheumatoid disorders		
Periodontal disease		

within 1 h of ejaculation and after at least 48 h of abstinence for consideration with the patient's hormonal data. The relationship of testosterone, LH, FSH, and prolactin helps to identify the specific clinical condition (Table 2.3). A normal serum FSH level does not guarantee intact spermatogenesis; however, an elevated FSH level even in the upper range of "normal" is considered suggestive of compromise to the capacity for spermatogenesis (Yialamas and Hayes 2003; Jarow et al. 2010). Additional discussion of male fertility is presented in Chap. 26.

Testosterone Deficiency-Associated Comorbidities

Testosterone deficiency (TD) has been associated with several common diseases or conditions. The HIM study noted the calculated odds ratios for conditions associated with TD and noted a correlation with known causes of erectile dysfunction, TD, and the top 10 leading causes of death in men (Table 2.4). To date it has not been conclusively determined that low testosterone levels are a consequence of the disease, connected with disease etiology, or have an identifiable and proven causal relationship. Further randomized controlled trials will be needed to determine if treating the TD is likely to improve the patient's identified disease symptoms.

Table 2.3 The relationship of testosterone, LH, FSH, and prolactin with clinical condition

Clinical condition	FSH	LH	Testosterone	Prolactin
Normal spermatogenesis	Normal	Normal	Normal	Normal
Hypothalamic pituitary disruption (HPD)	Low	Low	Low	Normal
Abnormal spermatogenesis	High/normal	Normal	Normal	Normal
Testicular failure (TF)	High	High	Normal/low	Normal
Prolactinoma	Normal/low	Normal/low	Low	High

Table 2.4 Male sexual health correlates

Causes of ED	Top 10 leading causes of death for men	Hypogonadism
Alcohol & drug abuse	Accidents	Asthma/COPD
Coronary artery disease (CAD)	Cancer	Diabetes
Diabetes	Diabetes	Hyperlipidemia
Hormonal problems	Heart disease (CAD)	Hypertension
Hypertension	Homicides	Obesity
Infections	Liver disease (cirrhosis)	Osteoporosis
Injuries	Lung disease (COPD)	Prostate disease
Nerve damage (RRP, MS, Parkinson's)	Pneumonia	
Stress, depression & anxiety	Stroke	
	Suicide	

Hypogonadism and Cardiometabolic Syndrome

Testosterone deficiency (TD) is associated with dyslipidemia (including low HDL and triglycerides), hypertension, obesity, diabetes mellitus, and insulin resistance. Testosterone has an inverse relationship with body mass index (BMI), waist circumference, low density lipoprotein, and triglycerides (Ebeling 2008; Shabsigh et al. 2005; Nettleship et al. 2009), but it has not been established that TD is the cause of or the consequence of these conditions. Physiologically, an increase in adiposity in adult males contributes to aromatization of testosterone in adipose tissue and results in elevated in estradiol and adipokine production in some men, in turn causing suppression of the hypothalamic-pituitary secretion of LH. This causes decreased testosterone production by Leydig cells in the testicles, and contributes to increased insulin resistance, further inhibiting testosterone production by Leydig cells (Aso 2008; Kapoor et al. 2005).

Experts reviewed the literature in search of evidence to support the claim that TRT increased cardiovascular risk. The researchers published their findings indicating that there were no studies conducted that produced conclusive evidence to support the claim that testosterone replacement therapy increased cardiovascular risk. Moreover, the data discovered by the researchers indicated that TRT in testosterone-deficient men decreased the risk of cardiovascular disease.

Testosterone Deficiency and Diabetes

The National Diabetes Statistics Report (Centers for Disease Control and Prevention 2017) reported that 15.3 million men (13.8–17.0, 95% CI) or 12.7% (11.5–14.1, 95% CI) had either diagnosed or undiagnosed diabetes in the United States. The estimated number of adult males aged ≥ 18 years of age reported as prediabetic was 44.5 million (40.5–48.7, 95% CI) or 36.9% (33.6–40.4, 95% CI), while the percentage of men aware of their prediabetes was 9.4% (6.6–13.3, 95% CI). Low testosterone concentrations occur in some men with type 2 diabetes, clinicians should be aware of the relationship between low testosterone and diabetes. Dhindsa et al. (2004) were the first to measure free testosterone and establish hypogonadism as a feature of type 2 diabetes in men (Dhindsa et al. 2004).

Diabetic men in the HIM study were twice as likely to be testosterone-deficient compared with a nondiabetic man (Mulligan et al. 2006). Overall prevalence of TD in diabetic men has been estimated at 33–50% (Dhindsa et al. 2004; Dandona et al. 2008), suggesting that TD is commonly seen with men diagnosed with type 2 diabetes.

The TD in type 2 diabetes is predominately the result of hypothalamic-pituitary disruption; there has been proven relationship between the degree of hyperglycemia and testosterone concentration (Tomar et al. 2006). However, markers of systemic inflammation (such as C-reactive protein) are commonly elevated in men with hypothalamic-pituitary disruption and type 2 diabetes. Concentrations of C-reactive protein in can be twice as high as those in eugonadal type 2 diabetics whose C-reactive protein levels are already elevated compared with nondiabetics. Men with elevated C-reactive protein have also been identifies as mildly anemic, osteopenic in the arms and ribs, and with increased adiposity compared with eugonadal type 2 diabetics (Bhatia et al. 2006; Dhindsa et al. 2007; Mascarenhas et al. 2017).

Interestingly, these findings are markedly like testosterone-deficient patients without diabetes; low testosterone concentrations can predict the development of type 2 diabetes. According to the NHANES III survey, men in the lowest free testosterone tertile were four times as likely to have diabetes as those in the highest free testosterone tertile (Selvin et al. 2007). However, studies have not determined a firm association with Type 1 diabetes and TD, suggesting that TD is specifically related to pathophysiologic features of type 2 diabetes and not specifically to hyperglycemia (Tomar et al. 2006).

Testosterone Deficiency, Obesity, and the Metabolic Syndrome

Obesity in adult men had a prevalence of 34.3% as reported by the 2011–2014 NHANES review (Ogden et al. 2015). Adults who have a body mass index (BMI) between 25 and 29.9 kg/m^2 are classified overweight, whereas adults with a BMI of 30 kg/m^2 or higher is considered obese. But BMI does not directly measure body fat, so people who have increased muscle mass may have a high BMIs even though they are not overweight, and may be quite lean.

The increased health risks associated with obesity have been well established, and include type 2 diabetes, hypertension, atherosclerotic diseases and coronary heart disease. Up to 83% of diabetic patients are overweight or obese (Ogden et al. 2015), and there is a clear association with obesity, low total testosterone, and reduced SHBG levels. There is also an inverse linear relationship between total testosterone, BMI, and free testosterone concentrations that decreases with increasing BMI. There also exists an inverse relationship between serum total and free testosterone concentrations and central obesity. Authors have confirmed that degree of hypogonadism is positively correlated to the degree of obesity in men with elevated BMI (Kapoor et al. 2005; Dandona et al. 2008).

Metabolic syndrome is a constellation of interrelated risk factors of metabolic origin—*metabolic risk factors*—that appear to directly promote the development of atherosclerotic cardiovascular disease (ASCVD). A patient with metabolic syndrome has three of these five risk factors: elevated waist circumference (≥102 cm (≥40 in.)); hypertension (≥130/80 mmHg) or antihypertensive drug treatment in a patient with a history of hypertension; reduced HDL (<40 mg/dl in males) or on drug treatment for reduced HDL; raised triglycerides (≥150 mg/dl) or on drug treatment for elevated triglycerides; and an elevated fasting plasma glucose (≥100 mg/dl) or on drug treatment for elevated glucose (Grundy et al. 2005). Men with metabolic syndrome are at increased risk for developing type 2 diabetes mellitus, and are additionally at high risk for developing coronary heart disease; there may also be an identifiable prothrombotic state and a pro-inflammatory state.

The elements of metabolic syndrome themselves have been correlated with testosterone concentrations, suggesting that TD is also associated with the metabolic syndrome, as has been shown in epidemiological studies (Morgentaler et al. 2015; Traish et al. 2009).

During the testosterone-deficient state, men are subject to increased deposition of abdominal adipose tissue containing high concentrations of aromatase; this increased aromatase activity starts greater formation of estradiol from testosterone. This conversion then further reduces both serum and tissue testosterone concentrations, increases deposition of abdominal fat, and creates progressive testosterone deficiency. Leptin, the adipocyte-secreted protein product of the *ob* gene may be a factor; it has been linked to obesity, and regulates weight and adipose tissue mass. Serum leptin levels correlate positively with age, BMI, serum insulin and fat mass and inversely with testosterone. Leptin levels are higher in aging males with lower testosterone; testosterone replacement therapy corrects this, although the precise mechanism is unclear, but may be related to the reduction in adipose tissue mass and direct suppression of *ob* gene expression (Foley 2019).

Estradiol negatively feeds back on the HPG system, reducing testosterone production by Leydig cells. Increasing adipose tissue also increases insulin resistance, which negatively impacts the Leydig cells as well as inhibiting the release of luteinizing hormone (LH) via the release of adipokines (inflammatory cytokines) such as TNF-a. Leptin, released in response to increased adiposity, also inhibits the release of LH via its effect on the release of gonadotropin-releasing hormone (Pivonello et al. 2019). As a result, testosterone-deficient, obese men with diabetes mellitus are at further risk of poor glycemic control, creating risk for the increased risk of development of complications of diabetes and an increased mortality risk.

Testosterone therapy has a role in ameliorating cardiometabolic risk. In a recent observational study conducted by the VA, participants were evaluated to establish the role of testosterone in improving overall mortality (Kapoor et al. 2005). Over the 4-year period of the study, overall mortality decreased by 10.3% in the treated group and 20.7% in the untreated group (Kapoor et al. 2005). In men with type II diabetes, researchers showed that over a 6-year period, all-cause mortality was 19.2% in untreated men and 8.4% in men treated with TRT (Muraleedharan et al. 2013).

Testosterone Deficiency and Opiates

The opioid crisis in the United States is attributed to increased use of prescription and illegal long-acting opioids such as heroin, methadone, morphine, fentanyl, oxycodone, and tramadol for both recreational use and for the treatment of chronic pain.

A lesser-known sequela of chronic use of opioids is opioid-induced androgen deficiency (OPIAD) or opioid-induced hypogonadism (OIH). Symptoms and side effects will happen with different duration and doses in each individual, suggesting that any male patient who has been using opioids for pain control be screened for hypogonadism. This syndrome is often associated with reduced libido, erectile dysfunction, fatigue, hot flashes, depression, mood alterations, and reduced quality of life (Basaria et al. 2015). These alterations in the hypothalamus-pituitary-gonadal (HPG) axis induced by exposure to opioids result in hypogonadotropic hypogonadism. Physical findings in men can include reduced facial and body hair, anemia, decreased muscle mass, weight gain, and osteopenia or osteoporosis (Raheem et al. 2017). Men taking opioid therapy equivalent to 100 mg of morphine daily should be monitored for development of hypogonadism (Brennan 2013). Identifying men who present with symptoms of hypogonadism must involve screening for current, past, or potential use of any opiates regardless of strength or potency (Howell et al. 1999; Daniell et al. 2006; Hashim et al. 2020).

Other Clinical Conditions

Testosterone Deficiency and Cancer Treatment

Men undergoing cancer treatment are at risk for developing testosterone deficiency (TD). Virtually all nonsurgical cancer treatment creates risk for changes to testosterone: radiation treatments, chemotherapy, corticosteroid, and opiates for pain can impair Leydig cell function or cause germinal epithelial failure and result in hypothalamic-pituitary disruption (HPD).

HIV
Testosterone deficiency in HIV+ men is strongly associated with AIDS wasting syndrome; 20–50% of HIV-infected men receiving highly active antiretroviral therapy may be testosterone-deficient. This is multifactorial in nature and includes testicular atrophy caused by opportunistic infection, HPG axis disruption due to malnutrition, and the effects of anti-mitotic medications that inhibit steroid biosynthesis. Testosterone replacement therapy (TRT), will increase in lean muscle mass, improve mood, and perceived well-being (Grinspoon et al. 1996, 1998, 2000).

Testosterone Deficiency and Hepatitis C
Hepatitis C Virus (chronic) infection is the most common bloodborne disease, according to analysis of the National Health and Nutrition Estimates Survey (NHANES). From 2013 to 2016, there were an estimated 4.1 million individuals living in the US who are HCV antibody positive and 2.4 million individuals who were HCV RNA positive representing, or approximately 1% of all US adults (Hofmeister et al. 2019). The CDC estimates that approximately three-fourths of all persons living with HCV infection in the United States were born during 1945–1965; this corresponds with the high HCV incidence (new infections) that occurred among young adults in the 1970s and 1980s, with 50% of those infected were unaware of their infection status (CDC 2017). Populations most at risk for HCV infection include persons who are currently or previously incarcerated, homeless, nursing home residents, hospitalized individuals, and individuals previously or currently on active military duty.

Hepatitis C virus (HCV) and hepatic dysfunction are associated with low total and free testosterone (TT and FT) and high sex hormone-binding globulin (SHBG) and are considered extrahepatic manifestations of chronic HCV infections.

Researchers conducted a large prospective study evaluating patients with active HCV infections or HCV/HIV coinfection who received treatment for HCV infections designed to yield a sustained virologic response (SVR). At baseline, the researchers observed the patients to have higher total testosterone (TT) and sex hormone binding globulin (SHBG) compared to patients who had achieved SVR. Interestingly, there was no statistical difference in FT between the groups. Further observation showed participants with SVR had a lower TT than those with active HCV; however, lower FT was observed to be nearly equal between groups (50% active HCV, 43% SVR). Study participants with longitudinal determinations showed significant decreases in TT and SHBG while FT remained unchanged post-SVR. Low FT persisted after SVR (pretreatment 58%, post SVR 54%). Researchers concluded that during active HCV infection, TD may be masked due to elevated SHBG and noted that despite patients reaching SVR and decreased SHBG post-treatment, low FT levels persisted (Chaudhury et al. 2019). This study clearly indicates the need to conduct careful evaluation and management of patients with HCV infection in either the active or posttreatment phases of the disease. Men that present with testosterone deficiency symptoms who are at high risk for HCV infection should be screened for HCV. Initiation of testosterone replacement therapy (TRT) in persons treated for HCV infection should be monitored carefully due to the variable effect on the levels of TT, FT, and SHBG.

Osteopenia and Osteoporosis

Osteoporosis remains largely underdiagnosed in males, mainly due to the infrequency of screening and controversies in BMD testing standards in men. Using the WHO diagnostic criteria, it is estimated that 1–2 million men in the US have osteoporosis and an additional 8–13 million have osteopenia (Gennari and Bilezikian 2007). Using data from 2002, researchers estimated that about 25% of the male Medicare population had osteoporosis based on 2002 data (Blume and Curtis 2011). In men with severe testosterone deficiency with or without low trauma fracture, measurement of bone mineral density by dual-energy x-ray absorptiometry (DEXA) scanning is also recommended (Bhasin et al. 2010; Mascarenhas et al. 2017). Because testosterone stimulates bone formation and inhibits bone resorption that involve both androgen and estrogen receptor-mediated processes, older men are at greater risk of low trauma fracture (Mascarenhas et al. 2017; Jackson et al. 1992; Ebeling 2008).

Diagnosis

There is no consensus establishing an absolute testosterone level below which a man can unequivocally be stated to be hypogonadal. The Endocrine Society recommends 300 ng/dl as a reliable level to consider as the lower threshold, while the American Association of Clinical Endocrinologists (AACE) suggests 200 ng/dl. Total testosterone represents the total of free, SHBG-bound, and albumin-bound testosterone.

The Endocrine Society recommends that the diagnosis of TD be made in men who have consistent signs and symptoms and low total testosterone levels. Serum total testosterone is the easiest and most common initial laboratory measurement to lead to a diagnosis of TD. Initial evaluation can include total and free testosterone, followed by a second confirmatory lab measurement. Testosterone is subject to circadian and circannual rhythms; lab values in the morning are recommended for accuracy. Most clinic and hospital laboratories can provide total testosterone measurements of good accuracy and reliability. Free testosterone may be more reliable to correlate with symptoms of TD due to variability in sex hormone binding globulin (SHBG). SHBG levels are easily affected by many conditions like diabetes, obesity, HIV infection, HCV infection, or the normal consequence of aging.

Total testosterone measurements may be misleading indicators of TD due to elevated or depressed levels of SHBG (Table 2.5). Obese or elderly men are not uncommonly seen in routine clinical practice; therefore it is prudent not to rely on total testosterone concentrations for diagnosing TD for these patients. It is important that clinicians use reliable laboratories and are aware of the lab reference ranges for testosterone. Where possible, calculate free testosterone reliably by using total testosterone, albumin, and SHBG concentrations using an online calculator (http://www.issam.ch/freetesto.htm) or smartphone app (T Calc, ViralMD). Some labs can accurately perform a free testosterone measurement by equilibrium dialysis.

As with total testosterone measurements, there is no general agreement as to what constitutes the lower limit of normal free testosterone levels; however, the Endocrine Society recommends 50 pg/ml for free testosterone measured by equilibrium dialysis and the ISA, ISSAM, EAU, EAA and ASA recommend 65 pg/ml for calculated free testosterone. The ISA/ISSAM/EAU/EAA/ASA guidelines recommend that subjects with total testosterone levels falling between 230 and 350 ng/dl (8–12 nmol/l) could benefit from having a repeat measurement of total testosterone with a measurement of SHBG concentrations, in order to calculate free testosterone levels, or free testosterone levels can be measured directly via equilibrium dialysis (Wang et al. 2009a, b).

Determining whether a patient has testicular failure or hypothalamic pituitary disruption (HPD) can be determined by measuring the serum LH and FSH. Elevated LH and FSH levels suggest testicular failure; low or low-normal LH and FSH levels suggest HPD. Normal LH or FSH levels with low testosterone suggest primary defects in the hypothalamus and/or the pituitary (secondary hypogonadism).

Table 2.5 Conditions that affect SHBG levels

Increased SHBG	Decreased SHBG
HIV	Opioids
Liver disease	Androgens
Hyperthyroidism	Hypothyroidism
Estrogens	Nephrotic syndrome
Anticonvulsants	Glucocorticoids
Low testosterone	Acromegaly
Age (1%/year)	Obesity

Treatment

Testosterone replacement therapy is indicated in men with primary or secondary hypogonadism (TF or HPD). The goal of testosterone replacement therapy is to treat the signs and symptoms of TD and achieve and maintain eugonadal serum testosterone levels. FDA approved testosterone replacement treatments are numerous and varied in their routes of administration and duration of action (Table 2.6), but access may be limited by an individual's insurance. The eugonadal range for adult men has been considered in most studies to be in the range of 300–1000 ng/dl (the AACE recommends 280–800 ng/dl), and it is usually considered best to aim for a testosterone level in the mid-normal range, avoiding excessive supraphysiologic peaks (Dean et al. 2015; Petak et al. 2002).

Intramuscular Injections

Testosterone injections have been available for at least 50 years and are usually the least expensive choice for treatment. The testosterone esters, testosterone enanthate or cypionate, are either administered in the office or self-administered at home by the patient or a caregiver. Injected testosterone esters reach peak concentration within 2–5 days after the injection, causing the serum testosterone levels to rise to supra-physiological levels followed by a gradual decline into the hypogonadal range by the end of the dosing interval (Shoskes et al. 2016). The usual frequency of injections is once every 10–14 days; peak serum testosterone levels can be reduced by decreasing the dose and/or frequency of injections to once a week.

Common side effects seen are variable and can include:

- breast tenderness,
- increase or decrease in sexual activity,
- emotional lability (anger or depression),
- and general well-being followed by fatigue as the testosterone levels change over time.

Men who are sensitive to injectable testosterone and report mood and sexual function changes in relation to time of dosing and duration of action may benefit from lower doses given more frequently and slowly titrated upward in dose with a reduction in frequency.

Testosterone undecanoate (Aveed™) is a long-acting depot preparation that carries some similar side effect profile as shorter acting injectable preparations. However, due to a reported increased risk of pulmonary oil microembolism (POME), clinicians in the United States are required to undergo Risk Evaluation and Mitigation Strategy (REMS) training prior to obtaining authorization to prescribe testosterone undecanoate. It also has a specific monitoring schedule (Table 2.7).

Clinicians have recently recommended subcutaneous injections as an alternative to intramuscular administration of testosterone cypionate and testosterone

Table 2.6 Testosterone preparations

Formulation	Dosage	Adverse effects	Benefits
Topical/transdermal			
Androgel 1%®, Androgel 1.62%®, Testim®, Fortesta®2%	5–10 g per day	Skin irritation, transference	Maintain T level concentration over a 24-h period High patient adherence
Transdermal patch Androderm®	2–4 mg patch QD	Skin irritation Transference	T levels mimic circadian rhythm Low incidence of polycythemia
Topical solution Axiron®	60–120 mg applied to axilla QD	Skin irritation Transference	Maintain T levels over 24-h period Unique administration presumed to minimize risk of transference
Buccal/oral			
Buccal system Striant®	30 mg q 12 h	Alterations in taste and irritation of gums and oral mucosa	Testosterone levels within physiologic range
Fluoxymesterone Halotestin®	5–40 mg daily	Hepatotoxicity	Pill form
Injectable			
Testosterone Cypionate Depo-Testosterone®	50–400 mg IM Q 10–14 days	Mood fluctuations or changes in libido, pain at injection site, excessive erythrocytosis	Effective in relieving symptoms, inexpensive
Testosterone Enanthate Delatestryl® Xyosted™	50–400 mg IM q 1 week 75–150 mg SQ weekly	Mood fluctuations or changes in libido, pain at injection site, excessive erythrocytosis	Effective in relieving symptoms, inexpensive Effective in relieving symptoms, auto-injector
Testosterone Undecanoate Aveed®	750 mg IM initial followed by second injection 4 weeks later, then Q 10 weeks (REMS certification required)	Mood fluctuations or changes in libido, pain at injection site, excessive erythrocytosis, pulmonary oil microembolism (POME)	Effective in relieving symptoms, inexpensive, long acting
Implantable			
Testopel® 75 mg pellets	6 pellets* implanted Q 3–4 months	Pain at insertion site, infection, expulsion, pain at insertion site, infection, expensive, requires OV	Long acting, convenient, consistent delivery for a prolonged period of time (3–6 months)

*Men may benefit from more or fewer pellets; 6 is listed a starting point for treatment. This number may also be limited by insurance.

Table 2.7 Testosterone undecanoate dosing schedule and monitoring

Week	Injection	Lab*	Office visit	Rationale
Testosterone undecanoate—initial series				
1	X			
4	X			
6		X		Monitor that loading dose was sufficient at 6 weeks (day 42)
14	X			
16		X		Check if reached steady state after 14 weeks (day 70) based on the pharmacokinetics statement: (*Steady state serum testosterone concentration was **achieved with the third injection of at 14 weeks***)
18			X	Review labs and assess symptoms
24	X			
34	X			
44	X			
54	X	X		
56			X	Review labs and assess symptoms. If stable order continued series of testosterone undecanoate injections
Testosterone undecanoate—continued series				
Initial	X			
10	X			
20	X	X		Routine monitoring
30	X			
40	X	X		
42			X	Review labs and assess symptoms. If stable order continued series of testosterone undecanoate injections

*Suggested

enanthate. This has been noted to produce stability of serum testosterone concentrations in individuals receiving subcutaneous testosterone injections in female-to-male (FTM) gender transition. Mean levels of total and free testosterone were stable and remained in the therapeutic range between injections (McFarland et al. 2017). Typically, patients receiving subcutaneous testosterone injections require lower doses than the typical IM dose. Currently there is one commercially available FDA approved testosterone subcutaneous injection (testosterone enanthate, Xyosted®).

Transdermal Patches

Transdermal testosterone patches are applied directly to the skin each night, and approximate normal circadian plasma testosterone concentrations. The first available testosterone patches were applied to the scrotum due to the 40-fold higher rate of absorption than the forearm; these are rarely prescribed as compliance is low due to the need to keep the scrotum clean-shaven to better ensure adherence of the patch.

More commonly used transdermal patches are applied once daily to the back, abdomen, thighs, or upper arms, preferably in the evening. Skin irritation is a common side effect of these delivery systems, making absorption unpredictable in some men. In cases of significant skin irritation, a preapplication of a weak corticosteroid cream to the skin can help reduce the skin irritation.

Transdermal Gels and Solutions

The most commonly prescribed therapy after injections are transdermal gels and solutions, and are usually applied in the morning. Gel preparations currently available in 1%, 1.62%, and 2% concentrations, whereas topical solutions are available in a standardized 30 mg of testosterone per pump actuation. Application sites for the gel products include the upper arms and shoulders, front and/or upper inner thigh, or the abdomen, while topical solutions are applied to the axilla. Advantages of topical gels and solutions are their relative ease of use, lower incidence of skin irritation, consistent delivery, and dosing flexibility.

Several reported issues with gels and solutions are related to transference from patient to partner or family member, particularly a child. Patients should be instructed to take necessary precautions to minimize the risk of transference by washing their hands with soap and water after applying the gel or solution, covering the application site with clothing after the gel or solution has dried, and by washing the application site when skin-to-skin contact is expected. Patients should also be given further instruction regarding proper and secure storage of the gel or solution to avoid accidental application of the gel or solution to a woman or child.

Buccal Tablets

These are adhesive tablets containing testosterone that are applied to the gum just above the incisor teeth. They release testosterone slowly, allowing for absorption through the gum and cheek surfaces and bypass first-pass hepatic metabolism. The tablet must remain in the mouth for a full 12 h, and two are needed for the 24 h dosing period. The incidence of adverse effects is low, although gum and buccal irritation and alterations in taste have been reported (Dandona 2010).

Subcutaneous Pellets

These are among the earliest effective formulations for administering testosterone, dating back to the 1940s. Although not frequently used, they remain available. The testosterone pellets are usually implanted under the skin of the lower abdomen using a trochar and cannula or are inserted into the gluteus muscle. Six to ten pellets are implanted at one time and they last 4–6 months, when a new procedure is required to implant more. Testosterone pellets currently are the only long-acting testosterone treatment approved for use in the United States. As a result of their long-lasting effect and the inconvenience of removing them, it is best to use pellets in men for whom the beneficial effects and tolerance for testosterone replacement therapy have already been established.

Oral Testosterone Tablets or Capsules

There are no FDA-approved orally ingested testosterone preparations currently available in the U.S. Concerns with hepatotoxic side effects and the development of liver tumors seen with previously available orally ingested testosterone preparations. Clinicians may encounter men who travel from other countries using oral preparations that are available in other areas of the world.

Contraindications and Precautions

The most important contraindications related to TRT are for prostate and breast cancer (Table 2.8). There is controversy surrounding testosterone's role in prostate cancer disease development, progression, and recurrence. However, due to the suspicion of "feeding a hungry tumor" with androgens is widely accepted, and no evidence to completely support or refute this claim have been elucidated, it is recommended that clinicians proceed with caution in these populations.

The evidence is much clearer regarding male breast cancer and the role testosterone plays in the development and progression of male breast cancer; men with breast cancer should never take testosterone because it causes breast cancer cells to grow (Osterberg et al. 2014). Testosterone is also contraindicated in pregnant or breast-feeding women, and children.

Further recommendations include performing a baseline digital rectal examination (DRE) and a baseline PSA level measurement before starting testosterone therapy for any man, regardless of age. Clinicians must inform and instruct patients on topical preparations to use the previously mentioned precautions to minimize transference to pregnant or breastfeeding women, or children.

Table 2.8 Contraindications and precautions with testosterone replacement therapy

Contraindications	Precautions
Male breast cancer	Benign prostatic hyperplasia (BPH)
Prostate cancer (known or suspected)	Lower urinary tract symptoms (LUTS)
Known or suspected sensitivity to	Eedema in patients with preexisting cardiac, renal,
ingredients used in the medication itself	or hepatic disease
	Gynecomastia
	Precipitation or worsening of sleep apnea
	Azoospermia
	Testicular atrophy

Monitoring Treatment

Once testosterone replacement therapy has started, patients need to be carefully monitored. The Endocrine Society recommends a PSA and DRE be performed initially and repeated during the course of treatment (Table 2.9). The clinical response to testosterone therapy typically occurs as early as 1 month up to 3 months; serum testosterone levels and hematocrit should be measured at baseline and at 1 and 3 months after initiating therapy. The clinical response of testosterone should be evaluated by assessing the serum testosterone levels, PSA levels, performing a DRE and correlating the testosterone levels with symptom relief. Should patients decline any part of this periodic evaluation, the providers is advised to clearly document which portion was declined by the patient. PSA levels and DRE can be performed at the recommended age and clinical history appropriate intervals thereafter. Any elevations in PSA should prompt the clinician to consider discontinuing testosterone replacement and either refer or conduct the recommended urological evaluation for elevated PSA. From then on PSA levels need to be checked according to the usual guidelines for prostate cancer screening.

Testosterone is a known stimulant of erythropoiesis and carries a 3–18% risk with elevated hematocrit values above 54% should prompt reduction or discontinuing TRT until the hematocrit decreases into the normal range; alternatively, men can be sent for phlebotomy while the hematocrit is monitored. Persistent elevations in hematocrit should prompt consideration for referral to a hematologist/oncologist for further evaluation.

Bone mineral density measurement can be carried out at baseline because TD is an important cause of male osteoporosis, although there is lack of consensus as to whether this is under the domain of urology or should be referred back to primary care for evaluation and management as needed. BMD measurement in a male with osteopenia/osteoporosis or low trauma fracture can be repeated in 1–2 years after testosterone replacement therapy is initiated (Bhasin et al. 2010; Mascarenhas et al. 2017).

Table 2.9 Endocrine Society Guidelines for the monitoring of testosterone therapy

	Start of treatment (baseline)	Each visit	3 Months	Annually	1–2 Years
Symptom response		√	√	√	
Adverse events		√	√	√	
Formulation-specific AEs		√			
Testosterone levels	√		√		
Hematocrit	√		√	√	
BMD of Lumbar spine Femoral neck					√
DRE	√		√		
PSA	√		√		

Men with benign prostatic hyperplasia (BPH) with or without lower urinary tract symptoms (LUTS) treated with androgens are at an increased risk for worsening of signs and symptoms of BPH and/or LUTS, especially in the first 6 months after staring treatment. While it is widely accepted that development of BPH requires androgens, studies have failed to show an association with testosterone treatment. Prostate volume has been shown to increase during TRT; however, this is usually to the normal volume seen in eugonadal men. Men may experience irritative voiding symptoms and should be counseled regarding the possible development of and/or worsening voiding symptoms (Wang et al. 2009a, b; Rhoden and Morgentaler 2004).

Testosterone Deficiency and Prostate Cancer

Use of testosterone replacement therapy (TRT) in men with prostate cancer remains controversial, although studies have shown that TRT can decrease the overall mortality risk in testosterone-deficient men with or without prostate cancer. Historically, it has been widely accepted that testosterone may potentiate the growth of prostate cancer cells resulting in the recommendation that TRT not be utilized or be used with extreme caution in men with a known diagnosis of prostate cancer regardless of treatment. However, recent data has provided evidence supporting that there is no increased risk of progression or recurrence of prostate cancer in men treated or untreated with a confirmed diagnosis of prostate cancer (Khera et al. 2009; Kaplan et al. 2015).

More recent data suggest that TRT may be safe in men with a known history of prostate cancer; however, researchers concluded that more studies are needed. Further evidence has shown low-serum testosterone levels has been associated with a greater risk of prostate cancer and higher grade of disease (Khera 2015). Furthermore, the rate of prostate cancer progression and recurrence in men treated for prostate cancer tends to be lower in hypogonadal men treated with TRT than in those men not treated with TRT. Contemporary data suggests that TRT may be protective against the development and recurrence of prostate cancer; the prostate saturation model explains the changes in prostate specific antigen (PSA) in response to TRT and androgen deprivation therapy (ADT) to treat prostate cancer.

Societal Issues

In cities across the nation, "Low T" centers have been established to treat men with presumed TD. Many of these establishments provide suboptimal evaluations, and often initiate inappropriate treatment which often leads to adverse reactions. Clear communication between the clinician and the patient is necessary to prevent unrealistic expectations about the benefits of testosterone replacement therapy.

Further clarification is important for both the clinician and the patient to understand the difference between testosterone *supplementation* and testosterone *replacement* therapy. Testosterone supplementation involves the addition of testosterone where the levels of testosterone are already in the normal range. This practice is recognized in bodybuilders or athletes to increase muscle mass or accelerate recovery from injuries. Testosterone replacement is the act of restoring abnormally low or deficient testosterone levels into the normal range.

Patient counseling defining these terms and the expected treatment outcomes is essential to helping the patient understand the true benefits of testosterone replacement therapy while setting realistic evidence-based treatment expectations. Clinicians should counsel patients with TD to make appropriate lifestyle modifications that support normal androgen production (such as weight loss) and/or improve response to therapy. Improving nutrition, increasing exercise, and decreasing or discontinuing medications contributing to TD will also support improvement in endogenous testosterone production and symptom relief.

Conclusion

Advanced Practice Providers (APP) caring for men with TD must be able to accurately diagnose, treat, and manage these patients effectively. The increased prevalence of TD and subsequent surge in treatment has forced experts to establish effective guidelines for the evaluation and treatment of hypogonadism. The International Society for Sexual Medicine (ISSM) guidelines, and most recently the AUA Guidelines on Evaluation and Management of TD, provide the most comprehensive and current data pertinent to patients who are more likely to present to a urology practice (Morgentaler et al. 2015). The ISSM guidelines contain information and guidance regarding patients with urologic disease including recommendations for patients with prostate cancer and benign prostatic hypertrophy (BPH). The ISSM guidelines also address the controversy surrounding cardiovascular risk associated with testosterone replacement therapy. Researchers further concluded that randomized controlled trials will be critical to accurately determine the efficacy and safety of testosterone replacement therapy with or without significant comorbidities.

Clinical Pearls

- The goal of testosterone replacement therapy is to treat the signs and symptoms of hypogonadism, and achieve and maintain eugonadal serum testosterone levels
- Men who participate in pain management programs, or are on long-term (>3 months) opioid therapy, should be screened for low testosterone.
- Men who are both diabetic and obese are at increased risk for low testosterone.
- The increased prevalence of TD and subsequent surge in treatment has forced experts to establish effective guidelines for the evaluation and treatment of TD.
- There are mixed opinions regarding free testosterone or bioavailable testosterone (BAT) measurements in all men other than healthy lean young men whose SHBG levels are presumably normal and whose measured total testosterone concentration is expected to be unaffected.
- Diminished libido and sexual function complaints are sensitive for the indication of hypogonadism.

- No thromboembolic events have been reported with men on testosterone replacement therapy.
- There is no increased risk for prostate cancer for men on testosterone replacement therapy.

Resources for Clinicians

Online free testosterone calculator: http://www.issam.ch/freetesto.html
    Smartphone apps: T Calc, ViralMD
    Men's Health Month: www.menshealthmonth.org/
    American Academy of Family Physicians curriculum for Men's Health http://www.aafp.org/dam/AAFP/documents/medical_education_residency/program_directors/Reprint257_Men.pdf

Resources for Patients

The Urology Care Foundation: www.urologyhealth.org
    Men's Health Network (MHN): www.menshealthnetwork.org
    Men's Health Month: www.menshealthmonth.org

References

Aso Y (2008) Cardiovascular disease in patients with diabetic nephropathy. Curr Mol Med 8(6):533–543
Basaria S, Travison TG, Alford D, Knapp PE, Teeter K, Cahalan C et al (2015) Effects of testosterone replacement in men with opioid-induced androgen deficiency: a randomized controlled trial. Pain 156(2):280–288. https://doi.org/10.1097/01.j.pain.0000460308.86819.aa
Bhasin S, Cunningham GR, Hayes FJ et al (2010) Task Force, Endocrine Society. Testosterone therapy in men with androgen deficiency syndromes: Endocrine Society clinical practice guideline. J Clin Endocrinol Metab 95(6):2536–2559. https://doi.org/10.1210/jc.2009-2354.x
Bhatia V, Chaudhuri A, Tomar R et al (2006) Low testosterone and high C-reactive protein concentrations predict low hematocrit in type 2 diabetes. Diabetes Care 29:2289–2294
Blume SW, Curtis JR (2011) Medical costs of osteoporosis in the elderly Medicare population. Osteoporos Int 22(6):1835–1844
Brennan M (2013) The effect of opioid therapy on endocrine function. Am J Med 126(3):S12–S18
CDC (2017) Surveillance for viral hepatitis—United States 2016. https://www.cdc.gov/hepatitis/statistics/2016surveillance/index.htm
Centers for Disease Control and Prevention (2017) National Diabetes Statistics Report, 2017. Centers for Disease Control and Prevention, U.S. Dept of Health and Human Services, Atlanta, GA
Chaudhury CS, Mee T, Chairez C, McLaughlin M, Silk R, Gross C, Kattakuzhy S, Rosenthal E, Kottilil S, Stanley TL, Hadigan C (2019) Testosterone in men with chronic hepatitis C infection and after hepatitis C viral clearance. Clin Infect Dis 69(4):571–576
Dandona P, Dhindsa S, Chaudhur A, Bhatia V, Topiwala S, Mohanty P (2008) Hypogonadotrophic hypogonadism in type 2 diabetes, obesity and the metabolic syndrome. Curr Mol Med 8(8):816–828

Dandona P (2010) Testosterone concentrations in diabetic and nondiabetic obese men. Diabetes Care 33(6):1186–1192

Daniell HW, Lentz R, Mazer NA (2006) Open-label pilot study of testosterone patch therapy in men with opioid-induced androgen deficiency. J Pain 7:200–210

Dean JD, McMahon CG, Guay AT et al (2015) The International Society for Sexual Medicine's process of care for the assessment and management of testosterone deficiency in adult men. J Sex Med 12(8):1660–1686

Dhindsa S, Prabhakar S, Sethi M et al (2004) Frequent occurrence of hypogonadotropic hypogonadism in type 2 diabetes. J Clin Endocrinol Metab 89:5462–5468

Dhindsa S, Bhatia V, Dhindsa G et al (2007) The effects of hypogonadism on body composition and bone mineral density in type 2 diabetic patients. Diabetes Care 30:1860–1861

Dobs A, Matsumoto A (2009) Klinefelter Syndrome. J Clin Endocrinol Metab 94(12):f2

Ebeling PR (2008) Osteoporosis in men. N Engl J Med 358(14):1474–1482

Foley J (2019) Driving expression of leptin. Sci Signal 12(578):eaax7601

Gennari L, Bilezikian JP (2007) Osteoporosis in men. Endocrinol Metab Clin N Am 36(2):399–419

Grinspoon S, Corcoran C, Lee K et al (1996) Loss of lean body and muscle mass correlates with androgen levels in hypogonadal men with acquired immunodeficiency syndrome and wasting. J Clin Endocrinol Metab 81:4051–4058

Grinspoon S, Corcoran C, Askari H et al (1998) Effects of androgen administration in men with the AIDS wasting syndrome. A randomized, double-blind, placebo-controlled trial. Ann Intern Med 129:18–26

Grinspoon S, Corcoran C, Stanley T et al (2000) Effects of hypogonadism and testosterone administration on depression indices in HIV infected men. J Clin Endocrinol Metab 85:60–65

Grundy SM et al (2005) Diagnosis and management of the metabolic syndrome: an American Heart Association/National Heart, Lung, and Blood Institute Scientific Statement. Circulation 112:2735–2752. https://doi.org/10.1161/CIRCULATIONAHA.105.169404

Hashim MA, El Rasheed AH, Ismail GAW, Awaad MI, El Habiby MM, Mohsen Ibrahim NM, Abdeen MS (2020) Sexual dysfunction in tramadol hydrochloride use disorder male patients: a case-control study. Int Clin Psychopharmacol 35(1):42–48

Hofmeister MG, Rosenthal EM, Barker LK, Rosenberg ES, Barranco MA, Hall EW, Edlin BR, Mermin J, Ward JW, Ryerson AB (2019) Estimating prevalence of hepatitis C virus infection in the United States, 2013–2016. Hepatology 69(3):1020–1031

Howell SJ, Radford JA, Ryder WD, Shalet SM (1999) Testicular function after cytotoxic chemotherapy: evidence of Leydig cell insufficiency. J Clin Oncol 17:1493–1498

Jackson JA et al (1992) Estradiol, testosterone, and the risk for hip fractures in elderly men from the Framingham Study. Am J Med Sci 304(1):4–8

Jarow J, Sigman M, Kolettis P, Lipshultz L et al (2010) The optimal evaluation of the infertile male: AUA best practice statement. American Urological Association. http://www.auanet.org/guidelines/male-infertility-optimal-evaluation-(reviewed-and-validity-confirmed-2011)

Kaplan AL et al (2015) Testosterone replacement therapy in men with prostate cancer: a time-varying analysis. J Sex Med 12(2):374–380

Kapoor D et al (2005) Androgens, insulin resistance and vascular disease in men. Clin Endocrinol 63(3):239–250

Khera M (2015) Testosterone replacement therapy: controversies versus reality. Grand Rounds in Urology. http://www.grandroundsinurology.com/TRT-Mohit-Khera-testosterone-replacement-therapy-controversies-versus-reality/. Accessed 27 June 2017

Khera M et al (2009) Testosterone replacement therapy following radical prostatectomy. J Sex Med 6(4):1165–1170

Kim W, Rosen MA, Langer JE et al (2007) US MR imaging correlation in pathologic conditions of the scrotum. Radiographics 27(5):1239–1253. https://doi.org/10.1148/rg.275065172

Mascarenhas MR et al (2017) Effects of male hypogonadism treatment on the bone mineral density. Endocr Abstr 49:EP1083

McFarland J, Craig W, Clarke NJ, Spratt DI (2017) Serum testosterone concentrations remain stable between injections in patients receiving subcutaneous testosterone. J Endocr Soc 1(8):1095–1103

Mohamed O, Freundlich RE, Dakik HK, Grober ED, Najari B, Lipshultz LI, Khera M (2010) The quantitative ADAM questionnaire: a new tool in quantifying the severity of hypogonadism. Int J Impot Res 22(1):20–24. https://doi.org/10.1038/ijir.2009.35

Morgentaler A, Khera M, Maggi M, Zitzmann M (2014) Commentary: who is a candidate for testosterone therapy? A synthesis of international expert opinions. J Sex Med 11(7):1636–1645

Morgentaler A, Miner MM, Caliber M, Guay AT, Khera M, Traish AM (2015) Testosterone therapy and cardiovascular risk: advances and controversies. Mayo Clin Proc 90(2):224–251

Mulhall JP, Trost LW, Brannigan RE, Kurtz EG, Redmon JB, Chiles KA, Lightner DJ, Miner MM, Murad MH, Nelson CJ, Platz EA, Ramanathan LV, Lewis RW (2018) Evaluation and management of testosterone deficiency: AUA guideline. J Urol 200(2):423–432

Mulligan T, Frick M, Zuraw Q, Stemhagen A, McWhirter C (2006) Prevalence of hypogonadism in males aged at least 45 years: the HIM study. Int J Clin Pract 60(7):762–769. https://doi.org/10.1111/j.1742-1241.2006.00992.x

Muraleedharan V et al (2013) Testosterone deficiency is associated with increased risk of mortality and testosterone replacement improves survival in men with type 2 diabetes. Eur J Endocrinol 169(6):725–733. https://doi.org/10.1530/EJE-13-0321

Nettleship J et al (2009) Testosterone and coronary artery disease. In: Advances in the management of testosterone deficiency, vol 37. Karger Publishers, Basel, pp 91–107

Ogden CL, Carroll MD, Fryar CD, Flegal KM (2015) Prevalence of obesity among adults and youth: United States, 2011–2014. NCHS data brief, no 219. National Center for Health Statistics, Hyattsville, MD

Osterberg EC, Bernie AM, Ramasamy R (2014) Risks of testosterone replacement therapy in men. Indian J Urol 30(1):2–7. https://doi.org/10.4103/0970-1591.124197

Petak SM, Nankin HR, Spark RF et al (2002) American Association of Clinical Endocrinologists Medical Guidelines for clinical practice for the evaluation and treatment of hypogonadism in adult male patients—2002 update. Endocr Pract 8:440–456

Pivonello R, Menafra D, Riccio E, Garifalos F, Mazzella M, de Angelis C, Colao A (2019) Metabolic disorders and male hypogonadotropic hypogonadism. Front Endocrinol 10:345

Raheem OA, Patel SH, Sisul D, Furnish TJ, Hsieh T (2017) The role of testosterone supplemental therapy in opioid-induced hypogonadism: a retrospective pilot analysis. Am J Mens Health 11(4):1208–1213. https://doi.org/10.1177/1557988316672396

Rhoden EL, Morgentaler A (2004) Risks of testosterone-replacement therapy and recommendations for monitoring. New England J Med 350(5):482–492

Seftel A (2006) Male hypogonadism. Part II: etiology, pathophysiology, and diagnosis. Int J Impot Res 18:223–228

Selvin E, Feinleib M, Zhang L et al (2007) Androgens and diabetes in men: results from the Third National Health and Nutrition Examination Survey (NHANES III). Diabetes Care 30:234–238

Shabsigh R, Katz M, Yan G et al (2005) Cardiovascular issues in hypogonadism and testosterone therapy. Am J Cardiol 96(12B):67M–72M

Shoskes J, Wilson MK, Spinner ML (2016) Pharmacology of testosterone replacement therapy preparations. Transl Androl Urol 5(6):834–843

Tomar R, Dhindsa S, Chaudhuri A et al (2006) Contrasting testosterone concentrations in type 1 and type 2 diabetes. Diabetes Care 29:1120–1122

Traish AM, Guay A, Feeley R, Saad F (2009) The dark side of testosterone deficiency: I. Metabolic syndrome and erectile dysfunction. J Androl 30:10–22

Wang C, Nieschlag E, Swerdloff R et al (2009a) Investigation, treatment, and monitoring of late-onset hypogonadism in males: ISA, ISSAM, EAU, EAA, and ASA recommendations. J Androl 30:1–9

Wang C, Nieschlag E, Swerdloff R et al (2009b) Investigation, treatment, and monitoring of late-onset hypogonadism in males: ISA, ISSAM, EAU, EAA, and ASA recommendations. Eur Urol 55:121–130

Yialamas MA, Hayes FJ (2003) Androgens and the ageing male and female. Best Pract Res Clin Endocrinol Metab 17(2):223–236

Evaluation and Management of Common Scrotal Conditions

3

Katherine Marchese

Contents

K. Marchese (✉)
Department of Urology, RUSH University Medical Center, Chicago, IL, USA

© Springer Nature Switzerland AG 2020
S. A. Quallich, M. J. Lajiness (eds.), *The Nurse Practitioner in Urology*,
https://doi.org/10.1007/978-3-030-45267-4_3

Objectives

1. Identify three conditions associated with acute scrotal pain, and criteria for referral.
2. Review the anatomy associated with hydrocele formation.
3. Discuss two percutaneous treatment options for varicoceles.
4. Outline the differences between a retractile testis and an undescended testis.

Introduction

In this chapter, a variety of common scrotal disorders will be discussed. Many of them are benign and require minimal evaluation and follow-up. Others present as emergent disorders and need immediate evaluation and treatment. Therefore, history taking needs to be comprehensive, structured, and relevant to the patients' stated chief complaint and current symptoms. The chief complaint points to the direction of your exam; the history of the present illness is where the NP collects pertinent information of where and what the symptoms are, the onset, and duration. It is important to listen to the patient and allow him to explain in his own terms. Obtaining the medical and surgical past history helps to focus on the possible differential diagnoses. The next step in evaluation of any scrotal disorder is the physical exam.

Review of the Components of a Scrotal Exam

Remember that the medical and surgical history just obtained helps to guide the examination of the scrotum (Table 3.1). Focus on the components of the scrotal exam that relate to the history given. Males, both adolescents and adults, experience anxiety and embarrassment about this genital exam. The practitioner can help to reduce this anxiety by teaching and explaining each step of the exam as it is being done. As the exam progresses, explain exactly what you are looking at and what you are seeing. This is also a good time to teach a patient how and when to do a testicular self-exam.

The best complement you can receive is when the patient says thank you and tells you that he has never heard that information before. Remember you will likely see this patient again, and this exam done properly helps to promote your therapeutic relationship with him.

Acute Scrotum (Acute Scrotal Pain)

Overview

Acute scrotal pain is defined as the sudden onset of pain, swelling, and/or tenderness in the scrotum with associated pain in the pelvis or abdomen. It requires a quick, efficient, and thorough assessment that includes an in-depth history and physical examination. Based on this immediate evaluation, further testing may be recommended or the patient may be scheduled for emergent surgery. Differential diagnosis for the adult with acute onset of scrotal pain includes testicular torsion, appendix torsion, epididymo-orchitis, idiopathic acute scrotal edema, Fournier's gangrene, testicular trauma, testicular tumor, or a strangulated inguinal hernia. These scrotal conditions range from benign and short term to complex, life-altering, malignant medical problems. The nurse practitioner must

Table 3.1 Scrotal examination review

Action	Structure	Comments
Inspection	Scrotal sac	Patient may be in a standing position or a lying down position and sometimes both positions are necessary
		Inspect the scrotum for overall size, shape, skin characteristics, and hair distribution
		May appear asymmetric with the left hemi-scrotum and left testes hanging lower than the right side
		Look for any visibly dilated veins; assess using the Dubin and Ametar's varicocele grading system
		Darker pigmentation is a normal variant
Palpation	Testicles	Using the thumb, middle, and index fingers, gently slide your fingers over the surface of each testicle, first one side then the other
		The size, preferably using an orchidometer, and consistency of each testis should be recorded. Normal testicular size is 4 cm in length and 2.5 cm in width, approximately 20 cc
		Gentle compression should not produce any discomfort
		The exam should demonstrate a smooth appearance with no lumps
		Any alteration in size, orientation, location, or texture should warrant further evaluation
	Epididymis	Located on the posterolateral aspect of each testes, the epididymal head, body, and tail should be palpated gently
		Assess for any area of increased size, tenderness, or induration
		Findings should demonstrate a smooth, nontender surface with some enlargement at the head of the epididymis
	Spermatic cord	Palpated at the opening of the inguinal canal and from the testes up to the inguinal canal
		Contents of the spermatic cord include arteries, nerves, and vas deferens. Thickness of the cord may vary if lipomas are present and do not resolve when the patient lies down
		During visual inspection and palpation, the presence/absence of dilated veins should be assessed and graded with the patient in a supine and standing position. A Valsalva maneuver will help with grading
		The term "bag of worms" is used to describe large varicoceles
	Vas deferens	Width of a pencil lead
		Should feel smooth, cord-like without lumps or beads
		Absence of the vas is an important finding in an azoospermic male
Reflex assessment	Cremasteric reflex	Brush the inner thigh with a finger in a light, upward movement
		Slight elevation of the testicle and scrotum on the ipsilateral side should be seen

be able to accurately triage these patients, plan a targeted workup, and implement the optimal treatment plan. The prime objective for the practitioner is to identify a true urologic emergency that, if not treated promptly, could result in the loss of a testis, testicular atrophy, infertility, and altered self-image. The four most common and serious causes of acute onset scrotal pain will be discussed in this section.

History

The initial history taken for acute scrotal pain can help the practitioner delineate the potential causes of the acute pain and provide a focus for the assessment and correct diagnosis.

1. What was the nature of the onset of pain (sudden, insidious), location, duration, and severity?
2. What makes the symptoms worsen and what helps them improve?
3. Have there been prior episodes, and how did they resolve?
4. Is edema present? What are the location, duration, and degree of severity?
5. Are there any associated symptoms such as nausea, vomiting, fever, chills, and urinary symptoms?
6. Is there a history of urinary tract infections, sexually transmitted infections, epididymitis, orchitis, or prostatitis?
7. Have there been any urologic traumas, procedures, instrumentations, or known urologic anomalies?

Testicular Torsion

Overview

Testicular torsion is defined as the twisting of the spermatic cord and testis and is considered a true urologic emergency that must be evaluated and treated in less than 6 hours for the best outcome. The torsion is related to inadequate fixation of the testis to the tunica vaginalis; this anomaly is called the bell clapper deformity. The twisting of the cord results in decreased arterial flow, venous outflow obstruction, and ischemic testicular tissue. This deformity is seen in intravaginal torsion. Intravaginal torsion of the testis and spermatic cord is the most common variant of testicular torsion.

The extravaginal testicular torsion is seen only in neonates. As indicated by its name, the twisting of the testis and gubernaculum occurs outside of the tunica vaginalis usually at the external inguinal ring. The entire cord and testis can become twisted resulting in ischemic testicular tissue noted at birth. The affected testis is usually not salvageable, appears atrophic, and does not require an emergent orchiectomy. At some point, a contralateral scrotal exploration and orchiopexy should be done. The infants may present as slightly restless and no acute pain and have a firm, nontender, discolored scrotum.

Testicular torsion can also be intermittent in nature and resolve on its own within an hour or two. It can present with sudden acute onset of pain, and by the time an examination happens, there are no signs or symptoms. This chronic intermittent torsion over time can still result in ischemic changes in the testis.

Incidence

The incidence of testicular torsion in males under the age of 25 is 4.5:100,000 and is the most common cause of testicular loss (Hazeltine et al. 2017). The incidence is bimodal with two peaks. The initial peak is in the neonate and the secondary peak is in the puberty period. Torsions in males under the age of 21 account for 61% of all torsions (Kapoor 2008). Torsions in the elderly male are rare but have been found in males as old as 69 years. Males with a history of cryptorchidism have a tenfold greater risk for torsion.

Pertinent Anatomy and Physiology

The bell clapper deformity, seen in about 12% of all males (Sommers and Jensen 2015), is a congenital anomaly that increases the risk for intravaginal testicular torsion. The bell clapper deformity is responsible for almost 90% of all cases. In this anomaly, the tunica vaginalis cloaks the entire testis and epididymis, preventing the tethering of the testis to the posterior scrotal wall allowing a twisting movement of spermatic cord. The testis floats freely within the tunica vaginalis, suspended by the spermatic cord. This anomaly is bilateral 80% of the time.

History

The general history discussed in the previous section provides the components needed to begin the evaluation. Given the presence of medical information on the Internet, it is possible for the history to include episodes of manual self-detorsion by the patient, after diagnosing his condition with the help of search engines.

Signs and Symptoms

The classic presentation of testicular torsion is sudden, severe, usually unilateral hemi-scrotal pain, possibly accompanied by nausea and vomiting. Abdominal pain may be the presenting symptom and should also raise the specter of suspicion for torsion. Scrotal edema, fever, and changes in urinary symptoms such as dysuria, frequency, and urgency may develop. Most torsions are left-sided.

Risk Factors

No specific risk factors have been identified but researchers have found a higher incidence of testicular torsion with certain anatomical anomalies. Males with a long mesorchium, bell clapper syndrome, or a history of cryptorchidism are linked to higher incidence of torsion. Term infants who underwent a prolonged, difficult labor were also at increased incidence. A possible link has been established with recent trauma and extreme physical workouts especially bicycling.

Physical Exam

Inspection: Observe the demeanor in the patient. Patients with torsion are anxious, have a difficult time sitting in one position, and look very uncomfortable. Observe the gait. If the gait is normal, torsion is unlikely.

A wide-based gait may be seen as the patient tries to avoid having contact between the scrotum and his legs.

During the exam, the practitioner should compare and contrast both testicles for size, symmetry, and consistency, although the extreme pain and edema experienced by the patient may preclude a thorough examination. Begin the exam with the normal testis. The affected testis and spermatic cord would be tender, possibly edematous, and warm. If the lower portion of the testis is painful, consider torsion of the testis. If the upper part of the testis is painful, consider torsion of the appendix and look for the "blue dot" sign. The torsed testis may present in a horizontal line and appear retracted or high riding due to the shortened spermatic cord. The degree of torsion can range between 180° and 720°.

A hydrocele may be present. The cremasteric reflex may be absent. This finding has a sensitivity of 88.2% and a specificity of 86.2% (Ta et al. 2015). Prehn's sign is negative but is not considered a definitive diagnostic sign for torsion but may help to rule out epididymitis. The epididymis may present in an anterior position. The ipsilateral skin may appear indurated or erythematous. After 12–24 hours, the edema and inflammation make it difficult to identify any anatomical structures in the scrotum.

Diagnostic Tests

Laboratory evaluation is not recommended for the diagnostic evaluation of testicular torsion but may help to identify an alternate differential diagnosis. A complete blood count (CBC) would be normal in the early phase of a torsion, but the white blood count (WBC) would be elevated in an infectious process. After 12–24 hours the WBC would become elevated due to the inflammatory response. A urinalysis (UA) would also be normal in torsion but pyuria might indicate a differential diagnosis of epididymitis or prostatitis and the C reactive protein.

If the history, symptoms, and physical findings are suggestive of torsion, ultrasonography should not be recommended, if it would delay the emergent need for scrotal exploration. A delay may result in further ischemia to the testicular tissue and adversely affect the salvage rates.

Color Doppler ultrasonography, the most commonly used imaging modality, has a high sensitivity and specificity for testicular torsion with only a 1% false-negative rate. A negative result alone should not rule out the need for surgical exploration. The Doppler flow study will assess the arterial flow patterns. If no flow pattern is noted, torsion is likely. Further, this imaging modality can identify testicular trauma, epididymitis, or an inguinal hernia that has prolapsed into the scrotum.

The "whirlpool effect" seen on the US study documents the spiral twist of the spermatic cord, notably at the external inguinal ring or at other sites along the inguinal canal.

Management

The gold standard for suspected testicular torsion is scrotal exploration with intra-operative detorsion of the testis, possible orchiectomy, and orchiopexy. Torsion is considered to be a urologic emergency that requires immediate surgical intervention. Delays to allow for further imaging or manual detorsion can result in lower salvage rates.

Manual detorsion can be attempted but this procedure should not delay preparations for the surgical intervention. The manual detorsion procedure is contraindicated if the onset of symptoms has been greater than 6 hours because of the strong likelihood of tissue ischemia and necrosis. Detorsion is very painful to the patient because the procedure needs to be done without local or general anesthesia. A mild analgesic may be given.

In torsion, the testis usually rotates medially toward the thigh but up to 33% will rotate laterally. Therefore, when attempting detorsion, the testis and cord are rotated laterally and based on the degree of twisting may need to be untwisted multiple times. Detorsion can be successful in 70% of attempts but scrotal exploration and orchiopexy are still required.

Sudden resolution of pain and return of the testis to the normal physiological location with good vascular reperfusion are the criteria for a successful manual detorsion. A Doppler study is usually done prior to the procedure and then post-procedure to document improved arterial flow to the tissue.

Surgical Options

The diagnosis of testicular torsion is an indication for an emergent scrotal exploration with best results achieved if done within 6 hours of the initial onset of symptoms.

Criteria for surgery is simply a clinical decision based mostly on history and physical exam that a testicular torsion is present and needs immediate surgical exploration.

The usual incisional approach for the scrotal exploration is trans-scrotal. After the detorsion of the affected testis and spermatic cord is completed, the testis is assessed for viability. If the testis is viable, an ipsilateral orchiopexy should be performed. An orchiopexy involves suturing the tunical albuginea to the dartos muscle in three points with nonabsorbable sutures. An orchiectomy is required if a clearly necrotic testis is uncovered. An orchiectomy will minimize the potential for possible injury to the contralateral testis related to postoperative swelling, inflammation, and infection. The contralateral, unaffected testis should also undergo an orchiopexy.

Delayed injury to the testis can be secondary to "testicular compartment syndrome." This is defined as increased pressure in the testis from the swollen inflamed testicular tissue. The structure of the tunica albuginea further increases this pressure and increases the potential for a later onset of testicular ischemia. A testicular fasciotomy with a small tunica vaginalis patch has been used to reduce the pressure and reduce the tissue injury.

In addition, some surgeons recommend concurrent removal of the testicular and epididymal appendices to prevent their possible torsion in the future.

Preoperative Considerations

The patient and the parents of a minor should always be counseled on the potential for an orchiectomy based on the ischemia found intraoperatively. Orchiectomy rates vary from 40 to 70% based on the age of the patient and time from first symptom to surgical exploration (Al-marzooq et al. 2018). The potential for immediate placement of a testicular prosthesis should also be presented. The bell clapper deformity, known to be bilateral in 80% of the patients, indicates a need to discuss a preemptive orchiopexy on the contralateral side.

Postoperative Management

This procedure may be done outpatient or may require an overnight stay in the hospital. Scrotal support, scrotal elevation, ice packs, and heat application will help to alleviate the swelling and discomfort. The scrotum and groin area may be bruised and swollen for 1–3 weeks. No heavy lifting or sports activities for approximately 4 weeks. No baths or showers until the practitioner gives clearance. Antibiotics, stool softeners, anti-inflammatory medication, and narcotics may be prescribed. No straining with bowel movements.

Complications/Risks

Postoperative complications can include hemorrhage, swelling, hematoma formation, infections, and pain. Recurrence of the torsion can occur.

Complications related to the torsion and related surgery can include testicular damage, testicular atrophy, contralateral testis injury, infertility, and a change in self-image related to an orchiectomy. Semen parameters following these procedures may be altered.

Long-Term Considerations

After recovering from surgery, there are no activity restrictions. Men should be advised that a male fertility evaluation may be appropriate if they are having trouble conceiving.

If the testes are preserved, the patient should be aware that a torsion can recur.

Torsion of the Testicular Appendage

Overview

The most important thing to know about the torsion of the testicular appendage is that it does not lead to loss of testicular function. This torsion is defined as a twisting of a vestigial testis appendage that has no function.

Incidence

This type of torsion is rare in adults. Children between the ages of 7–14 account for 80% of all torsion of the testicular appendage.

Pertinent Anatomy and Physiology

The testicular appendage is a remnant of the embryonic duct also called the Mullerian duct. Not all males will have a testicular appendix; it is seen in about 92% of all males. The appendix may be found on only one side. It is located on the upper pole of the testis, fitting between the testis and epididymal head. On an ultrasound image, it presents as an oval, sessile structure about 1–7 mm in length.

History

The initial history taken for acute scrotal pain is the same history used for torsion of the testicular appendage. It can help the practitioner delineate the potential causes of the pain or acute swelling and provide a focus for the assessment and correct diagnosis:

1. What was the nature of the onset of pain, location, duration, and severity?
2. What makes the symptoms worse and what helps them improve?
3. Have there been prior episodes of pain and how did they resolve?
4. Is edema present?
5. Are there any associated symptoms such as nausea, vomiting, fever, chills, and urinary symptoms?

6. Is there a history of urinary tract infections, sexually transmitted infections, epididymitis, orchitis, or prostatitis?
7. Have there been any urologic procedures, instrumentations, or known urologic anomalies?

Signs and Symptoms

The symptoms of scrotal pain have a more gradual onset than the pain associated with testicular torsion. The pain is one sided and can range from mild to severe and worsen with activity. The focus of the pain is on the superior aspect of the testis and a palpable nodule may be appreciated in that area. The "diagnostic sign" is the presence of a blue dot on the paratesticular nodule but it is seen in only about one-third of the cases. The blue dot is related to the infection of the testicular appendage. The cremasteric reflex remains present. The appendix torsion is not normally associated with nausea and vomiting. Reactive hydrocele, scrotal edema, and erythema may be present.

The symptoms of testicular appendage torsion mimic the symptoms of testicular torsion. The presentation of these symptoms helps to differentiate it from testicular torsion. In testicular torsion, the pain is more acute onset, more diffuse, and not isolated to the superior aspect. There is no "blue dot."

Risk Factors

A torsion is more likely to occur if the appendix is pedunculated.

Physical Exam

During the focused exam, the affected testis will be in the normal location. There may be focal tenderness at the superior aspect of the testis. The affected testicle should be pulled forward and out, stretching the scrotal skin. The "blue dot" may be seen on the superior aspect in this position; this "blue dot" is the necrotic appendix. Scrotal edema, erythema, and reactive hydrocele may be present.

Diagnostic Tests

Laboratory evaluation is not needed to diagnose this condition but a complete blood count (CBC), urinalysis (UA), and urine culture may be obtained to rule out an infectious process.

As with most of the other scrotal disorders, the color Doppler ultrasound is an invaluable diagnostic tool. Results of the study document the structures in the scrotum, the presence of a testicular mass, and signs of inflammation and most importantly demonstrate normal testicular blood flow. Images on the ultrasound show a small hypo- or hyperechogenic structure adjacent to the testis, frequently accompanied by the reactive hydrocele.

Management

If torsion of the testicular appendage occurs, it can lead to infection and necrosis of the appendix tissue. This tissue will become calcified and reabsorbed in 10–14 days with no complications. Conservative treatment options include observation, elevation of the scrotum, use of a scrotal support, and use of appropriate pain medication. NSAIDS would be first line but some patients may require a narcotic pain medication. Strenuous activity is discouraged until the symptoms abate. Application of heat and alternating with ice bags are comfort measures that may lessen the discomfort. The pain can persist up to several weeks. Long-term prognosis is good with no long-term complications or alterations in normal testicular function.

Surgical exploration of the scrotum should only be done emergently if there is an uncertain diagnosis about testicular torsion. The decision for delayed exploration of the scrotum is only done for poor tolerance of the pain, prolonged pain, concerns about an infectious process/abscess formation, or anxiety by the patient or parent. As discussed in earlier sections, the potential complications of scrotal exploration are severe, and the patients and parents need to be educated about the long-term complications.

Epididymo-Orchitis

Overview

Epididymitis and orchitis often occur concomitantly; rarely is orchitis seen as a single entity and, if seen, is associated with mumps. This chapter discusses the entities of epididymitis and orchitis together.

Epididymo-orchitis (EO) is one of the most common causes of acute scrotum with different studies citing an incidence of between 10 and 71%. This is much higher than originally thought and may be a result of better imaging modalities identifying the correct diagnosis. It is defined as an inflammation of the epididymis and testis, often accompanied by an infectious process, resulting from an ascending infection from the urinary tract.

Epididymo-orchitis is classified as acute or chronic. In the acute phase, the symptoms are present for up to 6 weeks. Most patients present to the emergency room or their primary care physician after 5 days of symptoms. Acute epididymo-orchitis may be further characterized as infectious or inflammatory in origin.

Acute *infectious* epididymo-orchitis (MO) is caused by a bacterial, viral, fungal (coccidioidomycosis and blastomycosis), or parasitic organism (*Schistosoma mansoni*). In the age group of males between 14 and 35, the common bacterial etiology is sexually transmitted infections, most frequently *N. gonorrhea* and *C. trachomatis*. Most cases of EO occur in this age group. Nonsexual transmission is most commonly seen in males less than 18 and older than 35. It is related to obstruction, urethral instrumentation, or a surgical procedure, and is primarily *E. coli*.

Acute *inflammatory* epididymo-orchitis (MO) is caused by an inflammatory or systemic disease, an obstructive condition, or a medication. Included in this group could be benign prostatic hyperplasia (BPH), recent urologic instrumentation, urethral stricture, or prostate cancer. The use of amiodarone, an antiarrhythmic, can cause an inflammatory EO because the medication accumulates in the head of the epididymis causing an inflammatory response and symptoms.

In the chronic phase, the symptoms are present for more than 3 months; men usually present with a more gradual onset and usually localized to the scrotum. Typically, the swelling, tenderness, and erythema are mild or not present. They may respond to treatment but still present with ongoing symptoms, including scrotal pain for months and even years.

Isolated orchitis is considered rare and is usually associated with a mumps viral infection in prepubertal and pubertal males who were not vaccinated or did not complete the vaccination cycle. Mumps orchitis may be unilateral or bilateral. Mumps orchitis is the most common complication of the mumps infection and has been linked to testicular atrophy in up to 50% of the affected testis. There is also a potential link to infertility or altered spermatogenesis.

Incidence

Each year there are over 600,000 cases of EO with the highest incidence in men between the ages of 18 and 35 (O'Reilly et al. 2016). The incidence is bimodal with the first group consisting of males between the age of 16 and 30. The second group is males between the ages of 51–70. Over 27% of patients will have a recurrence of EO.

Pertinent Anatomy and Physiology

The etiology of EO may be related to the retrograde flow of urine from the prostatic urethra, through the ejaculatory duct and up into the vas deferens and epididymis. The oblique angle that the prostatic ducts enter the urethra in theory should prevent this reflux. Males with an enlarged prostate, obstruction in the urethra, or a congenital anomaly are at risk for this reflux. But in males with bladder outlet obstruction, urethral stricture, BPH, the straining to void (Valsalva) overrides the integrity of the anti-reflux potential. Similarly, men who have urologic procedures that alter the angle of the duct or damage the integrity of the prostatic duct also increase their risk of reflux. Straining while doing strenuous exercise can also override this anti-reflux mechanism.

History

As with other conditions under the section of acute scrotum, testicular torsion must be considered first. The initial history taken for acute scrotal pain is the same history used for epididymo-orchitis with a few additions. This history can help the practitioner delineate the potential causes of the pain or acute swelling and provide a focus for the assessment and correct diagnosis. What was the nature of the onset of pain, location, duration, and severity? What makes the symptoms worse and what helps them improve? Have there been prior episodes of pain and how did they resolve? Is edema present? Are there any associated symptoms such as nausea, vomiting, headaches, fever, chills, general malaise, and urinary symptoms? Is there a history of urinary tract infections, sexually transmitted infections, epididymitis, orchitis, or prostatitis? Have there been any urologic procedures, instrumentations or known urologic anomalies? Have there been any viral illnesses within the past 2–6 weeks? Is there any swelling in the parotid glands? Has the patient been immunized with the MMR vaccine?

Signs and Symptoms

It may be difficult to differentiate between EO and testicular torsion (Table 3.2) and, in fact, torsion is often misdiagnosed as epididymo-orchitis. In EO, the onset of pain and swelling is more gradual than in a torsion and is expected to be localized posterior to the testis with possible radiation into the groin or flank. The

Table 3.2 Distinguishing acute epididymitis from testicular torsion

	Acute epididymitis	Testicular torsion
Onset	Gradual; can escalate quickly	Sudden Pain often begins during physical activity but can occur during sleep as well
Pain character	Mild to severe testicular or scrotal pain that is usually unilateral	Severe, unilateral scrotal pain and tenderness followed by scrotal swelling and erythema
Cause	Infectious (usually *Chlamydia trachomatis* and *Neisseria gonorrhoeae*)	Unknown
Common age group	Postpubertal (sexually active) males	Most common in boys between the ages of 12 and 18 years (but can occur at any age)
Ureteral discharge	Yes	No
Scrotal elevation	May decrease pain	Often causes intense pain
Treatment	Antibiotics, supportive symptomatic management	Surgery

epididymis may be swollen to ten times its normal size, with an accompanying reactive hydrocele and significant scrotal asymmetry. The testicular/epididymal pain is primarily unilateral. Symptoms of fever, chills, headaches, tachycardia, frequency, urgency, hematuria, and dysuria may be present. Symptoms of hematospermia, painful ejaculation, and prostatitis may also be seen. If a mumps diagnosis is in the differential, the scrotal pain and swelling develops days to weeks after the parotiditis.

Risk Factors

At-risk sexual behaviors increase the risk of epididymo-orchitis. Excessive physical activity, bicycle riding, and prolonged sitting increase the risk especially in males under 35. A history of prostatitis, urinary tract infections, recent urologic trauma, instrumentation, or surgery also increases the risk of EO. Uncircumcised males are at increased risk for genitourinary infections which also puts them at risk for EO. Risks are also increased for men with an enlarged prostate or blocked ejaculatory ducts that produces obstruction.

Physical Exam

Vital signs may demonstrate a fever or elevated pulse as an indication of an infection. Palpate for the parotid gland from the area in front of the ears down to below the jawbone. Record any nodule, swelling, or pain that may be present. This is indicative of mumps. Palpate the costovertebral angle for tenderness which could indicate a pyelonephritis. Suprapubic tenderness could indicate cystitis. The lower abdomen should be assessed for any indication of a hernia or enlarged inguinal nodes.

Inspect the penis, perineum, and anal area for signs of any rash, lesion, and open sores that could indicate a sexually transmitted infection. Inspect the meatus before and after a digital rectal exam and assess any urethral discharge.

Inspect the scrotum for erythema and scrotal edema. Normal cremasteric reflex should be present. Palpate the scrotum for a reactive hydrocele, testicular tenderness, epididymal tenderness, cord tenderness, and any unusual enlargement. As the swelling increases, it may become impossible to palpate the epididymis separate from the testis. The scrotum should also be examined for an indirect inguinal hernia. If indicated a stethoscope could be used over the scrotum to assess for potential bowel sounds. The testicle should be in the normal position. The above findings may be unilateral or bilateral. In most cases of EO, there will be a normal Prehn's sign.

A prostate exam may indicate a tender prostate asymmetrical with increased warmth, induration, and a change in consistency.

Diagnostic Tests

Laboratory evaluation should include a urinalysis and a subsequent culture if indicated. If an infection is present, the leucocytes, nitrites, and blood will be positive. First voided morning specimen should be sent to evaluate for a possible sexually transmitted infection. A UA would be positive for acute EO but is usually negative in chronic EO. A complete blood count (CBC) should be drawn and checked for leukocytosis. Some facilities would also order a C-reactive protein (CRP) and a sedimentation rate to further assess the inflammatory state versus a testicular torsion. If during the physical exam a urethral discharge is noted, a culture should be sent.

The imaging study of choice would be color Doppler ultrasonography. It has a high sensitivity (91.3%) and specificity (88.5%) for epididymo-orchitis (Yan et al. 2018). The Doppler flow study will assess the arterial flow patterns. If no flow pattern is noted, a torsion is likely. Further, this imaging modality can identify testicular trauma, epididymitis, or an inguinal hernia that has prolapsed into the scrotum. Epididymo-orchitis would be suspected if the epididymis is enlarged, thickened, and demonstrating an increase in the Doppler wave pulsations.

Management

Once the diagnosis of epididymo-orchitis has been made, antibiotics may be ordered based on the specific causative agent. If the etiology of the infection is a STI, both the patient and the partner need to be treated and counseling given about the use of condoms and other safe sex practices. Current CDC guidelines should be reviewed because of increasing drug resistance patterns. If the drug amiodarone is the cause of EO, simple dose reduction will resolve the symptoms.

Conservative medical care includes scrotal elevation, scrotal support, application of ice or heat, and the use of nonsteroidal anti-inflammatory (NSAIDS) agents. Bed rest during the acute phase is recommended. Improvement in symptoms should be seen within 2–4 days. Patients should be told to return to clinic if no improvement is noted. Short-term narcotic usage may be indicated during the acute phase but is not recommended long term. A nerve block into the spermatic cord using a long-acting local anesthetic may be tried. This may control the pain and indicate if permanent pain relief would be achieved if the nerves to that area were cut.

If chronic pain develops, the patient should be referred to the pain clinic for a nerve block. Some patients may respond to oral antiepileptic drugs such as Gabapentin or a tricyclic antidepressant amitriptyline or improvement in chronic pain symptoms. A recent adjunct to treatment for chronic scrotal pain is pelvic floor muscle rehabilitation. Some centers will have special physical therapists or nurses who are specifically trained to treat chronic pain without medications, focusing on the relaxation of the pelvic floor nerves and muscles.

Complications of acute epididymis-orchitis are abscess formation, chronic pain, testicular atrophy, testicular tissue damage, and the potential for infertility or decreased spermatogenesis. In the rare case where the conservative measures do not resolve the infection, the patient may be admitted to the hospital for IV antibiotics. Scrotal abscesses, unresponsive to IV or oral antibiotics, may develop and require an incision and drainage of the wound. The wound would be allowed to heal by secondary intention and would require daily wound care and dressing changes.

The surgical options of scrotal exploration should be considered only if there is a concern for testicular torsion, if chronic pain is not alleviated by any of the therapies, or if a scrotal abscess has not responded to antibiotics.

An epididymectomy with a small incision and removal of the affected epididymis can be done as an outpatient. Complications can include recurrent chronic scrotal pain, recurrent infections, wound infections, and most importantly testicular damage resulting in atrophy, infertility, and altered self-image if the testis is removed.

An orchiectomy, also an outpatient procedure, can be done if testicular injury has resulted in testicular death or if recurrent infections and abscess formations continue.

Long-Term Management

Men should be advised to avoid unprotected intercourse until their symptoms have resolved. Once the infection has resolved, further studies such as a uroflow and bladder scan to evaluate for retention should be considered if obstruction was the etiology of EO; a retrograde urethrogram and possible cystogram may be indicated.

Testicular Descent Problems (Maldescensus)

Cryptorchidism Overview

Cryptorchidism is a constellation of congenital or acquired anomalies in which the testis, unilateral or bilateral, does not descend completely and remain in the scrotum. Unilateral undescended testes are seen in almost two-thirds (Braga et al. 2017). The classifications of cryptorchidism include palpable and nonpalpable types. Palpable is further delineated into retractile, ectopic, and undescended. Nonpalpable is subdivided into canalicular, intraabdominal, and absent. The cryptorchid testis can be palpable in 70–80% of the cases or unpalpable in 20–30% (Cho et al. 2019).

Palpable
The undescended testis is defined as failure of a testis to descend into the normal scrotal position. The spermatic cord may be shorter than normal, thus limiting the natural progress into the scrotum. There is also the possibility that the ipsilateral scrotum may be underdeveloped.

Retractile testis is considered by some to be a normal variant and can be unilateral or bilateral. The retractile testes are usually fully descended at puberty but may move out of the scrotum and return spontaneously or with manipulation be brought to the base of the scrotum and remain in the scrotum for a finite period. The peak incidence of retractile testis is age 5 or 6. The site of the retractile testis can range from inguinal to low scrotum. The movement occurs with the strong cremasteric reflex. The affected testis is noted to have increased risk of impaired testicular growth, altered functioning, and increased infertility that is linked to the site with inguinal location being more affected. Annual or biannual examinations are recommended until puberty because as the male matures the cremasteric muscle weakens, the testicular size increases, and the force of gravity work together to keep the testis in the scrotal position.

The ectopic testes are located in regions that are not part of the normal pathway for descent into the scrotum. There are five common sites that are associated with ectopic testis. They include perineum, femoral canal, superficial inguinal pouch, suprapubic area, and contralateral scrotal pouch. The most common site of the ectopic testis is in the superficial inguinal pouch. The ectopic testis has normal development and normal spermatogenesis. Because of their location, they are prone to injury. They do not have increased risk of malignancy or infertility.

Unpalpable

The canalicular testis is located above the normal position in the scrotum in between the internal and external inguinal rings. Its descent into the scrotum is restricted by tension exerted by the external musculature of the body wall (Table 3.3).

The intraabdominal testes, as its name implies, are located in the abdominal cavity proximal to the internal inguinal ring. Its position makes difficult for examination and has increased risk of becoming cancerous.

The absent testis literally means no testis is present. This can be unilateral or bilateral. It is believed to be associated with in utero torsion, vascular insult, or agenesis.

Incidence

Cryptorchidism is seen in approximately 2–8% of full-term male infants (Cho et al. 2019) but as high as 30% in premature male infants (Leslie et al. 2020). Approximately 35% of undescended testes are nonpalpable.

Table 3.3 Classifications of Cryptorchidism

Palpable	Unpalpable
1. Retractile	1. Canalicular
2. Ectopic	2. Intraabdominal
3. Undescended (groin or abdominal)	3. Absent

Pertinent Anatomy and Physiology

The normal descent of the testis is usually complete by gestational week 32. The normal descent can be divided into three phases. The transabdominal phase begins by week 10–15 and is complete by week 22–25. This movement is assisted with the insulin-like hormone INSL3. The trans-inguinal phase occurs between weeks 25–30 in which the testis is moving down the inguinal canal. The final phase, the scrotal phase occurs in week 30–35 and is influenced by androgen production.

Signs and Symptoms

The predominant sign is an empty scrotum. The undescended testis may be unilateral or bilateral with 70% of the undescended testis noted on the right (Braga et al. 2017).

Risk Factors

Associated risk factors for cryptorchidism include preterm babies, low birth weight babies <900 g, twins, or a family history of cryptorchidism. Maternal issues such as gestational diabetes, alcohol, or tobacco use during pregnancy, preeclampsia, breech presentation, cesarean section, or a complicated delivery may increase the likelihood of cryptorchidism. Less understood mechanisms include hormonal imbalance, environmental factors, and genetics. Infants with a neural tube defect, prune belly syndrome, bladder exstrophy, trisomy 13 and 18, posterior urethral valves, or other abdominal wall defects also have a higher incidence of cryptorchidism. Hormonal imbalance as seen with the hypothalamic-pituitary-testicular axis disruption is also associated with cryptorchidism. An in-depth explanation of the various embryologic, hormonal, and mechanical causes is beyond the scope of this chapter.

Physical Exam

The testis should be examined and palpated at every infant well-being exam to assess for the position, mobility, size, and consistency. The focused examination to locate the undescended testis is done with the patient in a supine and cross-legged position. The external inguinal ring should be palpated, tracing the path of the inguinal canal. The ectopic testis may be palpated in the front of the pubis, in the perineum, or even in the medial aspect of the upper thigh.

During the exam, other abnormal findings may include a hypospadias or a hydrocele. Approximately 17–30% of males born with hypospadias will have undescended testes (Leslie et al. 2020). The examiner should also be assessing for a micropenis, ambiguous genitalia, and inguinal hernias. Epididymal anomalies may be seen in 36–79% and may impact fertility.

Specific Maneuvers

During the assessment of the testis, the examiner places the nondominant hand at the anterior superior iliac spine and slides his hand medially toward the groin. The use of a lubricant can assist this movement. The dominant hand is poised to capture and hold the testis and try to pull it into the scrotum. If the testis remains in the scrotum for 1 min after being released, it is termed a retractile testis. If it immediately ascends after release, it is termed an undescended testis.

Diagnostic Tests

The diagnosis is made primarily by the physical exam. Laboratory evaluation could include FSH, LH, and testosterone levels especially if bilateral undescended testis is suspected. Further testing could include Muellerian-inhibiting substance (MIS) or anti-Mullerian hormone (AMH) levels. The results of these labs can indicate the presence or absence of the testis.

Imaging studies are not usually required in the initial workup. The current AUA guidelines do not recommend the use of imaging as a component of a routine evaluation of undescended testes because it does not provide any new information that would guide the treatment choice. However, if bilateral undescended testes (UDT) are seen in a patient with ambiguous genitalia, an ultrasound would be able to assess for the Mullerian structures, including a uterus and cervix.

An ultrasound will identify the testis in the inguinal canal but has a low sensitivity for locating an intraabdominal testis, only 45% (Cho et al. 2019). Similar findings are noted with CT or MRI. Because the MRI would require sedation for the infant, it is seldom used. Due to the high number of false-negatives, imaging studies results should not be used to avoid the surgical approach for localization and fixation of the impalpable testis.

A laparoscopic surgery may be recommended as part of an initial workup if the testes in unpalpable.

Management

Medical

Medical treatment for undescended testis is controversial and is not currently recommended in the AUA guidelines. Hormones are used in some countries as a corrective measure for the disruption of the hypothalamic-pituitary-testis axis disruption. Hormones may help to promote the natural descent of the testis into the scrotum. The most commonly used therapy is hCG (human chorionic gonadotropin) with doses ranging from 250 to 1000 IU based on age. Patients are dosed twice each week, usually for 5 weeks, and may start therapy when less than 1 year old. Other therapies include the use of testosterone or combining hCG with a GnRH (gonadotropin-releasing hormone).

The goals of this therapy would be to encourage normal androgen-related responses including penile growth and onset of pubic hair development. Side effects could include painful erections and behavioral changes.

The AUA guidelines recommend that a patient with undescended testis, congenital or acquired, not in the scrotal position at 6 months should be referred to a pediatric urologist for follow-up. This patient may be a candidate for an orchiopexy.

Surgical

Treatment for the undescended testis whether palpable or unpalpable is an exam under anesthesia and localization of the testis followed by an orchiopexy. At this time the integrity of the testicular vessels and viability of the testis should be evaluated. An orchiectomy may be considered. Goals of surgery include prevention of further testicular damage, resumption of testicular growth, improvement in fertility, and reduction of the risk for testicular malignancy. The recommended age for the orchiopexy is between 6 and 18 months (Cho et al. 2019). The surgical approach may be open or performed laparoscopic. Short-term complications of orchiopexy include hematoma, infection, wound breakdown, and pain. Long-term complications include testicular damage, testicular atrophy, and damage to the vas deferens or epididymis.

Some physicians will suggest a testicular biopsy during the orchiopexy if genital disorders are present.

Treatment options for the retractile testis are still controversial. The retractile testis in the prepubertal males may be followed with annual or biannual evaluation, postponing surgical repair until puberty. If the testis is still highly mobile, an orchiopexy is warranted. Criteria for surgery for a retractile testis include no spontaneous return of the testis in a postpubertal male, the presence of a smaller and softer testis, or symptoms of rapid retraction and persistence of tightness of the spermatic cord.

Long-Term Complications of Cryptorchidism

Complications of cryptorchidism include infertility, increased risk of testicular cancer, testicular torsion, atrophy, trauma, and inguinal hernia. The incidence of infertility increases by more than 30% with bilateral cryptorchidism. There is also a significant psychological component related to abnormal scrotal structures, causing embarrassment and altered self-esteem.

Teaching Points

Parent of the child should be given information regarding the potential long-term risks and complications of cryptorchidism and monorchidism with a special focus on infertility and potential for cancer. Further, these boys as they mature should be reeducated regarding these risks.

Acute Idiopathic Scrotal Edema

Overview

Acute idiopathic scrotal edema (AISE) is part of the constellation of diagnoses that require immediate assessment because of the concern for testicular torsion, torsion of the appendix testis, or epididymo-orchitis. It is often a diagnosis of exclusion. Rapid, thorough evaluation is necessary to avoid an unnecessary scrotal exploration. This condition is usually self-limiting.

While the exact etiology of AISE is unknown, it is possible that it is related to a condition called angioneurotic edema. Angioneurotic edema presents as hypersensitivity, possibly allergic or nonallergic, to some unknown food, medication, or environmental exposure. This exposure results in the subcutaneous tissue swelling seen in the scrotum.

Incidence

Acute idiopathic scrotal edema is the fourth most common cause of acute scrotum in males under 20 years of age. It is less common than testicular torsion, torsion of testicular appendages, and epididymo-orchitis. The overall incidence rates vary from 20 to 69%. Acute idiopathic scrotal edema is typically seen in the prepubertal male less than 10 years old but has been noted in adults.

History

The initial history taken for acute scrotal pain (described in section "Torsion of the Testicular Appendage") is the same history used for AISE. It can help the practitioner delineate the potential causes of the pain or acute swelling and provide a focus for the assessment and correct diagnosis. In addition, the medical history should include a personal and familial history of similar episodes, current medications, exposure to known allergens (food, medication, or environmental), a sudden change in physical stimuli (heat, cold, exercise), and the timing of the exposure to the current episode.

Signs and Symptoms

Patients may present with rapid onset of painless scrotal edema that extends into the perineum and penis. However, some patients will present with pain in the scrotal or inguinal area. Superficial skin tenderness has also been noted. The edema may be unilateral (90%) or bilateral. Diffuse erythema is present and may extend into the perineum and inguinal area. The testis is nontender. A hydrocele may be present. Fever, urinary symptoms, or urethral discharge are not usually seen. The swelling resolves quickly over a period of 3–4 days.

Risk Factors

Since the etiology is unclear, it is difficult to predict risk factors. But if future studies support the theory about angioneurotic edema, exposure to the known allergens would be a significant risk factor.

Physical Exam

Inspection of the scrotum would demonstrate diffuse erythema on the scrotum with possible radiation to the inguinal area, perineum, and penis. Scrotal edema with similar radiation may be seen and may be unilateral or bilateral. Palpation would elicit possible scrotal skin tenderness, scrotal edema, and a hydrocele.

Diagnostic Tests

Laboratory evaluation is not indicated as a diagnostic tool for AISE, but a urinalysis (UA), urine culture, and complete blood count (CBC) could be ordered to rule out other pathologies.

Color Doppler ultrasound is the imaging modality of choice. Ultrasound images demonstrate a thickened, edematous scrotal wall with normal appearing testis and epididymis. The "Fountain Sign," a unique finding on a transverse image of the Doppler study, demonstrates an unusual pattern of hypervascularity in the scrotal wall that is suggestive of AISE. The ultrasound may also document a reactive hydrocele and enlarged lymph nodes. The use of the color Doppler ultrasound is associated with a reduction in unnecessary scrotal explorations.

Management

Since AISE is benign and usually self-limiting, there is no specific treatment algorithm. Conservative management is the initial approach and symptoms usually resolve in less than 5 days. The use of nonsteroidal anti-inflammatory drugs is the first choice. Some practitioners may choose to add an antibiotic. Comfort measures such as scrotal support, elevation, heating pads, and application of ice are included in the conservative management.

Surgical exploration of the scrotum should be avoided unless serious concern exists. Scrotal exploration may be considered if there was no response to the conservative measures discussed above. Other reasons to consider surgery would be extended duration and severity of pain, no resolution of the swelling and associated quality of life issues, or to alleviate the anxiety/fear of the patient or parent. Complications of the surgery should be carefully reviewed and include potential damage to testicular, epididymal, and vas deferens tissue. Potential long-term complications include testicular atrophy, infertility, and infections.

Spermatocele

Overview

A spermatocele is a fluid-filled cyst, most commonly seen in the caput of the epididymis but may also be located in the rete testis or vas deferens. The fluid is clear or opaque and may contain viable and nonviable sperm. Spermatoceles, sometimes located in the epididymis, may alternately be called epididymal cysts when smaller. The exact cause of the spermatocele formation is unclear, but some studies link it to a blockage in the tubules of the epididymis complicated by recent urological procedure, instrumentation, trauma, or inflammation. They are normally benign.

Incidence

Spermatoceles, rarely seen in children, increase with aging with the peak incidence in males between 40 and 50. They may be found as an incidental finding during an annual examination. Approximately 30% of males having a scrotal ultrasound will have an incidental finding of a spermatocele.

History

A patient or his partner is usually the one to discover the mass, although it can be noted because it can be quite tender or painful. This usually prompts a visit to the primary care provider. The detailed history should include onset, location, and any information regarding a change in size of the mass. Information about recent infections, trauma, or surgical procedures should be recorded. The patient should be asked about exposure to diethylstilbestrol (DES).

Signs and Symptoms

Often a spermatocele does not cause symptoms. A small lump or mass may be felt on the superior aspect of the testis, usually painless. Rarely, it will be accompanied by scrotal enlargement on the ipsilateral side, pain, redness, or sense of pressure. Spermatoceles by themselves do not affect fertility, but the corrective surgical procedure listed below can impair fertility by damaging the epididymal and vas deferens tissue.

Risk Factors

No significant risk factors for developing a spermatocele have been identified except for increasing age. While no clear link exists between Von Hippel-Lindau disease and spermatoceles, the incidence is higher in males with this disease. Some studies are suggesting a link between mothers taking DES and son's risk in utero. Most spermatoceles are idiopathic with no clear etiology.

Physical Exam

Palpation of a smooth, firm lump, freely mobile, located on the caput of the epididymis may indicate a spermatocele. Transillumination of the mass will differentiate between a fluid-filled cyst and a solid mass. The mass is separate from and above the testis. Because of the possible differential diagnosis, the groin should be palpated for an inguinal hernia. Unexpected findings during the exam would include a mass that does not transilluminate, scrotal edema, inflammation, or significant pain. Such findings would warrant additional workup and referral to a urology provider.

Diagnostic Tests

Laboratory Evaluation
No lab workup is necessary to diagnose a spermatocele. A urinalysis and a urine culture may be recommended to rule out an infection.

Imaging Studies
Scrotal ultrasound with Doppler: Highly sensitive in the diagnosis of a spermatocele. A scrotal ultrasound is indicated if the mass does not transilluminate or if other physical findings or patient history raise the concern for a more serious pathology. On ultrasound, a spermatocele should image as an anechoic cystic mass with posterior acoustic enhancement, usually 1–2 cm in size but can exceed 15 cm. It may appear as unilocular or oligolocular with thin-walled structure. These findings indicate a benign cystic mass.

Management

Most spermatoceles do not require treatment. Aspirin, acetaminophen, or anti-inflammatory drugs like ibuprofen may help if there is mild discomfort in the scrotum. Application of heat or ice packs may also provide symptomatic relief.

Surgical Options

If the size of the spermatocele is increasing and if the patient finds the associated pain burdensome, there are surgical options. Some infertile patients will undergo a spermatocelectomy in conjunction with a varicocelectomy to improve fertility. Patients should be counseled regarding the potential for infertility post-procedure due to injury to the epididymal tissue or vas deferens. Breach of the epididymis can also contribute to antisperm antibody formation, which can also contribute to lowered fertility.

Spermatocelectomy, an outpatient procedure, involves making a small incision in the scrotum and epididymis with removal of the spermatocele intact. This procedure is done either as an "open" procedure or with a microscopic approach.

Postoperative Management

Short Term: A drain may be in place for 1 day. A scrotal support and/or scrotal elevation is recommended for 1–2 weeks after surgery. Ice packs can be used for 2–3 days to help with swelling which is seen in 20–90% of the patients. Heating pads may also be used. Postoperative pain is managed with narcotics short term. To help prevent infections, no baths are allowed until the incision is completely healed but showers are permitted after 48 hours. No vigorous activity or contact sports for at least 2 weeks. Follow-up visit with the urologist is usually in 2 weeks. Other short-term complications include fever, infection (10%), hematoma (17%), and worsening pain.

Long Term: Long-term complications can include persistent scrotal pain, recurring spermatocele, hydroceles, and testicular atrophy. A more serious complication is possible injury to the epididymis or vas deferens which can lead to infertility.

Aspiration, with or without sclerotherapy, is also done as an outpatient. A needle is inserted into the spermatocele, and the fluid is aspirated. This procedure may be done in conjunction with a sclerotherapy procedure. Sclerotherapy involves injecting an irritating agent, sodium tetradactyl sulfate, into the spermatocele sac that will cause the sac to scar down.

Short-Term Complications: A scrotal support and/or scrotal elevation when erect is recommended for 1–2 weeks after surgery, but no direct pressure should be used. Ice packs can be used for 2–3 days to help with swelling. Heating pads may also be used. Postoperative pain is managed with narcotics short term. To help prevent infections, no baths are allowed until the incision is completely healed but showers are permitted after 48 hours. There are no restrictions on activity. Follow-up visit with the urologist is usually in 2 weeks. Other short-term complications include fever, hematoma, and worsening pain.

Long-Term Complications: Long-term complications can include persistent scrotal pain or recurring spermatocele. A more serious complication is possible injury to the epididymis or vas deferens which can lead to testicular atrophy or infertility.

Hydrocele

Overview

A hydrocele is defined as an abnormal collection of peritoneal fluid located between the parietal and visceral layers of the tunica vaginalis that surround the testicles. Hydroceles are classified as communicating or noncommunicating. Communicating hydroceles with incomplete closure of the tunica vaginalis are present at birth and allow fluid movement between the scrotum and the peritoneal space. The size of these hydroceles, aided by gravity and increased abdominal pressure associated with crying and coughing, may be smaller in the morning and increase during the day as activity levels increase.

Acquired, noncommunicating hydroceles, also called simple hydroceles, have no opening between the peritoneum and the scrotum. Acquired hydroceles are further classified as primary or secondary. Primary hydroceles are idiopathic, usually slow growing, perhaps over years, and have no abnormal pathology. Secondary hydroceles are caused by trauma, infectious process, or inflammation. The fluid in the acquired hydroceles, produced by an inflammatory response, may accumulate at a rate faster than the body can reabsorb it.

Incidence

It is a common finding in children but only 1% of adult males will develop a hydrocele. Worldwide, the most common cause for hydroceles in the adult males is related to a parasitic worm infection caused by the nematodes *Wuchereria bancrofti*. While rare in the United States, it is seen in over 70 countries, most predominantly Egypt and India. The incidence and prevalence in these endemic areas vary greatly by the country and the methods used to control the parasitic worm. In the endemic areas, filarial infection is acquired in early childhood but may not become clinically manifested until early adulthood. The adult worms are found in the intrascrotal lymphatic vessels causing lymphatic obstruction and formation of hydroceles as the most common manifestations. As the infection worsens, the hydroceles become very large and have significant morbidity including discomfort with walking and performance of other normal activities. As the disfigurement worsens, the patients experience social ostracism.

Differentiating filarial hydrocele from idiopathic hydrocele is difficult in many cases. A thorough history is necessary and often the key indicator is recent travel to the affected regions or exposure to recent travelers from those areas. The physical exam may demonstrate other symptoms of filariasis. The spermatic cord and epididymis may be thickened with multiple nodules. Excessive swelling of the scrotum and lymphedema in the pelvis and extremities may be seen. Precautions by the medical staff must be taken. Scrotal ultrasounds are used to diagnose and may demonstrate the filarial dance sign (FDS). The filial dance sign is the movement of the fluid in the hydrocele as the worms move. In this context, surgery is the treatment of choice. Filarial hydroceles are more difficult to excise surgically than idiopathic hydroceles, because of the effect of significant scarring and fibrosis associated with this disease.

Pertinent Anatomy and Physiology

In the last trimester of pregnancy, the testicles of the male fetus migrate from the abdomen through the inguinal canal and into the scrotum preceded by the processus vaginalis. In this early developmental stage, each testicle has a fluid-filled sac that encircles the testicles and allows fluid movement between the peritoneum and the sac. After passing through the inguinal ring, the processus vaginalis typically closes, and further fluid transfer between the peritoneum and the scrotum is impeded. A hydrocele may develop if this closure is not complete. Further, if the opening is significantly larger, a portion of the small intestine may also move into the scrotum causing an indirect inguinal hernia.

History

Information about the onset, location, size, and presence/absence of pain are the first components of the history. Medical history should include an updated list of any infections, trauma, and current medications. Surgical history should include any prior urologic procedure, any abdominal surgery, renal transplant, or AV shunt placement.

Signs and Symptoms

Frequently, hydroceles may be asymptomatic. They may change in size based on time of day or activity level, improving when lying down. Larger hydroceles may produce a feeling of "heaviness," "pulling," or "achiness" in the scrotum. This discomfort may radiate into the lower back and inguinal region. If GI symptoms of nausea, vomiting, constipation, or diarrhea are noted, the differential diagnosis includes an inguinal hernia.

Risk Factors

Prematurity and low birth weight are risk factors for hydrocele formation. Incomplete closure of the processus vaginalis is another risk factor. Exposure to the parasitic worm can predispose the individual to filarial hydrocele formation.

Physical Exam

In addition to the general scrotal exam recommended elsewhere in this chapter, there are some relevant findings specific to hydroceles. The hallmark presentation is a tense, smooth, usually nontender scrotal mass that transilluminates when a small penlight is placed against the scrotal skin. The size and the consistency of hydroceles can vary at different times of the day based on activity. Hydroceles may become smaller when recumbent, and as the day progresses it may become larger and more tense.

It may also be difficult to feel the testicle if the hydrocele is large. The hydrocele is located superior and anterior to the testis. Palpation of the spermatic cord and inguinal ring above the hydrocele should be normal. Since there is an association between inguinal hernias and hydroceles, have the patient perform a Valsalva maneuver in a standing position and then palpate the inguinal canal area for palpable bowel. Patients with an incarcerated hernia may present with fever, chills, nausea, vomiting, diarrhea, or constipation. Approximately 10% of testicular tumors may be accompanied by a hydrocele; therefore, assessment for lymphedema of the external genitalia and edema in the lower extremities may be indicated. See previous section for clinical findings related to filarial hydroceles.

Diagnostic Tests

Laboratory

Lab diagnostic testing is done to establish a differential diagnosis rather than for the definitive diagnosis of a hydrocele. Urinalysis and a urine culture would be done to rule out a urinary tract infection, epididymitis, or orchitis. Testing for sexually transmitted diseases (STD) could be ordered if the patient admitted to at-risk behaviors or recent STD infections, especially as the formation of a hydrocele may be reactive after epididymitis. Clinical findings concerning for a testicular tumor would suggest that AFP (alpha fetal protein), βHCG (human chorionic gonadotropin), and LDH (lactic acid dehydrogenase) should be added to the evaluation.

Imaging Studies

Imaging studies are not routinely needed and should only be ordered if the patient is symptomatic, if the scrotum did not transilluminate, if the diagnosis seems uncertain, or if abnormal findings during the exam raised concerns. A plain abdomen film would help to distinguish between a hydrocele and a hernia. If an incarcerated hernia were present, gas would be demonstrated over the groin area, but this is not ordered to definitively diagnose a hydrocele. A scrotal ultrasound with or without a Doppler study can help to diagnose a hydrocele and estimate the size. It can provide information about the testicular blood flow and differentiate between a hydrocele and a testicular torsion, a testicular tumor, a varicocele, or an incarcerated hernia. Increased epididymal blood flow can assist the clinician in associating a hydrocele with epididymitis.

Management

Hydroceles in infants usually resolve by the second year and no treatment is needed. If a hydrocele develops after age 1, 75% will resolve within 6 months (Dagur et al. 2016). These patients require closer observation and follow-ups. In certain cases, if there is concern about the viability of the individual testicle, an orchiectomy may be needed. Most hydroceles in adult men are benign and require no treatment.

Surgical repair, a hydroclelctomy, is considered the gold standard for symptomatic hydroceles. Indications for surgery include persistent pain, cosmetic concerns, disability due to the size of the hydrocele, or concern for an associated intratesticular mass. The approach may be inguinal or scrotal incision. Postoperative ultrasound imaging is recommended to assess structural integrity and testicular perfusion.

Another treatment option for hydroceles is the minimally invasive sclerotherapy, although this is used in only specifc circumstances, such a a ptaient that cannot tolerate any surgical procedure due to his comorbidities. This procedure usually includes aspiration of the hydrocele fluid and then instillation of the sclerosants which may remain in the sac or may be aspirated out prior to the end of the procedure. This procedure is done in the clinic or outpatient surgery using local anesthetic, and the patient is discharged shortly after the procedure. Agents used for sclerosing are tetracycline derivatives, a 95% alcohol-based solution, ethanolamine oleate, or other irritative agents. These agents may produce epididymal injury and obstruction; therefore, they are not recommended for males concerned about fertility.

Potential Complications: The practitioner should present all options of care for treating hydroceles. Included in this discussion should be the short-term and potential long-term complications. These early complications of a hydrocelectomy could include fever, acute and chronic scrotal pain, infection, and formation of a hematocele, hematoma, and edema. A hematoma is the most common complication following a hydrocelectomy. Sclerotherapy is associated with a high risk of recurrence. So, although the initial therapy is less costly than a hydrocelectomy, the need for repeat procedures lessens this benefit. Long-term complications include infertility related to injury to the epididymis or the vas deferens, the possibility of recurring hydroceles, and chronic pain.

Hematospermia

Overview

Hematospermia is defined as the macroscopic presence of blood in the semen. While usually a benign, self-limiting condition, it can be anxiety provoking for both the patient and the partner. Patients will present to their primary care provider with concerns about a malignancy or a sexually transmitted disease (STD). Hematospermia may present as a single incident or occur for weeks to months. The semen color can vary from bright red to coffee colored.

Incidence

The exact incidence and prevalence of hematospermia is unclear but it peaks in males between their 30s and 40s; it accounts for 1 in 5000 new patient visits in a urology clinic (Mathers et al. 2017). The cause of hematospermia was considered idiopathic in 70% of the cases, but improved imaging techniques are helping to reduce these numbers to about 10–20% (Mathers et al. 2017). In males under 40, it may be related to an infectious or inflammatory process. The list is quite extensive; the more common causes are epididymitis/orchitis, prostatic calculi, benign prostatic hyperplasia (BPH), or a sexually transmitted disease (STD). Common trauma-related causes include prostate biopsy, brachytherapy, and urethral instrumentation. There also has been an association with prolonged abstinence. In males older than 40, there is increased concern for a more serious pathology.

A new, emerging cause is linking hyperuricemia to hematospermia (Mathers et al. 2017). Uric acid crystals in the prostatic secretions and semen may produce an inflammatory response in the prostate or epididymis that results in mucosal inflammation, hyperemia, edema, and hematospermia.

Pertinent Anatomy and Physiology

Injury, inflammation, or obstruction at any point in the ejaculatory path can result in hematospermia.

History

A thorough detailed medical, surgical, and sexual history aids in the extent of the evaluation necessary. The sexual history should include the number of new partners, frequency of coitus (anal and vaginal), masturbation, and the prior history of and STD. Specifics about the ejaculate should include the character, color, timing, and frequency of the hematospermia. The examiner must rule out the female partner as a source of the blood in the semen. The blood could be related to micro-tears in the vaginal tissue, menstrual bleeding, or other gyne/anal pathology. This may include collecting an ejaculate specimen in a condom.

The medical history should include all comorbid conditions including hypertension, blood dyscrasias, liver disease, as well as the risk factors/symptoms for any inflammatory or infectious process. Travel to areas endemic for TB or schistosomiasis increases the risk for these infections. Urologic malignancy is not a common entity associated with hematospermia but it should be excluded. Medications such as aspirin and anticoagulants should also be recorded. The surgical history should include information about any recent prostate biopsy, brachytherapy, any invasive urologic procedure, and any at-risk sexual practices.

Signs and Symptoms

There are few symptoms associated with hematospermia but may include painful ejaculation, hematuria, dysuria, short-term urinary frequency, and scrotal discomfort. Symptoms associated with hyperuricemia associated with hematospermia also include foot arthralgia and chronic prostatitis.

Risk Factors

The risk factors listed are related to the pathologic conditions that may have hematospermia as a symptom. These include infections, inflammations, prostatic stones, and bleeding dyscrasias. Certain urologic procedures such as prostate biopsies, instrumentation, and brachytherapy can cause inflammation and infections that increase the risk for hematospermia.

Physical Exam

The physical exam should begin with the assessment of the vital signs especially looking for hypertension, fever, and recent weight loss. A focused abdominal exam should be done assessing for any abdominal mass including hepatomegaly, splenomegaly, or pelvis swelling. The genital exam should be very detailed. The patient should be examined in an upright and prone position to better identify any abnormality. The penis should be examined for any unusual skin lesion that could represent an STD, torn frenulum, or skin cancer. Any lesion, rash, and skin eruption warrants a further review of the medical-sexual history. After completing a digital rectal exam (DRE), the meatus should be examined for any bloody discharge. The spermatic cord, epididymis, and testis should be palpated for tenderness, induration, or swelling. Based on the finding of the physical exam and the pertinent history, the evaluation will progress to rule out specific processes.

Diagnostic Tests

The diagnostic tests that are ordered vary based on the personal history and exam findings and are usually ordered to help reassure the patient. Persistent hematospermia, associated hematuria, and males older than 40 require a more in-depth evaluation. Basic initial testing for all patients should include a urinalysis and urine culture and PSA. A first voided urine sample for an STD is necessary only if risk factors are present. Additional testing could include a fresh semen sample, prostatic secretion sample, and an additional urine sample for cytology, TB, or schistosomiasis. Blood samples for a CBC, urea, electrolytes, liver function studies, and clotting studies may be ordered to R/O conditions associated with hematospermia.

Imaging Studies

Transrectal ultrasound (TRUS) is the most common imaging study used to diagnose hematospermia. The TRUS can locate prostatic stones, cysts in the seminal vesicle, dilated seminal vesicles, and blocked ejaculatory ducts. These conditions are associated with hematospermia. Malignancy is a rare cause of hematospermia, but TRUS can also identify prostate, bladder, and seminal vesicle tumors. MRI is rarely used now in the initial workup of hematospermia but may be ordered if more significant pathology is suspected. Ultrasound of the scrotum may be ordered if the scrotal examination was abnormal. CT urogram may also be ordered.

Procedures

A cystoscopy may be ordered if hematuria is also present. The cystoscopy will allow for direct visualization of the ejaculatory ducts, the prostate, and the bladder and may allow confirmation of a friable prostate.

Management

Since this is normally a benign condition, early management is usually observation and reassurance. If an infectious process is then identified, appropriate antibiotics or antiviral medications should be ordered. If the prostate is friable, a limited trial of finasteride or dutasteride may address the hematospermia. If hyperuricemia has been diagnosed, allopurinol 300 mg tablets twice daily for 8 weeks and then reduced to once daily has been effective in reducing the incidence of hematospermia and reducing the serum acid level. A low purine diet and increased fluid volume were also encouraged. Other treatment algorithms for hematospermia are based on treating the pathological condition.

Testicular Microlithiasis

Overview

Testicular microlithiasis (TM) is calcium deposits seen within the seminiferous tubules of the testes that are found incidentally during an ultrasound of the scrotum (Balawender et al. 2018). They may develop because the Sertoli cells in the testes are unable to breakdown the calcium deposits of hydroxyapatite and the surrounding fibrotic tissue quickly enough. The accumulation of this debris and resultant irritation then induce an immune reaction that increases the permeability of the membrane and allows the deposits to remain in the tubules (Aoun et al. 2019).

The first cadaveric identification of testicular microlithiasis was in 1928 and not until 1987 was it detected by ultrasonic imaging studies. Testicular microlithiasis (TM) is a condition with uncertain etiology that is uncommon in adult males. TM has been associated with testicular malignancy but this is very controversial and there is insufficient data to confirm this.

In 2015 the European Society of Urogenital Radiology developed a classification system to characterize the findings of the US.

Advance practice practitioners who order ultrasounds of the scrotum will encounter this type of finding in many of their reports. As such, it is important to understand the significance of this diagnosis, its implications and current recommendations to follow.

Incidence

TM is seen in males of all ages: from prepubertal boys to elderly males. In the general population, it may exist in 5% of males between the ages of 17–35 but the true incidence is unknown because it is only detected when males undergo an imaging study. As the technology of ultrasounds improved, the incidental discovery of TM has increased. TM can be found in 0.6–9% of men who underwent scrotal imaging by ultrasound (Balawender et al. 2018). There is a higher incidence of TM identified in black males, followed by Hispanic males, then Asian or Pacific males and lastly by white males. Males with certain genetic disorders also have a higher incidence of TM than what is found in the general population. TM is found in 17.5% of men with Klinefelter syndrome and in 36% of men with Down syndrome (Balawender et al. 2018).

Pertinent Anatomy and Physiology

When conducting the testicular exam using the Prader orchidometer, a variance of >20% between the testicular sizes, indicates testicular atrophy. Remember that it is not uncommon for the left testis will be smaller than the right testis. Normal testicular volumes are between 12–30 ml with volumes <12 ml considered small (Richenberg et al. 2015).

History

The updated history for a male diagnosed with TM should include information about a prior history of testicular atrophy with a volume of less than 12 ml, testicular maldescent or a testicular orchiopexy. Other important additions to the history include a prior diagnosis of germ cell tumor or a first degree relative with a history of germ cell tumor.

Signs and Symptoms

There are no clinical manifestations of TM (Leblanc et al. 2018). Testicular microlithiasis can't be felt during a scrotal exam and do not cause any pain, swelling or discomfort.

Risk Factors

Some studies suggest that men with less physical activity and a diet that includes crisps (fries) and popcorn have a higher risk for development of TM because of the chemical called acrylamide which is contained in those foods. As mentioned before ethnicity and other medical conditions may also cause an increase. There is also a proposed link between socio-economic levels.

Probably one of the most concerning factors is a potential association between TM and testicular cancer. At this time, there is not enough strong high-quality research to substantiate a correlation between the two (Aoun et al. 2019). Some of the studies are identifying a higher prevalence of TM in males with cryptorchidism, infertility, family and personal history of a previously diagnosed testicular tumor which also independent factors for testicular cancer (Leblanc etal. 2018).

Physical Exam

There are no physical signs that the practitioner would detect. The microlights are not palpable.

Diagnostic Tests

Scrotal Ultrasound: These microcalcifications, as seen on the US, are characterized as small, uniform, echogenic, nonshadowing foci with a diameter of 1–3 mm that are distributed throughout one or both of the testicles (Richenberg et al. 2015). The number seen can vary from less than 5 per field of vision to 60 per field of vision.

The scrotal US should be conducted using a high frequency transducer of at least a 15 MHz because this identifies a higher volume of TM's (Richenberg et al. 2015). Testicular microcalcifications will not show up on an MRI.

Tumor markers: if there is clinical concern for a testicular mass.

Testicular biopsy or orchidectomy: if tumor markers or the ultrasounds are abnormal.

Management/Guidelines

While there are no clear consistent guidelines or protocols for management of a patient with microlithiasis (Brodie et al. 2018), there are some recommendations to guide (Table 3.4).

Table 3.4 European Society Urogenital Radiology Classification of Testicular Microlithiasis

Limited: <5 TM per field of vision
Classic: ≥5 per field of vision
Diffuse (Snowstorm): Multiple TM's per field of vision

The AUA guidelines suggested that the findings of TM in the absence of a solid testicular mass or other risk factors associated with developing a germ cell tumor (GCT) indicate that there is no increased risk of a malignant neoplasm, and therefore, no further evaluation is recommended.

The European Society of Urogenital Radiology (ESUR) also suggests that isolated TM in a patient with none of the associated risk factors does not require any additional follow-up including ultrasounds or a testicular biopsy (Balawender et al. 2018). The patient should be instructed on the technique for performing a monthly testicular self-exam and given home reference material on testicular microlithiasis (Aoun et al. 2019).

However, if TM presents with any of the above risk factors, the practitioner may consider this as a follow-up: annual follow-up with a scrotal ultrasound and a monthly self-testicular exam. Patients should be referred to a urologist if the repeat scrotal US documented any focal lesion. The EUA guidelines suggest follow-up for this group until age 55 years (Balawender et al. 2018).

Varicocele

Overview

A varicocele is a tortuous dilation of the pampiniform plexus and the internal spermatic veins. The pampiniform plexus is another term for the venous drainage system that consists of a deep and a superficial network. The deep network drains the testis, epididymis, and vas deferens. The superficial network drains the veins of the scrotum. These veins merge as they ascend the testicular cord forming a single testicular vein on each side. The right testicular vein drains into the right inferior vena cava and the left testicular vein drains into the left renal vein. The normal nondilated diameter of the vein is between 0.5 and 2.0 mm. With a varicocele, it dilates to greater than 3.5 mm with a Valsalva maneuver.

Varicoceles are problematic because they can lead to damage to testicular tissue resulting in testicular atrophy, altered spermatogenesis, Leydig cell dysfunction, and infertility. Some varicoceles are problematic because of persistent/chronic pain.

The proposed pathogenesis of a varicocele is multifactorial, and left varicoceles are more common. Left varicoceles may also be the result of a spermatic vein that is 8–10 cm longer than the right side combined with the right angle insertion into the left renal vein which can also increase the pressure and turbulence in the vein. Compression of the left renal vein between the aorta and the superior mesenteric artery (the nutcracker phenomenon) can occur and results in hypertension in the left renal vein causing increased venous pressure, turbulence, and backflow, resulting in a left varicocele. The right side drains into the vena cava which allows more direct flow with less pressure and less dilation. Absence of valves in the internal, external, and cremasteric veins or incompetent valves are another potential cause for varicoceles. Any retrograde flow into the pampiniform plexus is less in the sitting or recumbent positions but increases significantly when standing.

Testicular hyperthermia may result from the increased stagnant venous blood circulating around the testis. The normal temperature of the testicles is approximately 1–2 °C lower than normal body temperature. This cooler temperature is necessary for optimal spermatogenesis. Hormonal changes associated with puberty may also play a role. Changes in the testosterone levels may increase the flow of blood into testis promoting dilation of the pampiniform plexus and subsequent varicocele formation. Early detection of a varicocele is key. The longer the palpable varicocele is present and the greater the size of the varicocele, the more likely it is to have significant alterations in testicular functioning.

Incidence

Varicoceles represent a common entity in urologic assessments and are seen in 15–20% of the male general population but in 40% of males who present for infertility evaluations (Baigorri and Dixon 2016). Varicoceles are most frequently diagnosed in males between the ages of 13 and 30. There is a lower incidence in obese males possibly related to the increased abdominal fat that limits compression between the superior mesenteric artery and the aorta.

Pertinent Anatomy and Physiology

Ninety percent of varicoceles occur on the left side (O'Reilly et al. 2016); absence of valves is seen more commonly on the left side. The prevalence of bilateral varicoceles varies significantly by studies but ranges from 30 to 80% (Alsaikhan et al. 2016). The normal diameter of the veins in the pampiniform plexus range from 0.5 to 1.5 mm, whereas the main testicular vein will have a diameter of 2 mm (Prajapati et al. 2016). Palpable varicoceles (Grade I–III) can exceed 5–6 mm (Prajapati et al. 2016).

The finding of a right-sided varicocele, especially in men under 40, raises concern for a pelvic/abdominal malignancy. This could include a renal cell cancer, a retroperitoneal fibrosis, a retroperitoneal mass, a sarcoma, or a lymphoma. Further evaluation is always indicated.

Risk Factors

Congenital absence of veins in the spermatic veins is a significant risk factor. There appears to be a familial link to varicoceles, that is not well understood. Having a first-degree family member with a varicocele increases the risk for other members to develop a varicocele. Age is another common risk factor as mentioned above. The incidence of varicoceles increases in adolescents to 15% where it stabilizes into adulthood (Baigorri and Dixon 2016).

History

The pertinent history may vary, based on the reason the patient presents to the clinic. The visit could be a component of infertility evaluation, an evaluation for pain, or concern about the sudden occurrence of the varicocele. The age of the patient is another factor that can affect the history taking.

If the male of any age presents for infertility or is interested in fathering children at some future point, a reproductive and sexual history should be obtained and documented. Symptoms of androgen deficiency such as muscle loss ease of fatigability, low energy level, depressed mood, and low libido should be queried. Has there been a change in the position, the size, or consistency of the testicles, unilateral or bilateral? Has there been a change in erectile functioning? Obtain information about the onset, severity, and the outcomes of the different treatment choices. Is there a history of congenital anomalies, infections (mumps, orchitis, STDs), urologic surgery, or any known genital trauma? The patient should also be asked about past and current use/abuse of narcotics, alcohol, testosterone replacement therapy, or any other over-the-counter "hormonal" supplements.

If the patient presents primarily for pain, the onset, location, frequency, duration, and radiation of the pain should first be documented. Specifics about what makes the pain worse and what makes it better as well as previously tried comfort measures should be recorded. Based on the age of the patient, the questions about infertility may not be relevant but the provider should never make that assumption. The patient should always be asked if fertility is a concern. If the patient expresses concern, then the questions in the infertility section above should be reviewed. Sometimes a patient will present with no symptoms other than a concern about the appearance of the "lump" or new abnormal finding. The full history should be collected.

Signs and Symptoms

Patients with varicoceles may present as asymptomatic or symptomatic. Some patients with varicoceles have been identified through incidental findings on a physical examination or an imaging study.

If a varicocele is symptomatic, the patient may present with a pain described as a dull, aching, persistent, heavy sensation in the ipsilateral scrotum. Some men note that these sensations may radiate up into the inguinal region. The discomfort may worsen with standing, straining, or increased activity. The discomfort may lessen when he becomes supine with the resolution of the varicocele in this position. The patient may describe a soft mass above the affected testis as a "bag of worms." The duration of these symptoms prior to seeking medical care ranges from 3 to 18 months.

Patients may present with concerns about recent changes in the testis or laboratory results showing a low testosterone level or abnormal semen analysis. While many patients with varicocele remain asymptomatic, varicoceles have been implicated in male-factor infertility, testicular pain, and impaired testosterone production. It is the most common and treatable cause of male infertility; there is a large body of evidence indicating that varicocele is associated with abnormal semen parameters and testicular atrophy. Development of these symptoms may be the result of elevated scrotal temperature, hypoxia secondary to venous stasis, and/or reflux of renal and adrenal metabolites.

Obese patients have a lower prevalence of varicoceles detected by ultrasound. The lower prevalence is independent of physical examination and more likely due to another factor.

Physical Exam

The physical exam is the cornerstone for varicocele investigation. The patient should be examined in a warm room to promote relaxation of the cremasteric and dartos muscles. A cold room, an anxious or embarrassed patient, or an inexperienced clinician can result in retraction or elevation of the scrotum, making the varicocele more difficult to palpate. The patient should be examined in both the supine and standing positions.

Inspection: Assess the symmetry of the scrotum. Assess for symmetry of each testis. Observe for any visible swelling in the scrotum. Look for any visible tortuous veins.

Auscultate: Place the stethoscope on some of the larger varicoceles and the pulsing blood may be heard.

Palpation: Palpate the spermatic cord with the patient supine and while standing with and without a Valsalva maneuver. The Valsalva maneuver will facilitate increased engorgement of the varicocele and assist the clinician in locating the varicocele. Feel for "a bag of worms" above the testis but in the testicular cord. With full engorgement, a pulse may be felt at the varicocele. Grade the varicocele using the scale proposed by Dubin and Amelar (Table 3.1). Document the change in size or resolution of the varicocele with the change in position. If no reduction in size is noted when supine, further evaluation with a CT scan or pelvic ultrasound is required to evaluate for a retroperitoneal mass such as a sarcoma, lymphoma, or a renal tumor.

In addition, a right-sided varicocele as a solo finding is rare and should also suggest a more in-depth physical exam looking for pelvic lymphadenopathy, abdominal lymphadenopathy, or a kidney mass.

Palpate the testis using the Prader orchidometer assessing for ipsilateral or bilateral testicular atrophy.

Diagnostic Tests

As discussed before, the associated medical history and the physical exam are the main diagnostic criteria for varicoceles. Laboratory evaluation could be considered

Table 3.5 Dublin and Ameler (1970) varicocele grading system with the addition of color Doppler results

Grade of varicocele	Physical exam	US color Doppler results—median left gonadal vein diameter with Valsalva
Subclinical	Not palpable, found incidentally	
Grade I	Palpable only when standing and doing a Valsalva maneuver	3.65 mm
Grade II	Palpable when standing. Valsalva not necessary	3.75 mm
Grade III	Visible through scrotal tissue palpable when standing "Bag of worms"	4.7 mm

and would include testing to assess for possible complications of a varicocele. Semen analysis is recommended as a baseline; for men seeking observation only, periodic semen analyses are recommended. Serum testosterone (T) and follicle-stimulating (FSH) hormone levels may also be drawn.

If imaging studies are needed, scrotal ultrasonography is the modality of choice. However, scrotal ultrasonography is not recommended for the routine evaluation of every male with varicoceles, especially in males with subclinical varicoceles.

The American Urological Association and the American Society for Reproductive Medicine suggest limiting the use of scrotal ultrasonography to only the cases that are inconclusive after the history and physical examination are completed.

Pilatz et al. (2011) noted that color Doppler ultrasound has a greater than 80% sensitivity and specificity in linking the grade of the varicocele on exam with the findings on the Doppler study (Table 3.5). The use of the color Doppler may assist practitioners with determining the diagnostic grade of the varicocele and the optimal treatment choice. Posttreatment Doppler studies may be used to determine the success of the obliteration of the varicocele.

Although a retrograde spermatic venography study is highly sensitive for varicocele identification, it is rarely used unless coupled with the therapeutic occlusion procedure. In this procedure, a catheter is advanced into the testicular vein and a contrast dye is injected to identify the varicocele. A stainless steel coil is then placed which embolizes the varicocele. The venography in conjunction with the steel-coil embolization is indicated for persistent or recurrent varicoceles and has a success rate of 90–97% (Baigorri and Dixon 2016).

Management

Counseling: An adult male with a palpable varicocele, abnormal semen parameters, and a possible interest in future fertility should receive early counseling about the risks of infertility and the treatment options available (Chap. 2) and can be directed to the American Society of Reproductive Medicine for additional details. Similarly, a male with a palpable varicocele and normal semen parameters should be counseled that untreated varicoceles can result in potential testicular dysfunction. These patients should undergo yearly evaluation of the varicocele and the testicular size and its consistency. Consideration for repeat semen analysis and testosterone and FSH levels should be discussed. A review of the risks and complications of untreated palpable varicoceles should be presented each year.

Treatment Options

Conservative measures: Conservative, nonsurgical treatments are usually the first recommendation offered to men with varicocele-related pain. Conservative measures consist of application of heat or ice, scrotal elevation, use of a scrotal support, nonsteroidal anti-inflammatory medications, analgesics, and physical activity limitations. Physical activity limitations include restrictions on heavy lifting, sports activities, and strenuous exercises. While conservative measures may lessen the discomfort of the varicocele, they may not negate the need for surgical repair. Patients may also benefit from a referral for pelvic floor physical therapy or consultation with a pain medicine specialist. When conservative measures prove inadequate, definitive treatment of the varicocele can be offered, although patients should be counseled that surgery may not completely relieve their discomfort.

Medical therapy: Currently there is no conclusive study that indicates there is any medical therapy recommended to improve the outcomes or lessen the complications of varicocele formation and repair. A study conducted by Pourmand et al. (2014) proposed the use of daily oral dose of 750 mg of L-carnitine, an antioxidant, for 6 months for patients having the standard inguinal varicocelectomy, but the results did not discover any improvement in semen analysis parameters or DNA damage.

Radiologic Interventional Percutaneous Embolization

Varicoceles can be ablated by embolization of the spermatic veins using coils, balloons, or sclerosants in a minimally invasive outpatient procedure using local anesthetic or sometimes with addition of light sedation. These procedures are performed by an interventional radiologist with or without the assistance of a urologist. A venography is always done first in all three procedures to help identify the size of the varicocele as well as the venous anatomy. It can identify possible collateral venous systems. Patients are discharged after stabilization from the procedure.

Retrograde sclerotherapy is the most common percutaneous embolization procedure done. In retrograde sclerotherapy, a small incision is made into the brachial, femoral, or internal jugular vein. Using fluoroscopy and a contrast dye, the catheter is advanced into the internal spermatic veins. When the site of the refluxing flow is identified, the sclerosing agent is injected. Sclerosing agents used include N-butyl cyanoacrylate (N2BCA), sodium tetradecyl sulfate (STS) (a foam preparation), and polidocanol. The agent chosen is physician preference.

An alternate procedure is the antegrade sclerotherapy. This procedure is also outpatient, using local anesthesia and takes only 20 min. In this procedure, a small incision is made directly into the scrotum, directly visualizing and isolating the spermatic vein. A small catheter is similarly advanced to the refluxing flow and the sclerosant is injected.

Complications of sclerotherapy include scrotal hematoma, scrotal swelling, allergic reaction to the contrast dye, retroperitoneal leaking of the dye, fever, or rupture of the gonadal vein. There is a potential for an unresolved varicocele or a recurrent varicocele usually related to an alternate venous collateral system. Following the procedure, the scrotal pain noted preoperatively may be persistent. There may be a new pain associated with a recurrent varicocele.

Benefits of sclerotherapy include recurrence rates similar to surgical repair, less post-procedure pain, and earlier return to normal activities. Improvement in semen parameters are similar to outcomes noted with surgical repair.

Coil Embolization

During a coil embolization, a small incision is made in the groin and a catheter is advanced through the femoral vein and into the gonadal vein. A fluoroscopy with contrast dye is used to follow the path of the catheter to the site of the refluxing veins. The coil is deployed into the veins causing the varicocele, and the fluoroscopy is used to observe that occlusion of the appropriate vein is complete. The coils used today are MRI compatible. In addition, some radiologists will add a sclerosing agent to make sure that the collateral veins are also obstructed reducing the chances of recurrence.

Balloon Embolization

Balloon embolization is a similar procedure to coil embolization. This procedure is used mostly with large spermatic veins or in patients that have a bidirectional flow pattern. Again the fluoroscopy and administration of the contrast dye is used to tract the passage of the guide wire into the spermatic vein. Once the position has been confirmed, the balloon is used to occlude the retrograde blood flow. As with the coil procedure, some radiologists will add a sclerosing agent to improve success rates.

Complications of the coil and balloon embolization are similar to those seen with sclerotherapy. During the passage or adjustment of the coil or balloon, perforation of the vein may occur. An additional complication is migration of the coil or balloon. Hydrocele formation has not been seen with either procedure. Thrombophlebitis is another potential complication.

Advantages of the coil and balloon therapy include less discomfort, faster recovery, less infections, and comparable outcomes to surgery. An improvement in semen parameters were between 62 and 77% (Cayan et al. 2019). Embolization procedures have a success rate of 90–97% (Baigorri and Dixon 2016). Cost analysis of the embolization procedure and surgical costs associated with a varicocelectomy show no significant difference.

Varicocelectomy

Criteria for Surgery

The American Urological Association Best Practice Policy "Report on Varicocele and Infertility" outlined the conditions in which a varicocele should be treated.

1. Infertility: Their recommendations suggested that all four of these criteria be met before the male partner should be considered for a surgical repair:
   (a) The varicocele should be palpable. Subclinical varicoceles are not recommended for surgical repair.
   (b) Infertility is present.
   (c) The female partner has no infertility or has only a potentially treatable cause of infertility.
   (d) The semen analysis is abnormal on one or more semen samples.
2. Other situations that meet the criteria for surgical repair:
   (a) An adult male with a palpable varicocele, abnormal semen parameters, and a possible interest in future fertility.
   (b) Adolescent males with a varicocele and documented ipsilateral testicular atrophy. Some studies suggest that a 20% change in testicular size over a 1-year period constitutes adequate criteria. Semen analysis should be further evaluated in this population.
   (c) Males presenting with chronic scrotal pain longer than 3 months.
   (d) Males demonstrating abnormal testosterone levels on at least two occasions. Proposing a varicocelectomy for men with low testosterone levels is controversial, but multiple research studies indicate that progressive Leydig cell destruction and potential testicular atrophy result in impaired fertility and other complications of long-term hypogonadism.

Surgical

The goal of a surgical repair of a varicocele is to occlude the internal spermatic vein that is causing the varicocele, prevent any injury to the testicular artery, and minimize the risk of recurring varicoceles. There are multiple surgical approaches to the surgery. The scrotal approach for varicocele repair is outdated and has been replaced with procedures that cause less injury to the spermatic arteries and testicular tissues. The scrotal approach is associated with increased incidence of postoperative hydroceles.

Laparoscopic varicocelectomy is indicated for use in recurrent or bilateral varicoceles. It is used less frequently now since the advent of subinguinal microsurgical varicocelectomy, partly because of its association with a higher incidence of complications, increased operating room time, expensive equipment, and the need for general anesthesia. A laparoscopic Doppler probe is recommended during the surgery to identify the location of the spermatic artery. A port incision is made sub-umbilical for the working element and two smaller port incisions are made within inches of that site. Cautery, clips, or sutures are used to ligate the spermatic veins.

The open surgery techniques include retroperitoneal, inguinal (Ivanissevich), and subinguinal (Marmar) approach. In these procedures, the spermatic vein is accessed through a 2–3″ incision on the abdomen. The inguinal and subinguinal techniques are the most common approaches used. The Ivanissevich approach makes the incision superior and medial to the external ring. Caution must be taken to not injure the ilioinguinal nerve or the testicular artery.

The Marmar approach makes the incision where the spermatic veins are most superficial, right over the superficial ring. This subinguinal microsurgical varicocelectomy has an improved ability to preserve the testicular and cremasteric arteries and lymphatics minimizing the risks for significant side effects and testicular atrophy. This microsurgical technique is also associated with less postoperative pain, lower recurrence rates, and lower incidence of hydrocele formation.

Preoperative Considerations

The most important preoperative consideration for all patients is their understanding of why they are having this procedure. Patients need to have realistic expectations of the outcomes whether this is done for pain control, infertility, testicular changes, or hypogonadism. The risks and benefits should be presented in verbal and written format. Further discussion on the impact of varicocelectomy on infertility will be found in the chapter on infertility.

Postoperative Management

External dressings covering the incisions may be removed in 2 days. If steri-strips are used to cover the incision, they should be allowed to fall off themselves. No baths until the incision is completely healed. Showers may be started after 48 hours. Physical exertion is not recommended for 2 weeks. Sexual activity should be deferred for 1–2 weeks. If scrotal swelling or discomfort is noted, comfort measures of scrotal support, scrotal elevation, and application of ice should be employed. Most pain can be modulated with nonprescription medications. The patient should be instructed to call the physician if fever, unusual pain, bruising, swelling, or discharge is noted. An inability to urinate should prompt an immediate call. A postoperative visit should be scheduled from 2 to 8 weeks after the surgery and is likely to be surgeon and/or facility dependent. A second follow-up visit at 3–4 months is scheduled for evaluation of a recurrent varicocele and to collect a semen analysis. Additional visits are scheduled based on physician preference.

Complications of Surgery

Short-term complications can include scrotal swelling, bruising, postoperative pain, and infections. Long-term complications can include hydrocele formation which is one of the most frequent complications. A second long-term complication is the inadvertent ligation of the testicular artery that can result in testicular atrophy. Recurrence of a varicocele, a third complication, is related to type of procedure done. Subinguinal microscopic varicocelectomy has a less than 2% recurrence rate (Gomella 2010).

With newer surgical approaches, the resolution of scrotal pain is seen in 94% of the patients. New onset of scrotal pain after a varicocelectomy can be related to a recurrence of a varicocele in the collateral venous complex.

Clinical Pearls
- If a patient's gait is normal, testicular torsion is unlikely.
- Torsion of the testicular appendage is rare in adults.
- The acute phase epididymo-orchitis can result in symptoms for up to 6 weeks, and males may need symptomatic support that is not antibiotics, e.g., NSAIDs.
- Retractile testes are a normal variant and can be unilateral or bilateral; they fully descend at puberty but may move out of the scrotum and return spontaneously.
- Acute idiopathic scrotal edema is typically seen in the prepubertal male.
- <10 years old.
- Treatment for spermatoceles and hydroceles is almost always elective; unless an individual is not a surgical candidate, aspiration is rarely the treatment of choice due to rapid recurrence.
- A review of the risks and complications of untreated palpable varicoceles should be presented each year, especially in younger men with bilateral varicoceles.

Men's Health Month: www.menshealthmonth.org

Resources for the Nurse Practitioner

American Urological Association: The Optimal Evaluation of the Infertile Male: AUA Best Practice Statement http://www.auanet.org/common/pdf/education/clinical-guidance/Male-Infertility-d.pdf
    Men's Health Network (MHN): www.menshealthnetwork.org
    Men's Health Month: www.menshealthmonth.org

Resources for the Patient

The Urology Care Foundation: www.urologyhealth.org
    RESOLVE: The National Infertility Association: www.resolve.org
    American Society for Reproductive Medicine: www.reproductivefacts.org
    Men's Health Network (MHN): www.menshealthnetwork.org

References

Al-marzooq WA, Yahya SAE, Alhumairi AK (2018) Incidence of orchiectomy in patients with testicular torsion treated in the urology department in hilla teaching hospital. J Univ Babylon Pure Appl Sci 26(7):1–8

Alsaikhan B, Alrabeeah K, Delouya G, Zini A (2016) Epidemiology of varicocele. Asian J Androl 18(2):179–181

Aoun F, Slaoui A, Naoum E, Hassan T, Albisinni S et al (2019) Testicular microlithiasis: systematic review and clinical guidelines. Prog Urol 29(10):465–473

Baigorri BF, Dixon RC (2016) Varicocele: a review. Semin Intervent Radiol 33(3):170–176

Balawender K, Orkisz S, Wisz P (2018) Testicular microlithiasis: what urologists should know. A review of current literature. Cent European J Urol 71:310–314

Braga LH, Lorenzo AJ, Romao RLP (2017) Canadian Urological Association-Pediatric Urologists of Canada (CUA-PUC) guideline for the diagnosis, management, and follow up of cryptorchidism. Can Urol Assoc J 11(7):E251–E260. https://doi.org/10.5489/cuaj.4585. Epub 2017 Jul 11. PMID: 28761584; PMCID: PMC5519382

Brodie KE, Saltzman AF, Cost NG (2018) Adolescent testicular microlithiasis: a case-based, multinational survey of clinical management practices. J Pediatr Urol 14:151e1–151e8

Cayan S, Orhan I, Akbay E, Kadoglu A (2019) Systematic review of treatment methods for recurrent varicoceles to compare post-treatment sperm parameters, pregnancy and complication rates. Andrologia 51(11):e13419

Cho A, Thomas J, Perera R, Cherian A (2019) Undescended testis. BMJ 364:1926

Dagur G, Gandhi J, Suh Y, Weissbart S, Sheynkin YR, Smith NL, Joshi G, Khan SA (2016) Classifying hydroceles of the pelvis and groin: an overview of etiology, secondary complications, evaluation, and management. Curr Urol 10(1):1–14. https://doi.org/10.1159/000447145

Dublin L, Ameler RD (1970) Varicocele size and results of varicocelectomy in selected subfertile men with varicoceles. Fertil Steril 21:606

Gomella LG (2010) The 5-minute urology consult, 2nd ed. Wolters Kluwer/Lippincott Williams & Wilkins, Philadelphia

Hazeltine M, Panza A, Ellsworth P (2017) Testicular torsion: current evaluation and management. Urol Nurs 37(2):61–71

Kapoor S (2008) Testicular torsion: a race against time. Int J Clin Pract 62(5):821–827

Leblanc L, Lagrange F, Lecoanet P, Marcon B, Eschwege P, Hubert J (2018) Testicular microlithiasis and testicular tumor: a review of the literature. Basic Clin Androl 28:8. Published online July 9, 2018

Leslie SW, Sajjad H, Villanueva CA (2020) Cryptorchidism. [Updated 2019 Oct 8]. In: StatPearls [Internet]. StatPearls Publishing, Treasure Island, FL. https://www.ncbi.nlm.nih.gov/books/NBK470270

Mathers MJ, Degener S, Sperling H, Roth S (2017) Hematospermia—a symptom with many possible causes. Dtsch Arztebl Int 114:186–191

O'Reilly P, Le J, Sinyavskaya A, Mandel E (2016) Evaluating scrotal masses. J Am Acad Physician Assist 29(2):26–32

Pilatz A, Altinkilic B, Köhler E, Weidner W (2011) Color Doppler ultrasound imaging in varicoceles: is the venous diameter sufficient for predicting clinical and subclinical varicocele? World J Urol 29(5):645–650

Pourmand G, Movahedin M, Dehghani S et al (2014) Does L-carnitine therapy add any extra benefit to standard inguinal varicocelectomy in terms of deoxyribonucleic acid damage or sperm quality factor indices: a randomized study. Urology 84(4):821–825

Prajapati N, Ratogi SK, Kulshrestha V, Pandit A, Waheed N, Gupta A (2016) Varicoceles: co-relation of clinical examination with color Doppler sonography at a tertiary care hospital. Indian J Basic Appl Med Res 5(3):191–197

Richenberg J, Belfield J, Ramchandani P, Rocher L, Freeman S et al (2015) Testicular microlithiasis imaging and follow-up: guidelines of the ESUR scrotal imaging subcommittee. Eur Radiol 25:323–330

Sommers DN, Jensen J (2015) Sonographic findings of typical and atypical scrotal trauma. Ultrasound Q 31(2):99–108

Suh Y, Gandhi J, Joshi G, Lee MY, Weissbart SJ, Smith NL, Joshi G, Khan SA (2017) Etiologic classification, evaluation, and management of hematospermia. Transl Androl Urol 6(5):959–972. https://doi.org/10.21037/tau.2017.06.01

Ta A, D'Arcy FT, Hoag N, D'Arcy JP, Lawrentschuk N (2015) Testicular torsion and the acute scrotum: current emergency management. Eur J Emerg Med 8(11):37–41

Yan Y, Chen S, Chen Z, Pei X, Zhou P, Xiao Y, Wang X (2018) The applied value of medical history, physical examination, colour-Doppler ultrasonography and testis scintigraphy in the differential diagnosis of acute scrotum. Androl 50(4):e12973

Erectile Dysfunction: Identification, Assessment, Treatment, and Follow-Up

4

Penny Kaye Jensen and Jeffrey A. Albaugh

Contents

P. K. Jensen
Department of Veterans Affairs, Office of Nursing Services, Washington, DC, USA
e-mail: penny.jensen@va.gov

J. A. Albaugh (✉)
Sexual Health, John & Carol Walter Center for Urological Health, North Shore University
Health System, Glenview, IL, USA
e-mail: JAlbaugh@northshore.org

© Springer Nature Switzerland AG 2020
S. A. Quallich, M. J. Lajiness (eds.), *The Nurse Practitioner in Urology*,
https://doi.org/10.1007/978-3-030-45267-4_4

Objectives
1. Understand the incidence, prevalence, etiology, and risk factors associated with erectile dysfunction.
2. Identify the anatomy and physiology related to vascular, neurogenic, and hormonal components necessary for normal erectile function.
3. Identify the comorbidities associated with erectile dysfunction including cardiovascular disease, diabetes, obesity, metabolic syndrome, dyslipidemia, and hypertension.
4. Articulate that the linkage of ED symptoms is an early manifestation of endothelial dysfunction and should prompt further evaluation for cardiovascular risk.
5. Identify appropriate laboratory testing with interpretation of results.
6. Describe the role of both pharmacologic and nonpharmacologic treatment modalities.
7. Recognize that erectile dysfunction (ED) assessment can be a pathway for managing men's overall health, and
8. Describe the use of guidelines to assist in clinical decision-making, with integration into daily practice.

Introduction

Advances in the understanding of male sexuality have led to the development of a wide range of options for managing erectile dysfunction (ED). The availability of oral agents, particularly phosphodiesterase type-5 (PDE-5), inhibitors which are considered first-line treatment, has expanded the therapeutic choices for men with ED. Historically, ED was treated by urologists and mental health practitioners. Today ED is most often managed in the primary care setting initially with referrals to specialists as necessary when oral agents have failed. Primary care providers (PCPs) write approximately two-thirds of all PDE-5 inhibitors (Kuritzky and Miner 2004). Successful treatment with these agents requires attention to appropriate dosing and prescribing information. Furthermore, the association of ED with vascular disease risk factors, such as diabetes, hypertension, dyslipidemia, tobacco use, obesity, and coronary artery disease, may be initially identified by and treated by primary care providers. Thus, nurse practitioners (NPs) are in a unique position to identify men at risk for both vascular disease and ED.

Scope of the Problem

After decades as a problem considered off limits for discussion, erectile dysfunction is at the forefront of healthcare. The transformation from forbidden subject to well-publicized and accepted health problem began in 1993, when the National Institute of Health Consensus Development Panel on Impotence (1993) catapulted impotence into the limelight and labeled it an important public health problem. The panel proposed that the term "impotence" be replaced by the less disparaging and more acceptable term of "erectile dysfunction" (ED) to signify the inability to attain and/ or maintain a penile erection sufficient for sexual performance (NIH Consensus Panel on Impotence 1993). Erectile dysfunction is a common problem; an estimated 30 million men in the United States have some degree of erectile dysfunction (Bacon et al. 2003). ED occurs in approximately 1 out of 5 men in their lifetime and is more common in men 40 and older (Allen and Walter 2019).

Prevalence of Erectile Dysfunction and Aging

Prevalence studies demonstrate that, when controlling for other factors, increasing age is a risk factor for the development of erectile dysfunction, especially after 50 years of age (Allen and Walter 2019). The patients in these age groups make up the majority of patients evaluated in the adult primary care setting; thus, up to half of all men seen in primary care clinics will have some degree of ED. According to the United Nations, by 2025, there will be more than 356 million worldwide over the age of 65, an increase of 197 million from the current number. In 1995, the global proportion of men older than age 65 was 4.2%; this is expected to rise to 9.5% by 2025 (Shabsigh 2006). Due to the correlation between ED and age, global aging will bring an increase in the number of men with ED in the future. Aging alone does not explain the high prevalence of ED in older men. Rather, the high prevalence of ED is explained by normal age-related changes in combination with the accumulation of risk factors and health conditions that accompany aging (Seftel et al. 2004). Since the penis is a vascular organ, it is true that a man is as old as his penis. Kinsey's classical work revealed that aging is crucial risk factor for the development of ED. In his early works, he found that the prevalence of ED increased with age from 0.1% at 20 years of age to 75% at 80 years of age (Kinsey et al. 1948). Almost 50 years later, the MMAS revealed the same trend (Feldman et al. 1994). The aging process causes longer latent periods between sexual stimulation and attaining an erection. There is also a decrease in erectile rigidity and tactile sensitivity, diminished ejaculation, decrease in ejaculatory volume, and a longer refractory period. Patients and partners may be advised that men in their 50s and 60s and those with diabetes may benefit from additional stimulation because of increased tactile sensory thresholds (Rowland et al. 2005).

Physiology of an Erection

An erection begins with physical and/or mental stimulation. This information is processed and integrated in the frontal lobe of the brain. The message then travels down the spinal cord to the sacral area (S2–4) and the parasympathetic impulses contribute to smooth muscle relaxation and the inflow of blood. Chemical mediators activate smooth muscle relaxation and blood vessel dilatation leading to filling of the erectile cylinders. Nitric oxide and cyclic gua-nosine monophosphate (cGMP) are the primary noncholinergic-nonadrenergic and cholinergic mediators for the relaxation of the cavernosal smooth muscle (Gratzke et al. 2010). There are three erectile cylinders within the penis includ-ing the paired corpus cavernosa and the corpora spongiosum, and when these cylinders fill to capacity, they press against the superficial veins locking blood in the penis causing penile engorgement. Testosterone is the primary male andro-gen and is regulated via the hypothalamus-pituitary-testis axis. Testosterone is involved in the maturation and the maintenance of penile tissue architecture (Carson et al. 2009). Although testosterone plays a major role in normal libido, it also plays a smaller role in erectile function and ability to achieve ejaculation. There can be many underlying etiological factors associated with ED, and it may be multifactorial. Blood flow into the penis and nervous system communication between the brain and penis are essential to erections. Any disease process that impacts blood or nerve conduction may impact erectile function.

Etiology of Erectile Dysfunction

A general classification of ED by etiology is useful in evaluating patients with ED when choosing treatment options. Erectile dysfunction may be classified as organic, psychogenic, or mixed in origin (Lue 2000). Until the early 1980s, 80% of ED cases were attributed to psychogenic causes, and 20% were attributed to organic etiologies (Boyle 1999). The primary cause of ED in the large proportion of patients is now attributed to arterial disorders such as hypertension, diabetes mellitus, dyslipidemia, and peripheral vascular disease. Clinical research sug-gests that the penile vascular bed may be a sensitive indicator of early systemic endothelial cell and smooth muscle dysfunction (Jones et al. 2002). Organic dys-function is by far the most common form of ED and may be caused by multiple etiologies.

Psychogenic causes include performance anxiety, relationship problems, psy-chological stress, or depression, which causes a loss of libido, over inhibition, or impaired nitric oxide release. The most common psychogenic cause of ED is performance anxiety related to a man's fear that he will not be able to perform sexually. Anxiety may lead to an initial failure, which further increases anxiety, resulting in a cycle that leads to future failures to achieve an erection. Stress, tension, worry, guilt, and anger can also inhibit sexual performance. Sexual per-formance is closely associated with a man's self-esteem; therefore, erectile dys-function can be devastating not only to a man's sex life but also to his sense of self. Men with ED often develop feelings of inadequacy, embarrassment, or guilt. The psychological effects of ED can invade other areas of a man's life as well, such as social interactions and job performance. These psychological factors may occur secondary to and possibly as a result of the organic causes (Sachs 2003). Mixed etiologies can occur, and an organic etiology may become a sec-ondary psychogenic problem.

Organic Etiologies of Erectile Dysfunction

Vasculogenic: A common organic etiology of erectile dysfunction is vascular compromise, which can be either arterial or venous. Vasculogenic ED accounts for about two-thirds of patients with ED (Androshchuk et al. 2015). Vascular compromise may be related to hypertension, atherosclerosis, diabetes mellitus, pelvic irradiation, Peyronie's disease, and pelvic or perineal trauma, any of which can cause inadequate arterial flow or impaired venous occlusion. Traditionally, ED was viewed as an outcome of occlusive systemic vascular disease that occurred as a late consequence of atherosclerosis. Current and emerging clinical research investigators reveal that the penile vascular bed may be a sensitive indicator of early systemic endothelial cell and/or smooth muscle dysfunction. ED is likely among the initial signs of oxidative stress and subclinical cardiovascular disease (McCullough 2003). ED is becoming a barometer of overall cardiovascular risk factors and should be viewed in this context (McCullough 2003). In fact, the symptom of erectile difficulty, particularly the poor ability to maintain a firm erection, often occurs before the development of overt structural occlusive vascular problems that lead to adverse events such as myocardial infarction, stroke, or claudication (Kloner and Speakman 2002). The most important point of these findings is not that these comorbidities are related but that ED is an early end-organ manifestation of the disease process—one that manifests much earlier than a critical arterial stenosis of the coronary arteries, diabetic peripheral neuropathy, retinopathy, or hypertensive cardiomyopathy. ED is the body's "early warning system" (McCullough 2003). Because of its prevalence in CVD, diabetes, hypertension, and other systemic vascular illnesses, ED has traditionally been viewed as a secondary complication of these disorders. More recently, a growing body of clinical evidence has emerged to suggest that a paradigm shift is in order (McCullough 2003). Inman et al. (2009) have shown that when ED occurs in younger men, it is associated with a marked increase in the risk of future cardiac events and that overall ED may be associated with an approximately 80% higher risk of subsequent CAD.

According to the Massachusetts Male Aging Study (MMAS), erectile dysfunction is strongly associated with significant health risks, such as diabetes, dyslipidemia, hypertension, and cardiac disease (Feldman et al. 1994). Billups and Friedrich (2005) found that 60% of healthy men presenting ED had abnormal cholesterol levels, and over 90% of these men had evidence of penile arterial disease when Doppler ultrasound was performed. The Minneapolis Heart Institute Foundation study initially reported that ED may be one of the first signs of cardiovascular disease, because the narrow vessels of the penis appear more sensitive to atherosclerotic blockage than the larger vessels in the heart (Pritzker 1999). Studies that suggested a link between coronary artery disease (CAD) and erectile dysfunction (ED) began to appear in the literature in the late 1980s. Men with cardiovascular disease, diabetes mellitus, and metabolic syndrome have a higher prevalence of ED than men who do not have these diseases (Grover et al. 2006).

Neurogenic: A type of organic etiology, neurogenic etiologies include disorders such as Parkinson's disease, multiple sclerosis, Alzheimer's disease, stroke, spinal cord injury, and radical pelvic surgery, such as radical prostatectomy, diabetic neuropathy, or pelvic injury caused by failure to initiate nerve impulse or interruption of neural transmission. Injuries to the back, especially if they involve the vertebral column and the spinal cord, can cause erectile dysfunction. Diabetes mellitus, chronic renal failure, and coronary heart disease result in both neural and vascular dysfunction. A wide variety of operations performed for other conditions can cause incidental injury to the nerves of the penis resulting in ED.

Hormonal: Approximately 10% of erectile dysfunction is caused by hormonal imbalance. Testosterone declines with aging, with an average decrease in total serum testosterone levels of approximately 1.5% per year (Feldman et al. 2002). The prevalence of low serum total testosterone levels is approximately 20% by the age of 50 and 50% by the age of 80 (Matsumoto 2002). Androgen deficiency decreases nocturnal erections and libido. Symptoms of low testosterone include decreased muscle mass and bone mineral density, increased fat mass, central obesity, insulin resistance, decreased libido, low energy levels, memory loss, irritability, and depression. Hypogonadism and hyperprolactinemia cause loss of libido and inadequate nitric oxide release. Kidney and liver disease also may lead to hormonal imbalances that can cause erectile dysfunction.

Diabetes: The association between ED and diabetes is well established (Kolodny et al. 1974). The risk of ED in patients with diabetes approaches 50%. Diabetics are not only at risk for developing macrovascular and microvascular disease, but also these patients have an increased risk for neuropathies and hormonal abnormalities. These conditions have been found at higher rates in diabetics than in the general population (Corona et al. 2004). Poor glycemic control as demonstrated by elevated glycosylated hemoglobin levels correlates with severe ED (Rhoden et al. 2005).

Lower Urinary Tract Symptoms: It is now recognized that men with lower urinary tract symptoms (LUTSs) have a high prevalence of ED (Rosen et al. 2003). LUTS is most often caused by benign prostatic hyperplasia (BPH), which is comprised of multiple voiding symptoms, including urinary frequency, urgency, nocturia, and slow stream. Although the etiology remains unclear, findings from several studies suggest that LUTS is a risk factor for ED, independent of age and other comorbidities (Braun et al. 2003). There is a strong epidemiological evidence for a link between ED and LUTS supported by theories for their shared pathogenesis. The quality of life of men with BPH is reduced by its effects on sexual function (Carson and McMahon 2008). Investigators suggest that LUTS associated with BPH may be improved with phosphodiesterase (PDE-5) inhibitors (Liu et al. 2011). These medications are commonly prescribed for ED. The inhibition of PDE isoenzymes relaxes the smooth muscle in the prostate or bladder and can improve LUTS in BPH patients (Kaplan and Gonzalez 2007).

Sleep Apnea: Several studies have suggested a link between sleep apnea and ED; the correlation between the severity of sleep apnea and the severity of ED is strong (Jankowski et al. 2008; Teloken et al. 2006; Zias et al. 2009). Sleep apnea disrupts rapid eye movement or REM sleep; this is the time when men routinely experience nocturnal erections. It is hypothesized that decreased REM sleep means fewer nocturnal erections. Nocturnal erections are a necessary process for men to maintain healthy sexual function. APPs should consider concomitant sleep disorders when evaluating patients with ED, especially in those refractory to routine therapy (Jankowski et al. 2008). Further studies are necessary to clearly define the causative link between sleep disorders and ED.

Depression: When depression is the primary illness, erectile dysfunction can be considered a symptom of the depressive illness. However, if ED is the primary diagnosis, men may develop depressive symptoms due to the loss of erectile function. Regardless of whether ED is a symptom of depression or depression is a consequence of ED, these conditions are frequently comorbid. Araujo et al. (1998) concluded that the relationship between depressive symptoms and ED in middle-aged men is robust and independent of important aging confounders such as demographics, lifestyle, health status, medication use, and hormones (Araujo et al. 1998).

Risk Factors for Erectile Dysfunction

Risk factors for ED are any underlying disease process that can impact blood flow, nerve conduction, or hormonal imbalance. In addition to sedentary lifestyle, obesity, and tobacco use, recreational drug use is also a risk factor for ED. Many commonly prescribed medications can diminish erectile function. Medications that can impact erectile function are antihypertensives (the most common are diuretics and beta-blockers), antidepressants (the most common are serotonin reuptake inhibitors (SSRIs) and tricyclic antidepressants), anti-anxiety medications, anti-psychotics, anticholinergics, antiarrhythmics, antiandrogens, antihistamines (the most common is pseudoephedrine), narcotics (opioids), and analgesics. It is important to obtain a history to assess the patient's potential underlying medical issues that may impact erectile function, current medications both prescribed and over the counter (OTC), and drugs of habituation (alcohol, marijuana, cocaine) for potential effects on erectile function and lifestyle choices in terms of exercise/activity, diet, and sexual activity.

Obesity nearly doubles the risk of ED (Bacon et al. 2003). A Danish community-based cross-sectional study reported that ED was more prevalent in men with a body mass index (BMI) of 30 or more (Andersen et al. 2008). Esposito et al. found that men with a BMI above 25 are at a higher risk of ED (Esposito et al. 2004). One-third of men who were obese improved their erectile function with moderate weight loss and an increase in the amount and duration of regular exercise (Esposito et al. 2004).

A healthy lifestyle prevents the occurrence of ED. Derby et al. (2000) conducted a study to prospectively examine whether changes in smoking, heavy alcohol consumption, sedentary lifestyle, and obesity were associated with the risk of erectile dysfunction. Data were collected as part of a cohort study of a random sample of men 40–70 years old. In-home interviews were completed by 1709 men at baseline in 1987–1989 and 1156 men at follow-up in 1995–1997 (average follow-up 8.8 years). Analyses included 593 men without erectile dysfunction at baseline were free of prostate cancer and had not been treated for heart disease or diabetes. Obesity status was associated with erectile dysfunction ($p = 0.006$), with baseline obesity predicting a higher risk regardless of follow-up weight loss. Physical activity status was associated with erectile dysfunction ($p = 0.01$), with the highest risk among men who remained sedentary and the lowest among those who remained active or initiated physical activity (Derby et al. 2000). Changes in smoking and alcohol consumption were not associated with the incidence of erectile dysfunction ($p > 0.3$). The authors concluded that midlife lifestyle changes may be too late to reverse the effects of smoking, obesity, and alcohol consumption on erectile dysfunction. In contrast, physical activity may reduce the risk of ED even if initiated in midlife; therefore, early adoption of healthy lifestyles may be the best approach to reduce the risk of developing erectile dysfunction (Derby et al. 2000).

Management of Erectile Dysfunction

A consensus guidelines model was developed for managing erectile dysfunction (ED) for healthcare clinicians. The model emphasizes a systematic approach in identification, assessment, intervention, and follow-up in patients with ED. The guidelines are intended to provide a comprehensive care model for patients and their partners, which would be optimally cost-effective and clinically relevant. This model allows quality sexual healthcare to be provided to increasing numbers of patients and their partners (Albaugh et al. 2002).

Identification of Erectile Dysfunction

Traditionally, sexual health has not been a high priority for primary care providers, including NPs. Men are often reluctant to bring up sexual issues (Eardley 2013) and often look to their nurse practitioner (NP) to initiate discussion about sexuality and intimacy. To provide holistic care to patients, NPs should ask patients about problems with sexuality and intimacy.

ED has been viewed as a quality-of-life issue rather than a relatively common medical condition that increases in prevalence as men age. Although ED is not perceived as a life-threatening condition, it is closely associated with many comorbidities and shared risk factors for those comorbidities. ED is a widespread and significant condition that warrants further investigation and is considered a marker for current or future cardiovascular and metabolic disease, as well as diabetes, dyslipidemia, depression, hypogonadism, and other disorders. Identifying ED represents an opportunity to screen for serious concomitant conditions.

While various cultures may approach sex and intimacy differently, cultural sensitivity may be helpful in approaching each individual patient and their partner. There is cultural variation regarding eye contact; thus, providers must be mindful of cultural issues. In some cultures or religions, it may be unacceptable to engage in sexual activity within a certain number of days before or after menstruation. Assessing for and understanding any individual or cultural inhibition are important in order to best advise a patient in moving forward with ED treatment.

Men who should be screened include those over age 40, those with predisposing comorbidities, or patients who may have difficulties with physical intimacy. Patients with sexual concerns often feel the most comfortable discussing these issues with an NP. More than 70% of adult patients in a large sample considered sexual complaints an appropriate topic to discuss with their primary care clinician (Sadovsky and Curtis 2006). The rate of sexual dysfunction surveyed was 35% for adult men and 42% for adult women; evidence of discussion regarding these sexual complaints was documented in as few as 2% of the clinician's notes (Sadovsky and Curtis 2006).

Sexual inquiry is most often conducted by face-to-face interview with the patient, although partner interviews, paper-and-pencil questionnaires, or computer-based methods may also be of value. Each of these methods has distinct advantages and limitations. Perhaps the most important aspect of the interview is the manner in which inquiry is conducted. A high level of sensitivity for each individual's unique ethnic, cultural, and person background should be taken into consideration. Administering self-evaluation questionnaires such as the Sexual Health Inventory for Men (SHIM) (Cappelleri and Rosen 2005) is a discrete way of screening patients while they are waiting in the office. The SHIM was developed and validated as a brief, easily administered, patient-reported diagnostic tool. It is widely used for screening and diagnosis of ED as well as severity of ED in clinical practice and research (Cappelleri and Rosen 2005).

NPs can also approach patients using the PLISSIT model (Permission, Limited Information, Specific Suggestions, and Intensive Therapy) (Annon 1974). The approach begins with asking for and giving permission to discuss sexual concerns. Initiating discussion about sexual dysfunction opens the channels of communication and legitimizes the patient's concerns. The next step for the NP is to provide information about sexuality and sexual dysfunction. The information may include normal anatomy and physiology, dispelling myths about sexuality, and discussing common sexual problems. The next step is to provide specific recommendations on what may be helpful to improve the patient's sexual issue. These suggestions should be driven by the patient's sexual health goals. It is important to include the partner in the treatment plan and education process. The final step in the PLISSIT model is to guide the patient to intensive therapy (the IT of the model). The model should be instituted using a nonjudgmental and caring attitude while keeping in mind the patient's and partner's goals, feelings, and expectations. Including the partner in the visit can be very helpful and allow for sexual education of both the patient and their partner.

Sample Questions for Identifying ED
1. Do you have trouble achieving or maintaining an erection?
2. Do you have trouble all the time, some of the time, or infrequently?
3. Men with heart disease (or diabetes, high cholesterol, etc.) often have problems getting erections. Has this been a problem for you?
4. Did your erectile dysfunction begin suddenly or gradually?
5. Is erectile dysfunction (ED) global or dependent on circumstances, such as partner?

6. Are you having relationship conflicts with your partner not related to ED?
7. How often are intercourse attempts successful?
8. Is your interest still adequate?
9. Do you have early morning or nighttime erections?
10. Do you have any difficulties with ejaculation, too fast or too slow?
11. Are you able to achieve orgasm?
12. Have your tried any therapies to correct this problem?

Assessment of Erectile Dysfunction

A complete medical history should be obtained to evaluate for treatable organic and/ or psychogenic etiologies. The successful treatment of erectile dysfunction begins with a detailed medical history, including both psychosocial and sexual components. Due to the close association between cardiovascular risk factors and ED, searching for potential cardiovascular disease in these patients is critical. ED may be a warning sign of latent cardiac disease before symptoms of heart disease are present. The NP should assume underlying cardiovascular disease until proven otherwise because of the link between ED and cardiovascular disease (Nehra et al. 2012).

The history should include a comprehensive targeted sexual, medical, and psychosocial history (Shamloul and Ghanem 2013). History taking should be aimed at characterizing the severity of the symptoms, triggers that exacerbate symptoms, onset of symptoms, duration of the problem, as well as any concomitant medical or psychosocial factors. Contributing factors including all medical conditions that may impact sex and intimacy, prescription or nonprescription drug use, relationship issues, depression, anxiety, or other psychiatric disorders should be carefully assessed. Screening for depression can also be integrated into the history-taking process (Jensen et al. 2004). Depression, post-traumatic stress syndrome (PTSD), anxiety, and other psychiatric conditions may be responsible for ED. It is imperative to obtain a social history since stress surrounding a relationship or problems with alcohol or substance abuse including tobacco can have a direct impact on erectile function (Jensen et al. 2004).

A complete physical examination with special emphasis placed on the review of genitourinary, endocrine, vascular, and neurologic systems should be performed. The physical examination of the genitalia provides an opportunity for patient education and reassurance regarding normal genital anatomy. During inspection, the NP should note the patient's secondary sex characteristics (facial/body hair, normal/ abnormal breast tissue, deepness of voice), skin, scars from previous surgeries, and musculature development. Cardiovascular assessment should include blood pressure, heart sounds, and peripheral pulses in the lower extremities. The most useful physical finding is diminished femoral and/or popliteal pulses (LaRochelle and Levine 2006). This finding suggests that vascular disease, specifically arterial insufficiency, is the most likely cause or at least has a role in the patient's ED. If these large vessels have diminished pulsatility, it is likely that the cavernosal arteries, which are 0.5–1.0 mm in diameter, are also compromised (LaRochelle and Levine

2006). The neurologic evaluation may include muscle strength, muscle spasticity, assessment of gait, sensitivity to touch, and testing of the peripheral and genital reflexes. The genitourinary examination should involve assessment of the size of the penis, any indurations, nodules, fibrosis, lesions, or plaques along the penis or on the meatus. The scrotum and testicles should be evaluated for size and consistency. In addition, the NP should note any lesions, nodules, or abnormalities of the scrotum or testes. A digital rectal examination (DRE) should be performed to determine normal shape and consistency of the prostate and to determine the presence of any lesions, indurations, or abnormalities. The anal sphincter and the bulbocavernosus reflex may also be evaluated.

Laboratory Evaluation

Laboratory evaluation can range from simple to complex. Testing should be individualized to each patient and risk factors based on the patient history. Given the strong association between ED and vascular comorbidities, laboratory testing should be conducted for all patients who have not been evaluated in the past 6 months. Selective laboratory testing should be considered to evaluate potential endocrine or other systemic causes of the patient's ED and identify likely comorbidities contributing to ED, such as diabetes or hyperlipidemia. Standard serum chemistries including fasting blood glucose or glycosylated hemoglobin, CBC, and lipid profile should be evaluated. Serum thyroid-stimulating hormone (TSH) determination may also be of some value. Plasma testosterone varies diurnally and may be decreased by anxiety, stress, or depression. Free testosterone levels may be more accurate of tissue hormone status but tend to be much more expensive. Low libido is associated with low testosterone levels; therefore, testosterone levels should be drawn on those patients complaining of a diminished sex drive. A prolactin level should be evaluated if the testosterone level is low, if there is a history of loss of libido, or if there are symptoms of prolactinoma, such as visual field loss or headache (Akpunona et al. 1994). Elevated prolactin levels can be indicative of a pituitary tumor, which should be further evaluated by MRI if no other etiology can be identified. A serum PSA may be indicated based upon the patient's age and relative risk status according to the American Urological Association (AUA) guidelines (American Urological Association 2005).

Specialized Diagnostic Assessment

Erectile dysfunction is diagnosed and treated through history and physical exam. Treatment does not vary greatly or hinge upon specialized diagnostic testing. Some patients may need referral for specialized testing when medically indicated for consideration of reconstructive surgery, failure of conventional therapy, or medicolegal reasons specialized diagnostic procedures may be indicated. These tests may include nocturnal penile tumescence and rigidity (NPTR) testing, color Doppler cavernosal studies (penile blood flow studies), or other specialized vascular or neurologic procedures, and they may play a role in further understanding selected cases. For example, these procedures may be of value in assessing young patients with pelvic or penile trauma who may be candidates for reconstructive vascular surgery. The tests may also be performed for medicolegal reasons (documenting organic erectile dysfunction in cases of litigation) or because the patient wishes to establish arterial insufficiency or venous leakage, but in general these tests do not change or impact the course of treatment and therefore may not be necessary. Patient referral to urology, endocrinology, cardiology, neurology, and/or psychiatry may be appropriate depending on diagnostic findings.

Intervention and Treatment of Erectile Dysfunction

A wide variety of medical treatments are now available for patients diagnosed with erectile dysfunction. These treatment options are classified according to efficacy, degree of invasiveness, safety, ease of use, and cost. Every treatment has pros and cons, and each patient and partner should understand these factors. Treatment plans should be goal oriented and ideally aimed at satisfying the needs of the patient and partner to maximize the chance of achieving partner satisfaction. By presenting all information, including advantages and disadvantages of each, patients can then make an informed decision about which treatment option is best for them.

First-Line Therapy

Counseling
Comprehensive sexuality education is an essential element of successful ED treatment. Patients need to not only understand each treatment option to make informed decisions about treatment choice but also information on how to integrate treatment into love play with their partner. Discussion should center on factual information and focus on resolving the patient's ED. Teaching strategies should include written, video, model reference, and verbal communication.

The key to patient success with the therapy lies in the NP's ability to effectively work one on one with the patient and/or their partner to understand and safely use the treatment. The NP should identify appropriate lifestyle changes that are recommended including smoking cessation, regular exercise, weight loss, limiting alcohol, and following a cardiovascular low fat, low cholesterol plant-based (Mediterranean) diet. These changes can help improve erectile function, reduce one's risk of heart disease or cancer, and improve overall general health (Gupta et al. 2011). Although the majority of ED has an underlying physiologic etiology, there is often a psychological component as well. It is important to encourage patients to seek counseling for themselves and their partner. Counseling may include individual counseling, couples' therapy, or sex therapy.

Oral Agents
NPs play an important role in prescribing treatments medications for their patients, including treat ED. Since its arrival, the class of agents known as type-5 phosphodiesterase (PDE5) inhibitors has changed the management of ED. Type 5

phosphodiesterase (PDE5) inhibitors are considered first-line therapy in the treatment of ED, as recommended by the American Urological Association (AUA) (Montague et al. 2005) and the European Association of Urology (EAU) (Wespes et al. 2006). Four PDE-5 inhibitors are now available by prescription: Viagra® (sildenafil), Levitra® & Staxyn® (vardenafil), Cialis® (tadalafil), and Stendra® (avanafil). The approval of sildenafil in 1998 revolutionized the treatment of ED worldwide. These agents are competitive and selective inhibitor of cyclic guanosine monophosphate (cGMP) type 5 phosphodiesterase (PDE). This inhibition increases the level of intracellular cGMP and results in the efflux of calcium ions from the cell, which causes smooth muscle relaxation. Increased levels of cGMP act to enhance the effect of nitric oxide in the penis. PDE type 5 inhibitors prevent the breakdown of cGMP, which is the intracellular second messenger of nitric oxide. Nitric oxide is released following sexual stimulation; therefore, these agents are only effective when a male is sexually stimulated. Libido is not affected by PDE-5 inhibitors (Porst et al. 2013).

The majority of patients prefer oral medications due to ease and convenience of use (Hatzichristou et al. 2000). There are no compelling data to support the superiority of one agent over another. Comparisons of efficacy among various agents in this class are limited. The main difference in these medications is their duration of action; tadalafil produces longer lasting effects offering a longer time period in which sexual activity may occur and increased spontaneity, while the shorter lasting avanafil reaches peak blood levels twice as fast as the other oral agents allowing for a shorter wait time before intercourse can occur. All PDE-5 inhibitors are contraindicated in patients using organic nitrates, in any form or frequency.

NPs should consider activity tolerance as a guide to the cardiovascular status of their patients, since there is a degree of cardiac risk associated with sexual activity. Treatment of ED, including PDE-5 inhibitors, should not be used in men for whom sexual activity is inadvisable. Guidelines for managing ED in patients with cardiovascular disease developed by the Princeton Consensus Panel recommend categorizing patients to one of three risk levels (high, intermediate, and low) based on their cardiovascular risk factors. The guideline recommends that patients at high risk should not receive treatment for sexual dysfunction until their cardiac condition has stabilized. Patients at low risk may be considered for oral agents (Jackson et al. 2006). Overall, controlled trials have revealed no increase in myocardial infarction, worsening CVD, or death rates among patients using PDE-5 inhibitors. Preliminary research indicates that these agents may be cardioprotective (Sesti et al. 2007).

PDE-5 inhibitors potentiate the hypotensive effects of nitrates, and administration to patients who are using organic nitrates, either regularly and/or intermittently, in any form is contraindicated. PDE-5 inhibitors are contraindicated in patients with a known hypersensitivity to any component of the tablet. They should be used cautiously in patients with cardiovascular conditions who are sensitive to the vasodilatory effects of PDE-5 inhibitors such as left ventricular outflow obstruction and severely impaired autonomic control of the blood pressure. They should not be used in patients who have had a myocardial infarction, stroke, or life-threatening arrhythmia in the last 6 months, unstable angina, BP <90/50 or >170/110, or retinitis pigmentosa. The concurrent use of a protease inhibitor can greatly increase PDE-5 inhibitor levels. Caution should be used in patients on multiple antihypertensive agents because PDE-5 inhibitors can lower the blood pressure further. When used in conjunction with alpha-blockers, PDE-5 inhibitors may decrease blood pressure and should be used cautiously. They should be used with caution in patients with penile curvature or deformities or in patients with sickle cell anemia, multiple myeloma, or leukemia. Common adverse reactions to these medications may include headache, flushing, nasal congestion or stuffiness, and nausea. Sildenafil may be associated with color change disturbances, often described as a "blue halo" effect. Tadalafil and avanafil may be associated with muscle or back pain. Full prescribing information should always be reviewed for more detailed information.

Patients should notify his or her provider of any changes in vision or hearing, stop the medication immediately, and seek immediate medical treatment. Vision changes may be a sign of non-arteritic anterior ischemic optic neuropathy (NAION). NAION, a cause of decreased vision including permanent loss of vision, has been reported rarely postmarketing in temporal association with the use of PDE-5 inhibitors, including Viagra (Federal Drug Administration 2007). Most, but not all, of these patients had underlying anatomic or vascular risk factors for developing NAION, including but not necessarily limited to low cup to disk ratio ("crowded disk"), age over 50, diabetes, hypertension, coronary artery disease, hyperlipidemia, and smoking. It is not possible to determine whether these events are related directly to the use of PDE-5 inhibitors, to the patient's underlying vascular risk factors or anatomical defects, to a combination of these factors, or to other factors (VIAGRA® (sildenafil) New York, NY: Pfizer Inc. 2005).

A case report in the published literature of sudden hearing loss in a male patient using Viagra® prompted Federal Drug Administration (FDA) to search the Adverse Event Reporting System (AERS) for postmarketing reports of hearing loss for all PDE-5 inhibitors. The FDA identified a total of 29 reports of sudden hearing loss, both with and without tinnitus, vertigo or dizziness, in strong temporal relationship to dosing with Viagra® (sildenafil), Cialis® (tadalafil), or Levitra® (vardenadil). There have also been cases of hearing loss reported in patients using Revatio® (sildenafil) for the treatment of pulmonary arterial hypertension (PAH). Even though no causal relationship has been demonstrated, the FDA believed that the strong temporal relationship between the use of PDE-5 inhibitors and sudden hearing loss in these cases warranted revisions to the product labeling for the drug class (Federal Drug Administration 2007).

Patients should also avoid a high-fat diet for 2 h before administration, and be advised of onset of the particular medication prescribed. PDE-5 inhibitors do not affect ejaculation, orgasm, or libido. Guay et al. (2001) found that as testosterone levels fell, the response to sildenafil decreased and eventually became ineffective; therefore, it is important to evaluate testosterone levels if oral therapy is not effective.

In 2008, the FDA-approved once-daily use of tadalafil in a dose of 5 mg or a 2.5-mg dose for the treatment of ED. Theoretically, chronic dosing would result in continuous inhibition of PDE-5, therefore increasing a higher concentration of cyclic guanosine monophosphate, which may benefit men who have not responded to on-demand treatment. Once-daily tadalafil may be appropriate for men with ED who anticipate sexual activity more than twice per week and allow greater spontaneity in the patients' sexual encounters while improving tolerability, patient satisfaction, and adherence (Hatzimouratidis and Hatzichristou 2007; McMahon 2004; Porst et al. 2006). The majority of treatment failures with oral PDE-5 inhibitors can be salvaged with reeducation. Men who are not responsive may have issues with intimacy or establishing relationships, are not able to tolerate side effects, or have advanced endothelial dysfunction. Patients with advanced vascular disease or multiple comorbidities may have a poor response to PDE-5 inhibitors.

Vacuum Constriction Devices

Vacuum constriction devices (VCDs) are the least invasive and least expensive of all treatment options and can be used regardless of etiology. The efficacy and safety of vacuum constriction devices are well documented (Kohler et al. 2007; Pahlajani et al. 2012; Raina et al. 2006). VCDs are often used by individuals who wish to avoid taking medications or in combination with medications when the PDE-5 inhibitor is not completely or consistently effective. A VCD consists of a cylinder attached to a vacuum pump and tension rings. VCDs are noninvasive and may be a less least expensive treatment option. Medical grade devices have a pressure release valve on the pump or cylinder and may be either manual or battery operated. The devices produce an erection by creating negative pressure around the penis to pull blood into the penis. The erection is maintained by applying the tension band or ring around the base of the penis off the edge of cylinder. The band/ring does not completely constrict penile arterial blood flow but should be removed and should never be worn for greater than 30 min at a time maximum.

There are no major adverse effects reported when the vacuum device is used carefully and according to instructions. Adverse effects may include hematoma, ecchymosis, petechiae, numbness of the penis, pain, pulling of scrotal tissue, and blocked or painful ejaculation. The use of vacuum devices requires thorough one-on-one training for treatment success. The advantages of VCDs are that they are noninvasive and with proper instruction and practice have a high success rate. The disadvantages of VCDs are that they are cumbersome, awkward, and the resulting erection is often not viewed as natural. The erection must be maintained with a tension ring during intercourse.

A venous flow constriction loop/or ring alone can also be used to maintain erections. They consist of bands or rings of various designs and materials that are placed around the base of the penis to diminish venous return holding the blood within the penis. The device is placed on the penis after achieving an erection to assist in maintaining the erection. VCDs have been used successfully in combination with intracavernosal injection, intraurethral therapy, and PDE-5 inhibitors. A VCD can also be alternatively recommended for the initiation of programmed cavernosal oxygenation to accelerate penile erection recovery after prostatectomy (Kendirici et al. 2006).

Second-Line Therapy

Intracavernosal Injection Therapy

The introduction of intracavernosal injections (ICIs) revolutionized the diagnosis and treatment of erectile dysfunction in the mid-1980s. Before oral agents became available, intracavernosal self-injection was the most common medical therapy for ED. This therapy is effective in approximately 89% in most cases of ED, regardless of etiology (Coombs et al. 2012). These are vasoactive drugs that are injected directly into the corpora, causing erection as the smooth muscles of the arterioles and the cavernous trabeculae relax. Intracavernosal injections may be effective in those patients who have failed intraurethral or oral therapies.

Medications most commonly used in injection therapy are papaverine hydrochloride, phentolamine, prostaglandin (PGE1), and/or atropine. These agents are injected in bimix, trimix, or quadmix solutions and are available through compounding pharmacies and various urology clinics. Even though these agents have been available since the 1980s and documentation of efficacy is well established, they are not approved by the FDA and commonly injected mixtures are only available through an accredited compounding pharmacy. The injectable form of alprostadil (Edex® or Caverject®) is the only FDA-approved injectable agent for ED. All of these medications are used in parenteral form and require the patient to self-administer intracavernosal injections. Patient education is the key to penile injections. The patient must understand the need to rotate injection sites to prevent fibrosis or plaque. Adverse effects include penile pain, priapism, fibrosis, facial flushing, dizziness, hematoma, and ecchymosis. Injections are contraindicated in those patients with penile implants, have a hypersensitivity to prostaglandins, or have a condition that would predispose them to priapism (sickle cell anemia or trait, multiple myeloma, leukemia, hypervaricosity, thrombocytopenia, polycythemia, and those prone to venous thrombus) (Auxillium Pharmaceuticals Inc. 2011). The patient should press over the injection site for 5 min after removing the needle (especially if using any type of anticoagulant therapy or aspirin).

Penile injections may be used up to 3 times/week and never more than once in a 24-h period (even if the injection is not effective, the patient should be instructed not to reinject related to the risk of priapism). In some older patients, the effect of intracavernous agents seems to decline with time. The erection occurs with or without sexual stimulation. To decrease pain or burning associated with alprostadil, the patient may take acetaminophen 30–45 min before injection. It is important to teach patients what to do in case of priapism and to provide an information card to carry them in case of emergency (American Urological Association's Guidelines for treating priapism). One-on-one teaching and in-office trial of the first self-injection for the patient and/or partner is essential to success with penile injections. The APP should encourage partners to be involved in the learning process. Take-home educational materials should be utilized during face-to-face visits, as well as return demonstration of self-injection technique after instruction. Written and video instruction are available for both FDA-approved injectables via the website for each medication and can be accessed and studied before the self-injection visit to help the patient prepare for the process.

Intraurethral Therapy

Alprostadil may also be introduced intrauretrally in the form of a semisolid pellet that is partially absorbed into the surrounding corpora cavernosa. MUSE® is an intraurethral suppository containing alprostadil, which is a form of prostaglandin E1. It is inserted from within a special plastic applicator into the distal urethra. MUSE® is less invasive with a lower risk of priapism as compared to injection therapy. MUSE® is contraindicated in patients with a hypersensitivity to alprostadil or prostaglandins, and anyone who has a condition that would predispose them to priapism (sickle cell anemia, leukemia or multiple myeloma); patient with anatomical deformity of the penis (curvature, fibrosis, severe hypospadias).

MUSE® should not be used for sexual activity with pregnant women. Almost 10% of female partners report symptoms of vaginitis following exposure to intraurethral alprostadil. Adverse effects include urethral irritation, bleeding, or pain in pelvis or upper thighs (Meda Pharmaceuticals Inc. 2014).

Initial dosing should take place in the office setting. Patients should be monitored for syncope and hypotension secondary to orthostatis. The use of a Venoseal® band (constriction device) may increase absorption and help maintain the erection. Stress, anxiety, or the consumption of alcohol may reduce the efficacy of MUSE®. The patient should be given written, verbal, and video instructions prior to dosing. The NP should encourage partners to be involved in the patient education process.

Third-Line Therapy

Penile Implant

Penile prostheses were first introduced in the 1970s and are considered the final treatment for ED after less invasive treatments have failed. Penile prostheses are available in two forms: malleable or inflatable devices. The malleable implant is always semirigid, while the inflatable implant can be inflated or deflated. The inflatable implant is the most popular device and most consist of two cylinders that are implanted into the corpora cavernosa area, a reservoir for the fluid, and a pump mechanism which dwells within the scrotum. The pump is used to move the fluid into the chambers in the penis for intercourse and the release mechanism on the pump is used to deflate the chambers and return fluid to the reservoir after sex. This option is highly invasive, irreversible, and should be reserved for select cases failing other treatment modalities. Following surgery, other medical therapies will no longer be effective in producing erection due to the damage of the corporal bodies by the prosthesis. These devices produce a natural erection with a high degree of patient and partner satisfaction but are only available in specialized medical centers and costly. A 4–8-week postoperative recovery period is necessary before the prosthesis can be used for sexual intercourse (American Urological Association 2005). Outcomes are not guaranteed, and surgical risk is associated with this procedure.

The patient and his partner should be informed that penile prosthesis implantation may preclude subsequent use of a vacuum device or vasoactive injection therapy. Complications include erosion, infection, and mechanical failure. When these occur, the prosthesis must be surgically removed. After erosion or infection has resolved, a new prosthesis may be placed; however, a second surgery is technically more difficult and results may be less satisfactory.

Vascular Surgery

Young men with vascular insufficiency may benefit from surgical revascularization. Microvascular arterial bypass and venous ligation may increase arterial inflow and decrease venous outflow. Surgical revascularization is an expensive option and available only in large medical centers. Patients must be evaluated with specialized testing by an experienced surgeon.

Newer Experimental Treatments

There are several new rejuvenative therapies currently being performed on men even though they have not yet had enough research to support FDA approval. The American Urological Association, the Sexual Medicine Society of North America and the FDA have taken a very strong stance to say that these rejuvenation therapies are off-label, lack adequate research and are not approved. At present, they should only be performed under an institutional review board (IRB) approved study. These rejuvenation therapies may include stem cell therapy, low-intensity extracorporeal shock wave therapy and plasma rich protein therapy for erectile dysfunction. Each treatment is designed to possibly regenerate better blood flow, better nerve impulse conduction and/or healthier erectile tissue. Some represent exciting, new approaches to treating erectile dysfunction, but more research is needed to determine safety and effectiveness of each treatment.

Animal studies have shown promise for some of these treatments, but the human studies have been very small and limited and in some cases no human studies have been published. In particular, there are no randomized controlled human studies of plasma rich protein (PRP) therapy, which is sometimes referred to as the "P shot." There are a few small randomized studies for stem cell therapy and for short-term extracorporal shock wave therapy (LI-ESWL).

The exact mechanism of action of stem cell therapy is not understood, but it is thought to be due to immune modulation leading to secretion of cytokines and growth factors to decrease inflammation and promote healing. Animal studies have shown promise with stem cell therapy, but there are only four small studies published on using it for erectile dysfunction. In a recent systemic review of the literature, five studies of men with erectile dysfunction with 61 men in phase 1 and 2 clinical trials were found (Lokeshwar et al. 2020). The authors concluded that stem cell therapy as a restorative therapy for erectile dysfunction shows promise, but there is very limited data for the use of stem cell therapy for erectile dysfunction in humans and more research is needed (Lokeshwar et al. 2020). In men post radical prostatectomy, there are no randomized placebo-controlled studies, but only two small studies (Matz et al. 2019). Careful, methodic research is needed to determine both safety and efficacy to identify the best treatment protocol that may or may not help men with erectile dysfunction after prostate cancer treatment while minimizing harm. This research is just not accomplished yet.

Low-intensity shock wave therapy for erectile dysfunction is another treatment being investigated for treatment of erectile dysfunction. The mechanism is still being determined, but it is thought to decrease inflammation while causing cell membrane micro-trauma resulting in the release of blood flow promoting factors. It has been used for erectile dysfunction caused by blood flow problems (vaculogenic ED) specifically. From the limited small studies, it seems to work best in mild vasculogenic erectile dysfunction and younger patients do better with the treatment (Zhihua et al. 2017; Zou et al. 2017). There was only one study (not a randomized controlled study) using the therapy in men after radical prostatectomy with a small improvement in erectile function scores at 1 month after treatment and very minimal improvement in the average score 1 year after treatment (Frey et al. 2016). Given the lack of any randomized placebo controlled studies in men treated for prostate cancer, further research is needed to determine if this treatment will have any positive effect on erectile function in these men and there is no good evidence to support this to date.

It is exciting to know there are completely different treatments for erectile dysfunction currently under scientific investigation. Further research is needed through IRB approved studies with these new therapies experimental/investigational therapies.

Penile Rehabilitation

Men who undergo radiation therapy or surgical intervention such as radical prostatectomy for prostate cancer treatment will experience changes in erectile function. These changes can be attributed to a cascade of events that affect normal erectile function. The overall effect is a loss of smooth muscle tissue, increase in corporal collagen formation, and an increase in fibrosis leading to erectile dysfunction. Vascular changes caused by arterial injury result in ischemic and hypoxic insult, which may cause penile shortening up to 2 cm. Neuropraxia or damage to the cavernosal nerve is triggered by mechanical stretch during the procedure, thermal injury from cautery, and inflammation attributed to surgical trauma or ischemia from the vascular injury (Rabbani et al. 2010). Men post radical prostatectomy should understand that the erectile recovery may take up to 2 or more years (Rabbani et al. 2010).

Some recent studies have shown that most men continue to struggle with adhering to penile rehabilitation protocols and although they improve, the majority do not return to baseline function (Albaugh et al. 2019; Capogrosso et al. 2019).

Some men with prostate cancer undergo external beam radiation therapy (EBRT) or brachytherapy as opposed to surgical intervention. Both treatments are associated with delayed and progressive onset of ED (Stember and Mulhall 2012). Similar to radical prostatectomy, the most common long-term adverse effect of radiation therapy is ED. The mechanism of injury is due to damage done postradiation exposure leading to vascular changes, neurogenic injury and structural changes resulting in fibrosis, increased collagen formation, damage to the smooth muscle tissue, and ultimately an inability to obtain or maintain a rigid erection (Stember and Mulhall 2012). Very little evidence exists about penile rehabilitation in men undergoing radiotherapy and ADT (Doherty and Bridge 2019). The research focuses solely on PDE-5 inhibitors and the limited research shows that early ongoing intervention important for benefit (Doherty and Bridge 2019).

Treatment options for penile rehabilitation are similar for men undergoing radical prostatectomy or radiation therapy. Multiple factors should be taken into consideration when determining the likelihood of restoring erectile function after prostate cancer treatment. Most importantly, the NP must consider the patient's preoperative erectile function as previous erectile dysfunction is a factor in erectile recovery post treatment. In addition, other important factors are age and the presence of comorbid conditions, such as diabetes, hypertension, hyperlipidemia, cardiovascular disease, and neurological disorders. Pretreatment assessment of erectile function should be initially assessed through the use of the Sexual Health Inventory for Men (SHIM/IIEF5) or the international Index of Erectile Functioning (IIEF) (Rosen et al. 1999; Shamloul and Ghanem 2013). Men with comorbid conditions or those who have utilized medications for erectile dysfunction prior to prostate cancer therapy, such as an oral agent are at greater risk for worsened erectile dysfunction post prostate cancer treatment (McCullough 2001).

Penile rehabilitation involves early intervention with the PDE-5 inhibitors, vacuum constriction devices (VCDs), intraurethral suppositories, and penile injections to improve erectile function; however, further research is needed to validate long-term outcomes (Tal et al. 2011). The ultimate goal of penile rehabilitation is to preserve preoperative erectile function by establishing regular blood flow to the penis to enhance erectile response. During the period of neuropraxia following radical prostatectomy, the lack of blood flow and smooth muscle activity during erections and subsequent tumescence, can lead to atrophic structural changes. Penile rehabilitation is accomplished by trying to reduce the complications of prostate cancer therapies through preserving endothelial cell function, reducing the development of fibrosis, venous leakage, and penile shortening by encouraging regular erectile activity using medical treatments (McCullough 2008; Mulhall 2008; Padma-Nathan et al. 2008). The American Urological Association Guidelines on erectile dysfunction treatment conclude that men should be informed about the possible benefits of penile rehabilitation, that evidence does not support oral agents for penile rehabilitation, the other penile rehabilitation strategies and that there is not sufficient evidence to support one particular strategy (American Urological Association 2018). Further research with larger sample sizes to determine the best penile rehabilitation strategies.

PDE-5 inhibitors are considered first-line therapy and work at the cellular level to preserve endothelial cell function, improve cavernosal oxygenation, decrease apoptotic cell death, and decrease corporal fibrosis and collagen production (Tal et al. 2011). Many protocols recommend nightly use, while others suggest 2–3 times/week which is expensive and not often covered by insurance plans. The failure rate of PDE-5 inhibitors early after radical prostatectomy has been reported to be 69–80% (Blander et al. 2000; Mydlo et al. 2005). The use of oral agents for penile rehabilitation has produced mixed research results. Padma-Nathan et al. (2008) demonstrated in a study of 76 men after nerve-sparring radical prostatectomy that 4% of the men taking placebo reported an erection sufficient for sexual activity versus 27% of men taking sildenafil 50 or 100 mg. Another research demonstrated improvement in nocturnal penile tumescence with nightly sildenafil (Montorsi et al. 2000). Subsequent large, multicenter, placebo-controlled studies have failed to demonstrate benefit from regular use of PDE-5 inhibitors for penile rehabilitation (Montorsi et al. 2000, 2008; Pavlovich et al. 2013).

Vacuum constriction devices (VCDs) can be used for penile rehabilitation, the vacuum pulls venous and arterial blood into the corpora bringing the PO_2 levels to 80 mmHg, thus providing improved oxygenation of penile tissue and reducing the risk of collagen formation and fibrosis (Mazzola and Mulhall 2011). A systemic review and meta-analysis concluded that early use of vacuum device therapy has excellent therapeutic effects, may decrease penile shrinkage, with no serious side effects and larger quality studies are needed to further substantiate the penile rehabilitation benefits (Qin et al. 2018). Regular VCD use post prostatectomy may prevent penile shrinkage in both length and girth (Pahlajani et al. 2012). Post-prostatectomy patients reported improved erectile function and less penile shrinkage after using the vacuum device (Raina et al. 2006). An additional study by Kohler et al. revealed that early intervention with the vacuum constriction device was associated with a higher IIEF score and reduced penile shrinkage (Kohler et al. 2007). A study suggests improved results are achieved with a combination of sildenafil and a VCD; this combination resulted in almost a third of the men reporting return of spontaneous erections and improved satisfaction compared to therapy with oral medications or the vacuum device alone (Raina et al. 2005).

Alprostadil (MUSE) increases arterial flow to the corpora suppressing collagen synthesis and most likely preventing fibrosis. Rehabilitation protocols vary from nightly use to 3×/week with dose ranges of 125–250 µg. McCullough (2008) found that 125–250 µg of alprostadil improved cavernosal oxygen saturation, although these men often did not experience penile rigidity.

Intracavernosal injections increase blood flow to penile tissues resulting in increased oxygenation, preservation of endothelial cells, and reduction of permanent erectile damage. Intracavernosal injections produce an erection sufficient for sexual intercourse in men post prostatectomy, and also improve return of spontaneous erections. Montorsi et al. (1997) conducted a study in men who had undergone bilateral nerve-sparing radical prostatectomy. Fifteen men received intracavernosal alprostadil 3 times/week for a 12-week period and 15 men received no injections. The results revealed that men performing injection therapy experienced a 67%

return of spontaneous erections which were sufficient for intercourse versus a 20% return of spontaneous erections of those receiving no treatment (Montorsi et al. 1997). Raina et al. (2008) reported that 56% (10 of 18 patients) who had used a combination of either oral agents or injections of alprostadil experienced a return of partial erection at approximately 6 months, but required additional treatment in order to engage in sexual intercourse (Raina et al. 2008). Mulhall et al. (2005) conducted a study with a penile rehabilitation regimen that began with regular use of oral PDE-5 inhibitors. If oral agents were not working, the participants advanced to using penile injections regularly. If patients failed to respond to oral agents, they were treated with intracavernosal injections. The rehabilitation group was compared to a similar group of men who choose to not do penile rehabilitation. After 18 months, the men receiving rehabilitation treatment ($n = 58$) had a greater percentage of men able to engage in intercourse without medication compared to the men who did not do rehabilitation [$n = 74$, 52% versus 19%, $p < 0.001$] (Mulhall et al. 2005). There are no published reports of controlled trials using injection therapy.

A challenge when using penile injections for penile rehabilitation is convincing patients to self-inject 3 times/week, since injections are perceived as invasive and associated with pain early after radical prostatectomy. Although patients were told to do injections 3 times/week, Albaugh and Ferrans (2010) found that most men in their study did not follow the recommended protocol and only injected an average of once per week. Oral agents, intraurethral suppositories, VCDs, and penile injections all have pros and cons and may not be appealing to all patients. In addition, there is a high dropout rate related to various factors even when optimal results were achieved. The International Consensus of Sexual Medicine (ICSM) 2001 committee failed to recognize a specific regimen that is preferred for penile rehabilitation (Mulhall et al. 2010). Although current research shows that working closely with each individual man to encourage regular blood flow to the penis early after prostate treatment for erectile function preservation, further research is needed to evaluate each treatment option and the role it plays in penile rehabilitation.

Erectile dysfunction is a common adverse effect of radical prostatectomy or radiation therapy, the effects of which can be severe for both the patient and their partner. Penile rehabilitation can be initiated as an attempt to preserve preprostate cancer treatment erectile function. Several medical treatments can be used for penile rehabilitation to encourage improved erectile response and increased blood flow into the penis including oral agents (PDE-5 inhibitors), the vacuum constriction device, intraurethral alprostadil, and/or penile injections. The ideal strategy, personalized to the individual patient, would involve using various treatment modalities in both the peri and postoperative periods to maximally enhance erectile recovery. When counseling patients about treatment options, realistic expectations should be provided by the APP. Further research is needed to determine the best strategies to individualize rehabilitation regimens for patients.

Follow-Up of Erectile Dysfunction

As with any treatment plan, regular follow-up visits are necessary to evaluate the treatment and progress of therapy. Modifying risk factors may facilitate erection directly or improve response to ED treatments. Patients should be evaluated 1 month after initiation of treatment; during the visit, a brief history along with administration of standardized scales such as the SHIM may be used to evaluate erectile function. Although PDE-5 inhibitors are effective, safe, and well tolerated, they are often used suboptimally, and patient discontinuation rates are substantial. Patients may need additional assistance and information or wish to try another treatment option. Switching to a different PDE-5 inhibitor is another option for nonresponders. For example, a study revealed that one-third of patients who failed sildenafil therapy achieved normal erectile function after switching to vardenafil (Carson et al. 2004). Regular follow-up promotes long-term adherence and optimizes treatment outcomes (including patient and partner satisfaction) by assessing effectiveness and tolerability and making any needed "mid-course adjustments" in treatment expectations (Jensen and Burnett 2002). At follow-up visits, APPs should ask their patients (and/or partners) "Were you satisfied with your erection (or the sexual experience)?" Early success may increase the likelihood that a patient will continue treatment (Table 4.1).

Conclusion

ED is a common disorder that is frequently underreported and undertreated in clinical practice. It is important for APPs to screen for ED in at-risk patients to identify individuals who may benefit from treatment and/or have other serious conditions. APPs can play an integral role in the identification, assessment, treatment, and follow-up of erectile dysfunction. Diagnosis may lead to early recognition of other comorbidities, such as diabetes, vascular disease, and hormone deficiency. Most medical treatments can be initiated in the primary care setting; those patients requiring more complex treatment should be referred. The mounting body of clinical and basic science research strongly suggests that ED is a harbinger and very early warning sign of incipient endothelial dysfunction and associated vascular damage (Billups et al. 2005, 2008). The recognition of ED as a precursor of systemic CVD represents a significant opportunity for prevention. Future large-scale, longitudinal studies that prospectively monitor cardiovascular risk and emergent disease in young men with ED will ultimately support aggressive diagnostic and treatment recommendations.

There are multiple treatment options for men with ED, as with all therapies there are specific advantages and disadvantages inherent to the method of treatment. The APP can play a critical role in affecting treatment outcomes through patient education and facilitation of therapy.

Table 4.1 Erectile dysfunction treatment

Drug/onset/duration	Dosage	Contraindications	More common side effects	Teaching/instruction
Sildenafil (Viagra)®	25, 50, 100 mg PO	Absolutely contraindicated with nitrates including amyl nitrates (poppers) Contraindicated in patients with retinitis pigmentosa Known hypersensitivity to medication See full list of precautions and drug interactions in prescribing information	Headache, dyspepsia, visual changes (bright, blurred or blue), often described as a "blue halo," flushing, nasal congestion, dizziness	Take on empty stomach or 2 h after eating works only in presence of sexual stimulation Not approved for females Does not protect against STIs Use no more than once in a 24 h period Take at least 60 min or more prior to sexual activity May need multiple attempts for optimal results Excessive alcohol intake can cause orthostatic hypotension and tachycardia
Vardenafil (Levitra)® (Staxyn)®	5, 10, 20 mg PO 10 mg only (orally disintegrating tablet)	Absolutely contraindicated with nitrates including amyl nitrates (poppers) Use with caution in men with unstable angina and ischemic CV disease, QT interval: slight prolongation—precaution in labeling Contraindicated in patients with retinitis pigmentosa Known hypersensitivity to medication See full list of precautions and drug interactions in prescribing information	Headache, dyspepsia, flushing, nasal congestion, dizziness	Although it can be taken with food, food and fat may delay absorption Not approved for females Does not protect against STIs Use no more than once in a 24 h period Take 60 min or more prior to sexual activity May need multiple attempts for optimal results Works only in presence of sexual stimulation Excessive alcohol intake can cause orthostatic hypotension and tachycardia

Tadalafil (Cialis)® Long half-life Daily dosing with steady state within 5 days	5, 10, 20 mg 2.5–5 mg PO	Cannot be taken with nitrates or nitric oxide donor, patients with MI in last 90 days, unstable angina, class 2 heart failure, uncontrolled arrhythmias, hypotension, HTN, or stroke within 6 months Known hypersensitivity to drug See full list of precautions and drug interactions in prescribing information	Headache, dyspepsia, flushing, nasal congestion, dizziness, myalgias, back pain	Although it can be taken with food, food and fat may delay absorption Improved spontaneity Does not protect against STIs Do not use more than 20 mg in a 24 h period Take 60 min or more prior to sexual activity May need multiple attempts for optimal results No effect on libido, ejaculation, or orgasm Works only in presence of sexual stimulation Excessive alcohol intake can cause orthostatic hypotension and tachycardia
Avanafil (Stendra)®	50–200 mg PO	Absolutely contraindicated with nitrates including amyl nitrates (poppers) Patients taking CY3A4 inhibitors (ketoconazole, clarithromycin, ritonavir, nefazodone, etc.) Safety is unknown in patients with bleeding disorders and those with active peptic ulceration Known hypersensitivity to drug See full list of precautions and drug interactions in prescribing information	Headache, flushing, nasal stuffiness/congestion, back pain	No food restriction, large meals may decrease absorption, improved results if taken on empty stomach Not approved for use in females Provides no protection from STIs. Use no more than once in a 24 h Take 20–40 min prior to sexual activity may need multiple attempts for optimal results No effect on libido, ejaculation, or orgasm works only in presence of sexual stimulation excessive alcohol intake can cause orthostatic hypotension with hypotension and tachycardia
Venoseal® 30 min duration maximum	NA	Latex or rubber hypersensitivity Precautions: abnormally formed penis, sickle cell anemia, Leukemia, tumor of bone marrow or conditions that increase or decrease blood clotting	Ecchymosis, petechiae, numbness of the penis, pain, pulling of scrotal tissue, blocked or painful ejaculation	Remove after 30 min Allow 60 min period before reapplying

(continued)

Table 4.1 (continued)

Drug/onset/duration	Dosage	Contraindications	More common side effects	Teaching/instruction
Vacuum therapy	NA	No contraindications Precautions: history of priapism, sickle cell, bleeding disorders	Hematoma, ecchymosis, petechiae, numbness of the penis, pain, pulling of scrotal tissue, blocked or painful ejaculation	Requires thorough initial instruction, good dexterity, water-soluble gel and reconditioning for up to 2 weeks Do not use the tension ring for more than 30 min maximum
MUSE® Onset 5–10 min Duration 30–60 min	125, 250, 500, 1000 µg	Hypersensitivity to drug Abnormally formed penis Conditions causing prolonged erections like sickle cell, leukemia, tumor of bone marrow Not for intercourse with pregnant women without a barrier	Penile and urethral pain Warmth or burning in the urethra Erythema of the penis Hypotension Lightheadedness/dizziness Vaginal burning	First dose must be administered in clinic in accordance with prescribing information related to dizziness, lightheadedness, and hypotension Check HR and BP before and after trail dose. Physical activity is necessary to improve blood flow after dose is administered (i.e., walking) Refrigerate unopened package Can be kept at room temp for up to 14 days at <86°
Intracavernosal injection FDA-approved Alprostadil off label Compounded Trimix: papaverine/ phentolamine/ prostaglandin E1 or Bimix: papaverine/ phentolamine	2.5–40 µg Or as prescribed with compounds in units	Hypersensitivity to drug conditions that may lead to priapism like sickle cell, multiple myeloma, leukemia, deformed penis Penile implants Inability to visualize the penis for injections related to central obesity	Pain Injection site bleeding or bruising Priapism (prolonged erection) Peyronie's disease (curvature) due to fibrosis	Comprehensive one-on-one teaching In office titration of first dose; start low and titrate slow to avoid priapism Store at or below 77° single use item Rotate sites, avoid visible veins Press over injection site for 5 min after injection with alcohol wipe Once in 24 h, 3 times/week maximum use provide very specific instruction in case priapism occurs
Penile implant	NA	Poor surgical risk	Infection erosion Mechanical failure following surgery, other medical therapies will no long be effective due to damage of corporal bodies	Invasive Expensive Provide pre- and postoperative teaching 4–8 weeks postoperative recovery period Provide specific instructions for operating the device

Clinical Pearls

- Identification: Any man with common comorbid conditions such as diabetes, hyperlipidemia, hypertension, obesity, metabolic syndrome or obstructive sleep apnea should be evaluated for erectile dysfunction. These men should be counseled about the importance of getting and staying healthy with diet, exercise and weight control while controlling the comorbid conditions.
- Management: Multiple treatment options are available for erectile dysfunction and each treatment has pros and cons. The decision on treatment should be patient centered with the nurse practitioner empowering each man and his partner with the information they need to make an informed decision about the best treatment.
- Management: Men and their partners need more than a prescription for erectile dysfunction treatment. They need comprehensive education on how to integrate treatment into their love play and advocacy with helpful tips on how to make it all work during sex. The nurse practitioner is perfectly positioned to provide this comprehensive information either herself or from her nursing team members. Success with treatment with the vacuum device or injections is based on comprehensive individualized care.
- Evaluation and follow-up: Attrition rates can be high for many of the treatments for erectile dysfunction, men and their partners need continued help in determining what is and is not working for erectile dysfunction and how to continue moving forward with their trajectory to meet their goals for sex and intimacy.

Resources for the Nurse Practitioner and Physician Assistant

Erectile Dysfunction: AUA Guideline (2018) https://www.auanet.org/guidelines/erectile-dysfunction-(ed)-guideline

The Urology Care Foundation: http://www.urologyhealth.org and www.urology-health.org

Society of Urologic Nurses and Associates www.SUNA.org

Resources for the Patient

The Urology Care Foundation: http://www.urologyhealth.org and www.urology-health.org

Men's Health Network (MHN): http://www.menshealthnetwork.org and www.menshealthnetwork.org

Men's Health Month: http://www.menshealthmonth.org and www.menshealthmonth.org

Sexual Health Inventory for Men (SHIM)

Patient Instructions

Sexual health is an important part of an individual's overall physical and emotional well-being. Erectile dysfunction, also known as impotence, is one type of a very common medical condition affecting sexual health. Fortunately, there are many different treatment options for erectile dysfunction. This questionnaire is designed to help you and your provider identify if you may be experiencing erectile dysfunction.

Each question has several possible responses. Circle the number of the response that best describes your own situation. Please be sure that you select one and only one response for each question.

Over the Past 6 Months

1. How do you rate your confidence that you could get and keep an erection?

1	2	3	4	5
Very low	Low	Moderate	High	Very high

2. When you had erections with sexual stimulation, how often were they hard enough for penetration?

0	1	2	3	4	5
No sexual activity	Almost never/never	A few times	Sometimes	Most times	Almost always/ always

3. During sexual intercourse, how often were you able to maintain an erection after penetration?

0	1	2	3	4	5
Did not attempt	Almost never/never	A few times	Sometimes	Most times	Almost always/ always

4. How difficult was it to maintain your erection to the completion of intercourse?

0	1	2	3	4	5
Did not attempt	Extremely difficult	Very difficult	Difficult	Slightly difficult	Not difficult

5. How often was sexual intercourse satisfactory to you?

0	1	2	3	4	5
Did not attempt	Almost never/ never	A few times	Sometimes	Most times	Almost always/ always

Total Score:

Scoring Key

22–25: No ED	12–16: Mild-to-moderate ED	1–7: Severe ED
17–21: Mild ED	8–11: Moderate ED	

Used with permission from Rosen et al. (1999).

References

Akpunona AZ, Mutgi AB, Federman DJ (1994) Routine prolactin measurement is not necessary in the initial evaluation of male impotence. J Gen Intern Med 9:336–338

Albaugh JA, Ferrans CE (2010) Impact of penile injections on men with erectile dysfunction after prostatectomy. Urol Nurs 30(1):64–77

Albaugh J, Amargo I, Capelson R, Flaherty E, Forest C, Goldstein I, Jensen PK, Jones K, Kloner R, Lewis J, Mullin S, Payton T, Rines B, Rosen R, Sadovsky R, Snow K, Vetrosky D, University of Medicine and Dentistry of New Jersey (2002) Health care clinicians in sexual health medicine: focus on erectile dysfunction. Urol Nurs 22(4):217–231; quiz 232

Albaugh J, Adamic B, Chang C, Kirwen N, Aizen J (2019) Adherence and barriers to penile rehabilitation over 2 years following radical prostatectomy. BMC Urol 19(1):89. https://doi. org/10.1186/s12894-019-0516-y

Allen MS, Walter EE (2019) Erectile dysfunction: an umbrella review of meta-analyses of risk factors, treatment and prevalence outcomes. J Sex Med 2019(16):531–541. https://doi. org/10.1016/j.jsxm.2019.01.314

American Urological Association (2005) Management of erectile dysfunction, 3rd edn. http://www. auanet.org/content/guidelines-and-quality-care/clinical-guidelines.cfm?sub=ed. Accessed 15 Oct 2015

American Urological Association (2018) Erectile dysfunction: AUA guideline. https://www.aua-net.org/guidelines/erectile-dysfunction-(ed)-guideline

Andersen I, Heitmann BL, Wagner G (2008) Obesity and sexual dysfunction in younger Danish men. J Sex Med 5(9):2053–2060. https://doi.org/10.1111/j.1743-6109.2008.00920.x

Androshchuk V, Pugh N, Wood A, Ossei-Gerning N (2015) Erectile dysfunction: a window to the heart. BMJ Case Rep. https://doi.org/10.1136/bcr-2015-210124

Annon JS (1974) The behavioral treatment of sexual problems, 1st edn. Kapiolani Health Services, Honolulu

Araujo AB, Durante R, Feldman HA, Goldstein I, McKinlay JB (1998) The relationship between depressive symptoms and male erectile dysfunction: cross-sectional results from the Massachusetts Male Aging Study. Psychosom Med 60(4):458–465

Auxillium Pharmaceuticals Inc. (2011) Edex. http://www.edex.com/_assets/ pdf/prescribing_ information.pdf. Accessed 2015

Bacon CG, Mittleman MA, Kawachi I, Giovannucci E, Glasser DB, Rimm EB (2003) Sexual function in men older than 50 years of age: results from the health professionals follow-up study. Ann Intern Med 139(3):161–168

Billups K, Friedrich S (2005) Assessment of fasting lipid panels and Doppler ultrasound testing in men presenting with erectile dysfunction and no other medical problem. Am J Cardiol 96(Suppl):57M–61M

Billups KL, Bank AJ, Padma-Nathan H, Katz S, Williams R (2005) Erectile dysfunction is a marker for cardiovascular disease: results of the minority health institute expert advisory panel. J Sex Med 2(1):40–50; discussion 50–52. https://doi.org/10.1111/j.1743-6109.2005. 20104_1.x

Billups KL, Bank AJ, Padma-Nathan H, Katz SD, Williams RA (2008) Erectile dysfunction as a harbinger for increased cardiometabolic risk. Int J Impot Res 20(3):236–242. https://doi. org/10.1038/sj.ijir.3901634

Blander DS, Sanchez-Ortiz RF, Wein AJ, Broderick GA (2000) Efficacy of sildenafil in erectile dysfunction after radical prostatectomy. Int J Impot Res 12(3):165–168

Boyle P (1999) Epidemiology of erectile dysfunction. In: Carson C, Kirby RS, Goldstein I (eds) Textbook of erectile dysfunction. ISIS Medical Media, Oxford, pp 15–29

Braun MH, Sommer F, Haupt G, Mathers MJ, Reifenrath B, Engelmann UH (2003) Lower urinary tract symptoms and erectile dysfunction: co-morbidity or typical "Aging Male" symptoms? Results of the "Cologne Male Survey". Eur Urol 44(5):588–594

Capogrosso P, Vertosick EA, Benfante NE, Eastham JA, Scardino PJ, Vickers AJ, Mulhall JP (2019) Are we improving erectile function recovery after radical prostatectomy? Analysis of patients treated over the last decade. Eur Urol 75(2):221–228. https://doi.org/10.1016/j.eururo.2018.08.039

Cappelleri JC, Rosen RC (2005) The Sexual Health Inventory for Men (SHIM): a 5-year review of research and clinical experience. Int J Impot Res 17(4):307–319. https://doi.org/10.1038/sj.ijir.3901327

Carson C, McMahon C (2008) Fast facts: erectile dysfunction, 4th edn. Health Press, Oxford

Carson CC, Hatzichristou DG, Carrier S, Lording D, Lyngdorf P, Aliotta P, Auerbach S, Murdock M, Wilkins HJ, McBride TA, Colopy MW, Patient Response with Vardenafil in Slidenafil NonResponders Study Group (2004) Erectile response with vardenafil in sildenafil nonresponders: a multicentre, double-blind, 12-week, flexible-dose, placebo-controlled erectile dysfunction clinical trial. BJU Int 94(9):1301–1309. https://doi.org/10.1111/j.1464-410X.2004.05161.x

Carson CC, Kirby RS, Goldstein I, Wyllie MG (eds) (2009) Textbook of erectile dysfunction, 2nd edn. New York, Informa Healthcare

Coombs PG, Heck M, Guhring P, Narus J, Mulhall JP (2012) A review of outcomes of an intracavernosal injection therapy programme. BJU Int 110(11):1787–1791. https://doi.org/10.1111/j.1464-410X.2012.11080.x

Corona G, Mannucci E, Mansani R, Petrone L, Bartolini M, Giommi R, Forti G, Maggi M (2004) Organic, relational and psychological factors in erectile dysfunction in men with diabetes mellitus. Eur Urol 46(2):222–228. https://doi.org/10.1016/j.eururo.2004.03.010

Derby CA, Mohr BA, Goldstein I, Feldman HA, Johannes CB, McKinlay JB (2000) Modifiable risk factors and erectile dysfunction: can lifestyle changes modify risk? Urology 56(2):302–306

Doherty W, Bridge P (2019) A systematic review of the role of penile rehabilitation in prostate cancer patients receiving radiotherapy and androgen deprivation therapy. J Med Imaging Radiat Sci 50(1):171–178. https://doi.org/10.1016/j.jmir.2018.09.004

Eardley I (2013) The incidence, prevalence, and natural history of erectile dysfunction. Sex Med Rev 1(1):3–16. https://doi.org/10.1002/smrj.2

Esposito K, Giugliano F, Di Palo C, Giugliano G, Marfella R, D'Andrea F, D'Armiento M, Giugliano D (2004) Effect of lifestyle changes on erectile dysfunction in obese men: a randomized controlled trial. JAMA 291(24):2978–2984. https://doi.org/10.1001/jama.291.24.2978

Federal Drug Administration (2007) FDA announces revisions to labels for Cialis, Levitra, and Viagra: potential risk of sudden hearing loss with ED drugs to be displayed more prominently. www.fda.gov/NewsEvents/Newsroom/PressAnnouncements/2007/ucm109012.htm. Accessed 1 July 2015

Feldman HA, Goldstein I, Hatzichristou DG, Krane RJ, McKinlay JB (1994) Impotence and its medical and psychosocial correlates: results of the Massachusetts Male Aging Study. J Urol 151(1):54–61

Feldman HA, Longcope C, Derby CA, Johannes CB, Araujo AB, Coviello AD, Bremner WJ, McKinlay JB (2002) Age trends in the level of serum testosterone and other hormones in middle-aged men: longitudinal results from the Massachusetts Male Aging Study. J Clin Endocrinol Metabol 87(2):589–598. https://doi.org/10.1210/jcem.87.2.8201

Frey A, Sonksen J, Fode M (2016) Low-intensity extracorporeal shockwave therapy in the treatment of postprostatectomy erectile dysfunction: a pilot study. Scand J Urol 50(2):123–127. https://www.ncbi.nlm.nih.gov/pubmed/26493542

Gratzke C, Angulo J, Chitaley K, Dai YT, Kim NN, Paick JS, Simonsen U, Uckert S, Wespes E, Andersson KE, Lue TF, Stief CG (2010) Anatomy, physiology, and pathophysiology of erectile dysfunction. J Sex Med 7(1 Pt 2):445–475. https://doi.org/10.1111/j.1743-6109.2009.01624.x

Grover SA, Lowensteyn I, Kaouache M, Marchand S, Coupal L, DeCarolis E, Zoccoli J, Defoy I (2006) The prevalence of erectile dysfunction in the primary care setting: importance of risk factors for diabetes and vascular disease. Arch Intern Med 166(2):213–219. https://doi.org/10.1001/archinte.166.2.213

Guay AT, Perez JB, Jacobson J, Newton RA (2001) Efficacy and safety of sildenafil citrate for treatment of erectile dysfunction in a population with associated organic risk factors. J Androl 22(5):793–797

Gupta BP, Murad MH, Clifton MM, Prokop L, Nehra A, Kopecky SL (2011) The effect of life-style modification and cardiovascular risk factor reduction on erectile dysfunction: a systematic review and meta-analysis. Arch Intern Med 171(20):1797–1803. https://doi.org/10.1001/archinternmed.2011.440

Hatzichristou DG, Apostolidis A, Tzortzis V, Ioannides E, Yannakoyorgos K, Kalinderis A (2000) Sildenafil versus intracavernous injection therapy: efficacy and preference in patients on intracavernous injection for more than 1 year. J Urol 164(4):1197–1200

Hatzimouratidis K, Hatzichristou D (2007) Phosphodiesterase type 5 inhibitors: the day after. Eur Urol 51(1):75–88; discussion 89. https://doi.org/10.1016/j.eururo.2006.07.020

Inman BA, Sauver JL, Jacobson DJ, McGree ME, Nehra A, Lieber MM, Roger VL, Jacobsen SJ (2009) A population-based, longitudinal study of erectile dysfunction and future coronary artery disease. Mayo Clin Proc 84(2):108–113. https://doi.org/10.4065/84.2.108

Jackson G, Rosen RC, Kloner RA, Kostis JB (2006) The second Princeton consensus on sexual dysfunction and cardiac risk: new guidelines for sexual medicine. J Sex Med 3(1):28–36; discussion 36. https://doi.org/10.1111/j.1743-6109.2005.00196.x

Jankowski JT, Seftel AD, Strohl KP (2008) Erectile dysfunction and sleep related disorders. J Urol 179(3):837–841. https://doi.org/10.1016/j.juro.2007.10.024

Jensen PK, Burnett JK (2002) Erectile dysfunction. Primary care treatment is appropriate and essential. Adv Nurse Pract 10(4):45–47, 51–52

Jensen PK, Lewis J, Jones KB (2004) Improving erectile function: incorporating new guidelines into clinical practice. Adv Nurse Pract 12(4):40–50

Jones RW, Rees RW, Minhas S, Ralph D, Persad RA, Jeremy JY (2002) Oxygen free radicals and the penis. Expert Opin Pharmacother 3(7):889–897

Kaplan SA, Gonzalez RR (2007) Phosphodiesterase type 5 inhibitors for the treatment of male lower urinary tract symptoms. Rev Urol 9(2):73–77

Kendirici M, Bejma J, Hellstrom WJG (2006) Radical prostatectomy and other pelvic surgeries: effects on erectile function. In: Mulcahy JJ (ed) Male sexual function: a guide to clinical management, 2nd edn. Humana Press, Totowa, pp 135–154

Kinsey AC, Pomeroy WB, Martin CE (1948) Sexual behavior in the human male. W. B. Saunders, Philadelphia

Kloner RA, Speakman M (2002) Erectile dysfunction and atherosclerosis. Curr Atheroscler Rep 4(5):397–401

Kohler TS, Pedro R, Hendlin K, Utz W, Ugarte R, Reddy P, Makhlouf A, Ryndin I, Canales BK, Weiland D, Nakib N, Ramani A, Anderson JK, Monga M (2007) A pilot study on the early use of the vacuum erection device after radical retropubic prostatectomy. BJU Int 100(4):858–862. https://doi.org/10.1111/j.1464-410X.2007.07161.x

Kolodny RC, Kahn CB, Goldstein HH, Barnett DM (1974) Sexual dysfunction in diabetic men. Diabetes 23(4):306–309

Kuritzky L, Miner M (2004) Erectile dysfunction assessment and management in primary care practice. In: Broderick G (ed) Oral pharmacotherapy for male sexual dysfunction. Humana Press, Totowa, pp 149–183

LaRochelle JC, Levine L (2006) Evaluation of the patient with erectile dysfunction. In: Mulcahy JJ (ed) Male sexual function: a guide to clinical management, 2nd edn. Humana Press, Totowa, pp 253–270

Liu L, Zheng S, Han P, Wei Q (2011) Phosphodiesterase-5 inhibitors for lower urinary tract symptoms secondary to benign prostatic hyperplasia: a systematic review and meta-analysis. Urology 77(1):123–129. https://doi.org/10.1016/j.urology.2010.07.508

Lokeshwar SD, Patel P, Shah SM, Ramasamy R (2020) A systematic review of human trials using stem cell therapy for erectile dysfunction. Sex Med Rev 8(1):122–130. https://doi.org/10.1016/j.sxmr.2019.08.003

Lue TF (2000) Erectile dysfunction. N Engl J Med 342(24):1802–1813. https://doi.org/10.1056/NEJM200006153422407

Matsumoto AM (2002) Andropause: clinical implications of the decline in serum testosterone levels with aging in men. J Gerontol A Biol Sci Med Sci 57:M76–M99

Matz EL, Terlecki R, Zhang Y, Jackson J, Atala A (2019) Stem cell therapy for erectile dysfunction. Sex Med Rev 7(2):321–328. S2050-0521(18)30014-3

Mazzola C, Mulhall JP (2011) Penile rehabilitation after prostate cancer treatment: outcomes and practical algorithm. Urol Clin N Am 38(2):105–118. https://doi.org/10.1016/j.ucl.2011.03.002

McCullough AR (2001) Prevention and management of erectile dysfunction following radical prostatectomy. Urol Clin North Am 28(3):613–627

McCullough AR (2003) The penis as a barometer of endothelial health. Rev Urol 5(Suppl 7):S3–S8

McCullough AR (2008) Rehabilitation of erectile function following radical prostatectomy. Asian J Androl 10(1):61–74. https://doi.org/10.1111/j.1745-7262.2008.00366.x

McMahon CG (2004) Efficacy and safety of daily tadalafil in men with erectile dysfunction previously unresponsive to on-demand tadalafil. J Sex Med 1:292–300

Meda Pharmaceuticals Inc. (2014) MUSE full prescribing information. http://www.muserx.com/hcp/global/full-prescribing-information.aspx. Accessed 23 Oct 2016

Montague DK, Jarrow JP, Broderick GA, Dmochoski RR, Heaton JP, Lue TF, Milbank AJ, Nehra A, Sharlip ID (2005) Erectile dysfunction guideline update panel: the management of erectile dysfunction. J Urol 174(1):230–239

Montorsi F, Guazzoni G, Strambi LF, Da Pozzo LF, Nava L, Barbieri L, Rigatti P, Pizzini G, Miani A (1997) Recovery of spontaneous erectile function after nerve-sparing radical retropubic prostatectomy with and without early intracavernous injections of alprostadil: results of a prospective, randomized trial. J Urol 158(4):1408–1410

Montorsi F, Maga T, Strambi LF, Salonia A, Barbieri L, Scattoni V, Guazzoni G, Losa A, Rigatti P, Pizzini G (2000) Sildenafil taken at bedtime significantly increases nocturnal erections: results of a placebo-controlled study. Urology 56(6):906–911

Montorsi F, Brock G, Lee J, Shapiro J, Van Poppel H, Graefen M, Stief C (2008) Effect of nightly versus on-demand vardenafil on recovery of erectile function in men following bilateral nerve-sparing radical prostatectomy. Eur Urol 54(4):924–931. https://doi.org/10.1016/j.eururo.2008.06.083

Mulhall JP (2008) Penile rehabilitation following radical prostatectomy. Curr Opin Urol 18(6):613–620. https://doi.org/10.1097/MOU.0b013e3283136462

Mulhall J, Land S, Parker M, Waters WB, Flanigan RC (2005) The use of an erectogenic pharmacotherapy regimen following radical prostatectomy improves recovery of spontaneous erectile function. J Sex Med 2(4):532–540; discussion 540–542. https://doi.org/10.1111/j.1743-6109.2005.00081_1.x

Mulhall JP, Bella AJ, Briganti A, McCullough A, Brock G (2010) Erectile function rehabilitation in the radical prostatectomy patient. J Sex Med 7(4 Pt 2):1687–1698. https://doi.org/10.1111/j.1743-6109.2010.01804.x

Mydlo JH, Viterbo R, Crispen P (2005) Use of combined intracorporal injection and a phosphodiesterase-5 inhibitor therapy for men with a suboptimal response to sildenafil and/or vardenafil monotherapy after radical retropubic prostatectomy. BJU Int 95(6):843–846. https://doi.org/10.1111/j.1464-410X.2005.05413.x

Nehra A, Jackson G, Miner M, Billups KL, Burnett AL, Buvat J, Carson CC, Cunningham GR, Ganz P, Goldstein I, Guay AT, Hackett G, Kloner RA, Kostis J, Montorsi P, Ramsey M, Rosen R, Sadovsky R, Seftel AD, Shabsigh R, Vlachopoulos C, Wu FC (2012) The Princeton III

Consensus recommendations for the management of erectile dysfunction and cardiovascular disease. Mayo Clin Proc 87(8):766–778. https://doi.org/10.1016/j.mayocp.2012.06.015

NIH Consensus Panel on Impotence (1993) Impotence. NIH Consensus Development Panel on Impotence. JAMA 270(1):83–90

Padma-Nathan H, McCullough AR, Levine LA, Lipshultz LI, Siegel R, Montorsi F, Giuliano F, Brock G, Study Group (2008) Randomized, double-blind, placebo-controlled study of postoperative nightly sildenafil citrate for the prevention of erectile dysfunction after bilateral nerve-sparing radical prostatectomy. Int J Impot Res 20(5):479–486. https://doi.org/10.1038/ijir.2008.33

Pahlajani G, Raina R, Jones S, Ali M, Zippe C (2012) Vacuum erection devices revisited: its emerging role in the treatment of erectile dysfunction and early penile rehabilitation following prostate cancer therapy. J Sex Med 9(4):1182–1189. https://doi.org/10.1111/j.1743-6109.2010.01881.x

Pavlovich CP, Levinson AW, Su LM, Mettee LZ, Feng Z, Bivalacqua TJ, Trock BJ (2013) Nightly vs on-demand sildenafil for penile rehabilitation after minimally invasive nerve-sparing radical prostatectomy: results of a randomized double-blind trial with placebo. BJU Int 112(6):844–851. https://doi.org/10.1111/bju.12253

Porst H, Giuliano F, Glina S, Ralph D, Casabe AR, Elion-Mboussa A, Shen W, Whitaker JS (2006) Evaluation of the efficacy and safety of once-a-day dosing of tadalafil 5mg and 10mg in the treatment of erectile dysfunction: results of a multicenter, randomized, double-blind, placebo-controlled trial. Eur Urol 50(2):351–359. https://doi.org/10.1016/j.eururo.2006.02.052

Porst H, Burnett A, Brock G, Ghanem H, Giuliano F, Glina S, Hellstrom W, Martin-Morales A, Salonia A, Sharlip I, ISSM Standards Committee for Sexual Medicine (2013) SOP conservative (medical and mechanical) treatment of erectile dysfunction. J Sex Med 10(1):130–171. https://doi.org/10.1111/jsm.12023

Pritzker MR (1999) The penile stress test: a window to the hearts of man? Circ J 100(Suppl 1):3751

Qin F, Wang S, Li J, Wu C, Yuan J (2018) The early use of vacuum therapy for penile rehabilitation after radical prostatectomy: systematic review and meta-analysis. Am J Mens Health 12(6):2136–2143. https://doi.org/10.1177/1557988318797409

Rabbani F, Schiff J, Piecuch M, Yunis LH, Eastham JA, Scardino PT, Mulhall JP (2010) Time course of recovery of erectile function after radical retropubic prostatectomy: does anyone recover after 2 years? J Sex Med 7(12):3984–3990. https://doi.org/10.1111/j.1743-6109.2010.01969.x

Raina R, Agarwal A, Allamaneni SS, Lakin MM, Zippe CD (2005) Sildenafil citrate and vacuum constriction device combination enhances sexual satisfaction in erectile dysfunction after radical prostatectomy. Urology 65(2):360–364. https://doi.org/10.1016/j.urology.2004.09.013

Raina R, Agarwal A, Ausmundson S, Lakin M, Nandipati KC, Montague DK, Mansour D, Zippe CD (2006) Early use of vacuum constriction device following radical prostatectomy facilitates early sexual activity and potentially earlier return of erectile function. Int J Impot Res 18(1):77–81. https://doi.org/10.1038/sj.ijir.3901380

Raina R, Pahlajani G, Agarwal A, Zippe CD (2008) Early penile rehabilitation following radical prostatectomy: Cleveland Clinic experience. Int J Impot Res 20(2):121–126. https://doi.org/10.1038/sj.ijir.3901573

Rhoden EL, Ribeiro EP, Teloken C, Souto CA (2005) Diabetes mellitus is associated with subnormal serum levels of free testosterone in men. BJU Int 96(6):867–870. https://doi.org/10.1111/j.1464-410X.2005.05728.x

Rosen RC, Cappelleri JC, Smith MD, Lipsky J, Pena BM (1999) Development and evaluation of an abridged, 5-item version of the International Index of Erectile Function (IIEF-5) as a diagnostic tool for erectile dysfunction. Int J Impot Res 11(6):319–326

Rosen R, Altwein J, Boyle P, Kirby RS, Lukacs B, Meuleman E, O'Leary MP, Puppo P, Robertson C, Giuliano F (2003) Lower urinary tract symptoms and male sexual dysfunction: the multinational survey of the aging male (MSAM-7). Eur Urol 44(6):637–649

Rowland DL, Incrocci L, Slob AK (2005) Aging and sexual response in the laboratory in patients with erectile dysfunction. J Sex Marital Ther 31(5):399–407. https://doi.org/10.1080/00926230591006520

Sachs BD (2003) The false organic-psychogenic distinction and related problems in the classification of erectile dysfunction. Int J Impot Res 15(1):72–78. https://doi.org/10.1038/sj.ijir.3900952

Sadovsky R, Curtis K (2006) How a primary care clinician approaches erectile dysfunction. In: Mulcahy JJ (ed) Male sexual function: a guide to clinical management, 2nd edn. Humana Press, Totowa, pp 77–104

Seftel AD, Sundi P, Swindle R (2004) The prevalence of hypertension, hyperlipidemia, diabetes mellitus and depression in men with erectile dysfunction. J Urol 171:2341–2345

Sesti C, Florio V, Johnson EG, Kloner RA (2007) The phosphodiesterase-5 inhibitor tadalafil reduces myocardial infarct size. Int J Impot Res 19:55–61

Shabsigh R (2006) Epidemiology of erectile dysfunction. In: Mulcahy JJ (ed) Male sexual function: a guide to clinical management, 2nd edn. Humana Press, Totowa, pp 47–59

Shamloul R, Ghanem H (2013) Erectile dysfunction. Lancet 381(9861):153–165. https://doi.org/10.1016/S0140-6736(12)60520-0

Stember DS, Mulhall JP (2012) The concept of erectile function preservation (penile rehabilitation) in the patient after brachytherapy for prostate cancer. Brachytherapy 11(2):87–96. https://doi.org/10.1016/j.brachy.2012.01.002

Tal R, Teloken P, Mulhall JP (2011) Erectile function rehabilitation after radical prostatectomy: practice patterns among AUA members. J Sex Med 8(8):2370–2376. https://doi.org/10.1111/j.1743-6109.2011.02355.x

Teloken PE, Smith EB, Lodowsky C, Freedom T, Mulhall JP (2006) Defining association between sleep apnea syndrome and erectile dysfunction. Urology 67(5):1033–1037. https://doi.org/10.1016/j.urology.2005.11.040

Wespes E, Amar E, Hatzichristou D, Hatzimouratidis K, Montorsi F, Pryor J, Vardi Y, EAU (2006) EAU guidelines on erectile dysfunction: an update. Eur Urol 49(5):806–815. https://doi.org/10.1016/j.eururo.2006.01.028

Zhihua L, Guiting L, Amanda R-M, Chunxi W, Yung-Chin L, Tom FL (2017) Low intensity shock wave treatment improves erectile function: a systemic review & meta-analysis. Eur Urol 71:213–233

Zias N, Bezwada V, Gilman S, Chroneou A (2009) Obstructive sleep apnea and erectile dysfunction: still a neglected risk factor? Sleep Breath 13(1):3–10. https://doi.org/10.1007/s11325-008-0212-8

Zou Z et al (2017) Short term efficacy & safety of low-intensity extracorporeal shock wave therapy in erectile dysfunction: a systemic review & meta-analysis. IBJU 43(5):805–821

Benign Prostatic Hyperplasia

5

Gina M. Powley and Gail M. Briolat

Contents

Objectives

1. Define the pathophysiology, incidence, presenting symptoms, and risk factors of BPH.
2. Discuss assessment techniques associated with BPH.
3. Explain treatment options including pharmacologic, watchful waiting, and surgical.
4. Discuss complications and side effects of treatment options.

Incidence and Epidemiology

Benign prostatic hyperplasia (BPH) is a histologic diagnosis that refers to the proliferation of smooth muscle and epithelial cells within the prostatic transition zone (Foster et al. 2019). On autopsy studies BPH was not found in men less than 30 years

G. M. Powley (✉)
Urology of St. Louis, Chesterfield, MO, USA

G. M. Briolat
Michigan Institute of Urology, Michigan Institute of Urology, St Clair Shores, MI, USA

© Springer Nature Switzerland AG 2020
S. A. Quallich, M. J. Lajiness (eds.), *The Nurse Practitioner in Urology*,
https://doi.org/10.1007/978-3-030-45267-4_5

old (Vuichoud and Loughlin 2015) but is the fourth most common condition in men over 50 years old (Russo et al. 2014). It is estimated that greater than 70% of men between the ages of 60 and 69 suffer from BPH (Parsons 2014), and the incidence in men over 70 years of age is over 80% (Russo et al. 2014). In the United States, greater than 15 million men are affected leading to health-care cost of greater than 3 billion dollars annually (Bagla et al. 2014).

The etiology of BPH is not completely understood but appears to be endocrine controlled and multifactorial in nature (Cooperberg et al. 2013) BPH is not life-threatening but causes a significant impact on quality of life. Symptoms of BPH lead to loss of sleep, anxiety, depression, decreased mobility, increased falls, and impairment of activities of daily living as well as leisure activities and sexual activity (Gacci et al. 2014; Parsons 2014). In the last decade, hospitalizations in the United States for acute renal failure secondary to acute urinary retention from BPH have increased (Parsons 2014).

Risk factors for the development of BPH have not been well understood. Studies have suggested a genetic component, racial differences, and possibly half the men under age 60 undergoing surgery for BPH may have an inherited form of the condition. It is thought to be an autosomal dominant trait and first-degree male relatives carry a fourfold increased risk (Cooperberg et al. 2013).

Recent studies suggest correlations with obesity, increased animal protein in diets, and decreased exercise as risk factors for developing symptomatic BPH. Increased BMI, body weight, and waist circumference have been associated with increased prostate volume in ultrasound and MRI studies evaluating prostate volume (Parsons 2014). Moderate to vigorous physical activity has been associated with up to 25% decreased risk of BPH (Parsons 2014). Consuming at least four servings of vegetables daily, lycopene and green tea added to diets have shown a significantly lower risk of BPH (Espinosa 2013).

Pathophysiology

The prostate is composed of three zones of glandular tissue made of stromal and epithelial cells. The three zones are known as the transition, central, and peripheral zones. The prostate is attached superiorly to the bladder neck and inferiorly bound by the urogenital diaphragm, and posteriorly it is next to the rectum and the anterior surface lies against the pubis (Resnick 2003). BPH is a histological diagnosis that refers to an unregulated proliferation of glandular epithelial tissue, smooth muscle and connective tissue within the prostatic transition zone, also known as "stromo-glandular hyperplasia" (Vuichoud and Loughlin 2015; Foster et al. 2019). Testicular androgens are necessary for the development of BPH. Patients castrated prior to puberty, or who are affected by a variety of genetic diseases which impair androgen action or production, do not develop BPH (Walsh et al. 2002). At the end of puberty, the prostate gland is approximately 26 g and maintains that weight unless BPH develops (McConnell 1998). More recent studies are suggesting a role of inflammatory cells, whether local or systemic, in the development of BPH. BPH is an immune inflammatory disease, and that chronic prostatic inflammation has a role in the pathogenesis of this disease (Vuichoud and Loughlin 2015).

Presentation

Symptoms and presentation of patients suffering from BPH include various lower urinary tract symptoms (LUTS). Among the most common symptoms are decreased force of stream, hesitancy, intermittent stream, post-void dribbling, and nocturia. These symptoms typically occur in men over the age of 60. As BPH advances and bladder outlet obstruction (BOO) progresses, symptoms of overactive bladder (OAB) such as urgency and frequency may also develop (Wieder 2014). There is little correlation between the overall size of the prostate and the degree of symptoms. Frequency and urgency of symptoms vary from patient to patient. BPH is characterized by a spectrum of obstructive and irritative symptoms, referred to as lower urinary tract symptoms or "LUTS" (See Table 5.1).

History and Physical Examination

In making the diagnosis of BPH, care must be taken to rule out other pathologies of the urinary tract which can exhibit similar symptoms of LUTS. The first step is obtaining a detailed medical history from the patient. It is very important to inquire about sexual function. Determine if the patient has any preexisting neurologic disorders such as multiple sclerosis and Parkinson's disease or has had a stroke in the past. Determine if the patient ever experienced any urinary tract trauma or urethral stricture disease. Obtain a history of current prescriptions and over-the-counter medications, which may impact bladder emptying such as anticholinergics or regular use of muscle relaxants or narcotics. Determine if the patient has chronic constipation (Cooperberg et al. 2013; Vuichoud and Loughlin 2015).

Table 5.1 LUTS in BPH

Obstructive symptoms—secondary to the obstruction of the bladder outlet from the growing prostate	Irritative symptoms—caused by the effects on the bladder due to prolonged bladder outlet obstruction
Decreased force of urinary stream	Urgency
Hesitancy—trouble starting stream/straining to pass urine	Urge incontinence
Double voiding/post-void dribbling	Frequency
Acute or chronic urinary retention	Nocturia
Feeling of incomplete bladder emptying	
Prolonged micturition	
Overflow incontinence	

When assessing patients for BPH, it is important to ask very specific questions in history taking. BPH symptoms develop very slowly, and patients tend to adapt to the abnormal voiding pattern and lifestyle and do not consider their voiding pattern abnormal. Older patients tend to blame it on "getting older" and accept it as normal. Consider asking patients about details such as frequency of nocturia; evening fluid consumption or restrictions, fluid restrictions during the day to prevent interference with activities; strength of urinary stream; a need to push or strain to start the urinary stream; and quality of sleep.

Physical examination focuses on digital rectal exam (DRE), neurologic exam, and examination of the external genitalia. When performing DRE, note should be made of the anal sphincter tone; decreased tone may suggest neurologic etiology, while increased tone may suggest pelvic floor dysfunction. Physical exam of the prostate determines the approximate size of the gland, and particular attention is directed to examining for any indurated areas which could be concerning for malignancy. Exam of the external genitalia evaluates for meatal stenosis or palpable masses of the urethra which could contribute to abnormal voiding symptoms.

The international prostate symptom score (IPPS) is a seven-question tool used to quantitate the subjective symptoms of BPH. The tool asks patients to evaluate their sensation of incomplete bladder emptying, frequency, intermittency, urgency, stream strength, and nocturia on a scale of 0–5. The higher the number, the greater the urinary symptoms. The tool is very helpful for BPH management (Vuichoud and Loughlin 2015).

Abnormal Findings

Abnormal digital rectal exam (DRE) findings include a specific firm area or nodule which is of different texture from the rest of the gland or extreme tenderness on palpation of the gland. DRE does tend to underestimate the prostate volume. It is important to also assess for neurologic impairment which could contribute to lax or spastic anal sphincter tone found on DRE (Vuichoud and Loughlin 2015). External genitalia abnormalities include meatal stenosis, palpable ureteral mass, or phimosis. Other abnormal physical findings are a palpable bladder secondary to acute or chronic urinary retention (Silbert 2017).

Diagnostic Tests

A urinalysis must be done to rule out hematuria or a urinary tract infection both of which could suggest a non-BPH pathology for the symptoms. Serum creatinine is not recommended in the initial evaluation of BPH per the AUA guidelines and the International Consensus on New Developments in Prostate Cancer and Prostate Disease report (Silbert 2017). Serum creatinine may be performed if surgery is planned to assess renal function (Vuichoud and Loughlin 2015). See Resources. If the serum creatinine is elevated, imaging studies such as ultrasound should be obtained.

Prostate-specific antigen (PSA) should also be obtained in BPH evaluation and is directly proportional to prostate volume. Men with higher prostate volume will tend to have higher PSA. Many conditions other than BPH can elevate PSA and must be considered. Other causes for increased PSA include prostate cancer, infections, manipulation or trauma, and ejaculation within few days of obtaining sample. It is also important to note conditions which can lower PSA as well. Medications such as 5-α reductase inhibitors, androgen deprivation, or castration will reduce the PSA (Wieder 2014).

Much discussion has and continues to take place among the experts regarding PSA screening. In May of 2013, the American Urological Association (AUA) released a new guideline regarding PSA screening. The changes which are specific to BPH and PSA measurement include offering PSA testing to patients who have at least a 10-year life expectancy and for those in which the detection for prostate cancer would change the management plan or the plan for management of their voiding symptoms and shared decision-making (American Urological Association 2013). The AUA has developed a tool to guide practitioners in this process. Other useful diagnostic studies include uroflowmetry and post-void residual. Uroflowmetry is a noninvasive electronic recording of the urinary flow rate during voiding. Post-void residual is obtained immediately after the patient has voided and can be done noninvasively by transabdominal ultrasound or invasively by catheterization (Silva et al. 2014). Both studies have limitations and variability but decreased flow rates and increased post void residuals can be consistent with BPH. Another useful tool in determining the level of bother in a patient is the *international prostate symptom score (IPSS)*, an eight-question (seven *symptom* questions + one quality-of-life question) written screening tool used to screen for, rapidly diagnose, track the symptoms of, and suggest management of the symptoms of the disease BPH (see resources).

Management

Two goals in the management of BPH include decrease the bother of symptoms and prevent the delay of BPH related symptoms. The first treatment option for patient with BPH is watchful waiting. Patients with mild symptoms of LUTS (IPSS score of <8) or those with moderate to severe symptoms who are not bothered by the symptoms and are not experiencing medical complications (see Table 5.2) can opt for no intervention and be followed by active surveillance or watchful waiting.

Table 5.2 Long-term complications of bladder outlet obstruction	
	Formation of bladder diverticula(e)
	Bladder wall trabeculation
	Detrusor decompensation
	Hydroureteronephrosis
	Renal insufficiency
	Recurrent urinary tract infections
	Bladder stones

Often behavior modifications such as decreasing evening fluid intake, reducing alcohol or caffeine intake, weight loss or altering the timing of diuretics, and smoking cessation may improve mild symptoms (Vuichoud and Loughlin 2015). These patients should be evaluated annually with repeat of the initial exam. Symptom score via IPSS to determine subjective changes in voiding pattern should be repeated. It is important to remember the severity of urinary symptoms do not correlate with the prostates size, as well as, the severity of symptoms do not correlate with the degree of bladder outlet obstruction (Wieder 2014). Some patients never require further treatment and approximately 65% of patients continue to be satisfied at 5 years (Silva et al. 2014).

Many patients will seek nonprescription therapy for mild-to-moderate symptoms of BPH. The herbal product saw palmetto has been popular in the treatment of BPH. After review of several randomized trials involving over 3000 patients, no benefits of saw palmetto over placebo were noted (Espinosa 2013; Parsons 2014).

Medical therapies for moderate-to-severe BPH symptoms include α-blockers and 5-α reductase inhibitors (5ARIs) or a combination of the two classes of medication. Recent studies have investigated three other drug classes, antimuscarinics, β3-adrenoceptor agonists, and 5-phosphodiesterase inhibitors (PDE5i) in the treatment of LUTS in BPH when urine storage problems exist (Silva et al. 2014). Currently five α-blockers, doxazosin, terazosin, tamsulosin, alfuzosin, and silodosin, are available to treat BPH. Alpha-blockers inhibit α-1 adrenergic receptors relaxing smooth muscle tone in the prostate and bladder neck and improve voiding symptoms (Wieder 2014; Silva et al. 2014). Alpha-1 adrenergic receptors have three subtypes: α-1A, α-1B, and α-1D. Alpha-1A relaxes smooth muscle in the prostate, bladder neck, seminal vesicles, and vas deferens. These are the primary subtype of α-1 receptors in the prostate. Alpha-1B is mainly located in the vasculature; hypotension can be caused by blockage of this receptor. Alpha-1D is located in the nasal passages, bladder, and spinal cord; blocking this receptor often results in nasal congestion (Wieder 2014). The most common side effects of α-blockers are dizziness, headache, asthenia, postural hypotension, rhinitis, sexual dysfunction, and retrograde ejaculation. Studies have suggested all five of these drugs are statistically significant and better than placebo in improving flow and decreasing BPH symptoms. Silodosin is the only drug in the class to be selective to the α-1A receptor subtype. Due to being α-1A selective, silodosin has less incidence of cardiovascular side effects but increased incidence of ejaculatory dysfunction (Silva et al. 2014).

A significant side effect of α-blockers to be aware of is intraoperative floppy iris syndrome. This syndrome was described in 2005 by Chang and Campbell as miosis intraoperatively during cataract surgery, despite dilation preoperatively. The condition does not seem to occur with the older agents, doxazosin and terazosin. If a patient is planning a cataract surgery, it is recommended to avoid initiation of alpha-blockers until the surgery is completed; 5α-reductase inhibitors work to decrease BPH-related symptoms by preventing the conversion of testosterone to dihydrotestosterone. The two drugs currently available in this class are finasteride and dutasteride. Unlike the α-blockers the benefits of these drugs can take up to 6 months but reduce the prostate gland volume up to 25% (Wieder 2014). When taking either of these medications for 9–12 months, a 50% decrease in PSA is expected. Common side effects with these drugs include erectile dysfunction, decreased libido, and decreased volume of ejaculate (Silva et al. 2014). More recent studies have found additional potential side effects of the 5 α-reductase inhibitors include depression, suicidal attempts, persistent erectile dysfunction, gynecomastia and anxiety (Kim et al. 2018).

Two large long-term studies (the Medical Therapy of Prostatic Symptoms study (MTOPS) and Combination of Avodart® and Tamsulosin study (ComBat)) were conducted comparing α-blockers, 5 α-reductase inhibitors, and a combination of using both together. Conclusions of these studies suggested combination therapy works better on larger prostates. Combination therapy of an α-blocker and a 5 α-reductase inhibitor should be considered for patients with prostate gland volumes >40 ccs, PSA >4.0 ng/ml, moderate-to-severe voiding symptoms and advanced age. Combination therapy does increase the cost of medication for the patient and may increase the potential side effects the patient may experience (Silva et al. 2014; Wieder 2014).

Neither the MTOPS nor ComBat studies indicate when combination therapy should be initiated or how long the patient should remain on a single agent before adding combination mediations. Most clinicians begin with combination therapy in patients with severe symptoms and high risk for progression of BPH (Silva et al. 2014). The AUA guidelines support the use of combination therapy for patients with LUTS and demonstrated prostate enlargement (American Urological Association 2013).

Up to half the men suffering from BPH report detrusor overactivity, the more severe the obstruction, the greater the overactivity (Silva et al. 2014). The overactive bladder symptoms associated with detrusor overactivity may include nocturia, urgency, or frequency. Antimuscarinic therapy can be safe and helpful to these patients. Tolterodine 4 mg has been studied against placebo and found to reduce the associated symptoms. The incidence of increased post-void residual and acute urinary retention was similar to the placebo groups. Benefits of adding an antimuscarinic to patients already on α-blockers or 5 α-reductase inhibitors with detrusor overactivity symptoms were also found to be effective and well tolerated (Silva et al. 2014).

Another drug class having success with bladder capacity is the β3-adrenoceptor agonists. Mirabegron dosed at 50–100 mg showed a significant decrease in voiding frequency, and patients studied taking the 50 mg dose had a statistically significant decrease in urgency as well (Silva et al. 2014). The most common reported side effects of mirabegron were hypertension, nasopharyngitis, and urinary tract infections (Russo et al. 2014).

Several studies have suggested a strong correlation between BPH/LUTS and erectile dysfunction (ED) (Gacci et al. 2014). 5-Phosphodiesterase inhibitors (PDE-5) have been used for the treatment of ED and more recently studied in daily use for the treatment of BPH. The mechanism of action of the PDE-5 receptor is thought to relax prostatic smooth muscle, have antiproliferative effects, improve blood flow to the pelvis, and act on the afferent sensory nerves or the prostate and bladder (Paolone 2010). Of the PDE-5 products, only tadalafil 5 mg daily is approved for the treatment of BPH. At this time the efficacy of combining use of an α-blocker and tadalafil for BPH treatment is not recommended due to the risk of hypotension from combining these drugs. The most common side effects of tadalafil include headache, dyspepsia, back pain, nasopharyngitis, diarrhea, pain in the extremity, myalgia, and dizziness (Russo et al. 2014).

Surgical Management

The American Urological Association (AUA) updated surgical management of BPH in 2019. Surgery continues to be recommended in patients who have renal insufficiency, hydronephrosis or refractory urinary retention secondary to BPH. Surgery is also recommended in patients with recurrent urinary tract infections (UTI's), recurrent bladder stones or gross hematuria due to BPH, and those patients who experience LUTS attributed to BPH refractory to, or unwillingness to use other therapies (Foster et al. 2019; Wieder 2014).

Transurethral resection of the prostate (TURP) remains the gold standard by which other surgical approaches to treat BPH are compared and serves as a reference (Foster et al. 2019; Roehrborn et al. 2013; Shigemura and Fujisawa 2018).

Two types of TURP may be performed, monopolar or bipolar, depending on the experience of the clinician. The difference in procedures is how the energy transmission occurs. Contrary to monopolar TURP, the energy does not travel through the body to reach the skin pad. In bipolar TURP systems, the energy is confined between the active (resection loop) and passive pole situated on resectoscope tip (Foster et al. 2019). Monopolar TURP requires the use of either iso-osmolar solutions of sorbitol, mannitol or glycine, bipolar TURP may be performed with 0.9% NaCl solution. This reduces, or possibly eliminates, the risk for acute dilutional hypernatremia during prolonged resection, which may lead to the so-called TUR syndrome (Foster et al. 2019). Transurethral resection syndrome (TUR syndrome) is the excessive absorption of hypotonic irrigation fluid from the prostatic vascular bed resulting in hyponatremia, hypervolemia, hypertension, mental confusion, nausea, vomiting and visual disturbances. Treatment of TUR syndrome includes diuresis and fluid restriction (Wieder 2014).

When performing TURP a resection loop is used to remove "chips" of the prostate. The resection is performed circumferentially from the bladder neck to a location immediately cephalad to the verumontanum (Wieder 2014). TURP is most suitable for prostates <80 cc. Compared to monopolar TURP, bipolar TURP has a lower risk of bleeding, blood transfusion and TUR syndrome. There have been no differences in efficacy found on either mono or bipolar TURP (Foster et al. 2019).

Clinicians should consider open, laparoscopic or robotic assisted prostatectomy for the patients with large prostates (over 100 g). The choice is dependent on the surgeon's experience coupled with a potential need to perform other procedures, such as to treat a bladder diverticulum or bladder stone. Two approaches can be taken to perform open prostatectomies. The suprapubic approach is typically used if a secondary bladder procedure is intended, while the retropubic approach does not involve entry into the bladder (Cooperberg et al. 2013; Foster et al. 2019; Wieder 2014).

Transurethral incision of the prostate (TUIP) has been used to treat small prostates usually defined as <30 g for many decades. This procedure is achieved by using 1–2 endoscopic incisions in the prostatic urethra which are extended from the bladder neck to a location immediately cephalad to the verumontanum (Foster et al. 2019; Wieder 2014). TUIP has similar efficacy compared to TURP but has a lower rate of retrograde ejaculation (Wieder 2014).

Transurethral electrovaporization (TUVP) of the prostate is a technical electrosurgical modification of the standard TURP. TUVP can utilize a variety of energy delivery surfaces including rollerball, vaportrode or button (Foster et al. 2019). TUVP typically uses saline and is powered with a bipolar energy source. Compared to traditional resection loops, the different TUVP designs hope to improve upon tissue visualization, blood loss, resection speed and patient morbidity. Efficacy is similar to TURP, but TUVP has a higher rate of post-operative irritative voiding symptoms and urinary retention (Foster et al. 2019; Wieder 2014).

Photoselective vaporization of the prostate (PVP) is a transurethral form of treatment that uses a 600-μm side firing laser fiber in a noncontact mode. The laser wavelength is 532 nm which is absorbed by hemoglobin resulting primarily in tissue ablation/vaporization with a thin layer of underlying coagulation that provides hemostasis (Foster et al. 2019; Wieder 2014). The procedure is usually performed with saline irrigation, eliminating the possibility of TUR syndrome. The goal of the procedure is to vaporize the prostate adenoma sequentially outwards until the surgical capsule is exposed and a defect is created within the prostate parenchyma through which the patient can now void (Foster et al. 2019).

Prostatic urethral lift (PUL) is an option for patients with LUTS attributed to BPH with a prostate gland size of <80 g and verified absence of an obstructive median lobe (Foster et al. 2019). PUL was developed in 2004 as a treatment option for LUTS/BPH that works by altering prostatic anatomy without ablating tissue. PUL has shown to potentially offer rapid and significant improvement of LUTS while maintaining a morbidity profile considerably better than surgical resection or ablation while preserving sexual function (Roehrborn et al. 2013). Permanent intraprostatic implants are sutures that are delivered by a hand-held device through a cystoscope to mechanically open the prostatic urethra by compressing the prostate parenchyma. The sutures have "T-shaped" bars on the ends of them which are spring loaded and placed so the bars are set with one outside the prostate capsule and the other within the prostatic urethral lumen. The T-shaped sutures are placed so there is sufficient tension on them pulling the lumen of the prostatic urethra towards the capsule, compressing the tissue and opening the prostatic urethral lumen (Foster et al. 2019; Roehrborn et al. 2013). Single arm studies show an American Urologic Association Symptom Index (AUASI) reduction considerably larger than drugs, faster acting than thermal therapies and without serious complications associated with TURP or lasers (Roehrborn et al. 2013).

Transurethral microwave therapy (TUMT) heats the prostate to create thermal necrosis. The microwaves are delivered using an antenna embedded in a catheter. This is an office-based procedure, performed with local or oral pain medications avoiding spinal or general anesthesia. The ideal candidate has a prostate size between 30 and 100 cc, with no median lobe enlargement and a prostatic urethral length to accommodate the antenna. (Foster et al. 2019; Wieder 2014). Irritative symptoms can persist for several weeks after procedure. Patients should be aware the maximum effects of TUMT are likely to occur 3–6 months after the procedure (Wieder 2014).

Water vapor thermal therapy uses sterile water vapor (steam) to treat BPH by delivering targeted, controlled doses of thermal energy directly to the prostate gland, targeting and reducing the obstructive tissue that causes BPH. This is another office-based procedure performed with local or oral pain medications. The ideal patient has a prostate gland which is <80 g and does not exclude those with obstructing middle lobes or median lobes (Foster et al. 2019). Cystoscope lens is inserted into the delivery device. When the needle is deployed, a radiofrequency current generates a wet thermal energy in the form of water vapor is then injected into the prostatic transition zone or median lobe, in controlled 9 s doses. The vapor that is injected into the prostate tissue rapidly disperses through the interstitial space between the tissue cells. As the vapor cools, it condenses immediately on contact with tissue and the stored thermal energy is released, denaturing the cell membranes and causing cell death. The denatured cells are absorbed by the body, which reduces the volume of prostate tissue adjacent to the urethra. The vapor condensation process also causes a rapid collapse of vasculature in the treatment zone, resulting in a bloodless procedure (Mcvary et al. 2019).

Transurethral needle ablation (TUNA) is not recommended for the treatment of LUTS attributed to BPH. This is an office-based procedure performed with local or oral pain medications. The ideal candidate has a prostate size of <75 g and exhibits mainly lateral lobe enlargement of the prostate gland (Foster et al. 2019; Wieder 2014). This procedure is performed under direct visualization. The physician deploys two curved needles which extend from the tip of a special cystoscope sheath which delivers radiofrequency (RF) energy into the prostate to create thermal necrosis (Wieder 2014). Irritative symptoms can persist for several weeks. TUNA seems to require more sedation than TUMT (Wieder 2014).

Laser enucleation is used to resect (enucleate) or vaporize (ablate) prostate tissue. Due to the chromophore of water and minimal tissue depth penetration with both holmium and thulium, these two lasers achieve rapid vaporization and coagulation of tissue without the disadvantage of deep tissue penetration (Foster et al. 2019). They have better coagulative properties in tissue than either monopolar or bipolar TURP, and combined with their superficial penetration, both thulium and holmium are reasonable options depending on the clinician's expertise (Foster et al. 2019). Compared to TURP, laser therapies have lower risk of bleeding, shorter postoperative catheterization time, shorter length of hospital stay and decreased risk of TUR syndrome. However, laser therapies and TURP have comparable improvement in voiding symptoms (Foster et al. 2019; Wieder 2014).

Aquablation may be offered to patients with LUTS attributed to BPH with prostate volume >30 g and <80 g; however, long-term efficacy and retreatment rates remain limited. Patients must undergo general anesthesia for this procedure. This procedure utilizes a heat-free, robotically controlled water-jet to ablate the prostate. Pretreatment transrectal ultrasound is use to map out the specific region of the prostate to be resected with a focus on limiting resection in the area of the vermontanum. It is also used to monitor tissue resection in real time during the procedure. After completion of the resection, electro-cautery via a standard cystoscope/resectoscope or traction from a 3-way catheter balloon are used to obtain hemostasis (Foster et al. 2019; Saadat and Elterman 2019). Aquablation features a short ablation time independent of prostate size with good functional urinary and sexual outcomes (Saadat and Elterman 2019).

Prostate artery embolization (PAE) is not recommended for the treatment of LUTS attributed to BPH. PAE is a newer, largely unproven minimally invasive surgical treatment (MIST) for BPH (Foster et al. 2019).

Clinical Pearls
- Reviewing the IPPS score with men, helps them gain insight to their complaints. They many have been confused about how to best answer the question.
- "How is your stream today compared to 5 years ago?" can help men gain perspective on their present concerns.
- Some men may be embarrassed to ask for clarification regarding the IPSS questions.
- When discussing treatment plans with the patient, it is important to individualize the plan.
- Many patients cannot afford mediations and are embarrassed to tell the provider and therefore do not take the medications, resulting in symptom progression.
- The medications are considered long term, and if the patient will not be able to obtain them, an invasive procedure may be indicated sooner to address their BPH-related symptoms.

Resources for the Nurse Practitioner

http://www.auanet.org/education/guidelines/benign-prostatic-hyperplasia.cfm
https://www.youtube.com/playlist?list=PLF38D35BBEFD7740F&feature=plcp
AUA/IPSS Symptom Questionnaire www.urospec.com/uro/forms/ipss.pdf
NIH https://www.niddk.nih.gov/health-information/urologic-diseases/prostate-problems/prostate-enlargement-benign-prostatic-hyperplasia
https://nccih.nih.gov/health/providers/digest/BPH-science
UpToDate https://www.uptodate.com/contents/medical-treatment-of-benign-prostatic-hyperplasia?search

Resources for the Patient

http://www.uptodate.com/contents/benign-prostatic-hyperplasia-bph-beyond-the-basics

Society of Urological Nurses and Associates Patient Fact Sheet BPH https://www.suna.org/download/members/benign_prostatic_hyperplasia.pdf

Urology Care Foundation https://www.urologyhealth.org/search?term=bph

Men's Health Network www.menshealthnetwork.org

References

American Urological Association (2013). http://www.auanet.org/education/guidelines/benign-porstatic-hyperplasia.cfm. Accessed 21 Sept 2014

Bagla S, Martin CP, van Breda A, Sheridan MJ, Sterling KM, Papadouris D, Rholl KS, Smirniotopoulos JB, van Breda A (2014) Early results from a United States trial of prostatic artery embolization in the treatment of benign prostatic hyperplasia. J Vasc Interv Radiol 25(1):47–52

Cooperberg MR, Presti JC Jr, Shinohara K, Carroll PR (2013) Neoplasms of the prostate gland. In: McAninch JW, Lue TF, Smith DR (eds) Smith and Tanagho's general urology, 18th edn. McGraw-Hill Medical, New York, pp 350–379

Espinosa G (2013) Nutrition and benign prostatic hyperplasia. Curr Opin Urol 23(1):38–41

Foster HE, Barry MJ, Dahm P, Gandhi MC, Kaplan SA, Kohler TS et al (2019) Surgical management of lower urinary tract symptoms attributed to benign prostatic hyperplasia: AUA guideline. J Urol 200(3):612–619. https://www.auanet.org/guidelines/benign-prostatic-hyperplasia-(bph)-guideline. Accessed 30 Nov 2019

Gacci M, Carini M, Salvi M, Sebastianelli A et al (2014) Management of benign prostatic hyperplasia: role of phosphodiesterase-5 inhibitors. Drugs Aging 31:425–439

Kim JH, Baek MJ, Sun HY, Lee B, Li S, Khandwala Y et al (2018) Efficacy and safety of 5 alpha-reductase inhibitor monotherapy in patients with benign prostatic hyperplasia: a meta-analysis. PLoS One 13(10):e0203479. https://doi.org/10.1371/journal.pone.0203479. Accessed 30 Nov 2019

McConnell JD (1998) Epidemiology, etiology, pathophysiology, and diagnosis of benign prostatic hyperplasia. In: McConnell JD, Walsh PC (eds) Campbell's urology, 7th edn, vol. 2. W.B. Saunders Company, Philadelphia, pp. 1429–52

Mcvary KT, Rogers T, Roehrborn CG (2019) Rezūm water vapor thermal therapy for lower urinary tract symptoms associated with benign prostatic hyperplasia: 4-year results from randomized controlled study. Urology 126:171–179. https://doi.org/10.1016/j.urology.2018.12.041

Paolone DR (2010) Benign prostatic hyperplasia. Clin Geriatr Med 26:223–239

Parsons OA (2014) Associations of obesity, physical activity and diet with benign prostatic hyperplasia and lower urinary tract symptoms. Curr Opin Urol 24(1):10–14

Resnick MI (2003) Benign prostatic hyperplasia. In: Resnick MI (ed) Urology secrets, 3rd edn. Hanley & Belfus Inc, Philadelphia, pp. 98–101

Roehrborn CG, Gange SN, Shore ND, Giddens JL, Bolton DM, Cowan BE et al (2013) The prostatic urethral lift for the treatment of lower urinary tract symptoms associated with prostatic enlargement due to benign prostatic hyperplasia: the L.I.F.T. study. J Urol 190:2161–2167

Russo A, La Croce G, Capogross P, Ventimislia E et al (2014) Latest pharmacotherapy options for benign prostatic hyperplasia. Expert Opin Pharmacother 15(16):2319–2328

Saadat H, Elterman DS (2019) The role of aquablation for the surgical treatment of LUTS/BPH. Curr Urol Rep 20(8):65–100

Shigemura K, Fujisawa M (2018) Current status of holmium laser enucleation of the prostate. Int J Urol 25(3):206–211. https://onlinelibrary.wiley.com/doi/pdf/10.1111/iju.13507. Accessed 30 Nov 2019

Silbert L (2017) Benign prostatic disease. In: Newman DK, Wyman JF, Welch VW (eds) Core curriculum for urologic nursing, 1st edn. Society of Urologic Nurses and Associates, Pitman, NJ, pp 605–618

Silva J, Silva CM, Cruz F (2014) Current medical treatment of lower urinary tract symptoms/BPH: do we have a standard? Curr Opin Urol 24(1):21–28

Vuichoud C, Loughlin KR (2015) Benign prostatic hyperplasia: epidemiology, economics and evaluation. Can J Urol 22(Suppl 1):1–6

Walsh PC, Retik AB, Vaughan ED, Wein AJ (2002) Campbell's urology, vol 2. Saunders, Philadelphia

Wieder JA (2014) Pocket guide to urology, 5th edn. J. Wieder Medical, Oakland, CA, pp 210–223

Hematuria

6

Rebecca Thorne, Michelle J. Lajiness, and Susanne A. Quallich

Contents

Objectives
1. Distinguish between the clinical presentation of microscopic hematuria and gross hematuria.
2. Differentiate among potential causes for both conditions.
3. Determine the appropriate evaluation and management for the hematuria patient.

R. Thorne (✉)
Wooster Urology, LLC, Wooster, OH, USA

M. J. Lajiness
Department of Urology, University of Toledo, Toledo, OH, USA
e-mail: Michelle.Lajiness@utoledo.edu

S. A. Quallich
Division of Andrology, General and Community Health, Department of Urology, University of Michigan Health System, Ann Arbor, MI, USA
e-mail: quallich@umich.edu

© Springer Nature Switzerland AG 2020
S. A. Quallich, M. J. Lajiness (eds.), *The Nurse Practitioner in Urology*,
https://doi.org/10.1007/978-3-030-45267-4_6

Overview

Hematuria is the presence of blood in the urine; greater than 3 red blood cells per high-power microscopic field (HPF) is significant. Hematuria is a common problem seen in the urology office, one that cannot be ignored. Patients with gross hematuria (visible) are usually frightened by the sudden onset of blood in the urine and frequently present to the emergency department for evaluation. Hematuria of any degree should never be ignored and, in adults, should be regarded as a symptom of urologic malignancy until proven otherwise. Hematuria is classified by its site of origin: nephrologic, urologic, or pseudo-hematuria (origin from outside the urinary system, such as menstruation).

Studies have shown that the incidence of hematuria, both gross and microscopic, ranges from 2 to 30% (Lee et al. 2013; Harmanil and Yuksel 2013). Hematuria can be caused from urologic and nephrologic causes, and the clinician must have a thorough understanding of the causes, history, physical exam, and diagnostic studies to properly evaluate these patients. Any patient that presents with gross hematuria not related to recent surgery, trauma, or UTI in a female should complete a hematuria work-up. Patients with gross hematuria usually have an underlying pathology, whereas it is quite common for patients with microscopic hematuria to have a negative work-up (evaluation).

Microscopic hematuria is defined as one properly collected, noncontaminated urinalysis, with greater than 3 RBCs per 10 HPF (AUA Guideline 2016), that has no other attributable cause. Microscopic hematuria can result from both urologic and nephrologic causes; it can be the result of either anatomic issues or physiologic issues with the kidney (glomerular bleeding, Box 6.1). It is rarely the result of a patient complaint and is usually found incidentally during the evaluation for another condition. Long-term use of anti-inflammatory medications and other over-the-counter medications can result in medical renal disease that produces microscopic hematuria.

Box 6.1 Examples of Conditions Contributing to Medical/Renal Hematuria
- Berger's disease (IgA nephropathy)
- Bleeding disorder
- Bleeding dyscrasias/sickle cell disease
- Diabetes mellitus
- Drug-induced interstitial disease
- End-stage renal disease
- Exercise (marathon running)
- History of analgesic abuse
- HIV
- Infections (e.g., hepatitis)
- Postinfectious glomerulonephritis
- Systemic lupus erythematosus

Hematuria can be caused by menstruation, vigorous exercise, sexual activity, viral illness, trauma, kidney stones, or infection, such as a urinary tract infection (UTI). More serious causes of hematuria include malignancy (kidney or bladder); inflammation of the kidney, urethra, bladder, or prostate; polycystic kidney disease; blood clotting disorders, such as hemophilia; and sickle cell disease. Gross hematuria can be the only indication of urologic malignancy and is usually an indicator of an anatomic issue within the genitourinary tract or non-glomerular bleeding (Boxes 6.2 and 6.3).

Box 6.2 Examples of Conditions Contributing to Gross Hematuria
- Autosomal dominant polycystic kidney disease (ADPCKD)
- Benign prostatic hypertrophy (BPH)
- BPH regrowth post-transurethral resection
- Contamination from menstruation
- Hemorrhagic cystitis
- Interstitial cystitis
- Posterior urethritis
- Poststreptococcal glomerulonephritis
- Renal/ureteral/bladder stone
- Renal/ureteral/bladder tumor
- Sickle cell disease
- Trauma
- Tuberculosis
- Urethritis
- Urethral cancer
- Urethral stricture
- Vigorous exercise

Box 6.3 Medications That May Cause Red Urine
- Chloroquine
- Ibuprofen
- Levodopa
- Methyldopa
- Nitrofurantoin
- Phenacetin
- Phenazopyridine
- Phenytoin
- Quinine
- Rifampin
- Sulfamethoxazole

In evaluating hematuria, several questions should always be asked, and the answers will guide the work-up:

Is the hematuria gross or microscopic?
At what time during urination does the hematuria occur (beginning, end, or during entire stream)?
Is the hematuria associated with pain?
Is the patient passing clots?
If the patient is passing clots, do the clots have a specific shape?

Although inflammatory conditions may result in hematuria, all patients with hematuria, except perhaps young women with acute bacterial hemorrhagic cystitis, should undergo urologic evaluation. Older women and men who present with hematuria and irritative voiding symptoms may have cystitis secondary to infection arising in a necrotic bladder tumor or, more commonly, flat carcinoma in situ of the bladder. The most common cause of gross hematuria in a patient older than age 50 years is bladder cancer.

History

When obtaining the history from the patient it is very important to clarify the timing of the hematuria. The patient may note that the hematuria is at the beginning of the stream (initial) throughout the whole stream (total) or at the end of the stream (terminal). It is very helpful to establish the timing of blood in the urinary stream, which can help predict the source of bleeding and narrow the diagnostic evaluation (Table 6.1). Other items to consider are whether this is the first occurrence and were there any precipitating events and if duration of the hematuria has lasted (weeks, months).

Is there any associated pain? Hematuria is usually not painful unless it is associated with inflammation or obstruction. Thus patients with cystitis and secondary hematuria may experience painful urinary irritative symptoms, but the pain is usually not worsen with passage of clots. More commonly, pain in association with hematuria usually results from upper urinary tract hematuria with obstruction of the ureters with clots. Passage of these clots may be associated with severe, colicky flank pain similar to that produced by a ureteral calculus, and this helps identify the source of the hematuria.

The presence of clots usually indicates a significant urologic pathology. Usually, if the patient is passing clots, they are solid and of bladder or prostatic urethral origin. However, the presence of vermiform (wormlike) clots, particularly if associated with flank pain, identifies the hematuria as coming from the upper urinary tract.

There are certain distinct points that should be elicited from history, because they can indicate a higher risk factor for malignancy in the presence of microhematuria. This includes a history of smoking, chronic urinary tract infections, pelvic irradiation, irritative voiding symptoms, past episodes of gross hematuria, and male gender.

Table 6.1 Timing of blood in the urinary stream

Description of hematuria	Possible cause
Microscopic hematuria *Any site within the upper or lower urinary tract*	UTI, prostatitis, urethritis, medical renal disease, bladder/ureteral/renal malignancy, stone disease
Initial gross hematuria *Anterior urethra*	Stricture, meatal stenosis, urethral cancer
Total gross hematuria *Source above bladder neck: bladder, kidney, ureter*	Renal/ureteral/bladder stone or tumor; trauma, including vigorous exercise; hemorrhagic cystitis; interstitial cystitis; sickle cell disease; nephritis; ADPCKD; poststreptococcal glomerulonephritis
Terminal gross hematuria *Bladder neck, prostate, posterior urethra*	BPH or regrowth BPH post-transurethral resection, bladder neck polyps

ADPCKD autosomal dominant polycystic kidney disease, *BPH* benign prostatic hyperplasia, *UTI* urinary tract infection

Physical Examination

There is no specific physical examination for the patient with hematuria, unless associated with trauma or kidney stones (Chaps. 8 and 10). Physical examination should always include blood pressure. A routine genitourinary examination accompanied by a pelvic exam for female patients and a digital rectal exam for male patients is mandatory. Unfortunately, the physical exam tends to be unrevealing but can increase suspicion for other conditions, such as kidney stones, with a positive finding of costovertebral angle tenderness.

Other noted findings in the physical exam such as edema or cardiac arrhythmia may suggest nephrotic syndrome. Costovertebral angle tenderness suggests ureteral obstruction, such as due to stone disease. A careful history and physical examination will help stratify an individual patient's risk for underlying urologic disease.

Diagnostic Tests

Laboratory Evaluation

The urinalysis microscopic assessment is key to deciding how to proceed in a patient with hematuria; this should be obtained via a midstream voided clean-catch specimen, unless the patient is unable to void. Unless there is concern about compromise to renal function, or hematuria is present in a patient with known compromised renal function, the value of additional laboratory work is debatable but should include an estimation of renal function. Additional tests could include

CBC, serum electrolytes, serum creatinine and blood urea nitrogen, PT/PTT, or PSA testing. Choice of studies will be guided by the patient's presentation and risk factors.

Urine cytology may be considered part of the microscopic or gross hematuria evaluation to help eliminate low-risk patients from additional evaluation. A positive cytology may indicate that malignancy is present at any point in the genitourinary tract. Ideally the urine cytology should be obtained on a patient's first voided morning urine on three separate days, if possible, for the greatest degree of accuracy. It can also be obtained at the time of cystoscopy. Depending on the individual's risk factors, the provider may consider tumor markers as well.

Imaging Studies

The patient should also have the appropriate imaging study based on the suspected cause of the hematuria and will help establish an anatomic cause for hematuria. The appropriate imaging study will be selected based on patient's comorbidities and suspected causes for the hematuria. Other considerations will be influential as well, such as the speed with which the work-up is intended to be completed, coupled with available resources, as well as potential insurance coverage and preauthorization issues. CT urogram is the preferred initial imaging study because of its higher sensitivity and specificity for upper tract pathology. If this test is not available, an IVU and renal ultrasound is a suitable alternative.

Procedures

In a patient who presents with gross hematuria, cystoscopy should be performed as soon as possible, because frequently the source of bleeding can be readily identified. Cystoscopy will determine whether the hematuria is coming from the urethra, bladder, or upper urinary tract. In patients with gross hematuria secondary to an upper tract source, it may be possible to see red urine pulsing from the involved ureteral orifice. Ideally, the patient will also undergo a CT urogram, especially when there is a concern for malignancy.

In patients under age 35, without significant risk factors for malignancy a cystoscopy is considered at the discretion of the provider. Patients greater than age 35 and any patient with significant risk factors for malignancy will have a cystoscopy.

Management

The potential causes for both microscopic and gross hematuria are numerous and include such variable conditions as renal stones, interstitial cystitis, urothelial malignancy, radiation cystitis, and an enlarged prostate. Management depends on determining and treating the underlying cause of the hematuria and can include medical or surgical management. Conservative methods for managing these conditions include recommending that patients increase their fluid intake to help dilute their urine and stop taking analgesics that could potentially contribute to hematuria.

In the presence of renal insufficiency, hypertension, significant proteinuria, dysmorphic red blood cells, or red blood cell casts, the patient should be referred to the nephrologist for additional renal disease evaluation.

Initial management of gross hematuria will be determined by the suspected cause of the gross hematuria, such as reversing excessive anticoagulation. Frequently this involves placement of a three-way hematuria catheter for irrigation and may involve additional surgical procedures and possible inpatient stay. Placing the catheter on light traction may tamponade bleeding. Gross hematuria that is refractory to management can be managed in some instances with medication (5α reductase inhibitors for prostate bleeding) or surgical remedies (embolization of specific arteries or veins).

Long-Term Management

There is no specific long-term management for hematuria; rather its management is determined by cause. If after evaluation, no significant urologic or nephrologic disease is established, patients can be followed yearly with a routine urinalysis. If they have two consecutive negative annual urinalyses, no further evaluation is necessary. If a clear source of hematuria is established, the urinalysis should be repeated once treatment has been completed.

The exception to this is persistent microscopic hematuria, such as can be seen with diabetic patients and other patients with comorbidities that compromise their renal function. In this population, yearly urinalyses should continue to monitor for changes in the degree of microhematuria. The urinalysis is a low-cost test with little patient burden but may provide insight into patients who may be at risk for nonmalignant urologic disease. Serial urinalysis can be followed through an individual's primary care provider or through yearly visits with a urology provider.

Clinical Pearls
- Patients are often frightened and require reassurance. One drop of blood can color the urine and patients often believe they are hemorrhaging.
- Always include recent history of exercise with patients (male or female) who present with microscopic hematuria, especially those of a younger age.
- Gross hematuria must be evaluated urgently with accompanying studies arranged and, if possible, completed before the appointment.
- Therapeutic anticoagulation should not result in gross hematuria or microscopic hematuria. The anticoagulated patient presenting with either gross hematuria or microscopic hematuria needs to complete a urologic and nephrologic evaluation, beginning with coagulation studies.

- A patient is unlikely to lose enough blood through GU bleeding to compromise their hemodynamics, with a possible exception for gross hematuria that the patient has ignored.
- Helpful mnemonic: Pee ON TTTTHIS—Prostate, obstructive uropathy, nephritis, trauma, tumor, tuberculosis, thrombus, hematologic, infection/inflammation, stones.

Resources for the Clinician

Diagnosis, Evaluation and Follow-Up of Asymptomatic Microhematuria(AMH) in Adults: AUA Guidelines. https://www.auanet.org/guidelines/asymptomatic-microhematuria-(amh)-guideline

Resources for the Patient

Urology Care Foundation, What is Hematuria? 2019. http://urologyhealth.org/urologic-conditions?q=&filters=470

National Institute of Diabetes and Digestive and Kidney Diseases (NIDDK), Hematuria (Blood in the Urine), 2016. https://www.niddk.nih.gov/health-information/urologic-diseases/hematuria-blood-urine

References

American Urologic Association (2016) Diagnosis, evaluation and follow-up of asymptomatic hematuria (AMH). http://www.auanet.org/guidelines/asymptomatic-microhematuria-(amh)-guideline. Accessed 6 Nov 2019

Harmanil O, Yuksel B (2013) Asymptomatic microscopic hematuria in women requires separate guidelines. Int Urogynecol J 24:203–206

Lee Y, Chang J, Koo C, Lee S, Choi Y, Cho K (2013) Hematuria grading scale: a new tool for gross hematuria. J Urol 82(2):284–289

Orchialgia and Urologic Chronic Pelvic Pain Syndromes in Men

7

Susanne A. Quallich

Contents

S. A. Quallich (✉)
Division of Andrology, General and Community Health, Department of Urology, Michigan Medicine, University of Michigan, Ann Arbor, MI, USA
e-mail: quallich@umich.edu

© Springer Nature Switzerland AG 2020
S. A. Quallich, M. J. Lajiness (eds.), *The Nurse Practitioner in Urology*,
https://doi.org/10.1007/978-3-030-45267-4_7

Objectives
1. Discuss chronic prostatitis as a pain syndrome
2. Discuss treatment for chronic male pelvic pain from a pain perspective
3. Review the role of nonmedical interventions in urologic chronic pelvic pain syndromes in men

Overview and Introduction

Pain is one of the most common reasons that any patient seek care, and is the most expensive public health issue in the United States. Over 126 million Americans suffer from chronic pain (Kennedy et al. 2014) creating a cost of in excess of $635 billion both in direct medical care costs and decreased worker productivity (Institute of Medicine [IOM] 2011). Several factors can contribute to chronic pain and deciding whether or not he is a "pain patient". These include issues such as a trauma history, other chronic illness, legal concerns, financial concerns, grief, mental disorders, substance abuse, and healthcare access issues.

"Prostatitis" has historically been used as a nonspecific term to describe genital or pelvic discomfort in men; this has been a considerable disservice. A strict definition for prostatitis with a focus on inflammation of the prostate gland as a result of tissue response to infection or injury does not account for the associated symptoms clinicians may see when men present for prostatitis or pelvic pain. Because it is a nonspecific term, it is unclear what actual clinical symptoms "prostatitis" is meant to describe. Some men may experience lower urinary tract symptoms with or without functional sexual complaints. This in turn leads to management frustrations in the inability to describe a successful algorithm for successful or consistent treatment among men with this complaint.

Clinicians of all disciplines who treat men with "prostatitis" will recognize that there is not one homogeneous presentation or group of men that can be described clinically. This contributes to a management approach that combines using results of microbiological tests combined with clinical features to try and develop a plan that will best manage an individual patient. Some men benefit most from a multidisciplinary approach that can include input from physical therapists, psychologists, infectious disease specialists and even gastroenterologist in addition to a urology provider. Furthermore, many men may complain of a variety of symptoms in the pelvic, perineal, and rectal area, resulting in embarrassment or a lack of full disclosure about their actual symptom presentation which can in turn result in treatment lack of success.

Younger and middle-aged men present for evaluation more commonly, and is the presenting complaint responsible for up to 25% of all urology office visits (Nguyen 2014; Wagenlehner et al. 2013a). Prostatitis was classified into four categories by the National Institutes of Health (NIH) in 1999 (Krieger et al. 1999; Table 7.1). Many providers would simply provide men with antibiotics in the hopes that this

Table 7.1 NIH classification of prostatitis

Description	NIH designation	Clinical presentation
Acute bacterial prostatitis	Type I	Acute symptoms + bacterial infection Systemic infection
Chronic bacterial prostatitis (CP)	Type II	Recurrent symptoms + documented bacterial infection with same organism Prostatitis symptoms may or may not be present
Chronic prostatitis/ chronic pelvic pain syndrome (CPPS)	Type III	Chronic, intermittent or recurrent urogenital symptoms >3 months No evidence of urinary bacterial infection
	Type IIIa: inflammatory	Semen and prostate secretion leukocytes Inflammation, but no infection
	Type IIIb: noninflammatory (previous term: prostatodynia)	No semen and prostate secretion leukocytes No inflammation or infection
Asymptomatic	Type IV	No symptoms Incidental finding (e.g. with prostate biopsy) in the absence of genitourinary tract symptoms No treatment necessary

Adapetd from Krieger et al. (1999)

would provide some measure of relief. The majority of men with prostatic pain (approximately 90%) do not have an identifiable infective etiology, resulting in classification as chronic pelvic pain syndrome (CPPS) (Clemens et al. 2015).

Urologic chronic pelvic pain syndromes (UCPPS) were historically evaluated from only a urology perspective, with a resulting record of unpredictable results and poor treatment success (Clemens 2014), in part due to the failure to account for the multifactorial nature of pain. Large epidemiological studies (Multidisciplinary Approach to the Study of Chronic Pelvic Pain [MAPP]) revealed the role of underlying chronic pain syndromes in patients with UCPPS (Krieger et al. 2015). A shift away from a focus on only the urology component of UCPPS allowed for identification of the role of systemic syndromes that may have a relationship with UCPPS.

Application of the principles of chronic pain in the evaluation of men with UCPPS allowed for identification of characteristics that UCPPS patients shared with other chronic pain populations. Two phenotypes of UCPPS patients have been identified, one with bladder-focused symptoms and one with more systemic, centralized pain (Clemens 2014; Griffith et al. 2016; Krieger et al. 2015). Clemens et al. (2015) reported that perineal pain appears to be a defining characteristic in male UCPPS.

Acute Prostatitis

Clinical Presentation

Acute prostatitis affects all age groups of men, but tends to occur more frequently in young and middle-aged men, and has a rapid and severe onset. Etiology includes ascending urethral infection or intra-prostatic reflux, or as a complication of sexually transmitted infection. Men may be acutely ill, and may present because they are unable to void. They can report fever and chills, dysuria, urinary frequency, urgency, perineal/flank/low back pain, and possible generalized malaise that may have progressed over a few days. There may be a history of previous treatment with a short course of antibiotics for "epididymitis" that resulted in symptom improvement for a week or two.

Prompt diagnosis and treatment are critical to prevent complications of sepsis; the most common causative organisms are *Escherichia coli* (58–88%) and other Enterobacteriaceae species (*Klebsiella, Enterobacter, and Serratia;* 3–11%) (Kim et al. 2014). Prostate abscess is rare; it should be part of any differential if there is no improvement or if symptoms worsen on initial antibiotic therapy, and in men with decreased sensation to the pelvic region, such as men with spinal cord injuries.

Risk factors for acute prostatitis are multifactorial (Table 7.2), influenced by the overall health of the patient and his comorbidities, existing dysfunctional voiding, constipation, pelvic floor dysfunction, and potentially exercise habits. Anatomic issues that affect voiding, such as phimosis, enlarged prostate, or urethral stricture disease, increase the risk for prostate infection.

Table 7.2 Acute and chronic bacterial prostatitis: representative symptoms and risk factors

Common symptoms	Risk factors
Dysuria	Anatomical or functional GU tract abnormalities, e.g. urethral
Elevated PSA	stricture, prostate hypertrophy (BPH), bladder dysfunction
Erectile dysfunction	Chronic pain syndromes
Fever, chills	HIV
Hematospermia	Indwelling catheter or intermittent catheterization
Hematuria	Recent prostate biopsy or other GU instrumentation/procedure
Malaise or flu-like symptoms	Recurrent urinary tract infection
New onset urinary hesitancy	Sexually transmitted diseases
or dribbling	Trauma
Nonspecific back pain, can be	Possible: Marathon runners, cyclists, dehydration
unilateral or bilateral	
Painful erection or ejaculation	
Perineal, rectal, pelvic, groin	
or penis pain	
Prostate tenderness and/or	
enlargement on DRE	
Urge incontinence	
Urinary retention	
Urinary urgency or frequency	

Physical Examination

For all men with suspected prostatitis, a DRE must be attempted; the prostate may be soft, edematous, enlarged, and exquisitely tender. Prostate massage is not recommended with suspected acute prostatitis, to reduce the risk of urosepsis. Vitals may demonstrate fever, and blood pressure changes are possible. The bladder may be palpable, and there may be CVA tenderness; genital examination may be unhelpful, with any complaints of pain not reproduced on examination (examiner unable to provoke the pain that patient reports). The overall appearance may be toxic, especially if urinary retention is a concern.

Diagnosis/Evaluation

Obtain urinalysis, gram stain, urine culture, and complete blood count. Depending on the presentation, a basic metabolic panel, ESR, C-reactive protein and blood cultures can be added. PSA elevations are common during acute infection, and can be monitored over several weeks to confirm treatment success. Blood cultures are needed only if sepsis is suspected. Imaging is not usually indicated; however, if prostatic abscess is suspected, obtain transrectal ultrasound (TRUS) or CT. Ultrasound post-void residual should be obtained to evaluate for retention.

Laboratory results are likely to show elevated WBCs, pyuria/bacteriuria, and a positive urine culture. Cultured organisms are primarily gram-negative: *Escherichia coli* (~80%), *Klebsiella* (3–11%), *Proteus* (3–6%), and *Pseudomonas* (3–7%) (Wagenlehner et al. 2014). Instrumentation (prostate biopsy or resection) may be a factor in acute prostatitis with resistant pathogens, possibly secondary to periprocedure antibiotics (Meyrier and Fekete 2015a; Nguyen 2014; Sharp et al. 2010).

Treatment

Men who are in acute retention may need a suprapubic tube placed to avoid unnecessary manipulation of the prostate with catheter placement. Treatment requires antibiotics, but the recommendation may vary by facility community patterns of antibiotic resistance, society recommendations (Table 7.3) and must be based on culture results. Few men require hospitalization for hydration and IV antibiotics; the majority will be treated successfully as outpatients with oral antibiotics.

While the most common causative organism is *E. coli*, monitor culture/sensitivity results to be certain the patient is on appropriate antibiotic regimen. Treat for 4–6 weeks to avoid chronic prostatitis, emphasizing increased fluid intake and avoidance of pressure to the prostate. Men may benefit from a probiotic such as Align®, which can help prevent GI distress due to the lengthy course of antibiotics. Symptomatic management included NSAIDs or acetaminophen, stool softeners, and alpha blockers over for the first few weeks. Men should be advised that they will only notice gradual improvement for the first 2–3 weeks after starting treatment. If

Table 7.3 Prostatitis Treatment

Classification	Possible treatment	
Acute bacterial prostatitis[a] *Appears septic, potentially unable to urinate or unable to tolerate oral therapy Admit to hospital, offer parenteral therapy according to facility guidelines*	Sulfamethoxazole and trimethoprim 800–160 mg orally Fluoroquinolones orally Trimethoprim 300 mg orally Cephalexin 500 mg Amoxicillin and clavulanic acid 500 mg + 125 mg orally Appears septic, unable to urinate or unable to tolerate oral therapy Admit to hospital, offer parenteral therapy according to facility guidelines	
Chronic bacterial prostatitis[a] (CP) *Complaints include dysuria, hesitancy, urgency, perineal fullness, without toxic presentation*	Norfloxacin 400 mg orally every 12 h for 4 weeks, or Trimethoprim 300 mg orally daily for 4 weeks If *Chlamydia* or *Ureaplasma* noted • Doxycycline 100 mg orally every 12 h for 2–4 weeks	
Chronic prostatitis/chronic pelvic pain syndrome (CPPS) *Treatment aimed at both symptom relief and improving quality of life*	Type III Type IIIa: inflammatory Type IIIb: noninflammatory	Treatment for mental health issues, e.g., anxiety, depression Pelvic floor physical therapy Alpha1 adrenergic receptor antagonist (α blockers) NSAIDs 5α reductase inhibitors Pregabalin or other anticonvulsants PDE5I Trigger point injections Cognitive-based therapy/stress management Sitz baths Phytotherapy: pollen extracts, saw palmetto, quercetin Yin yoga
Asymptomatic	None required	

[a]Specific choice of antibiotic may be guided by facility guidelines, culture results, society guidelines

pain with erection or ejaculation was present, this may persist for a few weeks after treatment is started.

Complications such as abscess are uncommon, but may be seen at higher rates in men with neurologic compromise, diabetes, or HIV.

At a return clinic visit, there should be assessment of voiding function and bladder emptying, along with consideration for repeat UA/culture post-treatment (Meyrier and Fekete 2015a; Nguyen 2014). If the patient is not improving, he may require ultrasound-guided perineal puncture of any abscess to better identify causative organisms and update the antibiotic regimen. Assessment of bladder function may reveal preexisting voiding dysfunction that will benefit from management.

Chronic Bacterial Prostatitis

Clinical Presentation

Chronic bacterial prostatitis (CBP) can be due to inadequate treatment of a previous episode of acute prostatitis, and usually includes documented bacterial infections with the same pathogen(s). CBP is accompanied by urogenital symptoms similar to those in acute prostatitis, and with similar risk factors (Table 7.2) but presentation may lack the fever and acute symptoms, and rarely include concern for urinary retention. Younger and middle-aged men are again the most at-risk population. History may include waxing and waning of symptoms, especially if they had been treated with short courses of antibiotics. There can be a history of penis pain or pain with ejaculation. There may also be a history of repeated urinary tract infections, and left untreated, CBP can contribute to male factory infertility as the ejaculatory ducts can become obstructed, and chronic WBCs in the semen may be a contributor to decreased rates of fertilization. A history of "chronic epididymitis" may be noted, when the actual cause is recurrent bacterial migration from the prostate to the epididymis after inadequate treatment for acute prostatitis or previous CBP episode(s). Men with prostate or bladder calculi, diabetes, and tobacco abuse are at higher risk for chronic prostatitis.

Overall presentation can be very similar to that of the lower urinary tract symptoms seen with prostatic enlargement (dysuria, hesitancy, urgency, perineal fullness), but fever/chills are not typically part of the CBP presentation.

Physical Examination

The patient will be nontoxic, general examination is benign, and vitals will be normal. DRE may reveal hypertrophy, tenderness, irregularity or edema (soft to palpation), but the prostate may not be tender to examination. Genital examination may be unhelpful, with any complaints of pain not reproduced on examination (examiner unable to provoke the pain that patient reports). There may also be some suggestion of pelvic floor dysfunction on DRE.

Diagnosis/Evaluation

The historic gold standard of bacterial localization for CBP is the Meares & Stamey 4-glass test: first-voided urine, midstream urine, expressed prostatic secretions, and post-prostatic massage urine are sampled. While classic for diagnosis purposes, it is infrequently used in clinical practice.

Semen culture can be ordered, but it may identify pathogens in only about 50% of specimens. The laboratory evaluation for chronic bacterial prostatitis in usually normal, with negative results for the urinalysis and dipstick evaluation. But the most likely causative bacteria is *E. coli*. Post-void residual, either via bladder scan or bladder ultrasound, should be performed to confirm that urinary retention is not a concern. In the absence of proven bacterial infection, it is difficult to distinguish CBP from UCPPS (Meyrier and Fekete 2015b; Wagenlehner et al. 2013a).

Treatment

Table 7.3 discusses antibiotic treatment for prostatitis; the length of treatment should be a minimum of 4 weeks, but can range between 4 and 12 weeks depending on past episodes of treatment and their duration. Symptomatic management with NSAIDs or acetaminophen, stool softeners, probiotics, and alpha blockers will help with overall comfort levels and improve associated symptoms. Men may find non-pharmacologic options such as sitz bath, donut cushion, and hot/cold packs of some value. If chronic prostatitis is refractory to treatment, other options for evaluation can include a semen culture, a referral to infectious disease, and possibly consider-ation of laser treatment of the prostate to try and mechanically eradicate the infec-tions. It is rarely necessary to employ IV antibiotics for treatment of CBP, but if necessary, will be completed with the input of an infectious disease provider, and can usually be managed outpatient.

Follow-up

At the beginning of treatment, men should be advised that they may notice only modest improvement of symptoms over the first few weeks of treatment. Some men may benefit from assessment of preexisting voiding function, evaluation for urethral stricture disease or pelvic floor dysfunction, as these conditions can contribute to CBP. Men should be advised to avoid constipation and focus on adequate hydration.

Urologic Chronic Pelvic Pain Syndrome (UCPPS)

Urologic chronic pelvic pain syndrome (UCPPS), also described previously as chronic prostatitis, is a clinical syndrome defined as pelvic pain associated with urinary symptoms and/or sexual dysfunction, lasting for at least 3 of the past 6 months in the absence of other identified causes (NIH standardized definition). Contemporary thought has questioned to what extent the prostate is actually involved in creating and sustaining symptoms, and may be better characterized as chronic inflammatory condition. UCPPS remains a diagnosis of exclusion, and esti-mates suggest it is present in 2–10% of all adult men, although a precise incidence remains elusive (Nickel et al. 2013). Patient history, symptoms, and clinical presen-tation are similar to chronic prostate infection, yet without positive cultures.

In UCPPS, the term "prostatitis" may not be indicative that the source of symp-toms is the prostate, but some initiation of symptoms may have been the result of urine reflux into prostatic ducts. Krieger et al. (2015) report an association between nonurological somatic syndromes and the overall symptom severity of men with UCPPS. Recent research by the MAPP network has identified overrepresentation of

Burkholderia cenocepacia (gram negative bacteria) in the initial urine stream of men with chronic pelvic pain syndrome (Krieger et al. 2015; Nickel et al. 2015). The MAPP collaborative data also suggest that the term "urologic chronic pelvic pain syndrome" may, in fact, represent two categories of patients. Some patients demonstrate more focused pelvic and urinary symptoms, while some demonstrate both urological symptoms and nonurologic syndromes, suggesting a more systemic condition (Table 7.4) that may be influenced and possibly sustained by other chronic pain conditions.

Table 7.2 also distinguishes between traditional inflammatory (IIIA) and noninflammatory (IIIB) subtypes of chronic prostatitis.

Clinical Presentation

Men will provide a history of urologic and pelvic symptoms for greater than 3 months without a positive culture, although they may have had a positive culture at some point in the past if this condition has been present for several months, or years. A detailed history is essential: present urinary symptoms; pain sites and description of the pain; sexual history and current sexual activity; mental health history; attempt to elicit any history of physical, emotional, or sexual trauma; and nonurological somatic disorders. There may be reports of a variety of symptoms that can wax and wane (Table 7.5). Sexual dysfunction complaints may be present,

Table 7.4 Conditions associated with UCPPS

Associated nonurological somatic syndromes
Chronic fatigue syndrome
Irritable bowel syndrome or Crohn's disease
Fibromyalgia/chronic fatigue syndrome
TMJ disorder
Anxiety disorder
Widespread chronic pain
Interstitial cystitis/painful bladder syndrome (IC/PBS)

Krieger et al. (2015), Pontari (2015), and Wagenlehner et al. (2013b)

Table 7.5 Pelvic floor muscle examination via rectal examination

Rectal examination to determine pelvic floor muscle involvement
Notation (0:00) corresponds to clock face
Document presence/absence of pain with moderate pressure to each site; examiner may note "knot" at muscle site
Rectal sphincter tone: decreased, normal, increased, spasm
1. Suprapubic area pain?
2. Perineal body pain? (6:00)
3. Posterior levator muscle (2:00)
4. Posterior levator muscle (10:00)
5. Obturator internus muscle (9:00)
6. Anterior levator muscle (7:00)
7. Anterior levator muscle (5:00)
8. Obturator internus muscle (3:00)
Did the pelvic examination reproduce your pain or discomfort?

but pelvic floor tenderness, depression, and catastrophizing are more clinically significant and help determine treatment. Catastrophizing, in particular, is important; it is defined as an exaggerated negative mental set brought to bear during actual or anticipated painful experience (Sullivan et al. 2001; Sullivan 2009), which consists of three distinct components:

1. *Rumination*: repetitively going over a thought or a problem without completion. With repetition, feelings of inadequacy raise anxiety, and anxiety interferes with solving/understanding the problem;
2. *Magnification*: exaggerating the importance of (insignificant) events; and
3. *Helplessness*: behavior exhibited by a subject after enduring repeated aversive stimuli beyond their control, or perceived to be beyond their control.

Catastrophizing has been implicated as predictor of treatment success; the more time these symptoms have been present, the more this mindset may be a factor in an individual's willingness or lack of willingness, to try, and his compliance with, treatment suggestions.

Stress may also be implicated in flares of men diagnosed with UCPPS.

Physical Examination

General physical examination is typically unrevealing. Examination of the pelvic floor (Table 7.5) may demonstrate point tenderness and suggest trigger points; rectal examination may show tenderness or be benign, or suggest issues with the pelvic floor. Examination may reproduce complaints of pain (including genital pain) or fail to reproduce pain; there may be hyperesthesia (increased sensitivity to stimulation) and allodynia (pain from a stimulus that does not normally provoke pain) as well. Men more likely to have pelvic muscle spasms, increased pelvic tone, and tenderness to palpation of pelvic muscles.

Diagnosis/Evaluation

The following stepwise approach should be considered:

1. Rule out active bacterial infection of the prostate/bladder: urinalysis, culture, cytology (as indicated) and PVR;
2. Rule out other contributors to the same symptoms: constipation, untreated BPH, pelvic floor/radicular issues, undiagnosed/poorly managed diabetes, neurologic issues;
3. Confirm that symptoms and exams are representative of UCPPS: Table 7.6.
4. Acknowledge the limited role for imaging and other studies: scrotal ultrasound of pain localizes to testes, office cystoscopy, prostate ultrasound and/or biopsy, pelvic CT or MRI, abdominal imaging (Pontari 2015; Sharp et al. 2010; Stein et al. 2015).

Table 7.6 Complaints that may be associated with urologic chronic pelvic pain syndrome in men

Category	Complaint
Sexual	Erectile dysfunction
	Pain with erection
	Pain with ejaculation
	Decreased sensation with sexual activity, climax or erection
Urinary	Dysuria
	Nocturia
	Sensation of incomplete emptying
	Weakened urinary stream
	Bladder pain
	Urinary retention
	Urinary frequency
Genital	Pain at tip/glans of penis; can be localized to the meatal opening
	Generalized penis pain
	Scrotal pain
	Testicular pain
	Genital burning
Perineal or rectal	Rectal burning
	Rectal itching
	Constipation
	Sensation of perineal or rectal fullness
	Rectal pain before/after bowel movement
Musculoskeletal	Pain with prolonged sitting
	Pain with activity
	Radicular pattern of pain
	Low back pain
	Pain that is exacerbated moving from sitting → standing or the reverse

Table 7.7 UPOINTS classification for UCPPS

Domain	Evaluation
Urinary	Post-void residual measured by ultrasound
Psychosocial	Evaluate depression and catastrophizing
Organ-specific	Pain improvement with bladder emptying, prostate tenderness
Infection	Culture for mycoplasma and ureaplasma, urine culture
	Consider expressed prostatic secretions or a post-prostate massage urine
Neurologic/ systemic	Pain beyond the pelvis
	Investigate history of other chronic pain syndromes
Tenderness	Palpate the abdominal and pelvic skeletal muscles (via rectum)
	Check for spasm and trigger points
Sexual	Sexual dysfunction, pain with sexual activity

There are short, validated instruments that help assess symptoms and guide treatment, including the NIH Chronic Prostatitis Symptom Index (NIH-CPSI), AUA/IPSS Symptom Questionnaire and UPOINTS classification system (Table 7.7) (Nickel and Shoskes 2010; Shoskes and Nickel 2013).

Treatment

At present there is no universally accepted treatment regimen for UCPPS, and most medical treatments are largely ineffective with only low-grade evidence to support their use, contributing to the psychological distress of these men. No therapy will be effective in all cases, which is an important concept to emphasize to men undergoing treatment. Although the estimate is over 15 years old, Calhoun et al. (2004) estimated a cost of $4397 per man, per year, offering some perspective on the financial impact of UCPPS. Clemens et al. (2018) also reported that urinary symptoms were *not* the primary motivator for those men and women who frequently sought care for UCPPS, but that higher baseline pain and depression were more important contributors.

The UPOINTS screening tool can suggest domains in which to initially focus treatment or multimodal therapies, especially for providers who have limited experience managing men with UCPPS. Management goals should aim to improve the individual's functional status, quality of life and sexual function. Cognitive-based therapy or psychology/psychiatric evaluation may assist with identification and management of conditions such as anxiety and depression, help men identify stress and other triggers that may provoke or sustain pain episodes, and provide direction for stress reduction. Successful management of UCPPS involves introducing the concept that this condition has to be managed, like any other chronic condition; some men may benefit from referral to a multidisciplinary pain management program. Patients benefit from a "whole person perspective" when developing a plan of care (Table 7.8), and providers should have the following goals:

1. An individualized approach to management based on the symptom pattern. This can include treatment for pain itself, which can go undertreated.
2. Avoidance of recurrent courses of antibiotics unless clear evidence of infective etiology.

Table 7.8 Pain syndrome approach to management of chronic pain

Components to be considered in developing treatment plan	Pain mechanisms
	Visceral dysfunctions
	Emotional consequences
	Behavioral consequences
	Sexual consequences
	Social consequences
Sequelae that exacerbate, perpetuate, and facilitate the pain itself	Mood disturbances
	Sleep disturbances
	Anxiety/depression
	Reduced function in social and vocational roles
	Inability to maintain recreational activities
	Changes to feelings of self-worth and self-esteem
	Sexual dysfunction
	Increased stress
	Potential substance abuse

Table 7.8 (continued)

Management principles (progressive)	1. Identify multidimensional (biopsychosocial) factors that contribute to UCPPS/chronic orchialgia and address as comprehensively as possible	Common to establish physiologic basis for pain Behavior changes can result, such as posture and gait changes that sustain pain Issues such as anxiety, depression, sleep disturbance facilitate pain
	2. Treatment aims to resolve any facilitators of symptoms rather than simply treating them for greater long-term success	Difference between muscle relaxers and biofeedback Difference between anti-anxiety medications and cognitive behavioral therapy
	3. Engaging the patient in his/her abilities to self-care provides self-mastery and tools for long-term self-management	Discussion of patient's role in developing treatment plan Emphasis of individual's *role in own self-care* as chronic pain patient, such as acknowledging and redirecting stress Physical therapy for core strengthening and postural adjustment Cognitive behavioral therapy to help individuals cope with stress Instruction in relaxation techniques
	4. Carefully selected procedures and medications have a role chronic pain management	Not all invasive modalities have extensive evidence to support their use Many may be dependent on the patient's success with adjusting posture or muscle tension, for instance Explains some of the transient effectiveness of these modalities If centrally mediated pain is an issue, peripheral blocks, surgery, etc. will have questionable success rate

Coordination of referrals to other services, such as psychology or pain clinics

3. Education of the patient and his family/partners to address the gap between treatment expectations and available options. Patients must be active participants in their own care.
4. Early use of anti-neuropathic pain medication.
5. Early referral to a multidisciplinary specialist team/pain clinic.

6. Clear explanation of the condition to patients including the basis of the chronic pain cycle.
7. Consideration for including phytotherapies and adjunct treatment (saw palmetto, cernilton [bee pollen extract], quercetin [bioflavonoid], cannabis, acupuncture, yoga).

Asymptomatic Inflammatory Prostatitis

Clinical Presentation/Diagnosis

Asymptomatic inflammatory prostatitis is an incidental finding in men who undergo urological procedures, such as prostate biopsy, infertility, or cancer workup. It is a finding in the men who complain of chronic pelvic pain as well, and while never requires antibiotic management, it can help drive choices for generalized management.

Treatment

No treatment is required, with the possible exception of couples who are planning to proceed with an in vitro fertilization cycle, unless symptoms develop (see acute and chronic prostatitis earlier in this chapter). Little to no evidence exists to further describe the natural history or recommend treatment modalities for asymptomatic inflammatory prostatitis (Krieger et al. 1999; Sharp et al. 2010).

Chronic Unexplained Orchialgia

Chronic unexplained orchialgia (CUO) is "a subjective negative experience of adult men, perceived as intermittent or continuous pain of variable intensity, present at least three months, localizing to the testis(es) in the absence of objective organic findings, that interferes with quality of life" (p. 8, Quallich and Arslanian-Engoren 2014). It is a difficult clinical entity, as men may seek care episodically over its course. This is a male genital pain condition without a contemporary evidence-based treatment algorithm, and a lack of research into the condition (Quallich and Arslanian-Engoren 2013). Men seek repeated evaluation and treatment, as seen with many other chronic pain populations; evaluation includes elimination of causes of urgent and acute scrotal and testicular pain (Chap. 3).

Other terms used to describe chronic pain in the male genitals include such nonspecific terms as "chronic scrotal contents pain," which can make it challenging to compare among treatment recommendations among various publications.

Background and Risk Factors

No specific ethnic or genetic risk factors have been identified, and onset of CUO may be spontaneous or pain may linger after and infection or injury. Some men report constant pain, while the pattern may be intermittent for others, often without specific aggravating or alleviating factors. At times men may be able to identify a particular movement of activity that will provoke or increase their pain. Previous guidelines have suggested that CUO is a regional extension of male chronic pelvic pain syndrome (Engeler et al. 2013) but actual evidence for this is sparse, as despite the sparse representation the literature, reported symptoms in CUO do not typically involve voiding symptoms or pelvic floor complaints. Furthermore, the results of the MAPP study do not specifically support testicular pain as a predominant symptom of UCPPS.

A key piece in establishing potential etiologies is to directly ask men if they have had a vasectomy, to ensure this is not chronic epididymal congestion/post-vasectomy pain syndrome that has not been previously identified.

Clinical Presentation and History

Same as for urologic chronic pelvic pain syndrome. Individuals should be asked specifically about a history of vasectomy, as complaints of CUO can be improperly diagnosed post-vasectomy pain syndrome.

Physical Examination and Diagnostic Testing

A thorough examination of the male genitals must be performed, with attempts to precisely localize the source of pain. Similar to UCCPS, examination may reproduce complaints of pain or fail to reproduce pain; men may demonstrate hyperesthesia and allodynia as well.

A scrotal ultrasound is strongly suggested to rule out intrascrotal pathology that could be causing pain, if the patient has not undergone this imaging in more than 6 months, to avoid risk for missing intratesticular pathology that is contributing to pain. Depending on the specific history, screening for sexually transmitted infections can be added, along with cultures for *Ureaplasma* and *Mycoplasma*. In men with symptoms consistent with possible radiculopathy (e.g., testicular pain at the same time or after pain shoots down the leg, bladder/bowel control issues) imaging of the low back may be helpful.

Management

As men with CUO present like many other chronic pain populations, and similar to UCPPS, proceed from a noninvasive perspective, that benefits from a pain perspective approach (Table 7.7) or eventual referral to a multidisciplinary pain management program. Clinical management of symptoms can proceed as detailed for UCPPS (Table 7.3). Men can be referred to a urology provider for more focused evaluation, including a spermatic cord block.

Conclusions

While acute prostatitis and chronic prostatitis have straightforward plans for treatment, UCPPS and chronic orchialgia can significantly affect quality of life and social roles. Presently the evidence base for treating these conditions is low-grade evidence and expert opinion. Providers should proceed with an evaluation that screens for significant etiologies (such as testicular cancer) and proceeds with symptomatic management based on the individual's presentation. There is also value in treating these conditions in a multidisciplinary fashion by recommending a psychology evaluation or use of online tools to identify stressors and other psychosocial factors that may act as triggers that can provoke and sustain pain complaints.

Clinical Pearls
- Acute prostatitis is generally caused by the same organisms that cause urinary tract infections, most commonly gram-negative bacteria.
- If acute prostatitis is suspected, avoid vigorous DRE—may cause bacteremia.
- Imaging studies are not indicated for acute prostatitis unless prostate abscess is suspected.
- Recurrent episodes of chronic bacterial prostatitis are common. Consider patient compliance, antibiotic resistance, impaired absorption, and failure to complete prior treatment as factors.
- Most chronic prostatitis/urologic chronic pelvic pain syndrome is a diagnosis of exclusion.
- There is NO universally accepted treatment regimen for CP/UCPPS. Individual presentation should guide treatment regimen.
- This lack of defined process and diagnosis can be a source of frustration for men, and result in patients seeking evaluation with multiple providers in the same discipline.
- Only emerging, low-level evidence guides "best practice" for chronic orchialgia occurring in the absence of associated UCPPS symptoms.

Resources for the Nurse Practitioner and Physician Assistant

The Chronic Pain and Fatigue Research Center (CPFRC) at University of Michigan online tool for identifying pain triggers: https://fibroguide.med.umich.edu/aboutfibroguide.html

The National Institutes of Health Chronic Prostatitis Symptom Index (NIH-CPSI) http://www.proqolid.org/instruments/national_institute_of_health_chronic_prostatitis_symptom_index_nih_cpsi?private=yes&fromSearch

UPOINT clinical phenotyping system for CP/CPPS to guide multimodal treatment. http://www.upointmd.com/index.php

National Guideline Clearinghouse: Chronic Pelvic Pain. http://www.guideline.gov/content.aspx?id=38626#Section424

The Multidisciplinary Approach to the Study of Chronic Pelvic Pain (MAPP) http://mappnetwork.org/

AUA: Urology Care Foundation (2015). Prostatitis (Infection of the Prostate). http://www.urologyhealth.org/urologic-conditions/prostatitis-(infection-of-the-prostate)/symptoms

Resources for the Patient

The Chronic Pain and Fatigue Research Center (CPFRC) at University of Michigan online tool for identifying pain triggers: https://fibroguide.med.umich.edu/aboutfibroguide.html

Society of Urologic Nurses and Associates (SUNA): "Prostatitis—Patient Fact Sheet" (English and Spanish) https://www.suna.org/download/members/prostatitis.pdf

NIH: "What I need to know about Prostate Problems" (English and Spanish) http://www.niddk.nih.gov/health-information/health-topics/urologic-disease/prostatitis-disorders-of-the-prostate/Pages/ez.aspx

AUA: Urology Care Foundation (2015). Prostatitis (Infection of the Prostate). http://www.urologyhealth.org/urologic-conditions/prostatitis-(infection-of-the-prostate)/symptoms

References

Calhoun EA, McNaughton MC, Pontari MA, O'Leary M, Leiby BE, Landis JR et al (2004) The economic impact of chronic prostatitis. Arch Intern Med 164(11):1231–1236

Clemens JQ (2014) Update on the MAPP project (plenary session May 19). American Urologic Association annual conference, Orlando, FL

Clemens JQ, Clauw DJ, Kreder K, Krieger JN, Kusek JW, Lai HH et al (2015) Comparison of baseline urological symptoms in men and women in the MAPP research cohort. J Urol 193(5):1554–1558

Clemens JQ, Stephens-Shields A, Naliboff BD, Lai HH, Rodriguez L, Krieger JN et al (2018) Correlates of health care seeking activities in patients with urological chronic pelvic pain syndromes: findings from the MAPP cohort. J Urol 200(1):136–140

Engeler DS, Baranowski AP, Dinis-Oliveira P, Elneil S, Hughes J, Messelink EJ et al (2013) The 2013 EAU guidelines on chronic pelvic pain: is management of chronic pelvic pain a habit, a philosophy, or a science? 10 years of development. Eur Urol 64(3):431–439

Griffith JW, Stephens-Shields AJ, Hou X, Naliboff BD, Pontari M, Edwards TC et al (2016) Pain and urinary symptoms should not be combined into a single score: psychometric findings from the MAPP Research Network. J Urol, 195(4 Part 1), 949–954.

Institute of Medicine (2011). Relieving pain in America: a blueprint for transforming prevention, care, education and research. The National Academies Press: Washington, DC.

Kennedy J, Roll JM, Schraudner T, Murphy S, McPherson S (2014) Prevalence of persistent pain in the US adult population: new data from the 2010 national health interview survey. J Pain 15(10):979–984

Kim SH, Ha US, Yoon BI, Kim SW, Sohn DW, Kim HW, Cho SY, Cho YH (2014) Microbiological and clinical characteristics in acute bacterial prostatitis according to lower urinary tract manipulation procedure. J Infect Chemother 20(1):38. https://doi.org/10.1016/j.jiac.2013.11.004. Epub 2013 Dec 11. PMID: 24462423

Krieger JN, Nyberg N, Nickel JC (1999) NIH consensus definition and classification of prostatitis. JAMA 282(3):236–237

Krieger JN, Stephens AJ, Landis JR, Clemens JQ, Kreder K, Lai HH, Afari N, Rodríguez L, Schaeffer A, Mackey S, Andriole GL, Williams DA, MAPP Research Network (2015) Relationship between chronic nonurological associated somatic syndromes and symptom severity in urological chronic pelvic pain syndromes: baseline evaluation of the MAPP study. J Urol 193(4):1254–1262. pii: S0022-5347(14)04767-3. https://doi.org/10.1016/j.juro.2014

Meyrier A, Fekete T (2015a) Chronic bacterial prostatitis. In: Calderwood SB (ed) UpToDate. http://www.uptodate.com/contents/chronic-bacterial-prostatitis?topicKey=ID%2F86802&el

Meyrier A, Fekete T (2015b) Acute bacterial prostatitis. In: Calderwood SB (ed) UpToDate. http://www.uptodate.com/contents/acute-bacterial-prostatitis?topicKey=ID%2F8062&elaps

Nguyen N (2014) Treating prostatitis effectively: a challenge for clinicians. US Pharm 39(4):35–41

Nickel JC, Shoskes DA (2010) Phenotypic approach to the management of the chronic prostatitis/chronic pelvic pain syndrome. BJU Int 106(9):1252–1263. https://doi.org/10.1111/j.1464-410X.2010.09701.x

Nickel JC, Shoskes DA, Wagenlehner FM (2013) Management of chronic prostatitis/chronic pelvic pain syndrome (CP/CPPS): the studies, the evidence, and the impact. World J Urol 31(4):747–753

Nickel JC, Stephens A, Landis JR, Chen J, Mullins C, van Bokhoven A, Lucia MS, Melton-Kreft R, Ehrlich GD, The MAPP Research Network (2015) Search for microorganisms in men with urologic chronic pelvic pain syndrome: a culture-independent analysis in the MAPP Research Network. J Urol 194(1):127–135. pii: S0022-5347(15)00058-0. https://doi.org/10.1016/j.juro.2015.01.037

Pontari M (2015) Chronic prostatitis/chronic pelvic pain syndrome. UpToDate. http://www.uptodate.com/contents/chronic-prostatitis-chronic-pelvic-pain-syndrome?topic

Quallich SA, Arslanian-Engoren C (2013) Chronic testicular pain in adult men: an integrative literature review. Am J Men's Health 7(5):402–413. https://doi.org/10.1177/1557988313476732

Quallich SA, Arslanian-Engoren C (2014) Chronic unexplained orchialgia: a concept analysis. J Adv Nurs 70(8):1717–1726. https://doi.org/10.1111/jan.12340

Sullivan MJ, Thorn B, Haythornthwaite J, Keefe F, Martin M, Bradley L, Lefebvre J (2001) Theoretical perspectives on the relation between catastrophizing and pain. Clin J Pain 17(1):52–64

Sullivan MJ (2009) The pain catastrophizing scale user manual. McGill University: Montréal

Sharp V, Takacs E, Powell C (2010) Prostatitis: diagnosis and treatment. Am Fam Physician 82(4):397–406. http://www.aafp.org/afp/2010/0815/p397.html

Shoskes D, Nickel JC (2013) Classification and treatment of men with chronic prostatitis/chronic pelvic pain syndrome using the UPOINT system. World J Urol 31(4):755–760. https://doi.org/10.1007/s00345-013-1075-6. Epub 2013 Apr 16

Stein A, May T, Dekel Y (2015) Chronic pelvic pain syndrome: a clinical enigma. Postgrad Med 126(4):115–122. https://doi.org/10.3810/pgm.2014.07.2789

Wagenlehner F, Pilatz A, Bschleipfer T, Diemer T, Linn T, Meihardt A et al (2013a) Bacterial prostatitis. World J Urol 21:711–716. https://doi.org/10.1007/s00345-013-1055-x

Wagenlehner F, van Till J, Magri V, Perletti G, Houbiers J, Weidner W, Nickel JC (2013b) National Institutes of Health Chronic Prostatitis Symptom Index (NIH-CPSI) symptom evaluation in multinational cohorts of patients with chronic prostatitis/chronic pelvic pain syndrome. Eur Urol 63(5):953–959. https://doi.org/10.1016/j.eururo.2012.10.042

Wagenlehner FM, Weidner W, Pilatz A, Naber KG (2014) Urinary tract infections and bacterial prostatitis in men. Curr Opin Infect Dis 27(1):97–101

Kidney Stones

8

Marc M. Crisenbery and Suzanne T. Parsell

Contents

Objectives

1. Determine patients at risk for renal calculi and instruct regarding controlling risk factors.
2. Discuss management for patients with active renal calculi disease, including environmental and lifestyle factors.
3. Demonstrate knowledge of appropriate testing and imaging, and the indications.

M. M. Crisenbery (✉)
Department of Urology, University of Toledo Medical College,
Toledo, OH, USA
e-mail: marc.crisenbery@utoledo.edu

S. T. Parsell
Ann Arbor, USA
e-mail: sneboysk@med.umich.edu

© Springer Nature Switzerland AG 2020
S. A. Quallich, M. J. Lajiness (eds.), *The Nurse Practitioner in Urology*,
https://doi.org/10.1007/978-3-030-45267-4_8

Introduction

Kidney stones: for many, these two small words can trigger a horrific response. For some, the memory will be of unbearable pain similar to labor pains; others will recall surgery and time off work. The incidence of kidney stones has risen with >8% of the United States population being affected. The economic weight is outstanding with annual estimates exceeding $5 billion (Matlaga 2014). Research is being done to increase the quality of life for kidney stone patients and minimize their chance for recurrence. Research has been conducted on calcium supplements for women and has supported that calcium supplements do not contribute to renal calculi formation. This increase is closely related to lifestyle and diet factors (Scales et al. 2012).

Incidence

The prevalence of stone disease has increased in every age group and gender. The incidence of stone disease peaks in the fourth to sixth decades and is rare before age 20. Males have been historically at a higher risk for developing stones than their female counterparts, but recent data suggest that the gender gap is narrowing (Scales et al. 2012). Risk factors for stone formation also include increasing age and Caucasian race.

Anatomy

There are patient-specific conditions that increase the risk for stone formation. This includes the presence of a solitary kidney. Renal stones are considered a metabolic upper tract obstruction, although in large enough size they lead to mechanical obstruction of the urinary tract.

Risk Factors

Different areas of the United States can put individuals at an increased risk, such as the "stone belt," which is located in the Southeastern states, followed by the East, Midwest, and the West. This is influenced, to some extent, by exposure to excessive heat or other conditions that promote dehydration, such as a specific work environment. Additional risk factors include metabolic disease, i.e., gout, RTA, malabsorption disease, and Crohn's disease; there is also an increased incidence of stone disease seen with increasing body size, type II diabetes, family history, and metabolic syndrome. Obesity is a risk factor for stone formation; an increase in BMI in both males and females increases the chances of forming stones. SCI, spina bifida, and nonambulatory patients are at risk for stone formation.

There are a number of factors that can be controlled; dietary factors are one of them. Limiting salt and protein, mainly red meat, can decrease the risk for kidney stones. Staying well hydrated is key in preventing stone disease; drinking 2.5–3 l/

day is optimal. Low urine volume is an independent risk factor for stone formation. Low or high urine pH and high urinary excretion of calcium, oxalate, or uric acid also influence stone formation (Table 8.1). Diabetic patients are more likely to have uric acid stones due to low urine volume and acidic urine.

Table 8.1 Factors that influence stone formation

Hypercalciuria	Urinary calcium excretion >4 mg/kg/day or >200 mg/day on a calcium- and sodium-restricted diet
	Increased risk of both stone disease and osteoporosis
	Can result from issues with calcium handling in the gastrointestinal tract, kidney, or bone
	Renal hypercalciuria results from reabsorption of calcium from the proximal and distal renal tubules; creates calcium loss in the urine, increased PTH secretion, and stimulation of synthesis of 1,25 di-hydroxy vitamin D which increases intestinal calcium absorption and bone resorption
	Commonly due to primary hyperparathyroidism
Hyperuricosuria	Urinary uric acid excretion >700 mg/day
	Urine pH <5.5
	Promotes calcium oxalate stone formation
	Excessive purine intake from animal protein, most common etiology
	More likely to be seen with chronic diarrhea, myeloproliferative disorders, gout
	Can be addressed by moderating sodium intake and a low-purine diet
Hyperoxaluria	Can be the result of excessive intake of oxalate-rich foods (nuts, chocolate, spinach, beets, liver, brewed tea) or vitamin C (ascorbic acid)
	Can be due to vitamin B6 deficiency
	80% of cases are due to primary hyperoxaluria, an autosomal recessive disorder
	Intestinal malabsorption leads to enteric hyperoxaluria (ulcerative colitis, Crohn's disease, celiac disease)
	Presentation includes low urine volume, low urinary pH, decreased urinary calcium, elevated sodium and citrate in the urine
	Treated with pyridoxine, low-oxalate diet, low-fat diet, increased fluid intake, calcium supplementation
Hypocitraturia	Urinary citrate excretion <320 mg/day
	Risk factor for one in ten stone formers; acidic urine increases citrate metabolism and reduces citrate excretion, such as that seen with renal tubular acidosis
	Can also be a factor in chronic diarrhea, due to bicarbonate loss
	Thiazide diuretics also induce hypo-anemia and intracellular acidosis
	Cause is usually idiopathic
	Treated with potassium citrate
Low urine pH	Urinary pH <5.5
	Calcium oxalate stones may form
	Primary factor leading to uric acid stones
Hypomagnesiuria	Magnesium inhibits calcium stone formation, as it binds oxalate
	Associated with low urinary hypocitraturia
	Can be treated with a magnesium supplement

(continued)

Table 8.1 (continued)

Cystinuria	Urinary cysteine <400 mg/day
	Autosomal recessive defect resulting in impaired renal reabsorption of four amino acids
	Elevated urinary cysteine
	Cystine stones form in acid urine and may result in staghorn stones
	Treated with increased hydration, low sodium diet, low methionine diet (decreases cysteine production; limited intake of meat, eggs, wheat, milk, cheese)
	Oral potassium citrate can be added to alkalize the urine
	Cystine stones can be resistant to ESWL and are often treated with dissolution therapy

Cystine stones can form in patients with an autosomal recessive trait leading to a defective renal and intestinal transport of amino acids. Struvite stones can form in alkaline urine environments, as a result of the urease enzyme secreted by some bacteria (*Proteus mirabilis*, *Klebsiella pneumoniae*, *Staphylococcus aureus*, and *Staphylococcus epidermidis*).

History

Patients presenting to a urology office with kidney stones can present with a plethora of signs and symptoms. A provider should complete a screening evaluation, including detailed medical and dietary history, lsab studies and urinalysis (American Urological Association 2020). The "typical" renal calculus patient can present with flank discomfort, and a patient with a ureteral calculus may present with sharp flank/abdominal pain and N/V. Many patients may have already been seen by their PCP for hematuria before presenting to a urology office; others may have made a visit to the ED and will bring results of labs and imaging with them to their appointment. A detailed history should aim to determine the presence of any risk factors for stone disease (Box 8.1). The location of the stone, i.e., the kidney or ureter, obstructive or nonobstructive, and the creatinine results will help determine whether the patient will need surgery or the stone can pass without surgery.

Physical Examination

Conducting a physical exam on a patient with a kidney stone is largely unremarkable. Palpating the CVA region may elicit a positive response. Assess for fever, as this may be a sign of a possible infection. The patient may find it difficult to find a comfortable position; this can be a sign of active renal colic.

Box 8.1 Risk Factors for Urolithiasis
Bowel disease/intestinal malabsorption Diabetes mellitus Type II

- Family history of stone disease or gout
- History of bowel surgery (resection, gastric bypass/bariatric surgery, ileal conduit)
- Hyperthyroidism, obesity, and osteoporosis
- Personal history of stone disease
- Stone-provoking medications/supplements
- Furosemide
- High-dose vitamin C
- High-dose vitamin D
- Probenecid
- Protease inhibitors
- Salicylates
- Triamterene

Diagnostic Testing

Laboratory Evaluation

Labs and imaging assist with verifying the diagnosis of renal calculus. CBC and comprehensive panel may reveal elevated WBCs and elevated creatinine, which could indicate an emergent situation. Additional lab tests include serum electrolytes (see Table 8.2). creatinine, calcium, and uric acid. Parathyroid hormone levels may be considered.

Urinalysis can also be helpful in this context and help rule out a simple urinary tract infection. Patients may experience gross hematuria where approximately 85% of all patients demonstrate at least microhematuria. Urinalysis will also provide additional clues to the type of stones based on crystals within the urine. Urine pH

Table 8.2 Metabolic work up

24 h urine:	Total urine volume, pH, calcium, oxalate, uric acid, citrate, sodium, potassium, creatinine
Serum labs:	Uric acid, calcium, sodium, potassium, phosphorus, parathyroid hormone, vitamin D
Food diary:	72 h recall diary of all items ingested during 24 h urine collection period
UA:	Urine pH
Stone analysis:	Stone sent for analysis
Imaging study:	To evaluate stone burden status

can also be a clue as to what type of stones may be present. Urine culture may be helpful in the case of suspected infection; patient is febrile on presentation or if there is concern for infection by a urease splitting organism.

If the patient has been able to screen the urine and capture the stone, the stone should be sent for analysis. This will help establish any underlying pathophysiologic cause for their stone disease.

Recurrent stone formation should also be evaluated with 24-h urine testing, which can help distinguish the potential causes for stone formation, which closely mirror the risk factors seen in Box 8.1, but include pathologic fractures, gout, young age at onset of stone disease, and recurrent calcium stone formation.

The 24-h urine collection should be evaluated for total volume, calcium, pH, uric acid, oxalate, citrate, potassium, sodium, and creatinine (American Urological Association 2020).

Imaging

Each patient suspected of having kidney stones has a baseline imaging study, in order to better quantify potential stone burden and estimate metabolic activity. Ninety percent of kidney stones are radiopaque and can be demonstrated on imaging studies. This may include a KUB (rapid screening test but can miss many stones), ultrasound, or CT renal stone. If the patient was seen in the emergency department, commonly, a noncontrast CT renal stone is ordered; this is the most accurate test to evaluate for the presence of urolithiasis and in detail the collecting system anatomy. A renal ultrasound can identify hydronephrosis or can be used with patients that cannot tolerate a CT scan (See Chap. 21).

A CT urogram or IVU can identify the presence of stone and suggest whether obstruction exists. The CT urogram is considerably more detailed than the IVU.

Providers must attempt to decrease radiation exposure to as low as reasonably achievable (Brisbane et al. 2016).

Management

Once imaging has established the existence of a renal/ureteral calculus, the decision to treat the stone with surgery or provide medication for MET (medical expulsive therapy) is contemplated. The decision for surgery or MET depends on the size and location of the stone and the surgeon and the patient agreeing with the plan. MET with tamsulosin hydrochloride is commonly prescribed in the ED for patients with ureteral calculus. Patients will need prompt intervention for complete or high-grade unilateral urinary obstruction, bilateral urinary obstruction, obstruction in a solitary kidney, obstruction in the context of infection or sepsis, obstruction with an elevated creatinine, inability to tolerate oral intake, or pain that is not controlled by oral medications.

In patients with obstructing calculi and suspected infection, the provider must quickly drain the collecting system with a ureteral stent or nephrostomy tube and postpone stone treatment (American Urological Association 2020).

If the patient is asymptomatic, and the stone is nonobstructing, the patient will be observed and encouraged increase fluid intake to promote passage of the stone, if the stone is less than 10 mm. Stones are more likely to pass when they are located in the distal ureter and are small. Approximately 60% of stones less than 5 mm will pass spontaneously, usually within 40 days of symptom onset.

In the absence of these conditions, a referral is completed for the patient to be seen urgently by a urology provider. During the patient's urology visit, surgery is arranged in case the ureteral calculus does not pass with MET. But prior to beginning any treatment, any urinary tract infection should be adequately treated. Tamsulosin hydrochloride can decrease BP, so it is imperative to tell the patient regarding this risk and to take the medication at night.

In the case of a pregnant patient with an obstructing or renal calculus, the provider must coordinate pharmacological and surgical intervention with an obstetrician. Observation should be offered to patients that have well-controlled symptoms. Ureteroscopy may be offered if patient has failed observation. A ureteral stent or nephrostomy tube are options and with frequent stent or tube changes (American Urological Association 2020).

Surgical Management

If passage of the stone is not possible, the patient should be scheduled for a ureteral stent or nephrostomy tube placement to relieve the obstruction and prevent kidney damage. Open removal is rarely indicated for renal stones. A ureteroscopy with laser and possible stent is scheduled within 2 weeks. The details of the surgery are communicated with the patient; it is an outpatient procedure and the patient will need a driver. The potential problems with a ureteral stent placement necessitate a brief discussion on the value of maintaining a patent ureter. Potential side effects include, pain, dysuria, and hematuria; these can be controlled with medication. Providers may omit a ureteral stent following a ureteroscopy if there is no suspect of ureteric injury, no evidence of ureteral stricture or impediment anatomically of calculi clearance, and no plans of a secondary procedure (American Urological Association 2020).

For stones approximately 1 cm, outside of the lower pole and proximal calculus, shockwave lithotripsy (SWL) is the procedure of choice. Providers need to educate patients that SWL is the option with lowest morbidity and least complication rate, although ureteroscopy has the highest stone-free rate in a single procedure (American Urological Association 2020). This surgery is quite successful, with a rate of 74–90%. This surgery is also outpatient, and requires a driver, as the patient receives sedation. The patient must pass the fragments; tamsulosin hydrochloride is prescribed postoperatively to facilitate passage of stone debris. *Steinstrasse* describes obstructing stone fragments in the ureter following shock wave lithotripsy (SWL) and correlates with increased stone burden. It is seen in up to 10% of patients undergoing SWL (Matlaga and Lingeman 2010). Routine ureteral stenting should not be completed in patients undergoing SWL (American Urological Association 2020).

Percutaneous nephrolithotomy (PCNL) is recommended for patients with large lower pole renal calculi, staghorn calculi, or struvite calculi. The patient will have a general anesthetic and an overnight stay in the hospital. As with all surgeries, updated labs and additional testing may be ordered, i.e., CXR and EKG. Other treatment options that have been increasing in usage include dusting, and pop-dusting. The advantages of dusting seem to be reduced operative time, ureteral access sheath usage, fragment retrieval and less complications with basketing calculi. The high-power, high-frequency, long-pulse laser permits for dusting and pop-dusting, creating dust which can pass spontaneously. While studies have proven to be useful for small to medium calculi, the effectiveness of dusting and pop-dusting for large size calculi still remains unclear (Pietropaolo et al. 2018). Providers should order a non-contrast CT scan on patients before undergoing a PCNL (American Urological Association 2020).

Postoperative Surgical Management

Postoperatively, instructions are reviewed during the initial clinic visit, and handouts are provided. Instructions that are provided during the initial visit and reviewed may decrease the number of post-op phone calls. Medications that control pain, bladder spasms, and those that expedite stone passage need to be prescribed prior to discharge. Experienced urology phone triages RNs are crucial to the successful management of postoperative kidney stone patients.

Patients need education about their postoperative course, which includes the expectation of hematuria and that small clots are to be expected, pain/discomfort if a stent is left in the ureter, and diet instruction short-term, especially to increase fluid intake to promote passage of stone fragments. Specific instructions are tailored to the individual and are based on both the procedure and stone burden.

Postoperative return visits commonly happen 4 weeks after surgery. It is during this visit that the provider can examine the patient's need for metabolic evaluation. Every patient needs to be reminded that drinking 2.5–3 l/day and adhering to low salt/protein diet will now be a principal part of their everyday life. A modest calcium diet, 800–1200 mg daily is also recommended.

Long-Term Management

Pharmacologic therapies	Side effects indications
Thiazide diuretics (hydrochlorothiazide)	Dizziness, blurred vision, high or relatively high itching, stomach upset, urine calcium constipation, thirst recurrent calcium stone

Pharmacologic therapies	Side effects indications
Potassium citrate (Urocit-K)	Joint pain, stiffness, recurrent calcium skin rash, upset stomach, stones, low or nausea, diarrhea, drowsiness, relatively low changes in liver function test urinary citrate
Allopurinal (Zyloprim)	Abdominal discomfort, recurrent diarrhea, nausea/vomiting with confusion, anxiety, hyperuricosuria and irregular heart beat, abnormal urinary calcium

There is a lack of high-quality data that evaluates the utility of diet or pharmacologic therapy within the context of stone disease. However, patients are encouraged to maintain a high fluid intake. Providers should educate all stone patients that a fluid intake volume should be enough to produce a urine volume of 2.5 l or more every day (American Urological Association 2020). Patients at increased risk for forming additional renal calculi should be encouraged to complete a metabolic evaluation. Patient will feel empowered if they can assist with controlling their renal calculi disease. Serum labs include PTH, uric acid, phosphorus, Vitamin D, and a basic chemistry panel. Outside labs can arrange for a 24-h urine kit to be mailed to the patient's home. Twenty-four-hour urine results can assist with controlling stone disease through diet modifications and/or medications. Repeat 24-h urine may be suggested to assess changes that were implemented. Hard to control renal calculi patients are referred to nephrology. Some nephrology departments have an Registerd Dietician who can assist the patient with portion size and how to read labels.

Patients with recurrent renal calculi are seen every 6 months or every year with appropriate imaging, i.e., KUB, ultrasound, or CT renal stone (See Chap. 21). During this visit, a urinalysis can be completed, and a review of his medications can be assessed for compliance. Providers should order serum labs to evaluate for adverse effects in patients on pharmacological therapy (American Urological Association 2020). The frequency of follow-up can also be tailored to the frequency of stone formation.

NPs in rural areas may not have pamphlets and teaching materials to provide for their patients. AUA and SUNA provide specific information and guidelines regarding urology problems. Patient handouts can be extremely beneficial for patients; they are available in other languages. They can serve as a reminder to patients regarding diets and recommendations. Patients must recognize that recommendations for one individual may not pertain to them; they should listen to the suggestions of their provider.

Clinical Pearls
- Greater than 60% of stones less than 5 mm will pass spontaneously, usually within 40 days of symptom onset.
- Providers should be mindful of potential effects of ionizing radiation in patients undergoing repeated CT imaging, such as recurrent stone formers.

- Evaluation:
  - Obtain PTH level as part of screening evaluation if hyperparathyroidism is suspected.
  - Metabolic testing of one or two 24-h urine collections should be performed in the high risk, recurrent stone former, patients with a solitary kidney, young patients who present with bilateral renal calculi and family history, or interested first-time stone formers.
  - Nephrology can be beneficial, if available, for patients whose stone disease can be challenging to manage.
- Diet:
  - 72 h food diary should be kept during time of 24 h urine collection period for evaluation.
  - Fluid intake should be increased to 2.5 l a day.
  - Limit sodium intake.
  - Calcium stone formers should consume 1000–1200 mg/day of dietary calcium. It is okay for female patients to continue with their calcium supplements, as evidence-based articles have proven that calcium supplements do no play a role in forming renal calculi.
  - Calcium oxalate stone formers with high urinary oxalate intake should limit intake of oxalate-rich foods.
  - Low urinary citrate patients increase fruits and vegetables while decreasing nondairy animal protein.
  - High urinary uric acid should limit intake of nondairy animal protein.
  - Cystine stone patients should limit sodium and protein intake.
  - Obesity is linked to increase stone disease; advise patients on weight reduction.
  - Research into the link between sugar intake and renal calculi is being investigated.
- Follow-up:
  - 24-h urine specimen should be obtained 6 months after beginning a new treatment.
  - Yearly 24-h urine specimen can be considered for surveillance.
  - Periodic blood testing is recommended for those on pharmacologic therapy.
  - Recheck stone analysis to ensure appropriate treatment is being given or for patients who continue to form stones with treatment.
  - Sources of infection should be prevented in patients with struvite stones.
  - Imaging can be obtained occasionally for assessment and discovery of stones in the form of low-dose CT, plain abdominal imaging, or renal ultrasound.

Resources for the Nurse Practitioner

European Association of Urology 2014, Guidelines on Urolithiasis. http://uroweb.org/wp-content/uploads/22-Urolithiasis_LR.pdf

AUA Guidelines: Medical Management of Kidney Stones, 2014 http://www.auanet.org/education/guidelines/management-kidney-stones.cfm

National Institute of Diabetes and Digestive and Kidney Diseases (NIDDK)
www.niddk.nih.gov
National Kidney Foundation: www.nkfm.org

Resources for the Patient

National Institute of Diabetes and Digestive and Kidney Diseases (NIDDK) Diet for kidney stone prevention: http://www.niddk.nih.gov/health-information/health-top-ics/urologic-disease/diet-for-kidney-stone-prevention
www.urologyhealth.org
www.kidney.org
www.auanet.org/education
www.nkfm.org

References

American Urological Association (2020). https://www.auanet.org/
Brisbane W, Bailey MR, Sorensen MD (2016) An overview of kidney stone imaging techniques. Nat Rev Urol 13(11):654–662. https://doi.org/10.1038/nrurol.2016.154
Matlaga B (2014) Economic impact of urinary stones. Transl Androl Urol 3(3):278–283. https://doi.org/10.3978/j.issn.2223-4683.2014.01.02
Matlaga BR, Lingeman JE (2010) Chapter 48. Surgical management of upper urinary tract calculi. In: Wein AJ, Kavoussi LR, Novick AC, Partin AW, Peters CA (eds) Campbell-Walsh urology, vol 2, 10th edn. WB Saunders Elsevier, Philadelphia
Pietropaolo AK, Jones PK, Whitehurst LK, Somani BK (2018) Role of 'dusting and pop-dusting' using a high-powered (100 W) laser machine in the treatment of large stones (≥ 15 mm): prospective outcomes over 16 months. Urolithiasis 47(4):391–394. https://doi.org/10.1007/s00240-018-1076-4
Scales CD, Smith AC, Hanley JM, Saigal CS, Urologic Diseases in America Project (2012) Prevalence of kidney stones in the United States. Eur Urol 62(1):160–165

Idiopathic and Traumatic Male Urethral Strictures

9

Yooni Yi, Silvia S. Maxwell, and Richard A. Santucci

Contents

Abbreviations

DVIU	Direct vision internal urethrotomy
PFUDD	Pelvic fracture urethral distraction defect
PVR	Post-void residual
RUG	Retrograde urethrogram
VCUG	Voiding cystourethrogram

Y. Yi (✉)
Department of Urology/Michigan Medicine, University of Michigan, Ann Arbor, MI, USA
e-mail: yooniy@med.umich.edu

S. S. Maxwell
Department of Urology, Detroit Medical Center, Detroit, MI, USA

R. A. Santucci
Crane Center for Transgender Surgery, Austin, TX, USA

© Springer Nature Switzerland AG 2020
S. A. Quallich, M. J. Lajiness (eds.), *The Nurse Practitioner in Urology*,
https://doi.org/10.1007/978-3-030-45267-4_9

Objectives

1. Define stricture disease and discuss its incidence in the US
2. Review signs and symptoms that should raise concern for stricture disease
3. Provide an overview of surgical corrections and postopertaive care.

Overview

Incidence

Urethral stricture is defined as a narrowing of the urethra, which obstructs the flow of urine from the bladder to the urethral meatus as a result of fibrotic tissue. Scar tissue formation from traumatic injury, instrumentation, congenital malformations, malignancy, or infection can cause a narrowing of the urethral lumen. Although the actual incidence is unknown, urethral stricture disease represents a significant economic burden on the healthcare system. The economic burden of urethral stricture in the United States was last evaluated for the year 2000. The annual costs exceeded over $200 million and resulted in over 1.5 million office visits (Barbagli et al. 2014). Urethral strictures result in an extensive amount of office visits and procedures than some other common urologic problems.

True urethral stricture disease is considered to be a rare entity in females with reported estimates of prevalence to be 3–8%. Historically, treatment for female urethral strictures have included urethral dilations and self-catheterizations. However more recently, there is a trend towards treatment with a formal urethroplasty in reconstructive centers, but there is still a paucity of evidence available on long-term outcomes (Hampson et al. 2019). Given the rare incidence, this chapter will focus on male urethral stricture disease.

Anatomy

The urethra is about 20–25 cm in length and extends from the bladder neck to the urethral meatus (Brandes and Morey 2014).

The urethra can be broken down into different sections:

1. Fossa Navicularis: section of urethra located within the glans penis
2. Penile Urethra: section of urethra proximal to the fossa navicularis and distal to the bulbar urethra
3. Bulbar Urethra: section of urethra invested by the bulbospongiosus muscle; becomes larger in this segment
4. Membranous Urethra: section of urethra surrounded by the external urinary sphincter
5. Prostatic Urethra: section of urethra surrounded by the prostatic stroma
6. Bladder Neck: section of urethra surrounded by bladder neck musculature (McCammon et al. 2016)

Another way of describing the urethra is by distinguishing the anterior urethra vs. the posterior urethra. The anterior urethra consists of the bulbar urethra, penile urethra, and fossa navicularis. The posterior urethra consists of the bladder neck, prostatic urethra, and membranous urethra. When referring to a narrowing in the posterior urethra, these will often be indicated as a stenosis or contracture (Wessells et al. 2017).

Etiology

Most acquired urethral strictures are due to trauma, iatrogenic injury, or infectious processes, although truly the etiology of strictures (not including Pelvic Fracture Urethral Distraction Defects—PFUDD) is perhaps unimportant. The symptoms and treatments are usually the same no matter the cause (Santucci et al. 2007). In at least 50% of patients with stricture, the cause of the stricture is completely unknown.

Iatrogenic causes accounted for over 45% of all urethral strictures. Instrumentation from previous transurethral procedures such as a TURP, removal of kidney stones, previous urethral dilations, and traumatic urethral catheterization can cause urethral injury resulting in stricture. Most idiopathic and inflammatory urethral strictures occur in the bulbar urethra for reasons that are not known (Siegel et al. 2014).

Urethral catheterization is one of the most commonly performed procedures by healthcare providers. It may be an important cause of urethral stricture, especially when a Foley catheter balloon is inadvertently inflated in the bulbar urethra. Some researchers believe that prolonged catheterization can cause inflammation and urethral ischemia, which eventually leads to urethral stricture (Lumen et al. 2009).

Other causes of urethral stricture include:

- Gonococcal urethritis, or *Chlamydia,* may cause scarring, which results in a stricture formation, possibly years after the original infection. Post-inflammatory urethritis continues to be a common cause of urethral strictures in developing countries (Lumen et al. 2009).
- Lichen sclerosis (LS) is an inflammatory skin condition which can cause extensive genitourinary scarring. Strictures related to LS not only have a higher degree of treatment-related complications but also disease recurrence (Liu et al. 2014). Strictures secondary to LS will often affect the urethral meatus and fossa navicularis but can extend further into the urethra (McCammon et al. 2016).

Radiation damage can also be an important cause of strictures.

There is a special category of urethral obstruction, which is often referred to as a "stricture" but in fact results from complete distraction/tear of the urethra usually due to severe pelvic fracture trauma. Modern nomenclature refers to these as

PFUDDs. Pelvic trauma due to "straddle" injuries or pelvic fractures due to high-energy trauma such as motor vehicle accidents may partially or completely sever the posterior, membranous, or bulbar urethra.

Symptoms

Depending on severity of the stricture, patients may be completely asymptomatic or suffer extreme pain due to bladder distention or hydronephrosis. Most common symptoms include:

- Decreased force of stream
- Spraying with urination
- Urinary retention
- Urinary frequency
- Nocturia
- Recurrent urinary tract infections
- Dribbling
- Intermittency
- Bladder stones
- Straining to urinate
- Decreased force of ejaculation
- Dysuria

The history should also document the patient's preoperative erectile function and urinary continence.

Physical Exam

A physical exam may show the following:

- Decreased urinary stream
- Discharge from the urethra
- Enlarged or palpable bladder
- Enlarged or tender prostate
- Hardness on the under surface of the penis from a scarred urethra
- Redness or swelling of the penis

Often, the exam reveals no abnormalities.

If a procedure is indicated, it will be important to assess the lower extremity mobility for operative positioning especially in patients who have had a PFUDD.

Fig. 9.1 Uroflow pattern of patient with urethral stricture

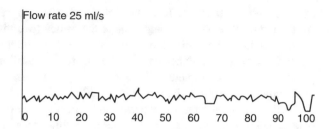

Flow rate 25 ml/s

0   10   20   30   40   50   60   70   80   90   100

Diagnostic Testing

- Uroflow: Generally, patients with severe stricture will have a decreased flow rate <10 ml/s. Instead of a bell-shaped curve, the flow pattern will be flat (Mundy 2006) (Fig. 9.1). http://www.medindia.net/articles/manual-urodynamics.asp
- Post-void residual (PVR): To determine if patient is retaining urine. The correct PVR varies from patient to patient and arbitrary limits for concern are PVRs >200 cc. Some patients with large, floppy, distended bladders from longstanding urethral stricture may have a large bladder capacity >1200 cc but are able to void large volumes >700 cc and leave large PVRs >400 cc without symptoms or problems.
- The existence of a stricture can be quickly determined by gently placing an 18 F urethral catheter. If the catheter passes into the bladder, significant stricture is not present. Cystoscopy can be used to determine the presence of stricture but does not indicate length. The definitive test for urethral stricture is the retrograde urethrogram (RUG), which will indicate length, location, and severity of any strictures present. Retrograde urethrogram is considered the gold standard for accurately diagnosing the true extent and location of the urethral stricture. A RUG is a study utilizing contrast and fluoroscopy. The patient is in the supine position with a modified positioning to capture the entire urethra as it traverses under the pubic symphysis and into the bladder. A RUG can often be paired with a VCUG to evaluate the proximal and distal anatomy more clearly.
- Renal/bladder ultrasound may show thickening of the bladder wall or hydronephrosis due to outflow obstruction but is not diagnostic for stricture. Some experts use urethral ultrasonography to determine the length and location of urethral strictures.

Management

Urethral strictures are an anatomical anomaly. There is no suitable medical treatment for this condition.

For centuries, urethral dilation and urethrotomy have been used to treat urethral strictures. Both of these procedures have been found to be effective mostly in the short term. The stricture recurrence rate after a single dilation is 88% and after an initial DVIU is about 50%. Only very short strictures ≤1.5 cm can expect cure from either procedure (Mundy 2006). Urethral dilations are a common procedure for treating urethral strictures. It can be performed using progressively larger dilators to stretch the urethral stricture and enlarge the lumen (Mundy 2006). Other forms of dilation include the utilization of a balloon dilator under direct visualization or under fluoroscopic guidance over a wire. A urethral dilation can be useful in emergency situations (complete urinary retention), but carries a high recurrence rate especially in recurrent strictures (Mundy 2006).

DVIU is another commonly performed procedure for the treatment of strictures. It is utilized to open the strictured area by cutting through the scar tissue without creating additional scarring. After the contracture is released, the urethral lumen is enlarged. A catheter is left in place for at least 3 days until healed. Some practitioners leave a Foley catheter longer than 3 days. There is no evidence that placement of a 16 F Foley for greater than 72 hours after DVIU is superior.

Unfortunately, repeat DVIU/dilation or DVIU/dilation on longer strictures has a very poor success rate, and in these cases, curative urethroplasty must always be considered. Recent research has shown that the initial success rate of DVIU may be as low as 8%. Repeated procedures eventually fail 100% of the time. Furthermore, it has been hypothesized that repeated treatments may actually contribute to increased scar formation, creating longer, more dense stricture (Santuccie and Eisenberg 2010). According to Anger et al. (2011), "repeat urethrotomy or dilation for urethral stricture is neither curative nor cost effective in the long term" (see Tables 9.1 and 9.2).

Some patients who are unable or unwilling to undergo urethroplasty procedures may choose to perform intermittent self-catheterizations in an attempt to keep the urethral lumen open. Unfortunately, the strictures will always recur once patients stop self-catheterizing (Broghammer et al. 2014). Patients generally find intermittent self-catheterizations painful, cumbersome, and difficult.

Another option for the management of a urethral stricture is the placement of a suprapubic cystostomy. This provides a safe means of urinary drainage. In addition,

Table 9.1 Complications from stricture disease

Short term (moderate)	Long term (rare)
LUTS	Acute urinary retention
Recurrent UTI	Renal failure
Need for repeat procedures	Urethral carcinoma
	Fournier's gangrene
	Bladder failure

Table 9.2 Postoperative complications of urethrotomy

Complication	Rate
Bleeding	4–6%
Infection	8–9%
Incontinence	1%
Impotence	1%
Failure after repeat procedure	Up to 100%

Adapted from Santucci et al. (2007)

a suprapubic cystostomy can be utilized to provide "urethral rest" prior to the evaluation of the stricture to ensure that the full extent of the stricture develops.

Beyond urethral dilation, DVIU, and intermittent self-catheterization, a patient may consider a formal urethroplasty. A urethroplasty should be considered in patients with a stricture in the penile urethra, a recurrent urethral stricture, or a long segment stricture (>2 cm). There are a variety of techniques for a urethroplasty that may or may not require tissue transfer.

Some of the major categories include:

– Anastomotic urethroplasty
– Buccal mucosal graft Urethroplasty
– Johanson urethroplasty (Staged approach)
– Fasciocutaneous flap urethroplasty
– Heineke-Milkuwicz

An anastomotic repair involves the complete excision of the fibrotic urethral stricture and joining the two healthy ends together. This technique is used for short <2 cm bulbar urethral strictures or PFUDD. This procedure has a 90% success rate for inflammatory/idiopathic stricture and a slightly lower success rate for PFUDD. Anastomotic repair is deservedly popular, although recent data suggests that even in expert hands, it can be associated with unacceptable sexual complications such as chordee (ventral bend in the penis), erectile dysfunction, and poor glans blood flow (Barbagli et al. 2007).

Buccal urethroplasty can be used anywhere in the urethra and is the treatment of choice for longer strictures >2 cm. Although non-hair-bearing tissue from the post-auricular, penile shaft or foreskin has been used, buccal mucosa is the preferred graft material today. This tissue is resistant to infection and trauma, "takes" well after placement, and is rich in elastin which decreases contraction of the graft. After incising the stricture (either ventrally—that is, the surface of the urethra closest to the skin, or dorsally—the surface of the urethral closer to the penis), the graft is then sutured to the edge of the urethra mucosa, creating a larger urethral lumen. This procedure has a variable reported success rate, generally accepted to be about 90% (Santucci et al. 2007). A newer modification of this procedure, using a dorsal buccal graft has been described for even very long strictures, and it has a good success rate of 80% despite being used against the worst and longest strictures (Santuccie and Eisenberg 2010).

The Johanson urethroplasty has been generally utilized for penile urethral strictures that are sequelae of a childhood repair of hypospadias. In hypospadias, the urethra is not formed properly, and the urethral meatus ends on the penile shaft, scrotum, or perineum. Given this abnormal development, there is aberrancy in the blood supply and often times a scarred environment requiring a staged procedure. The Johanson urethroplasty can also be used for patients who have failed several other repairs and have extensively damaged urethral tissue. The first stage involves the incising of the scar tissue and converting the tubular urethra into a flat "urethral plate" which is then sewn to the surrounding skin. Buccal grafts may be sewn into the urethral plate to enlarge it and make the second stage tubularization of the plate more successful. The second stage involves the tubularization of the urethral plate, restoring the patient to a normal urethral appearance. This is done after all healing is complete and all postoperative inflammation is resolved, usually 5–6 months after the first stage (Zimmerman and Santucci 2011).

While the Johanson urethroplasty is used to cure urethral stricture, some patients elect not to have a second stage procedure, as the first stage generally allows unobstructed urination. This may require sitting to void forever. In some patients such as the extreme elderly, unwell, or unwilling to undergo urethroplasty, a form of the Johanson urethroplasty called a perineal urethrostomy may be performed. With the perineal urethrostomy, the patient is able to void without difficulty in a sitting position. Patients who undergo a perineal urethrostomy have a reported high quality of life (Peterson et al. 2004; Barbagli et al. 2009).

Fasciocutaneous urethroplasty, a reliable but technically demanding form of urethroplasty, uses a penile skin fasciocutaneous (skin plus underlying tissue) flap to enlarge the urethra. The foreksin can also be utilized in this case. This technique is generally used for long, penile strictures but appears to have higher perioperative complication rates than other techniques. The high success rates and technical simplicity of the buccal urethroplasty has caused the buccal technique to largely replace the fasciocutaneous technique (Zimmerman and Santucci 2011).

PFUDD was introduced as a special case of urethral obstruction, which is not truly a "stricture" or narrowing of the urethra but generally a torn urethra with a wall of scar formed in between the torn ends. The major treatment of this is an anastomotic urethroplasty where the wall of scar is cut out and the two ends are sewn together. This procedure is technically demanding and may require transfer to a center of excellence for urethroplasty (Burks and Santucci 2010).

Postoperative Care

See details of immediate postoperative management in Box 9.1.

Box 9.1 Postoperative Management for Urethral Stricture
Patient Teaching
Pain/Swelling
- Avoid sitting directly on perineal area. Sitting at a 45° angle in a reclining chair is best.
- To decrease the pain and swelling, place an ice pack on the surgical area (between your legs) intermittently for 24 hours. Leave the ice pack in place for 20 or 30 min every 2 hours (a bag of frozen peas works well and can be refrozen between uses).

- When sitting or lying down, place a rolled-up hand towel under the scrotum. Elevating the scrotum also helps decrease the pain and swelling.
- If graft is taken from cheek, you may need to apply an ice bag to your face intermittently in the first 24 hours.
- If a buccal mucosal graft is harvested, the patient should utilize the mouthwash provided as needed for pain.
- No sexual intercourse for 6 weeks after surgery.

Hygiene
  - The dressings and jock strap may be removed after 24–48 hours. If they get soaked or very dirty, they may be removed early. No further dressings are needed.
  - Once dressings are removed, the patient may shower and let the water run over the incision. The patient should try to keep the area clean and dry.
  - No soaking in tub or pool for 6 weeks.

The postoperative follow-up time may vary by surgeon. The follow-up can range from 1–3 weeks with a postoperative RUG or VCUG to assess for urine leaks. If no extravasation of fluid is suspected, the Foley catheter may be removed. If extravasation is seen, the Foley catheter is reinserted and left in place for another week (Hosam et al. 2005).

Long-term management may also vary by the surgeon, but may include uroflow, PVR, symptom check, cystoscopy, or RUG more regularly within the first year and as needed beyond a year.

Clinical Pearls

- Reassure patient some bruising and swelling is normal after surgery
- Give patient "emergency" contact information to use when office is closed
- Reinforce all pre-op/post-op teaching regarding catheter and use of overnight and daytime drainage bags
- Normal activity is allowed, but no heavy lifting/strenuous activity until surgical site is healed

Intermittent Self Catheterization
- Teach patient to use correct dilation technique with 14 Fr. or 16 Fr. Catheter. This will keep the urethra open
- Lubricate catheter well
- Allow patient to choose catheter type
- Give patient samples of different styles of catheters: Lubricated, Silicone, Latex, Coude
- Assist patient with ordering needed supplies

Resources for the Nurse Practitioner and Physician Assistants

Litwin MS, Saigal CS, editors. Urologic Diseases in America. Society of Urologic Nurses and Associates www.suna.org. McAninch JW, Lue TF, editors. General Urology. American Urology Association www.auanet.org

Resources for the Patient

Urology Care Foundation: The official foundation of the American Urological Association www.urologyhealth.org

References

Anger JT, Buckley JC, Santucci RA, Elliott SP, Salgal CS (2011) Trends in stricture management among male Medicare beneficiaries: underuse of urethroplasty? Urology 77(2):481–485

Barbagli G, De Angelis M, Romano G, Lazzeri M (2007) Long-term follow up of bulbar end-to-end anastomosis: a retrospective analysis of 153 patients in a single center experience. J Urol 178(6):2470–2473. Epub 2007 Oct 15

Barbagli G, De Angelis M, Romano G, Lazzeri M (2009) Clincial outcome and quality of life assessment in patients treated with perineal urethrostomy for anterior urethral stricture disease. J Urol 182(2):548–557

Barbagli G, Kulkarni S, Fossati N, Larcher A, Sansalone S, Guzzoni G, Lasseri M (2014) Longterm followup and deterioration rate of anterior substitution urethroplasty. J Urol 192:808–813

Brandes SB, Morey AF (2014) Advanced male urethral and genital reconstructive surgery, 2nd edn. Humana Press, New York

Broghammer JA, Santucci RA, Schwartz BF (2014) Urethral strictures in males treatment & management. Medscape.com. Accessed 14 Oct 2014

Burks FN, Santucci RA (2010) Complicated urethroplasty: a guide for surgeons. Nat Rev Urol 7:521–528

Hampson LA, Myers JB, Vanni AJ, Virasoro R, Smith TG III, Capiel L, Chandrapal J, Voelzke BB (2019) Dorsal buccal graft urethroplasty in female urethral stricture disease: a multi-center experience. Transl Androl Urol 8(Suppl 1):S6–S12

Hosam HSQ, Cavalcanti A, Santucci RA (2005) Early catheter removal after anterior anastomotic (3 days) and ventral buccal mucosal only (7 days) urethroplasty. Int Braz J Urol 31(5):459–464

Liu JS, Walker K, Stein D, Prabhu S, Hofer MD, Han J, Yang XJ, Gonzalez CM (2014) Lichen sclerosus and isolated bulbar urethral stricture disease. J Urol 192:775–779

Lumen N, Hoebeke P, Williamsen P, De Troyer B, Pieters R, Oosterlinck W (2009) Etiology of urethral stricture disease in the 21st century. J Urol 182:983–987

McCammon KA, Zuckerman JM, Jordan GH (2016) Campbell-Walsh urology. Surgery of the penis and urethra, 11th edn. Elsevier, Philadelphia, PA

Mundy AR (2006) Management of urethral strictures. J Postgrad Med 82:489–493

Peterson AC, Palminteri E, Lazzeri M, Guanzoni G, Barbagli G, Webster GD (2004) Heroic measures may not always be justified in extensive urethral stricture due to lichen sclerosus. Urology 64(3):565–568

Santucci R, Geoffry J, Wise M (2007) Male urethral stricture disease. J Urol 177:1667–1674

Santuccie R, Eisenberg L (2010) Urethrotomy has a much lower success rate than previously reported. J Urol 183(5):1859–1862

Siegel J, Tausch TJ, Simhan J, Morey AF (2014) Innovative approaches for complex penile urethral strictures. Transl Androl Urol 3(2):179–185

Wessells H, Angermeier KW, Ellioo SP, Gonzalez CM, Kodama RT, Peterson AC, Reston J,
Rourke K, Stoffel JT, Vanni A, Voelzke B, Zhao L, Santucci RA (2017) Male urethral stricture:
AUA guideline. J Urol 197(1):182–190

Zimmerman WB, Santucci RA (2011) Buccal mucosa urethroplasty for adult urethral strictures.
Indian J Urol 3:364–370

Genitourinary Trauma

10

Anna Faris and Yooni Yi

Contents

A. Faris
Department of Urology, University of Michigan, Ann Arbor, MI, USA

Y. Yi (✉)
Department of Urology/Michigan Medicine, University of Michigan, Ann Arbor, MI, USA
e-mail: yooniy@med.umich.edu

© Springer Nature Switzerland AG 2020
S. A. Quallich, M. J. Lajiness (eds.), *The Nurse Practitioner in Urology*,
https://doi.org/10.1007/978-3-030-45267-4_10

Objectives
1. Highlight categories of genitourinary trauma—including kidney, ureter, bladder, urethra, and external genitalia
2. Review the methods of diagnosis and goals of repair.
3. Identify potential complications after trauma management.
4. Discuss priorities for patient follow-up.

General Principles

As with trauma of any anatomical system, individuals with injuries to the genitourinary tract must first be triaged and evaluated following the Advanced Trauma Life Support (ATLS) guidelines. A primary survey should follow the "ABCDE" protocol—airway maintenance, breathing and ventilation, circulation and assessment for bleeding, disability and neurological evaluation, and exposure to scan for further injuries (Galvagno et al. 2019). Once the primary survey is completed, a surgeon's decision-making process may be largely dependent on a patient's hemodynamic instability. For example, an individual with unstable blood pressure may not be appropriate to undergo a computerized tomography (CT) scan and instead may have to be expedited to the operating room. In addition, a clinician should always consider the mechanism of injury from the trauma as this may increase suspicion of certain types of injuries, though initially not suspected.

Renal Trauma

Overview

Incidence

The incidence of renal injury in all trauma patients is around 0.3% (Hotaling et al. 2012). Despite the relatively well protected position of the kidneys, they are the most commonly injured genitourinary (GU) organ in trauma—present in 24% of abdominal trauma cases compared to a total of 14% for the remaining GU organs (Smith et al. 2005). Patients with renal trauma are predominantly young males, with blunt trauma encompassing approximately twice as many renal injuries as penetrating trauma. The most common blunt injury mechanisms in select studied populations are motor vehicle accidents (63%), followed by patient falls (43%), and sports injury (11%). Penetrating mechanisms mainly consist of gun-shot wounds (65%) and stab wounds (35%) (Voelzke and Leddy 2014).

Evidence-based trends are driving the field of genitourinary (GU) trauma towards more conservative management. Large population studies have revealed that at high volume Level I trauma centers, conservative treatment had better outcomes with fewer nephrectomies (Hotaling et al. 2012). Thus, care providers in the outpatient setting may be more likely to see patients for follow-up after renal trauma who were managed nonoperatively.

Table 10.1 Revised injury staging classification

Grade of injury	Renal system component	Injury characterization
I	Parenchyma	Subcapsular hematoma and/or contusion
	Collecting system	No injury
II	Parenchyma	Laceration <1 cm in depth and into the cortex, small hematoma contained within Gerota's fascia
	Collecting system	No injury
III	Parenchyma	Laceration >1 cm in depth and into the medulla, small hematoma contained within Gerota's fascia
	Collecting system	No injury
IV	Parenchyma	Laceration through parenchyma and into the renal collecting system. Vascular segmental vein or artery injury
	Collecting system	Laceration, one or more into the collecting system with urinary extravasation. Renal pelvic laceration and/or complete ureteral pelvic disruption
V	Vascular	Main renal artery or vein laceration or avulsion, main renal artery or vein thrombosis

Adapted from Buckley JC, McAninch JW. Revision of current American association for the surgery of trauma renal injury grading system. *J Trauma - Inj Infect Crit Care*. 2011;70(1):35–37

The traditional grading system of renal injury severity is determined radiographically and is linked to patient outcomes and treatment recommendations. Many practitioners follow an updated classification system to that of the original AAST Organ Injury Severity Score created in 1989 aimed at delineating a more detailed classification system (Table 10.1) (Buckley and McAninch 2011). Patients can have features of multiple grades; however, ultimate classification is simplified to the highest grade features.

Pertinent Anatomy and Physiology

The kidneys typically reside on either side of the spine in the retroperitoneum. Posteriorly and superiorly they are protected by the ribs; however, the inferior portions are typically backed by paraspinal musculature. Anatomic differences between the right and left kidneys include proximity to the great vessels—the left kidney is closer to the aorta positioned and the right kidney is closer to the vena cava. The right kidney borders the duodenum, the right colonic flexure, and lies beneath the liver. The left kidney may overlap with the tail of the pancreas, the left colonic flexure, and lies below the spleen (Elkoushy and Andonian 2016).

History/Common Presentation

Renal injury should be considered in any patient with a rapid decelerating impact, trauma to the back, or penetrating injuries that involve the abdomen, flank, or lower chest. The trajectory of penetrating wounds such as bullets should also be considered (Morey et al. 2014).

Physical Exam

The medical provider should survey for such warning as:

- Hematuria (gross or microscopic)
- Contusions or lacerations on the flank or upper abdomen
- Flank pain or costovertebral angle (CVA) tenderness
- Swelling of the abdomen (retroperitoneal bleeding)
- Assess integrity of the ribs as their fracture can correlate with renal injuries

Diagnostic Tests

Laboratory Evaluation

Urinalysis—Microscopic hematuria can be indicative of renal injury in trauma patients, along with any distal anatomical injury from the ureter to the urethra. Microscopic hematuria or gross hematuria merits further investigation.

Imaging Studies

The CT urogram is the most commonly used imaging technique to evaluate the GU system after trauma. This entails injection of intravenous contrast and multiple stages of imaging. The early arterial phase can evaluate the integrity of the renal parenchyma and its vascular supply, while a "delayed" imaging phase represents the excretory stage in which the contrast transitions into the collecting system. It is within this phase that complications such as injuries to the renal pelvis or ureters are best revealed. A CT urogram is recommended in any hemodynamically stable patient with concerns for urogenital trauma (Morey et al. 2014). Imaging should then be referenced to either the AAST injury severity scale or its revised version as referenced above.

Scanning techniques such as a CT angiography target image acquisition to the late arterial contrast phase or early venous filling phase. This is useful if the kidney is not well visualized on initial scans as it can better characterize renal artery thromboses or avulsion injuries. However, such scans are time-consuming and may not be appropriate for hemodynamically unstable patients. Angiography is also used in real time during procedures such as angioembolization to control early or late bleeding of the renal vasculature (Hotaling et al. 2011).

Intravenous pyelography (IVP) is not used as commonly as a CT scan, as it has lower sensitivity detecting kidney and ureteral injuries. However, for patients that are unable to have a preoperative CT scan, IVP can be performed by injecting intravenous contrast and taking delayed X-ray films to assess renal excretion. This has great utility in critical situations to confirm presence and basic functionality of the contralateral kidney (Morey et al. 2014).

Management

Nonsurgical Management

Nonoperative management is appropriate for individuals with low-grade blunt renal injuries (Grade III or below) who remain hemodynamically stable (systolic blood pressure >90 mmHg) (Morey et al. 2014). Low-grade penetrating injuries can also be managed conservatively; however, patient selection is key. They must lack major injuries to the abdominal viscera, kidney parenchyma, or hilum vessels, and must not suffer from excessive blood loss. Angioembolization may be appropriate for individuals with bleeding present in a discrete segment of renal vasculature that can be targeted for embolization. However, this is limited to care centers where experienced interventionalists are available (Morey et al. 2014).

Patients who are conservatively managed should be followed carefully in the immediate posttraumatic injury period examining vitals, serial clinical exams, and serial labs (monitoring blood count and renal function). The American Urological Association (AUA) guidelines recommend follow-up CT imaging within 48 h of initial presentation for high-grade injury (Grade IV or V) or if their clinical status worsens (Morey et al. 2014).

The AAST recently released a nomogram to help predict whether an individual may require interventions by utilizing factors such as trauma mechanism (penetrating predicting higher risk), hypotension or shock, concomitant injuries, vascular contrast extravasation, para-renal hematoma, and hematoma size. This model was able to correctly predict risk of bleeding intervention in 83% of individuals in their cohort (Keihani et al. 2019). In the future, such models may continue to improve and help objectively guide providers with treatment decision-making.

Surgical Management

Surgery is indicated in instances of uncontrolled bleeding, persistent urinary extravasation despite drainage, compromise of renal vasculature, injury to a solitary kidney, or a failing kidney that appears nonviable. Potential surgical procedures include primary surgical repair, nephrectomy, and drainage of urine collections. Even after initial treatment or observation, patients may require subsequent intervention (Morey et al. 2014).

Surgical treatment or drainage interventions for urinary extravasation is generally indicated in individuals with signs of diffuse abdominal inflammation such as fevers, ileus, abdominal swelling/expanding urinoma, worsening pain, and/or fistula formation. Methods of drainage include ureteral stent, percutaneous nephrostomy tube, foley catheter, and percutaneous drain placement.

Short-Term/Long-Term Complications

In one cohort, approximately 20% of patients with a Grade 3 or 4 injury required readmission to the hospital for issues ranging from urinary tract infection, pyelonephritis, hematuria, and renal failure (Winters et al. 2016). Long-term complications of a renal injury include possible urinoma or strictures. A urinoma can become infected and form an abscess. Beyond pain and fever, an abscess can also have a mass effect on the collecting system causing impaired drainage and hydronephrosis. Scarring of the collecting system can also cause strictures. Strictures can increase the risk of kidney stones and pyelonephritis secondary to poor drainage of urine. More rarely, damaged renal vasculature can later manifest as an arteriovenous fistulas or renal vascular hypertension.

Follow-Up Care

If a patient undergoes a nephrectomy, much of their ongoing monitoring for renovascular hypertension and kidney function can be deferred to their primary care provider. Patients with lower grade injuries may not need follow-up imaging. Those with grade III or higher renal injuries are at higher risk for complications and re-interventions. They may benefit from functional kidney imaging such as radiographic scintigraphy, which serves as an estimation of kidney function.

Providers following patients after renal trauma should monitor for fevers or increasing flank pain. Repeat imaging may be considered to look for perinephric abscess, delayed bleed or continued urinary extravasation.

An abscess may require percutaneous drainage. If an abscess is caused by urine leakage, a placement of a ureteral stent or a percutaneous nephrostomy tube may be required tube. Delayed bleeding may be appropriate to refer to vascular or interventional radiology to determine if angioembolization is appropriate.

Ureteral Trauma

Overview

Incidence

Ureteral injury secondary to trauma is uncommon and has been observed in an estimated 3 per 10,000 traumas. However, it should always be considered with abdominal penetrating trauma or rapid deceleration events (Siram et al. 2010). Iatrogenic injuries during abdominal or pelvic dissection or endoscopic procedures also occur.

Pertinent Anatomy and Physiology

The ureter courses within the retroperitoneum from the ureteral pelvis (anteromedially) into the bladder (posteroinferiorly). It travels beneath the gonadal vessels and ascending/descending colon segments, traverses over the common iliac vessels, and dives under the vas deferens or uterine arteries to ultimately empty into the bladder. The bony pelvis serves as an anatomical landmark delineating the various segments of the ureter: proximal (above), mid (overlapping bony pelvis), and distal ureter (below) (Elkoushy and Andonian 2016).

History/Common Presentation

There are no definitive signs of ureteral injury, but patients with ureteral damage typically either had a rapid decelerating incident involving the pelvis/lumbar spine or a penetrating injury involving the retroperitoneum. Ureteral injury is frequently missed during initial survey, imaging, and/or surgical exploration, thus patients may present with a complication up to 7–10 days after initial presentation. Warning signs include fever, sepsis, flank or abdominal pain, and possibly poor bowel function with nausea/vomiting, if they develop a paralytic ileus secondary to urine spillage into the abdominal cavity (Siram et al. 2010).

Physical Exam

Warning signs of ureteral trauma include:

- Flank pain or ecchymosis
- Broken ribs or lumbar spine fractures
- Peritoneal signs from urine extravasation, such as guarding, diffuse tenderness, flank pain, or abdominal distension
- Watery vaginal discharge secondary to ureterovaginal fistula

Diagnostic Tests

Laboratory Evaluation

Urinalysis—Microscopic hematuria may indicate a possible injury to the GU system; however, its absence does not eliminate the possibility of ureteral injury (Elliott and McAninch 2003).

Blood chemistry—Increased levels of serum creatinine may be a sign of urine reabsorption within the body.

Body fluid analysis—Testing of vaginal fluid, cutaneous drainage, or abdominal fluid for creatinine can confirm urine content as creatinine levels would be markedly elevated compared to serum levels.

Imaging Studies

Just as with kidney injuries, an initial rapid trauma CT scan may not be able to properly evaluate the genitourinary system. Delayed excretory phase contrast sequences have a much better sensitivity for examining the ureter. Concerning signs for ureteral trauma on a CT scan include concomitant lumbar spine fractures, fluid collections in the retroperitoneum or adjacent to the kidney, inability to identify the ureters, ureteral dilation, or hydronephrosis (Siram et al. 2010).

Ureterography—Fluoroscopic evaluation of the ureter can be performed by injecting contrast either retrograde (injected from the ureteral orifice) or antegrade (from the kidney through a percutaneous nephrostomy tube). Operative planning for ureteral reconstruction depends on the location of injury, length of disruption, degree of laceration (complete versus partial transection), degree of injury and kidney function. An antegrade nephrostogram and retrograde pyelograms can help characterize the location, length, and degree of injury.

Radionucleotide scintigraphy (e.g. mercaptoacetyltriglycine or MAG 3 lasix scan) may also be used preoperatively. Quantitatively determining the level of kidney function may help weigh the risks and benefits for repairing the ureter of a complex injury. These scans can be critical to understand the distribution of kidney function. Laboratory studies alone may be insufficient to determine renal function.

Management

Surgical Management

Ureteral disruption, especially in the context of trauma, rarely takes precedence over more emergent surgical concerns. If a ureteral injury is discovered during a primary surgical exploration, the best treatment is to repair the ureter primarily if the patient is clinically stable. Repair during the initial encounter is favored as it can help the patient avoid subsequent procedures. Ureteral repair is commonly done over a ureteral stent to prevent stricture formation during the healing process. In some cases, a ureteral stent is sufficient for the management of a partial or small ureteral injury.

For patients who are either not clinically stable, have a delayed recognition of ureteral injury, or endured a severe ureteral transection, it is frequently appropriate to delay repair and temporarily divert urine with percutaneous nephrostomy tubes or ureteral stent. There are different techniques of ureteral repair dependent on the extent of injury; however, in-depth discussion of these techniques is beyond the scope of this chapter.

Short-Term/Long-Term Complications

Possible complications include extravasation of urine, stricture recurrence, or fistula formation.

Urine leak may lead to abscess or peritoneal inflammation with resultant ileus or peritonitis. Stricture recurrence could lead to flank pain, hydronephrosis, along with kidney injury. Fistula formation may lead to continuous urinary leakage dependent on type of fistula formation.

Follow-Up Care

If a ureteral repair was performed, practitioners will need to determine the timing of stent removal. Upon stent removal, follow-up imaging should be obtained about 4–6 weeks later. Follow-up imaging may include a Lasix renogram to assess for functionality along with drainage. An ultrasound may also be performed to assess for hydronephrosis.

If a ureteral repair was delayed, practitioners will need to perform work-up to determine the type of repair necessary. If a percutaneous nephrostomy tube was placed, consideration should be done to perform an antegrade nephrosto-gram or a retrograde pyelogram to determine the length and location of the stricture for operative planning. As some ureteral injuries may resolve with a stent placement alone, follow-up imaging may help to determine if a surgical repair is indicated.

Bladder Injury

Overview

Incidence

Traumatic bladder injury has been observed in approximately 1.6% of patients pre-senting with blunt abdominal trauma and 3.6% of those with pelvic fractures. The relationship between bladder injury and pelvic fractures is further demonstrated by the statistic of approximately 70% of individuals with bladder injury also having a pelvic fracture (McGeady and Breyer 2013). Blunt force can rupture a distended bladder either into the abdominal cavity (intraperitoneal) or in a separate space ante-riorly (extraperitoneal). Penetrating injuries are less common.

Pertinent Anatomy and Physiology

The bladder lies behind the pubic bone, well protected by the pelvic rim. Anteriorly it abuts the pubic symphysis and posteriorly lies atop either the rectum in men or the vagina and uterus in women. Important contiguous spaces include the abdominal cavity, marked by a peritoneal lining, which drapes over the posterior wall and the dome of the bladder. Anteriorly and laterally is the prevesical space. The ureters insert at a posterior and inferior edge of the bladder, creating the base of the trigone along with the bladder neck as the anterior apex. These landmarks are crucial to consider as the area of injury determines treatment recommendations (Rodriguez and Nakamura 2016; Chung et al. 2016).

History/Common Presentation

A classic presentation for a traumatic bladder injury is an individual with a pelvic fracture. One mechanism of injury is the displacement of a bony fragment, which can puncture through the bladder wall. Suprapubic blunt force can also rupture the bladder when the bladder is full. Other causes include iatrogenic/procedural inju-ries, for example, endoscopic transurethral procedures, gynecologic surgeries, and hernia repairs. Patients with a bladder injury will frequently present with hematuria and low urine output or inability to void. Certainly, any patient with combined pel-vic fracture and gross hematuria warrants evaluation of the bladder integrity (Morey et al. 2014).

Physical Exam

Examination signs concerning for bladder rupture include:

- Maneuvers for pelvic fracture include placing pressure on the lateral edge of the pelvis which may elicit pain or crepitus
- Suprapubic and/or abdominal tenderness
- Acute abdomen or peritonitis (a delayed presentation if a urine leak is present)
- Hematuria or passing clots
- Decreased urine output or inability to urinate
- Difficult catheter placement

Diagnostic Tests

Laboratory Evaluation

Urinalysis—Hematuria is not specific for bladder injury and could indicate injury along any area of the urinary tract.

Serum chemistry—increased serum creatinine can indicate reabsorption of leaked urine.

Imaging Studies

An abdominal X-ray may reveal a pelvic fracture or signs such as distortion or blurring of pelvic structures secondary to spilled urine or blood outside of the bladder consistent with bladder wall rupture.

X-Ray cystograms involve insertion of contrast into the bladder with films taken both at a maximally filled volume (typically around 300 cc by gravity) and a postvoid film to identify retained contrast in the bladder or extravasation. It is important to obtain multiple views to assess for extravasation in the posterior wall.

A CT cystogram, similar to an X-ray cystogram, also involves retrograde administration of contrast through a foley catheter prior to scanning. CT cystography has similar sensitivity and specificity as XR cystography for detecting bladder injury (Morey et al. 2014). Note a CT urogram may not be sufficient to assess bladder injury, as it may not have distended the bladder enough to detect a leak.

A retrograde urethrogram (RUG) should be considered if there is any clinical suspicion of urethral injury (see Urethral Trauma). This is particularly important, as a catheter, required for XR or CT cystography, should not be placed blindly until confirming that there is no urethral injury (Morey et al. 2014).

Management

Nonsurgical Management

The key determinant of management is the anatomical location of bladder injury. If the laceration is extraperitoneal (in the pre-vesicular space), then it may be appropriate to simply place a catheter and allow the bladder to heal while adequately drained. These catheters can typically be kept in place for 2–3 weeks.

Surgical Management

Intraperitoneal bladder injury typically indicates surgical repair. Intraperitoneal bladder injuries allow for urine to leak into the abdomen causing inflammation, peritonitis, ileus, and possibly sepsis.

There are very specific extra-peritoneal bladder injuries that require surgical treatment: bone fragments penetrating the into the bladder lumen, simultaneous injury to rectal or vaginal tissues, or simultaneous injury to the bladder neck (Morey et al. 2014). Each of these circumstances may prevent proper healing of bladder tissue on its own. For example, when there is an injury to the rectum or vagina even a small amount of urine can form fistulous connections impairing repair mechanisms.

Short-Term/Long-Term Complications

Soon after bladder injury or after surgical repair, there can be complications secondary to a urine leak. A continued leak can develop into a fistula, form an abscess, cause peritonitis or evens sepsis. Long-term complications include voiding dysfunction and incontinence. Injury to the pelvic nerves can present like a spinal cord injury and neurogenic bladder with poor compliance and/or urinary retention. Furthermore, there can be erosion of hardware from pelvic fractures into the bladder.

Follow-Up

As patients are healing from a bladder injury, they will frequently be sent home with a foley catheter or suprapubic (SP) catheter. This helps to drain the bladder and ensure proper drainage while the tissue layers heal. Crucial aspects of follow-up care include ensuring proper functioning of the catheter. Learning to trouble shoot proper drainage of an SP tube with techniques such as gentle irrigation is critical for both urologic providers and patients. Before removal of a catheter, radiographic evaluation of the bladder will typically be performed with either XR or CT cystography. Providers should then continue to follow these patients carefully screening for appropriate healing, signs of infection, along with proper urinary function and quality of life.

Urethral Trauma

Overview

Incidence

Urethral injuries make up only 4% of all genitourinary trauma cases and most patients are male (McGeady and Breyer 2013). Injury to the posterior urethra in men is often due to pelvic fractures, while straddle injury (trauma to the perineum and compaction of the urethra against the pubic bone) is associated with anterior urethral injury. Penetrating injuries to the penis such as stabs, gunshot wounds, or animal bites always warrant evaluation of the urethra as they can cause partial or complete disruption.

Pertinent Anatomy and Physiology

The urethra is broken up into contiguous segments, with two distinct sections referred to as the anterior and posterior urethra. Beginning distally at the urethral meatus, the anterior urethra consists of the fossa navicularis (within the glans penis), the penile urethra along the external length of the penis, and the bulbar urethra. The posterior urethra consists of the membranous urethra (at level of external urethral sphincter) and the prostatic urethra as it transitions to the bladder neck.

History/Common Presentation

Urethral trauma can be present in those with pelvic fractures or distinct injuries such as in straddle injury. Most patients are males as traumatic injury of the female urethra is very rare.

A harbinger of urethral injury is blood at the meatus. In this setting it is paramount that providers do not attempt to pass a catheter without further evaluation. Catheterization and other urethral instrumentations have the potential to cause additional bleeding, increase risk of infection, or potentially make a partial urethral injury into a more complete tear complicating surgical options and recovery. Patients may also report difficulty urinating. For penetrating injuries with concurrent injury to the corpus spongiosum there can be penile bleeding that is difficult to control.

Physical Exam

Providers should evaluate for signs of urethral injury such as:

- Blood at urethral meatus
- Suprapubic tenderness
- Instability of pelvis (pelvic fracture)
- High-riding prostate on rectal exam (possible posterior urethral disruption)
- Perineal or scrotal bleeding/ecchymosis (possible anterior urethra injury)

Diagnostic Tests

Laboratory Evaluation

Urinalysis—Hematuria is present in the majority of urethral injuries. However, as with other evaluations the blood could be additionally resulting from additional locations along the urinary tract.

Imaging Studies

Retrograde Urethrography (RUG) is recommended in any patient suspected of urethral injury. Proper execution of a urethrogram in a male requires the patient to be positioned laterally with the bottom leg flexed and the top leg straight, and the penis on stretch. The examiner can place a small catheter into the fossa navicularis, then while occluding the meatus can inject a mixture of contrast and water. This test is recommended before placing a urethral catheter in any patient with suspicion of urethral injury (Morey et al. 2014).

A direct visualization with a cystoscopy is an alternative option for evaluation based on the clinical situation.

Management

Nonsurgical Management

In the immediate setting, urethral bleeding can often be controlled initially by pressure. If a partial injury is suspected or a tear, a trial of passage of a catheter may be attempted. Some urologists may elect to perform an endoscopic realignment of the urethra with a cystoscopy and wire.

Surgical Management

In the case where an endoscopic realignment is unsuccessful, or if the patient has a significant posterior urethral disruption, a suprapubic tube catheter placement should be completed. This allows for bladder decompression and urethral rest. Surgical management of these injuries is usually done in a delayed fashion to allow for maturation of scar tissue within the urethra. As for a penetrating injury of the anterior urethra, an immediate exploration and repair is recommended (Morey et al. 2014). Given the high risk for later complications of incontinence, any injury to the female urethra is recommended to be repaired at primary presentation (Perry and Husmann 1992).

Short-Term/Long-Term Complications

Complications following urethral injuries include urinary tract infections (UTIs), urinary incontinence, urethral stricture and sexual dysfunction. More complex issues include fistulization or urethral diverticula. Patients who had catheters in place for a prolonged period of time may be at a particularly increased risk of developing UTIs and urethral erosion.

Follow-Up

In the immediate recovery period, patients with SP tubes or foley catheters should be followed closely to help determine when catheter removal is appropriate. A voiding cystourethrogram (VCUG) or RUG can help guide the decision for catheter removal. Patients with a posterior urethral injury and SP tube will require regular SP tube exchanges until a forma urethroplasty is planned.

Expert guidelines recommend that urologic providers continue to follow patients for at least 1 year following urethral or bladder injury to screen for urethral strictures, erectile dysfunction, and urinary incontinence (Morey et al. 2014). Signs of strictures can be determined by asking patients about difficulty with urination or changes in their stream over time. Clinic evaluation can include uroflowmetry or post-void residual scanning to determine urine flow and retention. Urodynamic testing may help evaluate voiding disorders especially if there is suspicion of nerve injury secondary to trauma. Patient reported symptoms of urinary tract infections such as dysuria, frequency, or urgency, warrants a prompt urinalysis, urine culture, and antimicrobial treatment as appropriate. Regarding sexual dysfunction, patients should be counseled that it may take 1–2 years prior to reaching optimal spontaneous recovery of the nerves contributing to sexual function.

External Male Genitalia Injury

Overview

Incidence

Population studies estimate that anywhere from 28 to 68% of GU injuries have involvement of the external genitalia, with scrotal and testicular injury more common than penile injury (McGeady and Breyer 2013). Around 85% of scrotal injuries result from blunt trauma, while blunt trauma to an erect penis can result in a penile fracture.

Pertinent Anatomy and Physiology

Key anatomical relationships of the male external genitalia include the different contiguous tissue layers. The scrotal skin envelopes the testicles with the remaining layers linked embryologically to the abdominal wall as the testicles descended in utero: the external spermatic fascia originated from the external oblique, the cremasteric muscle from the internal oblique, and the internal spermatic fascia from the transversalis muscle. The spermatic cord contains the gonadal vessels, vas deferens, and lymphatics. The innermost layer containing the testicle is a derivative layer of the peritoneum referred to as the tunica vaginalis which typically is obliterated superiorly to form a pouch no longer connected to the peritoneum. The outer layer of the testicle is called the tunica albuginea. As sperm develop within the testicle in the seminiferous tubules, the tubules eventually join together within the epididymis (which sits atop the testicle). This then merges into the vas deferens.

The erectile tissue of the penis includes paired, heavily vascularized, tubular structures called the corpus cavernosum running in parallel. The corpus spongiosum sits between the corpus cavernosa and includes the urethra, and expands into the glans penis (Kavoussi 2016).

History/Common Presentation

Blunt scrotal and testicular trauma is often observed in sporting accidents and the severity can range from bruising to loss of the testicle secondary to rupture. Injuries can also occur in motor vehicle accidents or from penetrating injuries. Penetrating injuries secondary to stabbing, gunshots, or animal or human bites can similarly affect the penis and urethra.

Penile fractures typically occur following impact to an erect penis during sexual intercourse. The impact to an erect penis results in tearing of the corpora, which

Table 10.2 Summary of penile fracture

Penile fracture	History:	Signs/symptoms:	True urologic emergency Evaluation:	Therapeutic interventions:

	• Erect penis became disengaged from the vagina and hits some impervious part of the female anatomy causing an acute bend in the penis
	• Rupture or tear to tunica albuginea
	  – Male patient (and partner) may report feeling and/or hearing a "pop," followed by pain to penile shaft and immediate loss of erection, and subsequent penile ecchymosis
	  – May also report bright red blood from urethra
		• Ecchymosis to site of injury, may extend to much of penile shaft
		• May result in deviation of the shaft
		• Edema
		• Pain
		• Urinary function typically unaffected
		Ecchymosis follows genital fascial barriers along the lines of those involved with trauma to the urethra
		This is a clinical diagnosis
			• Penile Doppler	• Immediate surgical repair of the tunica albuginea defect is necessary- ideally within 24–36 h after injury
				• Many men do not present within this time frame, due to embarrassment or belief that injury is less severe
				• If injury was minor (no loss of erection) and hematoma is confined to penile skin, supportive measures such as ice and (NSAIDs)
				• Reassurance this will improve with time

allows leakage of blood into the surrounding tissue layers. Patients typically present with a history of hearing a snap or pop associated with a sudden loss of an erection. Often penile pain, swelling, and bruising occur shortly after. Avulsion or burn injuries seen in trauma patients will also require evaluation for involvement of deeper structures (Table 10.2).

Physical Exam

Concerning signs on exam of the external genitalia that require further evaluation include:

- Scrotal or perineal bruising or hematoma
- Diffuse penile bruising and abnormal curvature could represent a penile fracture
- Blood at meatus or inability to void is suggestive of urethral involvement
- Loss of the cremasteric reflex can suggest compromised testicular blood flow

Diagnostic Tests

Urinalysis should be obtained to assess for hematuria, which may indicate concomitant urethral injury.

Imaging Studies

Ultrasound is a valuable imaging modality to evaluate external genitalia. It can evaluate the integrity of the corpora and assess for vascular compromise. In addition, it can screen for testicular rupture and determine blood flow to the testicles.

Magnetic resonance imaging (MRI) has also been utilized to assess the penile integrity in suspected cases of penile fracture where initial imaging results are equivocal (Morey et al. 2014).

Management

Nonsurgical Management

Some injuries to the external genitalia can be managed conservatively with pain control. However, many will require surgical exploration and possible intervention. Physical exam and imaging techniques must demonstrate intact structures with only superficial damage.

Surgical Management

Penetrating trauma from gunshot wounds, lacerations, or bites require surgical exploration. Foreign bodies should be removed, and the wound should be irrigated and debrided. Note that human bite injuries are not completely closed, as there is a risk of poor healing due to infections.

Perioperative considerations for the majority of penile injuries involve high suspicion and evaluation for urethral injury either by a RUG or cystoscopy. Large losses of penile or scrotal skin may require skin grafting for coverage. Severe cases of avulsion to the scrotal skin without enough left for coverage may even require surgical repositioning of spermatic cord and testes in the medial thighs while awaiting healing and reconstruction. If a testicle cannot be salvaged, aner an orchiectomy is performed. Penile fractures warrant urgent surgical repair to avoid long-term complications such as sexual dysfunction and poor cosmetic results such as penile curvature. A rare but serious injury of penile amputation can be seen. In these cases, the amputated member should be placed in a bag of saline and then within a bag of ice: referred to as the double bag technique (Morey et al. 2014).

Short-Term/Long-Term Complications

Trauma to the external genitalia can have impactful consequences to a person's life. Individuals can suffer from infertility, impaired sexual function, hormonal abnormalities, and there can be significant psychiatric afflictions.

Follow-Up

Most patients should refrain from sexual activity for several weeks following trauma to the genitalia. These individuals should also be followed carefully by clinical providers as their wounds heal. Visits can be arranged to assess tissue viability and wound healing. These follow-up visits are especially important for patients requiring delayed closure or future skin grafting. Each individual should also be provided care corresponding to any complications, such as reproductive counseling, sexual health counseling, and possibly psychiatric support.

Clinical Pearls
- Establish method of injury for suspected GU trauma, either from patient or paramedics.
- Urologic trauma is not usually the sole issue, but occurs in the context of multisystem trauma.
- Assess for presence and degree of hematuria.
- Staging upper tract injuries is vital.
- The kidneys are the GU organ most commonly damaged.

Resources

Resources for the Nurse Practitioner

American Urological Association Urotrauma Guidelines (updated 2017): https://www.auanet.org/guidelines/urotrauma-guideline.

Resources for the Patient

Urology Care Foundation:
   https://www.urologyhealth.org/urologic-conditions/urotrauma
   https://www.urologyhealth.org/urologic-conditions/kidney-(renal)-trauma
   https://www.urologyhealth.org/urologic-conditions/bladder-trauma
   https://www.urologyhealth.org/urologic-conditions/urethral-trauma
   https://www.urologyhealth.org/urologic-conditions/penile-trauma

References

Buckley JC, McAninch JW (2011) Revision of current American Association for the surgery of trauma renal injury grading system. J Trauma 70(1):35–37. https://doi.org/10.1097/TA.0b013e318207ad5a
Chung BI, Sommer G, Brooks JD (2016) Surgical, radiographic, and endoscopic anatomy of the male pelvis. In: Campbell-Walsh urology, 11th edn. Elsevier, Philadelphia, pp 1611–1630

Elkoushy MA, Andonian S (2016) Surgical, radiologic, and endoscopic anatomy of the kidney and ureter. In: Campbell-Walsh urology, 11th edn. Elsevier, Philadelphia, pp 967–977

Elliott SP, McAninch JW (2003) Ureteral injuries from external violence: the 25-year experience at San Francisco General Hospital. J Urol 170(4):1213–1216. https://doi.org/10.1097/01.ju.0000087841.98141.85

Galvagno SM, Nahmias JT, Young DA (2019) Advanced Trauma Life Support® update 2019: management and applications for adults and special populations. Anesthesiol Clin 37(1):13–32. https://doi.org/10.1016/j.anclin.2018.09.009

Hotaling JM, Sorensen MD, Iii TGS, Rivara FP, Wessells H, Voelzke BB (2011) Analysis of diagnostic angiography and angioembolization in the acute management of renal trauma using a national data set. J Urol 185(4):1316–1320. https://doi.org/10.1016/j.juro.2010.12.003

Hotaling JM, Wang J, Sorensen MD et al (2012) A national study of trauma level designation and renal trauma outcomes. J Urol 187(2):536–541. https://doi.org/10.1016/j.juro.2011.09.155

Kavoussi PK (2016) Surgical, radiographic, and endoscopic anatomy of the male reproductive system. In: Campbell-Walsh urology, 11th edn. Elsevier, Philadelphia, pp 498–515

Keihani S, Rogers DM, Putbrese BE et al (2019) A nomogram predicting the need for bleeding interventions after high-grade renal trauma: results from the American Association for the Surgery of Trauma Multi-institutional Genito-Urinary Trauma Study (MiGUTS). J Trauma Acute Care Surg 86(5):774–782. https://doi.org/10.1097/TA.0000000000002222

McGeady JB, Breyer BN (2013) Current epidemiology of genitourinary trauma. Urol Clin North Am 40(3):323–334. https://doi.org/10.1016/j.ucl.2013.04.001

Morey AF, Brandes S, Dugi DD et al (2014) Urotrauma: AUA guideline. J Urol 192(2):327–335. https://doi.org/10.1016/j.juro.2014.05.004

Perry MO, Husmann DA (1992) Urethral injuries in female subjects following pelvic fractures. J Urol 147(1):139–143. https://doi.org/10.1016/S0022-5347(17)37162-8

Rodriguez LV, Nakamura LY (2016) Surgical, radiographic, and endoscopic anatomy of the female pelvis. In: Campbell-Walsh urology, 11th edn. Elsevier, Philadelphia, pp 1597–1610

Siram SM, Gerald SZ, Greene WR et al (2010) Ureteral trauma: patterns and mechanisms of injury of an uncommon condition. Am J Surg 199(4):566–570. https://doi.org/10.1016/j.amjsurg.2009.11.001

Smith J, Caldwell E, D'Amours S, Jalaludin B, Sugrue M (2005) Abdominal trauma: a disease in evolution. ANZ J Surg 75(9):790–794. https://doi.org/10.1111/j.1445-2197.2005.03524.x

Voelzke BB, Leddy L (2014) The epidemiology of renal trauma. Transl Androl Urol 3(2):143–149. https://doi.org/10.3978/j.issn.2223-4683.2014.04.11

Winters B, Wessells H, Voelzke BB (2016) Readmission after treatment of Grade 3 and 4 renal injuries at a Level I trauma center: statewide assessment using the Comprehensive Hospital Abstract Reporting System. J Trauma Acute Care Surg 80(3):466–471. https://doi.org/10.1097/TA.0000000000000948

Diagnosis and Management of Urinary Tract Infections, Asymptomatic Bacteriuria and Pyelonephritis

11

Michelle J. Lajiness and Laura J. Hintz

Contents

M. J. Lajiness (✉)
Department of Urology, University of Toledo, Toledo, OH, USA
e-mail: Michelle.Lajiness@utoledo.edu

L. J. Hintz
Saginaw, MI, USA
e-mail: laurahintz@mpui.org

© Springer Nature Switzerland AG 2020
S. A. Quallich, M. J. Lajiness (eds.), *The Nurse Practitioner in Urology*,
https://doi.org/10.1007/978-3-030-45267-4_11

Objectives

1. Define urinary tract infection, and differentiate its presentation in men and women.
2. Identify causes and the presentation of pyelonephritis.
3. Discuss asymptomatic bacteriuria

Diagnosis and Management of Urinary Tract Infections

The purpose of this chapter is to assist nurse practitioners and physician assistants, particularly those specializing in urology, on how to recognize and manage urinary tract infections. Unfortunately, the lack of knowledge in assessing both a urine specimen correctly and the inability to correlate this information with a patient's presenting signs and symptoms is cause for frequent misdiagnosis of urinary tract infections. In addition, the misuse and overuse of antibiotics in today's society has made treating urinary tract infections more complicated. This chapter will review the different types of infections, the diagnostic testing required, as well as population-specific guidelines for proper management.

Definitions

Urinary tract infection (UTI) is an inflammatory response of the urothelium to bacterial invasion that is typically associated with bacteriuria and pyuria. The term acute cystitis is often used interchangeably.

Bacteriuria is the presence of bacteria in the urine and it may be symptomatic or asymptomatic.

Asymptomatic bacteriuria (ASB) is the isolation of bacteria from the urine with or without pyuria but in the absence of local or systemic urinary tract symptoms (greater than 100,000 colony forming units per milliliter CFU/mL).

Pyuria is the presence of white blood cells in the urine. This typically indicates an inflammatory response secondary to an infectious process caused from bacteria. Pyuria without bacteriuria warrants evaluation for tuberculosis, stones, or cancer. Pyuria in the presence of bacteriuria is not always indicative of an infection.

Acute pyelonephritis is the presence of bacteriuria and pyuria, in addition to the presence of specific symptoms (i.e., fever, chills, and flank pain), indicating an interstitial inflammation of the renal parenchyma.

Incidence and Epidemiology

Urinary tract infections (UTIs), also referred to as acute cystitis, are the most common bacterial infection and are responsible for between four and eight million clinic visits (Hanno 2014). Therefore, this ranks UTIs as the most common cause for ambulatory care visits in the United States. The direct costs are more than $1.6

billion per year (Hanno 2014). Medina and Castillo-Pino (2019) note that the life-time incidence of UTI in adult women is 50–60%.

Urinary tract infections affect men, women, and children. In women, the incidence is higher in the younger population, typically at the onset of sexual activity. The risk factors relevant to the premenopausal woman are the use of spermicides and sexual frequency. The incidence will increase slowly again after menopause due to the changes in the vaginal tissues and the increased pH of the vagina as a result of estrogen deficiency. Medina and Castillo-Pino (2019) note that the lifetime incidence of UTI in adult women is 50–60%.

Of the millions of UTIs reported, women account for approximately 85% of them. Eleven percent of women will report having had a UTI during any given year (Hanno 2014). Fifty percent of all women will report having had at least one infection in their lifetime. By the age of 24, one in three women will have had a urinary tract infection. UTIs in men are less common until after the age of 50 when the incidence of enlarged prostate increases, contributing to bladder outlet obstruction and urinary retention.

Nearly 30–44% of women with a first UTI will have a recurrent UTI and 50% will have a third UTI if they have had 2 UTI's in 6 months (Brubaker et al. 2018). Whether the infection is left untreated, or treated with short-term, long-term, or prophylactic antibiotic therapy, the risk of reoccurrence remains unchanged. Therefore, the symptomatic episodes are more of a nuisance than a health threat in the healthy population.

Asymptomatic Bacteriuria

The incidence of ASB in healthy nonpregnant adult women ranges from 1 to 8.6%. The incidence increases with age and is noted to be 10.8–16% in women in the community over age 70 and 25–50% for women in long-term care (LTC) (Nicolle et al. 2019). In men, the incidence ranges from 3.6 to 19% in the community and 15–50% for those in LTC. Women with diabetes have an incidence of 10.8–16% and men of 0.7–11%. *E. coli* is the most common organism isolated from patients with ASB (Zalmanovici et al. 2015). Despite current practice guidelines many patients are routinely screened and treated for ASB (Nicolle et al. 2019).

Catheterized Urinary Tract Infections (CAUTI)

Catheter-associated urinary tract infection (CAUTI) has also become of great concern over the past several years. They are the most common cause of nosocomial infection (Stamm and Norrby 2001). The end result is an increased risk for falls, delirium, and immobility in the older population and an increased financial burden on the health care system. Most of the uropathogens responsible for CAUTIs gain access by extraluminal (direct inoculation when inserted) or intraluminal (reflux of uropathogens from failure to maintain a closed system). As soon as the catheter is inserted, bacteria will start to develop colonies known as biofilms (living layers).

These biofilms are collections of microorganisms with altered phenotypes that adhere to a medical device, such as the catheter and/or collection bag. The biofilm is protective against antimicrobials and the host–immune response. The risk of colonization increases in relation to the duration of catheterization and reaches nearly 100% at 30 days (Hanno 2014).

Risk factors for UTIs include:

- Sexual intercourse;
- A new sex partner within the past year;
- Use of spermicides;
- Use of diaphragm/cervical cap;
- Estrogen deficiency;
- Previous UTI;
- History of UTI in first-degree female relative;
- Urinary retention;
- Benign prostatic hyperplasia;
- and steroid use.

Subpopulations at increased risk for UTIs:

- Pregnant women;
- Elderly;
- Spinal cord injury;
- Indwelling catheters;
- Diabetes;
- Muscular sclerosis;
- Acquired immunodeficiency disease;
- and those with underlying urological abnormalities.

Pathophysiology

The model for uncomplicated UTIS is that bacterial virulence is crucial for overcoming normal host defenses (Hanno 2014). However, in complicated UTIs the paradigm is reversed; the bacterial virulence is not as critical as the host factors. UTIs are typically initiated by a potential urinary pathogen migrating from the bowel. In some cases the pathogens arise from the vaginal flora, as a direct result of inoculation during sexual activity. These pathogens then begin to colonize the vagina and perineum with enteric organisms. As the organisms move to the periurethral mucosa, they ascend through the urethra into the bladder (urethritis and/or cystitis) and in some cases through the ureter to the kidney (pyelonephritis).

Most infections in women represent an ascending infection, and this process of infection is related to the relatively short length of the female urethra. UTIs are less common in the younger male, with the incidence increasing in the aging male. The male urethra is considerably longer than the female, which makes ascending infections less common. Most UTIs in older men are typically related to a voiding dysfunction that puts them at risk for acquiring an infection (i.e., urinary retention secondary to an enlarged prostate), or they may acquire it after some form of instrumentation.

Classification

Urinary tract infections may be classified by several different categories: complicated or uncomplicated, upper tract or lower tract, and first infection, unresolved bacteriuria, or recurrent infection. Recurrent infections can be separated into two separate classifications of "reinfection" or "bacterial persistence." On occasion, UTIs may be classified by the type of organism.

Uncomplicated UTIs may be defined as a UTI in the setting of a functionally and structurally normal urinary tract, in a patient that is typically afebrile. This type of infection typically occurs in women, and the uropathogen is one that is susceptible to and eradicated by a short course of an inexpensive oral antimicrobial therapy. Complicated UTIs are typically defined as pyelonephritis and/or a structural or functional abnormality that decreases the efficacy of antimicrobial therapy. In most cases, complicated UTIs are caused by bacteria that are resistant to many antimicrobials. CAUTIs are classified as complicated and the rate of innoculation of bacteria averages about 5% per day (Nicolle et al. 2019).

The diagnosis of upper UTI refers to an infection of the kidney (pyelonephritis). The lower urinary tract (LUT) refers to infections of the bladder (cystitis) or urethra (urethritis). As for the organism responsible for the infection, it may be caused by bacterial, fungal, viral, or parasitic organisms.

The majority of uncomplicated UTI's (95%) are monobacterial (only one organism) and typically caused by a gram-positive organism. It is estimated that 75–95% of uncomplicated UTIs are caused by *E. coli*, followed by *Klebsiella pneumoniae*, *Staphylococcus saprophyticus*, *Enterococcus faecalis*, group B streptococci and *Proteus mirabilis*. *E. coli* can cause both complicated and uncomplicated UTI's. *Pseudomonas aeruginosa*, *Enterococcus*, and *P. mirabilis* are typically seen in complicated UTIs. *Corynebacterium urealyticum* is a nosocomial infection typically associated with catheter use.

UTIs categorized as first infections are typically new or an isolated infection that is separated by a previous infection of at least 6 months, such as the "honeymooners' UTI." Unresolved bacteriuria occurs during therapy and implies that the urinary tract is not sterilized during the treatment period. Recurrent UTIs are defined as two episodes of acute bacterial cystitis within a 6 month period or three infections in a 12 month period. This definition includes episodes that are different in nature with resolution of symptoms in between. The definition does not include those that require more than one treatment or multiple antibiotic courses as a result of inappropriate initial or empiric treatment (Anger et al. 2019).

Presentation

In most patients, the presenting signs and symptoms may include dysuria (pain with urination), frequency, urgency, nocturia (nighttime voiding), suprapubic pain, gross hematuria, and low back pain. Fever with an uncomplicated UTI is unusual (see Table 11.1). Therefore, acute pyelonephritis should be considered when fever, tachycardia, and/or costovertebral angle pain are present. Cloudy urine and foul smelling urine can be indicative of many other conditions (dehydration, food intake) and are not considered indicative of a UTI by itself. A UTI's number one symptom is burning with urination and is key to diagnosis (Anger et al. 2019). In addition, patients with suspected pyelonephritis may present as ill appearing and seem uncomfortable.

History and Physical Examination

The patient's history is the most important tool for diagnosing an uncomplicated UTI. Always include an evaluation of the patient's current urinary tract symptoms, past history of urinary tract infections, and any other urinary tract problems or conditions include episodes of dysuria, frequency, urgency, nocturia, incontinence hematuria and constipation, diarrhea, or bowel incontinence. Use and frequency of antibiotics should be obtained. Vaginal discharge and irritative symptoms should be assessed. Follow that with a routine family history and social history (specifically looking at smoking history) prolapse, rectocele or atrophic vaginitis. In addition, one should also inquire into the patient's sexual history, with a special focus on any known history of sexually transmitted infections (STIs). Finally, one should support the detailed history with a focused physical exam and urinalysis.

Female Examination
- Temperature
- Check post void residual
- Evaluate the possibility of pregnancy and history of reproductive issues

Table 11.1 Signs and symptoms

Uncomplicated UTI	Pyelonephritis
Dysuria	Fever (temp >38 °C)
Urgency	Chills
Frequency (voiding smaller amounts)	Nausea
Gross hematuria	Vomiting
	Flank pain
	Any combination of uncomplicated UTI signs and symptoms
Low back pain	Costovertebral angle tenderness with palpation
Suprapubic pain and tenderness with palpation	

- Include pelvic exam, assessing for and if symptoms indicate a possible pelvic infection or urethritis
- Examine low back, abdomen, and suprapubic area for tenderness, pain, or abnormalities

Male Examination
- Temperature
- Check postvoid residual
- Evaluate any history of prostate problems
- Examine genitals, low back, and abdomen for tenderness, pain, or abnormalities
- Examine rectum and prostate for prostate enlargement, growths, inflammation, or pain

Abnormal Findings
- Pain or discomfort in response to pressure on the lower back, abdomen, or the area above the pelvic bone (10–20% of patients have suprapubic tenderness in uncomplicated UTIs)
- Costovertebral angle tenderness is typically indicative of pyelonephritis
- Growths or abnormalities detected during the pelvic or rectal exam
- Enlarged or tender prostate gland (men only)
- Discharge from the urethra

Differential Diagnosis

Among the female population, interstitial cystitis (IC) and sexually transmitted infections (STIs) are the most common diagnoses that present with similar symptoms. Dysuria is common with cystitis, urethritis, and vaginitis. However, cystitis is more likely when the signs and symptoms also include frequency, urgency, and/or hematuria. If the symptoms are of severe or sudden onset and in the absence of vaginal irritation and/or discharge, then cystitis is also more likely. The probability of acute UTI is greater than 50%, in women with any one of the signs or symptoms. It increases to more than 90% when there is a combination of symptoms, such as dysuria and frequency, without vaginal irritation or discharge. A urine culture is typically positive with bacterial cystitis.

Urethritis is typically caused by *Chlamydia trachomatis*, *Neisseria gonorrhoeae*, or the herpes simplex virus. Vaginitis is caused by *Candida* species or *Trichomonas vaginalis*. Pyuria is commonly seen in cystitis and urethritis but is less likely in vaginitis. The symptoms of urethritis also tend to be mild, gradual in onset, and include vaginal discharge. Vaginal irritation or discharge, if present, is a symptom suggestive of vaginitis and reduce the likelihood of the diagnosis of bacterial cystitis by 20%. In a patient that has a documented history of bacterial cystitis, as evidenced by a positive urine culture, and they present again, with similar symptoms, the likelihood of true infection approaches 90% (Hanno 2014).

In the male population, prostatitis, epididymitis, and STIs are the most common diagnoses that present with similar symptoms when compared to acute cystitis. However, with acute bacterial prostatitis, in addition to the typical dysuria, frequency, urgency, and nocturia, additional constitutional symptoms, such as fever, chills, and malaise, may also occur. Patients may also report complaints of perineal and/or low back pain. On exam, the prostate may feel enlarged and boggy, with acute tenderness. Epididymitis occurs more commonly in the adolescent and elderly male population but can affect men of all ages. In the population of men under the age of 35, the form of transmission is sexual and is typically caused by *C. trachomatis* and *N. gonorrhoeae* pathogens. In the elderly population, *E. coli* and *Pseudomonas* are the most common offending pathogens. Indwelling catheters, in the elderly population, are also responsible for the development of epididymitis, through a retrograde mechanism. In patients, with epididymitis, the presenting symptoms may include a tender hemiscrotum, in addition to a swollen epididymis. The scrotum may be warm, erythematous, and swollen. Fever, chills, voiding symptoms, and pain that radiates to the ipsilateral flank may also occur.

Diagnostic Testing

Commercially available dipsticks that test for leukocyte esterase (an enzyme released by leukocytes), and for nitrites (which is reduced from nitrates by some bacteria), are an appropriate alternative to urinalysis and urine microscopy, to diagnose cases of acute uncomplicated cystitis. When obtaining a urine specimen for evaluation, it is recommended that in order to avoid contamination, with skin flora the patient should obtain a midstream, clean-catch urine specimen. Since nitrites and leukocyte esterase are the most accurate indicators of uncomplicated cystitis in symptomatic patients, the urine dipsticks are convenient and cost effective. However, critical evaluation of each individual patient's case needs to be evaluated cautiously since even negative results for both tests do not reliably rule out the presence of infection.

An urinalysis is often used to detect UTI's and a clean-catch dipstick leukocyte esterace is a rapid screening test for detecting pyuria, however, the presence of pyuria is nonspecific and does not always indicate clinical UTI. And the presence of bacteriuria alone without symptoms is nonspecific and should not be treated (Nicolle et al. 2019).

The only true diagnosis of a UTI is symptoms associated with a positive urine culture.

Imaging

Typically, no further studies beyond urinalysis and urine cultures are needed to diagnose acute uncomplicated cystitis. In those patients that present with atypical symptoms of acute uncomplicated cystitis, those who do not respond to initial antimicrobial therapy, those with a history of recurrent UTIs, or those with suspected pyelonephritis may need imaging studies to rule out complications and other disorders (see Table 11.2).

Table 11.2 Imaging Considerations

Imaging studies should be considered in the following
Women with febrile infections
Men
If urinary tract obstruction is suspected and with history of
Calculi
Ureteral tumor
Ureteral stricture
Congenital ureteropelvic junction obstruction
Previous urologic surgery or instrumentation
Diabetes
Persistent symptoms despite several days of appropriate antibiotic therapy
Rapid recurrence of infection after apparently successful treatment

Ultrasound (U/S) Ultrasonography is the recommended initial screening tool if testing is indicated. It is noninvasive, is cost effective, has no risk of contrast reaction, and has no risk of radiation exposure. Ultrasonography is able to identify calculi, obstruction of the upper urinary tracts, abscess, and other congenital abnormalities. Renal ultrasounds are the most cost-effective treatment option.

Intravenous Pyelogram (IVP) IVP is useful for visualizing the ureters, the details of calyceal anatomic structures and the presence of calyceal dilatation, and the presence of stricture, stones, or obstruction. The calyceal details are necessary for diagnosis of reflux nephropathy as well as papillary necrosis.

An IVP is usually done in the operating room and requires anesthesia.

Computed Tomography (CT Scan) CT scan offers the best anatomic detail but its cost prevents it from being used for screening. It is more sensitive than ultrasound in the diagnosis of acute focal bacterial nephritis and renal and perirenal abscess (it may demonstrate stones or obstruction).

It is useful if a patient has an abnormal ultrasound.

Patients with known pyelonephritis should have a CT scan with contrast or a U/S to assess the presence of foci of pyelonephritis in the renal cortex or cortical or perinephric abscesses. Immediately after a CT scan with contrast, it is possible to obtain the equivalent of an IVP by taking a KUB (X-ray of kidney, ureter, and bladder) film of the patient in the prone position and observe the anatomic structures of the collecting system and ureters, as the contrast is cleared into the bladder.

Magnetic Resonance Imaging (MRI) MRI provides much greater contrast between different soft tissues than a CT scan. It relies on obtaining a radiofrequency (RF) signal from alignment and subsequent relaxation of protons in hydrogen atoms in water in the body. It should never be utilized in routine practice or as a first-line diagnostic test. It is typically used in follow-up when the ultrasound has already been performed and has been unable to fully answer the diagnostic question. The CT and magnetic resonance imaging (MRI) provide the best anatomic data as well as the cause and extent of the infection.

Risk Factors

Some of the risk factors for UTIs, along with the causes of bacterial persistence, and the factors that increase the risk of complications from UTIs are shown in tables below Table 11.3.

Management of Urinary Tract Infections

Behavioral Modifications

The majority of behavioral interventions are aimed at prevention. Based on a meta-analysis by Smith et al. (2018), there are few recommended behavioral interventions that have shown to reduce recurrent UTIs. These include voiding before or after sexual relations, delaying voiding, wiping from front to back, frequency of urination, douching, tampons, use of hot tubs or bubble baths, body mass index, use of tight clothing, type of clothing, bicycle riding, and volume of fluid consumed. The meta-analysis did find a correlation between spermicide use with or without a contraceptive diaphragm and recurrent UTI among sexually active women. Smith et al. (2018) found that certain prevention strategies were supported by indirect

Table 11.3 Causes of bacterial resistance

Infected stones
Chronic bacterial prostatitis
Unilateral infected atrophic kidney
Vesicovaginal fistula
Intestinal fistula
Ureteral anomalies
Infected diverticula
Foreign bodies (stent or catheters)
Infected urachal cyst
Infected medullary sponge kidney
Infected papillary necrosis
Ureteral stump after nephrectomy
Factors that increase the risk of complications from UTIs
Urinary tract obstruction
Infection from urea-splitting bacteria
Diabetes
Renal papillary necrosis
Neurogenic bladders
Factors that increase the risk of complications from UTIs
Pregnancy
Congenital urinary tract anomalies
Elderly patient with acute bacterial prostatitis
End-stage renal disease on hemodialysis
Immunosuppression after a renal transplant

data; patients with diabetes having good glucose control, normal vaginal pH by avoiding harsh cleaners, limit antibiotic use to under five days, and avoiding broad spectrum or unnecessary antibiotics. The authors felt that though not supported in the literature preventing recurrent UTI through the following practices are advised, maintaining adequate hydration, voiding after intercourse, avoiding delayed voiding, and avoiding sequential anal and vaginal intercourse.

Oral Supplements

There have been several studies looking at the use of cranberry juice to prevent urinary tract infections. Cranberry juice does inhibit bacterial attachment to and pills epithelial cells. Based on a meta-analysis done in 2012, it was concluded that adults that consumed cranberry juice or pills on a regular basis were 38% less likely to develop symptoms of UTI. In addition, the cranberry may reduce the symptoms of UTI by suppressing the inflammatory response. A Cochrane review in 2012 found no evidence of cranberry being effective in the prevention of UTI. It remains unclear which ingredients in cranberry products may be responsible for the overall benefit. Cranberry is essentially safe and inexpensive and is recommended for the prevention of UTI. However, it is not currently recommended as a treatment for acute cystitis.

Pharmacological Treatment

The management of UTIs has become quite complicated due to the increasing prevalence of antibiotic-resistant uropathogens. Symptomatic relief is a high priority in the majority of patients with UTIs. With appropriate antibiotic treatment relief should be obtained within 24 h for an uncomplicated cystitis. Complicated nosocomial UTIs were primarily responsible for antibiotic resistance in the past. However, as things change the resistance has spread to uncomplicated community-acquired UTIs. It is important to try and understand the antibiotic resistance rates within the area that one is practicing (see Table 11.4). Urine levels are more important than serum levels in relation to the efficacy of antibiotics treating UTIs.

Current guidelines in the treatment of acute uncomplicated cystitis with antibiotics recommend nitrofurantoin, fosfomycin, trime thoprim sulfamethoxazole and fluoroquinolones as first-line antibiotics. However, fluoroquinolones have become more of a second-line treatment in the past 10 years due to resistance patterns as

Table 11.4 Antibiotic Stewardship

Choose antibiotics based on the following:
1. Likelihood that it will be active against enteric bacteria that commonly produce UTIs
2. High concentration level of the antibiotic in the urine
3. Tendency not to alter the bowel or vaginal flora
4. Selection for resistant bacteria
5. Limited toxicity
6. Available at a reasonable cost/covered by patient insurance

Table 11.5 Antimicrobial Agents for the Management of Uncomplicated UTI

Tier	Drug	Dosage	Pregnancy category
First	Fosfomycin (Monurol)	3-g single dose	B
	Nitrofurantoin (macrocrystals)	100 mg BID for 5 days	B
	Trimethoprim-sulfamethoxazole (Bactrim/Sulfa)	160/800 BID for 3 days	C
Second	Ciprofloxacin (Cipro)	250 mg BID for 3 days	C
	Ciprofloxacin, extended release (Cipro XR)	500 mg QD for 3 days	C
	Levofloxacin (Levaquin)	250 mg QD for 3 days	C
Third§	Ofloxacin	200 mg QD for 3 days Or 400 mg single dose	C
	Amoxicillin/clavulanate (Augmentin)	500/125 mg BID for 7 days	B
	Cefdinir (Omnicef)	300 mg BID for 10 days	B
	Cefpodoxime	100 mg BID for 7 days	B

well as side-effect profiles (Brubaker et al. 2018). At the writing of this publication the Infectious Disease Society of American was updating their 2010 guidelines.

When treating with nitrofurantoin, or sulfamethoxazole patients with renal impairment especially the elderly must be monitored carefully (see Table 11.5). Although nitrofurantoin is on the BEERS criteria short-term usage has not been shown to be detrimental to patients. Although nitrofurantoin is on the BEERS criteria short term usage has not been shown to be detrimental to patients. Routine monitoring of patient's renal function is recommended in all patients over 65 years of age. Nitrofurantoin is well tolerated, has good efficacy, and does tend to be effective against *Pseudomonas* and *Proteus* species. If symptoms persist after 2–3 days of therapy, one can always consider changing the antibiotic to a more expensive, broad-spectrum antibiotic. However, the recurrence of symptoms after the initial short-course therapy would indicate the need for culture and sensitivity testing, and retreatment should be for a 7–10-day period.

Fluoroquinolones have a very broad spectrum of activity against the majority of uropathogens, including *Pseudomonas*. However, it is not recommended to use this drug class in treating uncomplicated UTIs. This class has limited gram-positive activity and is not effective in treating *Enterococcus*. Fluoroquinolones are very expensive agents and should be reserved for the treatment of complicated UTI, pseudomonal infections, or treatment of resistant organisms.

Recurrent Bacterial Cystitis

Women with recurrent UTIs need a complete history that includes symptoms of dysuria, frequency, urgency, nocturia, incontinence, and hematuria. Include any bowel symptoms such as diarrhea, bowel incontinence, or constipation. Note previous or current antibiotic use, allergies, and prior antibiotic-related problems such as *Clostridium difficile*.

Any vaginal symptoms such as discharge or irritation should be noted. Note the frequency of UTI's and any associations with the UTI such as intercourse or menses. Menopausal status and use of localized estrogens or spermicides should be noted. Obtain surgical history of any previous urinary tract or pelvic surgery. Note urgency, frequency, nocturia, and incontinence between episodes of infection. Document what the patient considers symptoms of a UTI, and relationships of acute triggers to episodes.

Physical exam should include an abdominal and detailed pelvic examination.

Document culture proven symptomatic uncomplicated acute cystitis episodes in the last year. As discussed in uncomplicated cystitis rule out, interstitial cystitis, OAB, kidney or bladder calculi, pelvic floor hypertonicity, bacterial or fungal vaginitis, and dermatitis.

Each recurrent episode must have a urine culture prior to treatment. Obtain a repeat culture when contamination is suspected. Consider a catheterized specimen if unable to get a clean catch. The vaginal flora of a women contains many bacterial species that are considered pathogens in urine (*S. aureus, S. viridans, Enterococci,* and Group B *Streptococci*).

Routine screening of patients should not be initiated. Only screen when a patient is symptomatic. Do not treat ASB.

Over the years, patients have also been treated with long-term prophylactic use of antibiotics. This therapy may have been utilizing nitrofurantoin (50–100 mg every night) or TMP-SMZ (1/2 tab every other night). Typically after 6–12 months, the therapy could be stopped in the hopes that the colonization with uropathogenic gram-negative organisms has resolved. Over the next 6 months, if a patient develops 2–3 episodes of UTI, then another course of prophylaxis would be initiated (Anger et al. 2019).

The current goal in treating UTIs is to decrease the overall use of antibiotics while maintaining a quality of life. Several studies have looked at different strategies that can be used to achieve this goal. One of these strategies is the "self-start" strategy. This relies on the patient to make the clinical diagnosis of UTI, which is typically not difficult for these patients, when the previous infections have been confirmed by a positive culture. These patients are given a prescription for an antibiotic (i.e., TMP-SMZ, cephalexin, or nitrofurantoin), to be taken for 2–3 days at the onset of symptoms. If symptoms persist or reoccur beyond this initial therapy, then an office visit is recommended for culture and sensitivity testing. Self-start therapy works very well in the patient who has been well educated.

Special Situations

There are certain populations in which an otherwise uncomplicated UTI requires more attention. There are physiologic changes that take place during pregnancy that have important implications in regard to ASB and the progression of infection. During pregnancy there is an increased renal size, altered renal function, hydroureteronephrosis, and anterosuperior displacement of the bladder. The rate of pyelonephritis in pregnant females is much higher than that of the nonpregnant female and a 20–40% increase in acute pyelonephritis if ASB is left untreated in the pregnant population (Nicolle et al. 2019). In turn, it is associated with higher rates of prematurity and perinatal mortality. In a pregnant woman with acute uncomplicated UTI, one could consider treating with amoxicillin (250 mg every 8 h), ampicillin (250 mg every 6 h), nitrofurantoin (100 mg every 6 h), or even an oral cephalosporin. As previously noted, amoxicillin and ampicillin are no longer first-line recommendations due to their ability to interfere with the fecal flora.

Young healthy men with no complicating risk factors may be treated with a 7–10-day course of antibiotics. The recommended course of treatment is TMP-SMZ (double strength every 12 h), trimethoprim (100–200 mg every 12 h), or a fluoroquinolone, and a pretreatment culture and sensitivity is recommended in this population. In the middle-aged and elderly population, who are sexually active, no further workup is needed if the infection is eradicated with antibiotic therapy. However, in the younger, nonsexually active, population or when there is a high clinical suspicion, then further workup can be done to look for an abnormality of the urinary tract. One might obtain imaging studies to assess the kidneys, ureters, and bladder, a cystoscopy, and a post-void residual.

Patients with indwelling catheters, whether short term or long term, pose a risk for infection. It should be noted that for every day that a catheter is left indwelling, the risk of colonization is 5–10% per day (Nicolle et al. 2019). The Center for Disease Control (CDC) has completed studies evaluating the majority of circumstances where an indwelling catheter may be utilized. The recommendations can be reviewed at http://www.cdc.gov/hicpac/pdf/CAUTI/CAUTIguideline2009final.pdf and a brief summary of the recommendations are as follows:

- Limit long-term use, especially for the treatment of incontinence, unless the patient has a stage 3 decubitus.
- Limit use in nursing home patients and consider intermittent or external catheter if possible.
- Only use for specific surgical procedures when necessary, not as a routine surgical intervention and remove the catheter within 24 h or as soon as possible.
- Only treat patients with symptoms.
- Do not do routine urine cultures.

In addition, the CDC guidelines support the use of indwelling catheters when attempting to promote comfort and quality of life for the terminal patient and those patients whom will be experiencing prolonged immobilization (i.e., spinal surgery or traumatic injuries, such as pelvic fractures).

Pyelonephritis

Incidence

Acute uncomplicated pyelonephritis is much less common than cystitis. There is an estimated ratio of 1:28 cases of pyelonephritis to that of cystitis, with an annual incidence of 25 cases per 10,000 women between the ages of 15 and 34 years (Hooten 2012).

Presentation

As previously shown in table below Table 11.6, the classic symptoms of pyelone-phritis are any combination of cystitis symptoms, accompanied by bacteriuria, pyuria, fever, chills, flank pain, and/or nausea and vomiting. One should remember that patients with flank pain and UTI do not necessarily have pyelonephritis, and the reverse is true in that patients may actually have a case of pyelonephritis in the absence of local and systemic symptoms. The majority of patients with acute pyelo-nephritis will be ill appearing and may have additional symptoms such as malaise or hypotension. It should create a high level of suspicion if a patient has any of the known risks factors, listed in the table below.

Classification

Pyelonephritis may be caused by several different routes:

1. Ascending: Bacteria reach the renal pelvis through the collecting ducts at the papillary tips and then ascend through the collecting tubules. The presence of urinary reflux from the bladder or increased intrapelvic pressures caused by lower urinary tract obstruction can also cause upper urinary tract infection.
2. Hematogenous: This tends to be the result of *Staphylococcus aureus* septicemia or *Candida* in the blood stream. Hematogenous causes are uncommon.
3. Lymphatic: This is an intraperitoneal infection (i.e., abscess) caused by an unusual form of extension to the renal parenchyma.

The majority of acute uncomplicated pyelonephritis cases can be managed in the outpatient setting. However, if one has diabetes, a renal stone, hemodynamic instability, or is pregnant, then they should be hospitalized for the initial 2–3 days of parenteral therapy. Pyelonephritis can lead to sepsis, hypotension, and even death, especially if the infection is caused by an unrecognized upper tract obstruction.

Flank tenderness is a prominent finding on physical exam. In addition, an infected urine with large amounts of granular or leukocyte casts in the sediment is also indic-ative for the diagnosis. Eighty percent of the cases of pyelonephritis are caused by *E. coli*. In patients who have undergone a form of urinary tract instrumentation, who

Table 11.6 Risk factors for pyelonephritis

Vesicoureteral reflux
Obstruction of the urinary tract (congenital ureteropelvic junction obstruction, stone disease, pregnancy)
Genitourinary tract instrumentation
Diabetes mellitus
Voiding dysfunction
Age (renal scarring rarely begins in adulthood; this is typically related to reflux in children)
Female gender

have had a previous indwelling catheter, or those that have developed a nosocomial infection, the microorganism responsible for the infection in these situations is typically *Pseudomonas, Serratia, Enterobacter, and Citrobacter*. In patients with stone disease, one should suspect *Proteus* or *Klebsiella*. Both of these microorganisms contain the enzyme urease, which has the ability to split urea with the production of ammonia and an alkaline environment. This leads to the precipitation of the salt struvite (magnesium ammonium phosphate), which form branched calculi. These calculi harbor bacteria in the interstices of the renal calculi. These types of stones are referred to as staghorn calculi, which can lead to chronic renal infection.

Diagnostic Testing

Laboratory testing and radiology studies can assist in differentiating the cause. One should order both urine and blood cultures to rule out sepsis. An intravenous urogram may demonstrate normal results or it may show renal enlargement secondary to edema. It is necessary to distinguish whether focal enlargement is a result of a renal mass or abscess. A delayed appearance of the pyelogram or a diminished nephrogram may be caused by inflammation. When assessing an imaging study, the most important thing to rule out is the presence of obstruction and/or urolithiasis. Both of which could lead to a life-threatening situation if left undiagnosed and untreated. Ultrasound is useful in some cases; however, CT may demonstrate the patchy decreased enhancements that suggest focal renal involvement.

Complications

Abnormal findings and complications associated with pyelonephritis are:

(a) Xanthogranulomatous pyelonephritis (XGP)—severe and chronic renal infection that destroys the kidneys.
(b) Chronic pyelonephritis—rare in the absence of an underlying functional or structural abnormality of the urinary tract.
(c) Renal insufficiency—rare complication.
(d) Hypertension—is noted in over 50% of patients.
(e) Renal abscess—collection of purulent material confined to the renal parenchyma.
(f) Infected hydronephrosis—bacterial infection of a hydronephrotic kidney and can often be associated with destruction of the renal parenchyma.
(g) Perinephric abscess—typically results from a rupture of a cortical abscess or hematogenous seeding from another infection site.
(h) Emphysematous pyelonephritis—acute necrotizing parenchyma and perirenal infection caused by gas-forming uropathogens.

Management

In the majority of cases, acute uncomplicated pyelonephritis can be treated on an outpatient basis. However, the patient should be hospitalized in the following situations:

- Nausea or vomiting.
- Dehydrated.
- Pregnant.
- History of non-adherence to medical therapies.
- Evidence of septicemia.

Urine cultures should be obtained on all suspected cases of pyelonephritis. On all hospitalized patients, one should obtain blood cultures and baseline labs to check renal functioning. The results of the blood cultures tend to be positive in approximately 15–20% of patients (Bastani 2001).

Initial treatment for uncomplicated pyelonephritis should be started using a fluoroquinolone pending cultures results. It is becoming a more common practice to administer a single parenteral dose of ceftriaxone (1 g), a consolidated 24 h dose of an aminoglycoside (i.e., gentamicin), or a fluoroquinolone before initiating oral antibiotics (Hanno 2014).

In the outpatient setting, it is recommended to treat with a 10-day course of antibiotics using a fluoroquinolone or trimethoprim-sulfamethoxazole. In the presence of sepsis, it is recommended to treat for 14 days. According to the Infectious Disease Society of America (IDSA), the recommendation is to treat with ciprofloxacin 500 mg BID for 7 days or levofloxacin 750 mg QD × 5 days (2011). If the patient demonstrates improvement within 72 h, then continue the oral antibiotic therapy and obtain a repeat urine culture at 4 days on and 10 days off of the medication. If no improvement is noted, then the patient should be hospitalized and one should review the culture and sensitivity results. In the presence of an obstruction or abscess, treatment and/or drainage of the causative factor would be recommended. Complicated cases of pyelonephritis requiring hospitalization or a procedure may also require up to 3 weeks of antibiotic therapy.

Clinical Pearls

- In uncomplicated UTIs, there is no association between recurrent infections and renal scarring, hypertension, or renal failure.
  - Methenamine or hexamine hippurate are used as urinary antiseptics for chronic therapy, which reduces the risk of antibiotic resistance and efficacy may be increased if used as adjuvant therapy to cranberry supplements. Asymptomatic bacteriuria, in the elderly population, should not be treated.

- In uncomplicated UTIs, there is no association between recurrent infections and renal scarring, hypertension, or renal failure.
- Methenamine or hexamine hippurate are used as urinary antiseptics for chronic therapy, which reduces the risk of antibiotic resistance and efficacy may be increased if used as adjuvant therapy to cranberry supplements.
- Asymptomatic bacteriuria, in the elderly population, may be unjustified and is typically ineffective.
- It is a challenge clinically to differentiate between upper and lower UTI; however, it is most often not necessary because management and treatment are similar.
- Recurrent UTI tends to be biological in nature and not necessarily related to personal hygiene.
- When investigating UTIs, the best overall screening tool remains the retro-peritoneal ultrasonography.
- Due to the risk of pulmonary fibrosis with nitrofurantoin use, it is not recommended as a long-term prophylactic antibiotic of choice. However, it remains an excellent option for short-course treatment of recurrent UTI.
- If a male patient has no culture documented history of a UTI, then it is unlikely that he will have a diagnosis of chronic bacterial prostatitis.

References for Clinicians

AUA Guidelines (https://auanet.org/guidelines)

- Recurrent uncomplicated urinary tract infections in women

AUA White papers (https://auanet.org/whitepapers)

- Beers criteria
- Catheter-associated urinary tract infections

Infectious Disease Society of America Clinical practice guideline for the management of Asymptomatic Bacteriuria retrieved from: https://www.idsociety.org/practice-guideline/asymptomatic-bacteriuria/

Resources for Patients

Urology Care Foundation https://www.urologyhealth.org/educational-materials?product_format=466l&language=1122l
    NIDDK https://www.niddk.nih.gov/search?s=all&q=uti

Bibliography

Anger J, Lee U, Ackerman L, Chou R, Chughtai B, Clemens Q et al (2019) Recurrent uncomplicated urinary tract infections in women: AUA/CUA/SUFU Guideline. J Urol 202(2):282–289. Retrieved from: https://www.auanet.org/guidelines/recurrent-uti

Bass-Ware A, Weed D, Johnson T, Spurlock A (2014) Evaluation of the effect of cranberry juice on symptoms associated with a urinary tract infection. Urol Nurs 34(3):121–127

Bastani B (2001) Urinary tract infections. In: Noble J, Greene HL II, Levinson W, Modest GA, Mulrow CD, Scherger JE, Young MJ (eds) Textbook of primary care medicine, 3rd edn. Mosby, Inc., Missouri, pp 1364–1371

Bernard MS, Hunter KF, Moore KN (2012) A review of strategies to decrease the duration of indwelling urethral catheters and potentially reduce the incidence of catheter-associated urinary tract infections. Urol Nurs 32(1):29–37

Brubaker L, Carberry C, Nardos R, Carter-Brooks C, Lowder L (2018) American Urogynecologic Society best-practice statement: recurrent urinary tract infection in women. Female Pelvic Med Reconstr Surg 24(5):321–323

Center for Disease Control and Prevention (2005) Urinary tract infections [Disease Listing]. Retrieved from http://www.cdc.gov/ncidod/dbmd/diseaseinfo/urinarytractinfections_t.htm

Center for Disease Control and Prevention (2009) Guideline for prevention of catheter associated urinary tract infections 2009. Retrieved from http://www.cdc.gov/hicpac/pdf/CAUTI/CAUTIguideline2009final.pdf

Colgan R, Williams M (2011) Diagnosis and treatment of acute uncomplicated cystitis. Am Family Phys 84(7):771–776. Retrieved from http://www.aafp.org/afp/2011/1001/p771.html

Ellsworth P, Onion DK (2012) The little black book of urology, 3rd edn. Jones & Bartlett Learning, Sudbury, pp 68–71

Goldman HB (2001) Evaluation and management of recurrent urinary-tract infections. In: Kursch ED, Ulchaker JC (eds) Office urology: the clinician's guide. Humana Press Inc., Totowa, pp 105–111

Gould CV, Umscheid CA, Agarwal RK, Kuntz G, Pegues DA, Healthcare Infection Control Practices Advisory Committee (HICPAC) (2009) Guideline for catheter associated urinary tract infections 2009. Center for Disease Control and Prevention. Retrieved from http://www.cdc.gov/hicpac/pdf/cauti/cautiguideline2009final.pdf

Gupta K, Hooton TM, Naber KG, Wullt B, Colgan R, Miller LG, Moran GJ, Nicolle LE, Raz R, Schaeffer AJ, Soper DE (2011) International clinical practice guidelines for the treatment of acute uncomplicated cystitis and pyelonephritis in women: a 2010 update by the Infectious Diseases Society of America and the European Society for Microbiology and Infectious Diseases. Clin Infect Dis 52(5):e103–e120

Hanno PM (2014) Lower urinary tract infections in women and pyelonephritis. In: Hanno PM, Guzzo TJ, Malkowicz SB, Wein AJ (eds) Penn clinical manual of urology, 2nd edn. Elsevier Saunders, Philadelphia, pp 110–132

Harlow HF (1983) Fundamentals for preparing psychology journal articles. J Comp Physiol Psychol 55:893–896

Hooten TM (2012) Uncomplicated urinary tract infection. N Engl J Med 366:1028–1037. Retrieved from http://www.nejm.org/doi/full/10.1056/NEJMcp1104429

Jepson RG, Williams G, Craig JC (2012) Cranberries for preventing urinary tract infections. Cochrane Database Syst Rev 10(10):CD001321. https://doi.org/10.1002/14651858.CD001321.pub5

Macfarlane MT (2013) Urology, 5th edn. Lippincott Williams & Wilkins, Philadelphia, pp 86–110

Medina M, Castillo-Pino E (2019) An introduction to the epidemiology and burden of urinary tract infections. Ther Adv Urol 11:3–7. https://doi.org/10.1177/1756287219832172

Nicolle LE, Gupta K, Bradley S, DeMuri GP, Drekonja D et al (2019) Clinical practice guidelines for the management of asymptomatic bacteriuria: 2019 Update by the Infectious Disease Society of America. Italicized Clin Infectious Dis 68:e83–e109

Sandock DS, Kursh ED (1995) Urinary tract infections in adult females. In: Resnick MI, Novick AC (eds) Urology secrets. Hanley & Belfus, Inc., Philadelphia, pp 205–207

Smith AL, Brown J, Wyman JF, Berry A, Newman DK, Stapelton AE (2018) Treatment and prevention of recurrent lower urinary tract infections in women: a rapid review with practice recommendations. J Urol 200(6):1174–1191

Society of Urological Nurses Association (2010) Prevention & control of catheter-associated urinary tract infection (CAUTI) [clinical practice guidelines]. Retrieved from https://www.suna.org/sites/default/files/download/cautiGuideline.pdf

Stamm WE, Norrby SR (2001) Urinary tract infections: disease panorama and challenges. J Infect Dis 183(Suppl 1):S1–S4. Retrieved from http://www.ncbi.nlm.nih.gov/pubmed/11171002

Uphold CR, Graham MV (1998) Clinical guidelines in family practice, 3rd edn. Barmarrae Books, Gainesville, pp 601–607

Zalmanovici TA, Lador A, Sauerbrun-Cutler MT, Leibovici L (2015) Antibiotics for asymptomatic bacteriuria (review). Cochrane Databases Syst Rev 4:1–27

Basics of Pre and Postoperative Management Specific to Urology Patients

12

Tasha M. O. Carpenter, Marc M. Crisenbery, and Michelle J. Lajiness

Contents

T. M. O. Carpenter (✉)
University of Michigan Health System, Pre-Operative Clinic,
Ann Arbor, MI, USA
e-mail: tharr@med.umich.edu

M. M. Crisenbery · M. J. Lajiness
Department of Urology, UTMC, Toledo, OH, USA
e-mail: Michelle.Lajiness@utoledo.edu

© Springer Nature Switzerland AG 2020
S. A. Quallich, M. J. Lajiness (eds.), *The Nurse Practitioner in Urology*,
https://doi.org/10.1007/978-3-030-45267-4_12

Objectives
1. Discuss the key points to consider in the preoperative evaluation of patients
2. Explain the process for preoperative risk stratification
3. Considerations for patient education and lifestyle modifications
4. Discuss postoperative care of the urological patient
5. Discuss interventions for common urological postoperative complications

Introduction

Placing patients into an operating room can be a life-altering experience, complicated by both the adaptable and unadaptable comorbidities and lifestyle habits of the individual. Classically, patients have been evaluated and "cleared" by their general practitioner for an upcoming procedure. While involvement of a routine provider is essential to the long-term success in patient outcomes, further workup that involves a focus on categories of airway assessment, medication management, and risk stratification play an important role in the safety and success of the perioperative setting. This chapter aims to educate the clinician on guidelines for a preoperative assessment of a surgical candidate.

History Specifics

When assessing a patient prior to surgery, the first step is to determine medical comorbidities. Patients may present with a variety of medical conditions that, without appropriate preoperative management, can lead to such perioperative complications as bleeding, infection, poor wound healing, and negative anesthesia outcomes. While the following is not an exhaustive list of comorbidities, these common diagnoses require thorough documentation and management.

Cardiac History and Examination

- Arrhythmias: Document onset and duration of arrhythmia, type of arrhythmia, in addition to related medical and surgical interventions.
- Coronary stents versus coronary artery bypass grafting (CABG): Placement of coronary stents versus CABG may change anticoagulation management in the preoperative setting. In addition to procedural type, attempt to document placement of stents. In general, patients are given an implant card to be kept on them, of which documents type and placement of stent. In setting of CABG, document where grafting was taken, i.e., mammary versus lower extremity.
- CHF: Ask patient about associated hospitalizations, and obtain cardiac testing. Upon obtaining most recent echocardiogram, document left ventricular ejection fraction. If there are no recent cardiac studies, and/or patient has been lost to cardiac follow-up, consider cardiology referral and repeat imaging.
- Cardiac valve repairs versus valve replacements: Documenting a valvular repair versus replacement can also alter anticoagulation plan. This is once again a good opportunity to ask patient for their implantable device card, should they have undergone a valve replacement. Look for information on porcine versus bovine versus mechanical valve.

Pulmonary History and Examination

- Smoking history: Quantify your patient's smoking history as a pack year history, and be sure to ask about cigarette replacement products. In addition to tobacco products, be clear in asking patient about modalities that are advertised as tobacco-free, such as E-cigarettes and vaping.
- Supplemental oxygen: Question patient on use of supplemental oxygen. It is helpful to document chronic versus prn status, and typical settings when in use.
- Asthma/Chronic Obstructive Pulmonary Disease (COPD): Ask patients about their inhaler regimen, if applicable. In patients that utilize inhalers, ask about frequency of use for the prn products, which can provide a picture for how well-managed their lung function is. Question patients on whether they have required either hospitalization and/or intubation for their pulmonary diagnosis.

History and Examination Specifics for Patients with Diabetes

A diabetic patient should have thorough documentation on last Hemoglobin A1C, foot exam, and ophthalmology consult, as applicable. Individuals who appear to lack routine diabetic care may be a candidate for referral to endocrinology, or consult placed to follow up with their primary provider before surgery.

Both non-insulin and insulin-dependent diabetics provide an opportunity for careful medication reconciliation in the preoperative setting. A constant influx of new diabetes pharmaceutical options, in addition to frequent fluctuations of patient insulin demands, can rapidly alter the medication directions given to your surgical candidate.

History and Examination Specifics for Patients with Rheumatology

Documenting rheumatologic conditions in any surgical candidate should include applicable medications, history of exacerbations, and certainly associated surgical history. These individuals, depending on condition, may be of increased risk for postoperative infections and disease flares. Consider involving the patient's rheumatologist, or placing rheumatology consult for those without routine care.

Physical Examination Specifics for Patients Who Have a History of Previous Surgery

Obtaining a thorough surgical history is essential to the preoperative planning. While it is important to document the patient's past procedures, this is of upmost importance in the surgical setting, as it can dramatically change the approach and possible complications of a pending case.

When asking the patient about their surgical history, consider a more detailed documentation than only the title of the procedure. For example, a patient with a past surgical history of hysterectomy: Was this an abdominal approach or a vaginal approach? If abdominal incisions are in place, document whether the surgery was performed laparoscopic or open. Depending on your medical institution, the capacity for robotic or laparoscopic cases on your patient may be altered based on presence of previous incisions. Such incisions can lead to adhesions, and complicate minimally invasive approaches, leading to the need to convert to open incisions

In addition to documenting patient-reported surgical history, remember to perform a complete physical exam. While patients may not intend to falsely provide all surgical history, it has been a frequent experience that additional surgical scars are identified on exam that are not consistent with the patient-provided history. Common misnomers have been that the procedure was as a child and does not need to be mentioned; or simply that the undocumented surgery was on a different organ system, and patient assumes that it is not pertinent. Ask patients the following:

- ALL surgeries from birth to present. Consider asking specifically about procedures that may not be considered "surgery," such as vasectomy or hernia repair as an infant.
- Laparoscopic versus hand-assisted versus open procedures
- Presence or history of herniations

In addition to asking patients about incision sites, it is important to ask about mesh and other implantable devices. As with the aforementioned complications of adhesions, the presence of these objects can alter the surgical plan. Ask patients specifically about the presence of the following:

- Mesh (slings, hernia mesh);
- and implantable devices (baclofen pumps, nerve stimulators, penile implants, artificial sphincters).

Medication History

Relying on what may be previously entered as the patient's medication list may not be thorough enough in the preoperative setting. It is important to consider all categories of medications, including the following:

- Prescription tablets and capsules;
- Topical medications;
- Injectable medications (insulin, disease-modifying antirheumatic drugs [DMARDS]);
- Implantable medications (baclofen pumps, intrauterine device [IUD]);
- Inhaled medications (nebulizers, inhalers);
- Use of over-the-counter medications (proton-pump inhibitor drugs [PPIs], antihistamines);
- and vitamins and mineral supplements.

Establishing Functional Capacity

Surgical optimization of your patient should include assessment of their functional capacity. Questions about the patient's ability to perform activities of daily living, exercise regimen, and ambulatory aids can provide valuable information for guidance of intraoperative outcomes and postoperative care needs. A useful tool to guide you on a patient's functional capacity is the Duke Activity Status Index (DASI) (Hlatky et al. 1989; Coutinho-Myrrha et al. 2014). This screening tool incorporates a range of questions that provide a summary of the patient's ability to perform small effort tasks of eating and dressing themselves, to rigorous tasks that involve yard work and participation in sports. Each item carries a score, and by adding all "yes" answers, clinicians are able to estimate a patient's METs (metabolic equivalents). Adding the points and dividing by 3.5 will provide a METs score. For consideration of further workup, a score of 4 or under may justify further preoperative testing (Table 12.1).

Table 12.1 Example of Duke Activity Status Index

Activity	METS
Able to engage in self-care such as eating, dressing, bathing, toileting	2.75
Walk indoors around the house	1.75
Walk at least a block on level ground	2.75
Climb a flight of stairs or walk up a hill	5.50
Run a short distance	8.00
Do light housework, such as washing dishes	2.70
Do heavier housework such as moving furniture	8.00
Do moderate housework such as carrying groceries	3.50
Do yard work such as pushing a mower	4.50
Participate in sexual activity	5.25
Exercise such as golfing or tennis	6.00
Exercise such as swimming or basketball	7.50

Preoperative Testing

Electrocardiogram

Follow institutional and surgical center guidelines on obtaining ECG, possibly based on age, body mass index (BMI) and/or comorbidities (Fleisher et al. 2014). This is a routine study performed on males 45 year old and older, and females 55 year old and above. When protocols are not in place for your surgical facility, useful guidelines can be found within the American College of Cardiology/American Heart Association Task Force on Practice Guidelines (2014).

Laboratory Studies

Routine blood tests can include a complete blood count, comprehensive panel and coagulation studies (PT/PTT) in patients without recent studies, particularly those being evaluated for inpatient postoperative courses. This will provide assessment for preoperative clinicians, but also provide a baseline for inpatient providers.

The surgical candidate may benefit from preoperative type and screen, particularly in the setting of open surgical approaches and inpatient stays. Consider patient history of hematologic conditions such as anemia and thrombocytopenia, prompting increased risk of requiring perioperative blood products.

Consider ordering a baseline A1C in patients that lack recent testing. This can guide you on necessity of preoperative endocrinology evaluation, medication management, and risk stratification of the pending surgery.

Both symptomatic and asymptomatic bacteriuria have the potential to complicate a urology procedure. Obtain a urine culture in the preoperative setting, and treat per institution and/or surgeon guidelines.

Studies have shown that colonization of *S. aureus* is the biggest predictor of invasive *S. aureus* infection (Septimus 2019). Dependent on hospital guidelines, consider a preoperative staph swab particularly in patient populations that will be undergoing a procedure that includes an implantable device.

Chest X-ray

A preoperative chest X-ray can be helpful when evaluating patients that are at a higher risk of postoperative pneumonia, difficult extubation, or require oncologic staging. Depending on your institutional guidelines, consider an AP and Lateral view in the following patients:

- Recent asthma/COPD exacerbation
- Recent pneumonia
- Current tobacco use
- Pulmonary physical exam changes from baseline
- Department protocols on staging

Additional Cardiac Testing

When obtaining patient history and performing a physical exam, utilize this valuable information to determine whether the patient warrants further cardiac testing. Items to review when considering an additional workup:

- METs <4 (see Duke Functional Capacity Index)
- New murmur on exam
- Exertional chest pain
- Shortness of breath at rest
- New EKG findings, i.e., left bundle branch block

Anesthesia Assessment

Anesthesia assessment has traditionally occurred in the preoperative holding area on the day of surgery. The concern of such delayed assessment is multifactorial; depending on the surgical center, some outpatient facilities may not have the capacity to handle difficult airways. Additionally, undiagnosed conditions such as obstructive sleep apnea may cause unnecessary complications in extubating your patient. Screening of potential difficult airways can help to avoid last-minute delays or cancellations of cases, and can be quickly added as part of the history and physical exam. One of the key questions to ask patients, and family members if available, is whether or not patients have had difficulty in the past with anesthesia and or being intubated.

Table 12.2 Mallampati score

Score	Description
Class I	Soft palate and uvula fully visible
Class II	Uvula partially obscured by base of tongue
Class III	Only soft palate can be visualized
Class IV	Soft palate not visible; only hard palate is visualized

Reproduced from the reference (Nuckton et al. 2006) with permission

The Mallampati airway evaluation (Table 12.2) is helpful in identifying patients with a potential difficult airway. This rapid assessment is performed on physical exam, and determines whether the patient may be a complex intubation. The patient should sit upright with their head in a neutral position. By asking the patient to open their mouth and stick out their tongue, the clinician is able to grade their airway from a Class I to a Class IV. This information is obtained by how much of the soft palate and uvula are visible. This score helps predict sleep apnea and the ease with which a patient can be intubated. Other factors to be considered are previous issues being intubated, whether or not his patient has in high palate, a short neck, configuration of the teeth/buck teeth, reduced mouth opening, a small mouth, and mandibular protrusion.

Cervical Spine Range of Motion

A surgical candidate's physical exam should include evaluation of their cervical spine range of motion. Less invasive cases that may require only IV sedation, i.e., cystoscopy, are less concerning than an abdominal case that requires general anesthesia and intubation, i.e., cystectomy. Regardless, documentation of flexion, extension, and rotation will be helpful for the anesthesia team.

A unique demographic that may warrant cervical spine imaging is in the Trisomy 21 population. These individuals are at a higher risk of atlantoaxial instability. If previous X-ray views have not been obtained, consider cervical spine X-rays as part of your preoperative testing.

Sleep Apnea

Sleep apnea patients carry increased complications during surgical procedures, particularly those that are either noncompliant with their mask or those that remain undiagnosed/untreated. These risks may include (but are not limited to) hypertension, pulmonary hypertension, heart failure, nocturnal cardiac dysrhythmias, myocardial infarcts, and ischemic stroke (Brenner et al. 2014). Statistically, sleep apnea may remain undiagnosed in up to 80% of patients at the time of surgery. Such perioperative complications of sleep apnea include an increased sensitivity to anesthetic agents, hemodynamic fluctuations, and altered requirements for pain management. Ask patients and screen for the following:

Table 12.3 STOP Bang Questionnaire

S	Snoring loudly, enough to be heard through closed doors?
T	Feeling tired and fatigued or sleepy during the daytime?
O	Being observed stopping breathing or gasping during your sleep?
P	High blood pressure?
B	Body Mass Index >35?
A	Age >50
N	Neck circumference greater than 15.7 in.?
G	Male gender
Obstructive Sleep Apnea (OSA)—Low Risk: Yes to 0–2 questions	
OSA—Intermediate Risk: Yes to 3–4 questions	
OSA—High Risk: Yes to 5–8 questions	
or Yes to 2 or more of 4 STOP questions + male gender	
or Yes to 2 or more of 4 STOP questions + BMI >35 kg/m^2	
or Yes to 2 or more of 4 STOP questions + neck circumference 17 in. /43 cm in male or 16 in./41 cm in female	

Reproduced from the reference (Chung et al. 2008) with permission

- Do you have a known difficult airway?
- Do you have limited range of motion in your neck? Is this related to a past procedure or to pain?
- STOP BANG questionnaire (Table 12.3)

A helpful screening tool for sleep apnea is the STOP BANG questionnaire, which involves both subjective and objective analysis of the patient's candidacy for a polysomnogram. A score of 3 or greater is considered high risk, and warrants referral to sleep medicine.

American Society of Anesthesiologists Physical Status Classification System

The American Society of Anesthesiologists (ASA) Physical Status Classification System (Table 12.4) was developed over 60 years ago as method to assess and communicate a patient's pre-anesthesia medical comorbidities (Hurwitz et al. 2017). The advantage of being familiar with this classification system is that more and more advanced practice providers (APP) may be involved in pre-op evaluation of patients. This classification system can help determine whether it is safe for patient to be scheduled at an outpatient surgery center, or an off-site surgery center as opposed to the main hospital with its full contingent resources. Most APP is working in urology clinics will come across patients that can be classified as ASA Class 1–4; this may involve preoperative scheduling decisions regarding outpatient surgery center versus full hospital operating room.

However, the ASA classification system alone cannot fully predict the perioperative risks for patients, but when used as a metric with other factors that can include age, specific type of surgery (e.g., open versus laparoscopic), and anticipated length of surgery, it can be helpful in establishing the most appropriate surgical facility at

Table 12.4 Examples of the American Society of Anesthesiologists Physical Status Classification System

ASA Class	Explanation
CLASS I	Normal healthy patients with no significant systemic disease: fit, nonobese patient
CLASS II	Patients with mild to moderate systemic disease (examples include but are not limited to): A. Mild, stable angina B. Diabetes mellitus—well controlled C. Controlled essential hypertension D. Stable, mild degree of pulmonary insufficiency—COPD, asthma, chronic bronchitis E. Minimally decreased renal function F. Mild to moderate obesity
CLASS III	Patients with moderate to severe systemic disease (examples include but are not limited to): A. Poorly controlled insulin-dependent diabetes mellitus (BS >300, <500) B. Immunosuppressed (HIV with CDH4 <200, PMN <500) C. Moderate degree of pulmonary insufficiency (Saturation <85% room air) D. Previous myocardial infarction with frequent angina E. Compensated congestive heart failure F. Moderate renal failure G. Chronic hepatic disease H. Extreme obesity (BMI >40) I. Poorly controlled hypertension J. One or more moderate to severe systemic diseases
CLASS IV	Patients with severe systemic disease that is a constant threat to his/her life (examples include but are not limited to): A. Coronary artery disease with unstable angina or recent MI B. Acute and/or uncompensated CHF with pulmonary edema and/or decreased cardiac output C. Advanced degree of pulmonary, hepatic, renal, or endocrine insufficiency with severe metabolic and electrolyte abnormalities
CLASS V	Patient not expected to survive without the operation
CLASS VI	Brain-dead patient being prepared for organ donation

which to schedule a patient, which in turn can affect facility reimbursement. It can also potentially provide insight into the potential for postoperative complications.

Venous Thromboembolism (VTE) Risk Stratification

The combination of surgical trauma with a postoperative decrease in activity level places your surgical candidate at an increased risk of a venous thromboembolic event. By performing a risk stratification assessment in the preoperative setting, a clinician is able to determine whether their patient is a candidate for pneumatic compression devices and chemoprophylaxis.

While the Caprini assessment is a valuable tool to screen patients, make sure to consult with the patient's surgeon before proceeding with preoperative and intraoperative anticoagulation. Depending on the procedure, the risk of bleeding and hematoma may outweigh the concern for thrombus formation. Institutional guidelines may vary for administration of these medications, but a score of 5 or greater, particularly in-patient cases, warrants consideration of chemoprophylaxis (Table 12.5).

Table 12.5 Venous Thromboembolism (VTE) Risk Stratification

1. Point risk factors	• Abnormal lung function such as COPD • Acute MI • Age 41–60 years • Body mass index greater than 25 • CHF diagnosed within the past month • Early on bed rest • History of inflammatory bowel disease • History of prior major surgery within the preceding 4 weeks • History of unexplained still more and or recurrent spontaneous abortion • Minor surgery • Oral contraceptive or hormone replacement • Pregnancy or postpartum in past 4 weeks • Premature birth with toxemia or growth restricted infant • Sepsis within the last 4 weeks • Serious lung disease diagnosed within the previous 4 weeks • Swollen legs • Varicose veins
2. Point risk factors	• Age 61–74 years • Arthroscopic surgery • Central venous access • Confined to bed for greater than 72 h • Immobilizing cast within the previous month • Laparoscopic surgery less than 45 min • Major surgery lasting more than 45 min • Past or present malignancy
3. Point risk factors	• Age 75 or greater • Elevated anticardiolipin antibodies • Elevated serum homocysteine • Family history of thrombosis • Heparin induced thrombocytopenia • Other congenital or acquired thrombophilia • Personal history of DVT/PE • Positive factor V Leiden • Positive lupus anticoagulant • Positive prothrombin 20210A
4. Point risk factors	• Acute spinal cord injury within the preceding 4 weeks • Elective major lower extremity arthroplasty • History of a hip, pelvis, or leg fracture within the preceding 4 weeks • History of multiple traumas within the preceding 4 weeks • STROKE within the preceding 4 weeks

Adapted from Caprini et al. 1991.

Patient Education for Optimizing Outcomes

The importance of patient education is essential for preoperative optimization, intraoperative safety, and postoperative success. This section will focus on opportunities to ensure that patients are aware of all medication instructions, but also provides suggestions for patient involvement that may provide short- and long-term health benefits.

The reconciliation and management of a patient's medications in the preoperative setting can decrease such surgical complications as bleeding, poor wound healing, infection, and length of stay. The following provides some general guidelines to adjustment and manage your patient's medications. Know that these are guidelines only, and specific medication adjustments may depend on your institutional protocols and a patient's prescribing providers.

Diabetes Medication Management

Preoperative management of diabetes is a vital piece of ensuring a good surgical outcome. This means a reduction in morbidity and mortality, avoidance of hyper- or hypoglycemia, promotion of good fluid and electrolyte balance by prevention of ketoacidosis less than 140 mg/dL in a healthy stable diabetic patient (Sudhakaran and Surani 2015). A natural extension of this goal of management is to cancel emergency procedures if the patient presents with diabetic ketoacidosis or a glucose reading above 400 mg/dL.

Provided below are guidelines for a variety of diabetes medications (Table 12.6).

Table 12.6 Guidelines for diabetes management

Night before procedure	Guide
Oral medications	Take usual dose
Insulin at night: NPH, mixed	Take usual dose
Regular insulin	Take usual dinner dose
Glargine insulin alone	50% usual dose
Glargine insulin + additional insulin at meals	70% usual dose
Non-insulin injectables	Take usual dose
Insulin pump	Basal rate stays constant pre-op
	Additional adjustments in consultations with endocrinologist /PCP
Morning of procedure/surgery	**Guide**
Oral medication	Hold dose
Morning insulin: NPH, mixed, glargine	50% usual dose
Morning insulin: Glargine insulin + additional insulin at meals	70% usual dose
Regular insulin or Non-insulin injectables	Hold dose
Insulin pump	Basal rate reduced to 70%

Adapted from: Bodnar, T.W. & Gianchandani, R. (2014) Preprocedure and Preoperative Management of Diabetes Mellitus, *Postgraduate Medicine, 126*:6, 73–80

Anticoagulation Medication Management

Below are guidelines for a number of common anticoagulation medications (Table 12.7) other. When assessing the capacity and duration for preoperative holding of anticoagulants, factor in the following questions:

1. Can my patient safely stop their anticoagulation, given its indication?
2. How does their renal function factor into length of hold?
3. Does my patient need to be bridged off of their anticoagulant?
4. Has prescribing clinician provided feedback or agreement on the anticoagulation plan?

Additional Medication Management

Basic guidelines for preoperative management of cardiac medications, with the caveat that there can always be exceptions:

- Beta-blockers—continue
- ACE-Inhibitors and ARBs—hold for 18 h before surgery
- Diuretics—hold on the morning of surgery
- Anti-arrhythmic—continue
- Calcium channel blockers—continue

Table 12.7 Guide for preoperative anticoagulation management

Medication	Interval between last dose and procedure
Apixaban	2 days with creatinine clearance >60 mL/min 3 days with creatinine clearance 50–59 mL/min 5 days with creatinine clearance <30 to 49 mL/min
Aspirin	7 days
Clopidogrel	7 days
Dabigatran	1–2 days with the creatinine clearance greater than 50 mL/min 3–5 days with creatinine clearance less than 50 mL/min
Lovenox	24 h; consider Lovenox bridge
Prasugrel	7 days
Rivaroxaban	Greater than 1 day with normal renal function 2 days with creatinine clearance 60–90 mL/min 3 days with creatinine clearance 30–59 mL/min 4 days with creatinine clearance 15–29 mL/min
Warfarin	1–8 days depending on INR

Adapted from Baron et al. 2013.
NOTE. Anticoagulation plan includes discussion with prescribing provider on indication for use, in addition to consult with surgery team. Type of planned anesthesia administration (general versus neuraxial) can affect the duration for preoperative hold of these medications

Vitamins and Supplements: The market for herbal supplements and vitamins is booming, and is commonly portrayed to the general public as safe. On the contrary, it is important to educate your patient that many of these OTC products can be as risky or more risky than their prescription medications. There is limited regulation of these products, and dosing standards can vary greatly. As a result, they must be carefully managed along with a patient's prescribed items. Below is not an exhaustive list of supplements, but provides guidelines on some commonly used items. When in doubt, unless prescribed for specific dietary purposes, it is safer to hold these medications for a minimum of 7 days before surgery.

- Multivitamins—hold for 7 days
- Fish Oil—hold for 7 days
- Garlic, ginger, cinnamon, green tea (tablet form)—hold for 7 days
- Glucosamine-chondroitin—hold for 7 days
- Creatine—hold for 7 days
- CoQ10—hold for 14 days

Additional medication instructions for other classes of medications:

- NSAIDS—hold for 7 days
- Stimulants (i.e., ADHD medications)—hold for 2 days
- Aromatase Inhibitors—hold on the day of surgery
- Tamoxifen—hold for 14 days before surgery
- Weight loss products (i.e., Adipex)—hold for 7 days
- Niacin—hold on the day of surgery
- Disease-modifying antirheumatic drugs (DMARD)—consult rheumatology
  - Discussion with patient's rheumatologist will provide information on risk versus benefit of holding medication. Depending on indication for use, there may be greater concern for disease flare than for immunosuppression. One must also factor in the type of surgical procedure, and whether concern for postoperative wound healing necessitates the hold.

Bowel Preps:
- Yogurt prep—Research on yogurt preps before cystectomy procedures have identified multiple positive outcomes, to include decreased surgical site infections, decreased postoperative diarrhea and decreased length of postoperative antibiotics (Kasatpibal et al. 2017). The suggested benefit of probiotics in the preoperative setting encourages balance of healthy gut flora, which can play a beneficial role in these high-risk procedures.
- The yogurt prep may be started as soon as patient education can be provided, and continued until 2 days before day of surgery (patient is generally switched to a clear liquid diet on the day before surgery). This prep suggests that patients consume a probiotic yogurt daily.

Carbohydrate loading: Providing education on carbohydrate loading can be an inexpensive and readily accessible modality to improve patient experience and surgical outcomes in a variety of ways. It has been proven to stimulate the return of post-op bowel function by several days (>2 days), decreasing incidence and duration of post-op ileus (Noblett et al. 2006). It also deters the catabolic response to surgery by conserving lean tissue mass and reducing nitrogen losses (Yuill et al. 2005). Additional benefits include decreasing length of stay (>3 days) (Melis et al. 2006) and increasing capacity to cope with hemorrhagic and endotoxemic stressors. Furthermore, there is evidence of both subjective and objective improvements in postoperative nausea and vomiting (Hausel et al. 2001). Suggested patient instructions may be as follows:

- Buy at least 36 oz of 100% pure, no sugar added white grape juice (no substitutions) You may need to buy a 64 oz bottle or 2–32 oz bottles of this juice.
- After dinner and before midnight the night before surgery, drink 24 oz of the juice.
- On the morning of surgery, drink 12 oz of the juice. You need to finish this 2–3 h before your scheduled surgery time. This means you may need to drink it on your drive to the hospital, depending on what time surgery is.
- If you are on a fluid restriction, include this amount of juice in your restriction.
- If you need a bowel prep the day before surgery, this must be completed after your bowel prep.

Lifestyle Modifications

A discussion on modifiable factors of your patient's lifestyle can provide tools that will improve surgical outcomes, but also provide patients with knowledge on healthy habits that can benefit their well-being long after the perioperative interim. The following should be included when assessing lifestyle modifications, but consider all behavioral factors when evaluating the patient in the preoperative setting. When available, include the patient's support system in these discussions, as encouragement from their loved ones can provide structure and routine.

- Exercise: Encourage your patient to increase their physical activity where possible. A common misnomer heard among patients is that they should decrease their activity prior to surgery, when in fact it is the opposite. By maintaining muscle mass and flexibility, patients can decrease their risk of falls, loss of lean muscle mass, even loss of independence as present in the preoperative setting.
- In an era of smart watches and phones with built-in pedometers, talk to your patient about logging their steps or minutes of exercise to obtain a baseline. Encourage even the smallest increases in activity leading up to their surgery day.
- Tobacco cessation: Your surgical patient has presumably been educated on tobacco cessation in some capacity, whether in their primary care setting or specialty office. Take the opportunity to further educate your patient on the surgical

complications of tobacco use, to include but not limited to increased postoperative infection rates and decreased wound healing. Keep in mind that some department guidelines may consider tobacco use as a reason for cancellation or delay of elective procedures.
- Options to discuss with your patient:
  - Support groups
  - Nicotine-replacement products to wean use, such as Bupropion, Varenicline
- Dietary changes: Discuss your patient's current food choices, and find room to encourage an increase in whole fruits and vegetables, lean meats, and healthy fats. There are a variety of excellent websites to provide to your patient, including Centers for Disease Control, Food and Drug Administration, and the American Diabetes Association.
- Relaxation/Stress: Decreasing stressors and improving relaxation before a surgery can provide both subjective and objective improvements to patient outcomes. Some topics to consider:
  - Sleep hygiene
  - Mindfulness and meditation
  - Participating in hobbies
  - Deep breathing
  - Developing/maintaining a support system

Clinical Pearls
- Do not rely on patient-entered medication lists, ask directly about all medications, including non-prescription. It has been found that without asking such a question directly, patients will not recognize them as items to disclose, or items that may complicate surgery.
- On physical exam, always assess the surgical site. Both inaccuracies of historical information on the area from patient reports (i.e., past surgeries) or acute information, such as rashes or wounds, can delay or cancel a case on the day of surgery.
- A pending surgery is one of the best times to discuss lifestyle changes, as patients are oftentimes more motivated for a successful surgical outcome than they are during a routine appointment. Take advantage of discussions on smoking cessation, alcohol consumption and exercise routines.
- Have a discussion with the anesthesiology team about intended type of anesthesia. Some protocols or providers may request longer preoperative holds of anticoagulation (i.e., neuraxial)
- These visits entail a significant amount of patient education (Table 12.8). Make sure to send the patient home with written instructions, and even ask ahead of the pre-op visit to have friends/family join them. Another set of ears can make a huge difference in adhering to preoperative instructions

Table 12.8 Urology preoperative education for patients

Surgery/procedure	Drains/ catheters/ incisions	Instructions to patients
Cystoscopy	None	• Hematuria common should clear spontaneously within 48 h • Dysuria common should clear spontaneously within 48 h • Call to EC with fever >101.5, more blood than urine or inability to urinate

Cystectomy + neo-bladder	• Incisions
	• Foley
	• Will have drains usually removed prior to discharge
		• Will require 2–3 day hospital stay (bring loose clothes to wear home)
		• Diet progress from clear liquids to soft slowly. Ensure adequate protein liquid initially
		• Foley care
		  – Keep urethra site clean and dry—if bothersome ok to use A&D ointment or antibiotic ointment
		  – Secure catheter with security device to prevent movement
		  – Bladder spasms possible—call if bothersome
		  – Keep bag below the bladder
		  – How to change from leg bag to overnight bag
		• Bowel prep per institution/surgeon guidelines/preference
		• Discuss potential for ISC
		• Post-op appointments
		  – Foley removal
		  – Staple removal
		  – Pathology results
		• To EC/call with:
		  – Fever >101.5
		  – Uncontrollable pain
		  – Incision cite redness, inflammation warmth to touch
		  – Wound drainage that is purulent and continuous or getting worse
		  – Inability to have a bowel movement or pass gas

(continued)

Table 12.8 (continued)

Surgery/procedure	Drains/ catheters/ incisions	Instructions to patients

Cystectomy + ileal conduit	• Incisions
	• Stoma
	• Foley
	• Will have drains usually removed prior to discharge
	• Stents out through stoma
		• Will require 2–3 day hospital stay (bring loose clothes to wear home)
		• Diet progress from clear liquids to soft slowly. Ensure adequate protein liquid initially Bowel prep per institution/ surgeon guidelines/preference
		• Stoma care
		  – Should be pink/red
		  – Stents will be present
		  – Will learn to apply the bag in hospital
		  – It is normal for the stoma to shrink in the initial post-op period
		• Post-op appointment
		  – Staple removal
		  – Pathology results
		• To EC/call with:
		  – Fever >101.5
		  – Uncontrollable pain
		  – Incision cite redness, inflammation warmth to touch
		  – Wound drainage that is purulent and continuous or getting worse
		  – Inability to have a bowel movement or pass gas
		• Marking for stoma preoperatively (some institutions do this pre-op morning of surgery, if available an appointment to discuss stoma care with the ostomy nurse before surgery is preferable)

Extracorporeal shockwave lithotripsy (ESWL)	None	• Hematuria common especially if passing stone fragments
		• May pass small fragments or dust
		• Filter urine for stone fragments
		• LUTS possible
		• Call to EC with
		  – Fever >101.5
		  – More blood than urine
		  – Inability to urinate

Nephrectomy	Incisions Often have drains	• May require overnight stay or longer depending on the surgery (open vs. robotic, partial vs. radical)
		• Early ambulation
		• Keep incision(s) clean and dry
		• If robotic will have some air in abdominal area that will need to be reabsorbed
		• If open splinting incision with cough/deep breathing
		• Increase activity level as tolerated
		• Increase food as tolerated
		• Call to EC with
		– Fever >101.5
		– More blood than urine
		– Inability to urinate
Penile prosthesis (IPP)-3 piece *Similar care instructions for 2-piece or malleable*	None	• Implant to be partially inflated to prevent scarring—men should be counseled not to try and deflate it
		• Penis will be positioned upright against lower belly in order to promote proper healing
		• Prescription for 7–14 days of antibiotics at discharge
		• Keep incision(s) clean and dry
		• Swelling is expected; minimize activity as much as possible for 10–14 days
		• Call with
		– Fever >101.5
		– Redness, warmth to touch or drainage.
		• Scrotal support/athletic underwear can be helpful
		• After 48 h: Ok to shower and gently clean incision after 48 h
		• 7–10 days after your surgery: Alternate anti-inflammatory medications such as ibuprofen with any remaining pain medication
		• 14 days after your surgery: first preoperative visit, where provider will ensure proper healing
		• 6 weeks after your surgery: cleared for sexual activity and taught how to use the implant

(continued)

Table 12.8 (continued)

Surgery/procedure	Drains/catheters/incisions	Instructions to patients

Prolapse repair vaginal	• Vaginal packing
	• Foley if unable to void post-op
	• Vaginal incisions
		• Usually out patient
		• Vaginal bleeding is normal (like a period) can last 3–4 weeks
		• If still in childbearing years no tampons for 6 weeks
		• Will be stiches in vagina usually dissolvable and will take 4–5 weeks to dissolve
		• Avoid baths for 4 weeks
		• Ok to shower
		• No sex for 6 weeks
		• Avoid heavy lifting 1 gallon of milk for 4 weeks ok to gradually increase after
		• No strenuous workouts for 6 weeks, ok to walk
		• To EC/call
		  – Vaginal drainage that is purulent/foul smelling
		  – Bleeding greater than normal period or bright red blood after 2 weeks
		  – Fever >101.5
		  – Inability to urinate
		• Post-op appointments per individual surgeon/institution guidelines/preference

| Prostatectomy (open or robotic) | Foley catheter JP Drain/Penrose drain Incisions | • Overnight stay required
  – Bring pads for men to wear home
  – Bring loose fitting pants to wear home
• Kegel exercises (do not do while catheter in place)
• Urinary incontinence is normal and starts to get better after 2 weeks after the catheter is removed (Kegels best way to return to baseline)
• Hematuria
  – Maybe common for up to 6 weeks post-op but should not be continuous
  – Increase fluids and decrease activity
  – To EC/call more blood than urine, catheter not draining
  – If increasing activities and start bleeding rest increase fluids
• Foley care as above
• JP empty and record
• Penrose drain keep covered with gauze, change as needed
• Reintroduction of food
• To EC/call with:
  – Fever >101.5
  – Uncontrollable pain
  – Incision cite redness, inflammation warmth to touch
  – Wound drainage that is purulent and continuous or getting worse
  – Inability to have a bowel movement or pass gas
• Post-op appointments for
  – Catheter removal
  – Staple removal
  – Drain removal
  – Pathology review |

Table 12.8 (continued).

Surgery/procedure	Drains/ catheters/ incisions	Instructions to patients

Sling procedure	• Incisions/ puncture sites
	 • Foley prn
		• Usually out patient
		 • Foley care as above
		 • No sex for 6 weeks
		 • If childbearing age no tampons for 6 weeks
		 • No lifting greater than 10 lb for 2 weeks
		 • No lifting greater than 20 lb for 6 weeks
		 • Vaginal spotting and discharge normal for upto 6 weeks
		 • To EC/call with
		   – Excessive bleeding
		   – Inability to urinate for 6 h
		   – Redness/inflammation/drainage from incision site
		   – Fever >101.5

Stone procedures (invasive)	• Stent(s) possible
	 • Nephrostomy tube possible
		• Stent expectations
		   – LUTS common if bothersome can be treated
		   – Hematuria common, increase fluids
		   – Bladder spasms common if bothersome can be treated
		 • Nephrostomy tube
		   – Keep secured
		   – Leg bag instructions
		 • To EC/call with
		   – More blood than urine
		   – Fever >101.5
		   – Inability to urinate

Testicular and scrotal procedures	Incisions; may have a drain placed	• Keep incision(s) clean and dry
		• Any drain will be pulled after 24–48 h
		• Swelling is expected; minimize activity as much as possible for 10–14 days
		• Call with
		   – Fever
		   – Redness
		   – Warmth to touch or drainage.
		• Scrotal support/athletic underwear can be helpful

Transurethral resection of a bladder tumor (TURBT)	Foley catheter possibility	• Hematuria
		   – Common up to 6–8 weeks
		   – Increase fluids and decrease activity
		   – To EC/call more blood than urine, catheter not draining
		• Foley care as above
		• Post-op appointments
		   – Foley removal
		   – Pathology results

Transurethral resection of the prostate (TURP)	Foley catheter	• Hematuria
		   – Common up to 6–8 weeks
		   – Increase fluids and decrease activity
		• Urinary incontinence is common post-op for 2–3 weeks if older than 70 may last longer
		• LUTS maybe common
		• Foley care as above
		• Post-op appointments
		   – Foley removal

Vasectomy	none	See Chap. 26 for post-procedure care guidelines

Postoperative Management

Introduction

The key to postoperative (post-op) care is to minimize complications while optimizing recovery to improve surgical outcomes. Postoperative care can be broken down into three categories, in hospital considerations, transition/discharge, and follow-up and surveillance. This discussion will focus on the follow-up and surveillance. Postoperative pain management is covered in Chap. 20. Post-op long-term surveillance of the oncologic patient is found in the appropriate chapter. Postoperative follow-up immediately after discharge centers around preventing complications, emergency visits, and hospital readmissions.

Arpey et al. (2019) did a retrospective review of 488 adult patients involving 10 surgeons (527 surgeries) for postoperative unscheduled clinical encounters (UCE) over a 3-month time period. UCE included telephone calls, emergency visits, hospital readmission, e-mails, patient portal messages, and office visits. They determined that 40% of postoperative patients had an UCE. The majority of the encounters were telephone calls (68%) followed by emergency visits (9%) and visits outside the medical system (9%). The UCE occurred on a median of 9 days after surgery. The most common reason for the UCE was medical reasons (68%) and included pain (22.3%), wound concerns (15%), and voiding complaints (13%). Krishnan et al. (2016) determined that the optimal time frame for follow-up for a cystectomy after discharge was 4–5 days. They determined that the type of model to follow up (in office vs. phone call) was not as important as the timing. Preoperative education and post-op scheduling may lead to decreased UCE (Arpey et al. 2019).

Many post-op complications can be prevented if patients are encouraged to monitor for early signs and symptoms; patients need to be educated prior to surgery about these common signs/symptoms (Table 12.8).

The importance of adequate fluid intake, early and frequent ambulation, rest with leg elevation as needed and pain control should be stressed to promote appropriate healing. Maintenance of bowel regimen should be stressed. This will need to be balanced with accurate descriptions of restrictions including lifting and activity. Include family members significant others and caregivers in the explanations (AUA 2019).

There is little documentation on care of post-op complications. There is information on types of complications based on individual surgeries but no recommendations for evidence-based interventions. Below are some of the common post-op complications/patient concerns and basic interventions (Table 12.9).

Table 12.9   Selected examples of postoperative complications specific to urology patients[a]

Post-op complication	PT education/discussion	Intervention
Catheter • Leakage • Not draining • Discomfort	• Ensure catheter is below the level of the bladder and tubing is not kinked • Appropriate fluid intake • Secure catheter	• Anticholinergics • Irrigate catheter • Possible catheter replacement (collaboration with surgeon, may need to be done with cystoscopy)
Drains (Penrose/passive; Jackson Pratt/active) • Leaking • Change in amount and type of drainage	• Monitor output • Teach activation of bulb • Keep clean and dry • Secure tubing	• Consider fluid for creatinine if high volumes for several days post-op • Consider wound culture if signs/symptoms of infection • Treat as appropriate
GI • Nausea • Vomiting • Diarrhea • Constipation	• Discuss progression of diet • Discuss signs of ileus (no bowel movement, pain, not passing gas, vomiting bile) • Review medications (take with food prn) and compliance (stool softeners)	• Consider antiemetic • Consider stool softener, bulking agent, enema • If persistent diarrhea on antibiotics consider stool for *C. Diff* • If Ileus will require hospitalization with NG tube, IV fluids
Hematuria • Expected and light • Clot retention/heavy	• Encourage hydration • Avoid straining events/heavy lifting • Elevate legs/rest • Reassurance	• PVR—if high consider clot retention • If more blood than urine or clot retention irrigate until clear • If unable to clear may consider admission for continuous bladder irrigation (CBI)

Infection
• UTI
• Wound
• Surgical Site Infection (SSI)
  – Drainage
  – Redness
  – Inflammation
  – Warm to touch
	• Discuss LUTS which are normal in many urological surgeries
	• Fever >101.5 is never normal
		• Culture as indicated
		• If UTI treat
		• SSI may require opening and packing
		• Antibiotics as indicated

LUTS	• Reassure -LUTS is a complication of stents, bladder surgeries etc… • Encourage fluids • Call? EC with inability to urinate or fever >101.5	• R/O UTI and treat appropriately • Anticholinergics/bladder pain spasms medications RX and OTC
Vaginal	• Some bleeding is normal • Pain is normal	• Check PVR if elevated consider Foley • Persistent vaginal bleeding may require packing/consult surgeon

Note. Specifics of any interventions will be determined by facility policy and procedures.

Non-urological Surgery Post-op Retention (POUR)

Introduction

According to the AUA (2020) acute urinary retention is the most common urology emergency. It is thirteen more times likely in men than women and the incidence increases with age. Patients with obstructive symptoms prior to general anesthesia are at increased risk for POUR. The patient's preoperative urological symptoms should be assessed. Patients with LUTS prior to surgery are at greater risk for post-op retention and difficulty with passing a trial of void.

Incidence

Mason and colleagues (2016) did a systematic review and meta-analysis of patient related factors for urinary retention after general surgery. They included 21 studies with a total of 7802 patients and determined the incidence of POUR was 14%. The risk increased with age and symptoms of LUTs prior to surgery, there was no gender differences noted. These authors also looked at pre-op use of α-adrenergics and determined use was associated with decreased POUR however, there is a need for adequately powered random clinical trials in this setting. The Michigan Spine Surgery Improvement Collaborative (MSSIC) monitored post-op retention in patients undergoing lumbar surgery and found 7.4% of patients experienced POUR. This included 26 hospitals in the state of Michigan with over 190 surgeons with 25,769 patients. They determined POUR was associated with older age, male gender, lower BMI, diabetes, osteoporosis, and history of deep vein thrombosis (DVT) (Zakaria et al. 2020).

Diagnosis

According to Baldini et al. (2009) the diagnosis of POUR is made by three different methods; clinical examination, bladder catheterization or ultrasound assessment.

Clinical examination notes suprapubic pain and discomfort, often these maybe masked by anesthesia and are not reliable. Palpation and percussion of the suprapubic area is commonly used but dependent on the skill level of the assessor and are not recommended. Catheterization is often used based on clinical assessment and is an invasive procedure that can cause complications of CAUTI, urethral trauma, prostatitis, and patient discomfort. Urinary catheterization should be used to treat POUR not diagnose POUR. Ultrasound assessment has shown good reliability in appropriately trained personnel, and can be used to diagnose POUR (Baldini et al. 2009). Management of POUR is fairly straightforward. The goal is to decompress the bladder to avoid long-term damage to bladder integrity and function. Immediate catheterization is always the first step. This may be performed either with in-and-out catheterization or with placement of an indwelling Foley catheter. Although placement of an indwelling Foley catheter is easier, there are several drawbacks to prolonged use of this method. Indwelling catheters lead to increased rates of UTI compared to intermittent catheterization.

Management

Urology is often consulted after the decision to put in a Foley is made (inpatient) or the patient is sent home with a catheter and shows up in the office for clinical management. Management of POUR in the office has not been researched or described well in the literature. Often alpha blockers are given prior to the office visit. Patients with LUTS, BPH, neurological disease preoperatively are at higher risk for post-op POUR and often are difficult to manage in the office. POUR is discussed in the literature for immediate post-op complications but little information is available on discontinuing the catheter post-op after the patient has gone home. Intermittent self-catheterization (ISC) is an excellent method of monitoring post-op retention but is rarely taught in the post-op period. In the office a trial of void is indicated. There is no agreement in the literature on the amount to fluid to place in the bladder a general rule of thumb is to put in enough fluid that the patient can't hold it any longer. If the patient is able to void at least 50% of the volume placed it is usually ok to send home with close follow-up. The patient should be instructed to monitor to go to EC with inability to void, more blood than urine or fever. The patient should be scheduled for a follow-up appointment to check PVR, appropriate laboratory tests (PSA in men, creatinine and GFR as indicated) and exam based on underlying cause (see appropriate chapter). Patients who are unable to void can be taught ISC as it is an excellent way to monitor for return of function.

Clinical Pearls
- Patients who initially have less than 50% can be monitored closely and given a chance to continue urinating. Often patients with LUTS prior to surgery especially the elderly have high residuals and allowing them to urinate will return to baseline in 1–2 weeks.
- If not on alpha blockers, initiating a course maybe helpful.

Resources for the Nurse Practitioner and Physician Assistant

See appropriate chapter for surgical intervention

AUA White paper on optimizing outcomes in urological surgery preoperative. https://www.auanet.org/guidelines/optimizing-outcomes-in-urological-surgery-pre-operative-care-for-the-patient-undergoing-urologic-surgery-or-procedure

AUA White paper on optimizing outcomes in urological surgery postoperative https://www.auanet.org/guidelines/optimizing-outcomes-in-urologic-surgery-postoperative

AUA university for medical students https://www.auanet.org/education/auauniversity/for-medical-students/medical-students-curriculum/medical-student-curriculum

---

Resources for the Patient

See appropriate chapter for surgical intervention

Urology Care foundation has several sources for patients https://www.urologyhealth.org/educational-materials?product_format=466|&language=1122|

References

Arpey NC, Sloan MJ, Hahn AE, Polgreen PM, Erikson BA (2019) Unscheduled clinical encounters in the postoperative period after adult and pediatric urologic surgery. Urology 124:113–119

AUA (2019) AUA white paper on optimizing outcomes in urological surgery post-operative. Retrieved from https://www.auanet.org/guidelines/optimizing-outcomes-in-urologic-surgery-postoperative

AUA (2020) Medical student education acute urinary retention. Retrieved from https://www.auanet.org/education/auauniversity/for-medical-students/medical-students-curriculum/medical-student-curriculum/urologic-emergencies

Baldini G, Bagry H, Aprikian A, Carli F, Phil M (2009) Postoperative urinary retention. Anesthesiology 110(5):1139–1157

Baron TH, Kamath PS, McBane RD (2013) Management of antithrombotic therapy in patients undergoing invasive procedures. N Engl J Med 368:2113–2124

Brenner MJ et al (2014) Obstructive sleep apnea and surgery: quality improvement imperatives and opportunities. Curr Otorhinolaryngol Rep 2:20–29

Caprini JA, Arcelus JI, Hasty JH, Tamhand AC, Fabreg F (1991) Clinical assessment of venous thromboembolic risk in surgical patients. Semin Thromb Hemost 17(Suppl 3):304–312

Chung F, Yegneswaran B, Liao P et al (2008) STOP questionnaire: a tool to screen patients for obstructive sleep apnea. Anesthesiology 108(5):812–821

Coutinho-Myrrha MA, Dias RC, Fernandes AA, Araújo CG, Hlatky MA, Pereira DG, Britto RR (2014) Duke Activity Status Index for cardiovascular diseases: validation of the Portuguese translation. Arq Bras Cardiol 102(4):383–390. https://doi.org/10.5935/abc.20140031

Fleisher LA et al (2014) 2014 ACC/AHA guideline on perioperative cardiovascular evaluation and management of patients undergoing noncardiac surgery: a report of the American College of Cardiology/American Heart Association Task Force on Practice Guidelines. Circulation 130:e278–e333

Hausel J et al (2001) A carbohydrate-rich drink reduces preoperative discomfort in elective surgery patients. Anesth Analg 93:1344–1350

Hlatky MA, Boineau RE, Higginbotham MB, Lee KL, Mark DB, Califf RM et al (1989) A brief self-administered questionnaire to determine functional capacity (the Duke Activity Status Index). Am J Cardiol 64(10):651–654

Hurwitz EE, Simon M, Vinta SR et al (2017) Adding examples to the ASA-physical status classification improves correct assignments to patients. Anesthesiology 126:614–622

Kasatpibal N et al (2017) Effectiveness of probiotic, prebiotic, and synbiotic therapies in reducing postoperative complications: a systematic review and network meta-analysis. Clin Infect Dis 64(Suppl 2):S153

Krishnan N, Liu X, Lavieri MS et al (2016) A model to optimize follow-up care and reduce hospital readmissions after radical cystectomy. J Urol 195(5):1362–1367

Mason SE, Scott AJ, Mayer E, Purkayastha S (2016) Patient related risk factors for urinary retention following ambulatory general surgery: a systematic review and analysis. Am J Surg 211:1126–1134

Melis GC et al (2006) A carbohydrate-rich beverage prior to surgery prevents surgery-induced immunodepression: a randomized, controlled, clinical trial. JPEN 30(1):21–26

Noblett SE et al (2006) Pre-operative oral carbohydrate loading in colorectal surgery: a randomized controlled trial. Colorectal Dis 8(7):563–569

Nuckton TJ, Glidden DV, Browner WS, Claman DM (2006) Physical examination: Mallampati score as an independent predictor of obstructive sleep apnea. Sleep 29(7):903–908

Septimus EJ (2019) Nasal decolonization: what antimicrobials are most effective prior to surgery? Amer J Infect Control 47S:A53–A57

Sudhakaran S, Surani SR (2015) Guidelines for perioperative management of the diabetic patient. Surg Res Pract 2015:284063. https://doi.org/10.1155/2015/284063

Yuill KA et al (2005) The administration of an oral carbohydrate containing fluid prior to major elective upper-gastrointestinal surgery preserves skeletal muscle mass postoperatively- randomized clinical trial. Clin Nutr 24:32–37

Zakaria HM, Lipphardt M, Bazydlo M, Xiao S, Schultz L, Chedid M et al (2020) The preoperative risks and two-year sequelae of postoperative urinary retention: analysis of the Michigan Spine Surgery Improvement Collaberitive (MSSIC). World Neurosurg 133:E619–E626

Neurogenic Bladder/Underactive Bladder

13

Michelle J. Lajiness

Contents

M. J. Lajiness (✉)
Department of Urology, University of Toledo, Toledo, OH, USA
e-mail: Michelle.Lajiness@utoledo.edu

© Springer Nature Switzerland AG 2020
S. A. Quallich, M. J. Lajiness (eds.), *The Nurse Practitioner in Urology*,
https://doi.org/10.1007/978-3-030-45267-4_13

Objectives
1. Discuss the definition and incidence of underactive bladder (UAB).
2. Describe assessment techniques in UAB.
3. Discuss appropriate interventions for the treatment of UAB.

Definition, Incidence, and Epidemiology

Underactive bladder (UAB) is a chronic, complex, and debilitating disease that is not well known and has few options for treatment. UAB is closely related to detrusor underactivity (DU), a urodynamic definition; however, few clinicians, scientist, or researchers agree on a definition (Chappele et al. 2018). UAB is more correctly defined as a constellation of clinical symptoms or clinical syndrome that includes or clinical syndrome that includes the symptoms and signs of DU. The International Continence Society (ICS) defines DU as "a contraction of reduced strength and/or duration, resulting in prolonged bladder emptying and/or failure to achieve complete bladder emptying within a normal time span" (Chapple et al. 2018). UAB is a multifactorial condition that may be caused by myogenic (muscle denervation) and/or neurogenic (nerve denervation) conditions, aging, and medication side effects. Dewulf and colleagues (2017) suggest the definition of UAB as "reduced voiding efficiency characterized by a decreased detrusor contraction with decreased or absent flow on urodynamics."

Lower urinary tract dysfunction is especially prevalent in the elderly. As the population continues to age, the number of affected people and the associated costs will escalate (Chancellor and Diokno 2014). Solid epidemiology is dependent on accurate and precise definitions of a disease studied; as a result UAB is thought to be misrepresented (Chancellor and Diokno 2014).

Prevalence of UAB varied across clinical studies and patient populations. Diokno et al. (1986) concluded that 22% of men and 11% of women over 60 years had difficulty emptying their bladders. A study by Taylor et al. in 2006 found detrusor underactivity in two-thirds of incontinent institutionalized patients. Valente et al. (2014) did an epidemiological study and had 633 subjects return questionnaires. It was determined that 23% of the respondents reported difficulty emptying his/her bladder and only 11% had ever heard of the term underactive bladder.

Pathophysiology

The exact cause of UAB is not always known; known causes include myogenic, neurogenic, and medication side effects. Theories have been postulated to account for the signs and symptoms associated with UAB (see Table 13.1). These hypotheses include but are not limited to overactive bladder (OAB) to UAB model and the aging bladder model (Miyazato et al. 2013). Comorbidities can also increase the risk of OAB (see Table 13.2).

Table 13.1 Signs/symptoms of UAB
Hesitancy
Weak stream
Interrupted urine flow
Straining to void
Feeling of incomplete emptying
Frequent small volume urination
Urinary tract infections
Nighttime leakage
Flank pain (bilateral, rare—related to hydronephrosis)
Incontinence
Diminished stream
Rely on abdominal straining to urinate

Table 13.2 Comorbid conditions that predispose patients to retention and incomplete emptying
BPH
Cognitive impairment
Diabetes
Mobility impairment
Neurological diseases
Pelvic organ prolapsed
Spinal cord injury
Spinal stenosis
Stroke
Urethral stricture

A myogenic basis for DU may result from abnormality of the myocytes to generate contractile activity in the absence of external stimuli, or the problem may lie with the extracellular matrix, resulting in impaired contractility. Bladder outlet obstruction (BOO)-related DU has been well studied in numerous animal models where sequential changes were described leading to decompensation of bladder contraction (Osman et al. 2014). Disruption to the efferent nerves may result in reduced neuromuscular activation that may manifest as an absent or poor detrusor contraction. This is typically seen with diseases causing direct neuronal injury such as multisystem atrophy and other autonomic neuropathies. In DU of non-neurogenic origin, the exact contribution of efferent dysfunction is unknown. The decline in autonomic nerve innervation in normal human bladders with aging, as well as BOO, may contribute to insufficient activation for adequate contraction to occur in individuals without overt neurologic disease (Osman et al. 2014).

DHIC, or detrusor hyperactivity with impaired contractility, was first characterized by Resnick and Yalla in 1987 in a series of women with both urge urinary incontinence and elevated post-void residual volumes associated with poor bladder contractility. Men with DHIC or even pure detrusor underactivity may have their symptoms incorrectly attributed purely BPH alone and undergo unnecessary surgical procedures to relieve obstruction (Griebling 2015).

Neurogenic cause is well known to those working with UAB patients (see Table 13.3). Neurogenic bladder dysfunction happens when the efferent and/or afferent pathways or the lumbosacral spinal cord is damaged. The afferent system is integral to the function of the efferent system in the neural control of micturition during both the storage and voiding phases. The afferent system monitors the volumes during storage and also the magnitude of detrusor contractions during voiding. Urethral afferents respond to flow and are important in potentiating the detrusor contraction. Bladder and urethral afferent dysfunction may lead to DU by reducing or prematurely ending the micturition reflex, which may manifest in a loss of voiding efficiency (Osman et al. 2014).

OAB may over time lead to the development of UAB. Chancellor (2014) postulates that in OAB the bladder wall thickens, and a rise in nerve growth factors occurs resulting in structural changes leading to alteration of the muscle and connective tissue structure and function that results in impaired contractility. Chapple and colleagues (2018) believe that it is during the storage phase patients note overactivity and during the voiding phase underactivity.

The causes of detrusor underactivity as a result of the typical aging process are not well understood. The bladder should remain adequately elastic and contractile despite a patient's age, and urinary incontinence should not be considered either an inevitable or normal part of aging (Griebling 2015). Animal studies suggest that as the bladder ages, there is a reduction in the strength of contraction; however, the few urodynamic studies done on older humans have differing results. There are age-induced morphology changes noted in the bladder which include a decrease in the ratio of detrusor muscle to collagen as well as a decrease in M3 receptors. This may all lead to decreased ability of the bladder to contract (Miyazato et al. 2013). The simple fact remains not every person over the age of 70 is affected by UAB. The true

	Neurogenic	Myogenic
Table 13.3 Predisposing/ risk factors for neurogenic bladder	Spinal cord injury	Excessive fluid intake with infrequent voiding
	CVA	BOO
	Parkinson's disease	Aging bladder
	Multiple sclerosis	Diabetes
	Spina bifida	
	Diabetic neuropathy	
	Guillain–Barre syndrome	
	Multisystem atrophy	
	Herniated disk	
	Cauda equina syndrome	
	Aids	
	Neurosyphilis	
	Herpes zoster/herpes simplex	
	Pelvic radiation	
	Pelvic/sacral fracture	
	Pelvic surgery	

relationship between microscopic and cellular changes to clinically significant bladder behavior is unclear, and the associate between aging and detrusor underactivity is likely multifactorial (Griebling 2015).

History

An accurate assessment of voiding symptoms is essential in UAB (see Table 13.1). Include onset and duration of symptoms. A voiding diary, a daily record of the patient's bladder activity, is an objective documentation of the patient's voiding pattern, incontinent episodes, and inciting events associated with urinary incontinence and can be helpful in eliciting voiding patterns (see Chap. 14 for an example). For those who present with acute urinary retention, attempts should be made to obtain potential precipitating factors that led to urinary retention (see Table 13.2). For those who present with an indwelling Foley catheter, doing intermittent catheterization, or with significant voiding symptoms and a high post-void residual urine, attempt should be made to determine any predisposing/risk factors factor/s such as neurologic disorders including spinal cord injury and cerebrovascular accidents (see Table 13.3) that lead to the problem. In patients with spinal cord injury history should include current sexual functioning and reproductive plans.

Obtain history of previous surgical intervention related to the GU tract. Obtain an accurate list of current medications to evaluate drugs that can lead to detrusor weakness (Table 13.4). However, the diagnostician must also be aware that UAB may be completely silent, meaning that the person with UAB may be totally asymptomatic (Diokno 2015).

Physical Examination

A focused physical examination is essential in a comprehensive evaluation of a patient suspected of having an UAB. This should include an overall general assessment of the physical and cognitive ability of the patient. Include a functional assessment and a neurological assessment. Abdominal examination must include inspection and palpation of the suprapubic area to identify any signs of distended bladder. The lumbar area must also be palpated for any evidence of any masses or tenderness that may indicate hydronephrosis.

Genital and perineal examination is mandatory for suspected cases of UAB. The skin of the genitalia and the perineum may indicate significant irritation manifested by erythema or even excoriation and ulceration from chronic urinary leakage and wearing of undergarments/diapers. For men, the penis and scrotum and its content must be evaluated. Digital rectal examination should elicit the anal sphincter tone and the voluntary ability to contract the sphincter. The prostate is palpated to assess the size and evidence of any tenderness or masses/nodules. One must remember that the size of the prostate on digital rectal examination does not necessarily correlate to the voiding symptoms. A small-size prostate may present with more intense lower urinary tract symptoms than one with a large prostate palpated on digital examination (Diokno 2015).

Table 13.4 Medications that can cause detrusor weakness

Class	Drug
Antipsychotics (anticholinergic effects)	Chlorpromazine (Thorazine)
	Clozapine (Clozaril)
	Mesoridazine (Serentil)
	Olanzapine (Zyprexa)
	Promazine (Sparine)
	Quetiapine (Seroquel)
	Thioridazine (Mellaril)
Antiarrhythmics (anticholinergic effects)	Disopyramide (Norpace)
	Procainamide (Pronestyl)
	Quinidine (Quinaglute, Quinidex)
Antiemetics (anticholinergic effects)	Dimenhydrinate (Dramamine)
	Meclizine (Antivert, Bonine)
	Trimethobenzamide (Tigan)
	Prochlorperazine (Compazine)
Antihistamines (anticholinergic effects)	Azatadine (Optimine)
	Chlorpheniramine (Chlor-Trimeton)
	Clemastine (Tavist)
	Diphenhydramine (Tylenol PM, Sominex, Benadryl)
Hydroxyzine (anticholinergic effects)	Atarax, Vistaril
	Promethazine (Phenergan)
Antiparkinson agents (anticholinergic effects)	Benztropine (Cogentin)
	Biperiden (Akineton)
	Procyclidine (Kemadrin)
	Trihexyphenidyl (Artane)
Antispasmodics (anticholinergic effects)	Atropine (Sal-Tropine)
	Belladonna alkaloids (Donnatal, Bellatal, Barbidonna)
	Dicyclomine (Antispas, Bentyl)
	Flavoxate (Urispas)
	Hyoscyamine (Anaspaz, Levbid, Cystospaz, Levsin/SL)
	Oxybutynin (Ditropan)
	Scopolamine
	Tolterodine (Detrol)
	Solifenacin succinate (VESIcare)
	Darifenacin (Enablex)
	Trospium (Sanctura)
	Fesoterodine (Toviaz)
Skeletal muscle relaxants (anticholinergic effects)	Carisoprodol (Soma)
	Chlorzoxazone (Parafon, Forte)
	Cyclobenzaprine (Flexeril)
	Methocarbamol (Robaxin)
	Orphenadrine (Norflex)

Table 13.4   (continued)

Class	Drug
Tricyclic antidepressants (anticholinergic effects)	Amitriptyline (Elavil)
	Desipramine (Norpramin)
	Doxepin (Sinequan)
	Imipramine (Tofranil)
	Nortriptyline (Aventyl, Pamelor)
Opiate analgesics	Codeine (Atasol, Tylenol 2,3,4)
	Morphine
	Methadone
	Meperidine (Demerol)
	Hydromorphone (Dilaudid)
	Oxycodone (OxyContin, Percocet)
NSAIDs	

For women, a vaginal inspection, including speculum examination and bimanual examination, must be performed. Inspection should identify the health of the vaginal mucosa to identify signs of atrophy and signs of skin irritation suggestive of atrophic vaginitis. Pelvic organ prolapse is identified visually for any organ protruding outside of the vaginal introitus and provoked by asking the patient to strain and cough to determine the extent of the prolapse. One must also look for evidence of urine leakage during coughing and straining. The lack of leakage does not eliminate urinary incontinence; however, the presence of urine leakage during straining or coughing is a positive sign for stress urinary incontinence. The vaginal speculum is used to inspect the cervix and the vaginal mucosa and to assess the level of the individual pelvic organ prolapse if one is present. The prolapsing organ must be identified such as cystocele (anterior), rectocele (posterior), uterus, or intestine/enterocele (central/vaginal vault). The severity of prolapse must be established (See Chap. 13). This is important because in severe vaginal prolapse, chronic obstruction from the prolapsing pelvic organ could lead to chronic urinary retention. Digital examination of the anal canal must also be performed to assess the anal tone and voluntary strength as well as assess the status of the rectovaginal wall (Diokno 2015).

In both men and women, the perineal sensation must be tested for sensory deficiency by testing the ability to perceive a gentle pinprick applied to the saddle and the perianal area. Without performing this maneuver, one may miss saddle perineal anesthesia that may be the only neurologic sign that may suggest sacral cord lesions that may be contributing to an underactive bladder (Diokno 2015).

Diagnostic Testing

Urinalysis should look for signs of pyuria and bacteriuria and if infection is suspected, urine culture and sensitivity should be ordered. Asymptomatic bacteriuria (see Chap. 20) is highly prevalent in this population do not send a culture if there are no symptoms of infection. Urinalysis should also seek to check the presence of glucose as this may correlate to diabetes and its potential consequence, diabetic neuropathy, and for albumin for possible kidney disease. Specific gravity should also be tested to provide a hint of the ability of the kidney to concentrate the urine. Nephrogenic diabetes insipidus causing excessive diuresis can lead to chronic bladder overdistention and underactive bladder (Diokno 2015).

Urine Cytology

Carcinoma in situ of the urinary bladder causes symptoms of urinary frequency and urgency. Irritative voiding symptoms out of proportion to the overall clinical picture and/or hematuria warrant urine cytology and cystoscopy. Blood tests that may contribute to the overall assessment of UAB include the renal panel (BUN, creatinine, GFR rate), serum protein, electrolytes, and glucose/Hgb A1c levels.

Almi and colleagues (Alimi et al. 2018) did a systematic literature search of 220 records and included 15 studies that looked at screening patients with neurogenic bladder with urine cytology. They determined there is insufficient data to make recommendations; however, urine cytology had a screening sensitivity of 71% out performing cystoscopy.

Imaging Tests

The portable bladder scanner has made it easier to quickly measure post-void residual (PVR) urine volume and establish the efficiency of bladder emptying. It also obviates the risk of trauma, pain, and potential contamination with the use of catheter to measure the post-void residual urine (Diokno 2015). In UAB, there is no consensus on what PVR amount requires intervention. The AUA (2016) white paper on chronic urinary retention defines it as greater than 300 cc documented on 2 or more occasions lasting at least 6 months. Other imaging techniques that have led to identifying large distended bladder are abdominal and/or pelvic ultrasound, CT, and MRI imaging.

Endoscopic Assessment

Cystourethroscopy is an optional procedure performed to confirm the presence or absence of anatomical obstruction including enlarged occluding prostate gland, bladder neck contracture, or presence of urethral strictures. The presence of obstruction may indicate that the underactive bladder may be secondary to the obstruction. Cystoscopy may confirm the presence of bladder wall trabeculations, and even diverticula formations, noted in cases of obstruction. Relieving the obstruction may allow the patient to void spontaneously. However if there is no evidence of any detrusor contractility, relieving the obstruction may not benefit the patient's ability to void. Endoscopy is helpful if the study revealed no evidence of any urethral stricture and the prostatic fossa appeared wide open especially after a previous TURP. Likewise, in UAB not caused by chronic obstruction, cystoscopy may reveal a large bladder with smooth lining (Diokno 2015).

Urodynamic Tests

Uroflowmetry can provide useful indirect information as to the strength of the detrusor contraction based on the measurement of the maximum or peak flow rate, the time it took to complete the act of voiding, and the average flow rate. However, it in itself will not be sufficient to make a diagnosis of underactive bladder (Diokno 2015; Bok et al. 2018).

Cystometry can provide a hint of underactive bladder with observation of a large capacity bladder, poor sensation or perception of bladder distention, abnormally high compliance, and lack of detrusor contractility. Although in underactive bladder, the post-void residual urine is usually abnormally elevated, the fact that the bladder is empty post-void does not rule out underactive bladder (Diokno 2015).

Combined pressure-flow test is the only legitimate test that can diagnose underactive detrusor and therefore confirm underactive bladder suspected on the basis of clinical symptoms (see Table 13.1) (Diokno 2015). The basic principle in this test is to simultaneously measure the intravesical pressure, the abdominal pressure, intraurethral pressure, bladder volume, urine flow rates, and post-void residual urine volume. When properly done, the detrusor pressure can be ascertained by subtracting the intravesical pressure from the abdominal pressure. The detrusor pressure at the height of the maximum urine flow rate will determine the presence of underactive, overactive, obstructive, or normal detrusor function. The most common accepted tenets of pressure-flow abdominal pressure diagnosis include the following results:

- Obstructed outlet when there is high detrusor pressure associated with poor urine flow rate.
- Underactive bladder when there is abnormal low or absent detrusor voiding pressure associated with poor urine flow rate.
- Overactive bladder may be diagnosed when involuntary detrusor contractions are noted during the filling phase of the study.
- Normal study when the detrusor pressure and the urine flow rate are within the limits of accepted normal rates.

Unfortunately, except for the obvious case of extreme pressures of high detrusor and poor flow or extremely low detrusor pressure and poor flow, there are many cases that are somewhere in between. This may be due to the severity of the dysfunction or technicalities of the procedure as performance of pressure-flow abdominal pressure test demands great precision and patient cooperation (Diokno 2015).

Musco and colleagues (2018) screened 5348 records from 49 studies and they determined that patients with spinal cord injury have an increased risk of hydrone-phrosis when compared to MS patients long term. They believe that detrusor leak point pressure and reduced compliance are the best predictors of upper urinary tract disease.

Behavioral/Conservative Therapy

The treatment for underactive bladder (UAB) is to protect the upper urinary tract, to improve continence and quality of life, and whenever possible to improve lower urinary tract functioning (Bok et al. 2018). Regular bladder emptying reduces intravesical bladder pressure and overdistention, which improves blood flow to the bladder and reduces the risk of infection (Lapides et al. 1972).

The objectives of conservative therapy in the underactive bladder are to provide low-pressure storage, preserve continence, avoid renal deterioration, minimize complications, and maintain quality of life. Conservative therapy in the underactive bladder patient includes behavioral management, incontinence products, and catheters.

Behavioral Treatment

There is a lack of information in the literature that discusses behavioral therapy for underactive bladder, other than discussing catheters and incontinence products. A PubMed search in utilizing the term "underactive bladder" after limits set to the last 5 years revealed 126 articles available for review, utilizing "behavioral interventions" found in 46,707 articles available for review, but these terms combined yielded only one article.

According to the European Association of Urology (EAU) guidelines on neurogenic lower urinary tract dysfunction, there are few prospective, randomized, controlled studies supporting conservative treatment. The guidelines state that lower urinary tract rehabilitation might be beneficial. Rehabilitation techniques include prompted voiding, timed voiding (bladder training), and lifestyle modifications (See Chap. 15). The EAU guidelines do not recommend assisted bladder emptying such as Valsalva maneuver, crede, or triggered reflux. The authors state these procedures may create high pressures and are potentially hazardous.

Tubaro and colleagues (2012) completed a systemic review on the treatment of lower urinary tract symptoms in patients with multiple sclerosis. A meta-analysis could not be performed secondary to the multiple and differing outcome criteria. The authors concluded the nature of bladder dysfunction and the course of the disease make it difficult to standardize treatments or create guidelines.

Patil and colleagues (2012) completed an open arm pre-post study on 11 patients with multiple sclerosis (MS). The MS patients underwent a 21-day yoga intervention with statistical improvement noted in post-void residual, total micturition, and quality of sleep. Prior to that McClurg and colleagues (2006) compared electromyography (EMG) feedback and neuromuscular electrical stimulation, alone or in combination with pelvic floor muscle training, and were able to reduce the amount of leakage in the MS population. Later McClurg et al. (2008) taught 11 patients with MS pelvic floor training for lower urinary dysfunction and found the participants quality of life (QOL) was enhanced after completing the 9-week training course.

Behavioral therapy has been extensively studied in the overactive bladder population and authors have concluded that it may work in the UAB population. Other than those discussed above, no clinical studies are available to determine the effectiveness of behavioral therapy in the UAB population.

Incontinence Products

Patients may choose incontinence pads or diapers as their first initial method to remedy the loss of urine or may use them as a last resort. These items tend to be for long-term usage with UAB patients. The main goal of incontinence products is to minimize, conceal, and control urinary leakage. There are a variety of options available from pads to undergarments. Patient preference, comfort, and level of incontinence, shape, and contour of the product will determine which products to use (AUA 2014; Newman and Wein 2009). Patients should be counseled that incontinence products are *management strategies* and not treatment options (Newman and Wein 2009; Blok et al. 2018).

Catheterization

Intermittent Catheterization (IC) Versus Indwelling

The best treatment for neurogenic bladder remains controversial. Clean intermittent catheterization (CIC) was first introduced in 1972 by Lapides and colleagues. The authors concluded that CIC aids the treatment and prevention of urinary tract infections. Prevention is a direct result of reducing intravesical bladder pressure and improving blood flow to the bladder wall. Tubaro and colleagues (2012) in a comprehensive review discussed the importance of bladder emptying but were unable to make a recommendation on intermittent catheterization (IC) vs. indwelling catheter and felt the decision should be based on lifestyle.

Weld and Dmochowski (2000) retrospectively reviewed medical records, upper tract imaging, and video urodynamic of 316 posttraumatic spinal cord-injured patients looking at their rate of urologic complications. They compared indwelling catheters, IC, spontaneous voiding, and suprapubic catheterization. Their results indicated that IC is the safest management option for spinal cord-injured patients.

Cochrane reviews concluded that there is a lack of compelling evidence from clinical trials that the incidence of UTI is affected by use of aseptic or clean technique, coated or uncoated catheters, single- (sterile) or multiple-use (clean) catheters, self-catheterization or catheterization by others, or by any other strategy. There is no evidence to support any method above another; however, patient preference is noted throughout the clinical trials. More well-designed trials are strongly recommended and should include analysis of cost-effectiveness data, because there are likely to be substantial differences associated with the use of different catheter designs, catheterization techniques, and strategies (Jamison et al. 2013; Prieto et al. 2014). Evidence-based guidelines suggest CIC is preferable to indwelling or suprapubic catheters for patients with bladder-emptying dysfunctions (AUA 2014).

Indwelling catheters can be used for short-term and long-term use; for the purposes of underactive bladder, only long-term use will be discussed. Indwelling catheters can be urethral or suprapubic. The complications of indwelling catheters include bacteriuria, catheter-associated urinary tract infections (CAUTI), catheter-associated biofilms, encrustations, urosepsis, and urethral damage (see Table 13.5). Indwelling catheters should be considered when anatomical, functional, or familial limitations prohibit intermittent catheterizations. A suprapubic tube is an attractive alternative to long-term urethral catheter use. The most common use of a suprapubic catheter is in individuals with spinal cord injuries and a malfunctioning bladder.

Table 13.5 Complications of indwelling catheterization

Complication	Prevention
Bacteriuria—Most patients with long-term catheterizations develop bacteriuria. The incidence is 3–8 % per day and duration of catheter is the most important risk factor	1. Ensure sterile technique
	2. Maintain a closed system
	3. Do not treat unless patient is symptomatic
Catheter-associated urinary tract infections (CAUTI)—Incidence varies based on definitions used. The Center for Disease Control (CDC) has come out with new definitions for use http://www.cdc.gov/nhsn/PDFs/pscManual/7pscCAUTIcurrent.pdf	1. Ensure proper insertion technique
	2. Use sterile technique
	3. Use ample lubrication
	4. Following aseptic insertion, maintain a closed drainage system
	5. Maintain unobstructed urine flow
	6. Practice good hand hygiene
Biofilms and encrustations—Biofilms are a result of colonization with uropathogens creating adhesions and adhering to the catheter wall. Encrustations are formed by organisms in biofilms and usually associated with alkaline urine. Encrustation can cause catheter blockage	1. Maintain natural pH
	2. Ensure sterile technique
	3. Maintain a closed system
	4. Change catheters when blockage occurs; it is not recommended to irrigate
Urethral damage—Occurs primarily in men. Risk increases with the length of catheterization	1. Ensure proper technique is used
	2. Ensure liberal lubrication
	3. Ensure stability of catheter to leg
	4. May use antibiotic ointment at tip of meatus

Both paraplegic and quadriplegic individuals have benefited from this form of urinary diversion. Suprapubic tubes should be changed once a month on a regular basis.

Suprapubic catheters have many advantages. With a suprapubic catheter, the risk of urethral damage is eliminated. Multiple voiding trials may be performed without having to remove the catheter. Because the catheter comes out of the lower abdomen rather than the perineal area, a suprapubic tube is more patient friendly. Bladder spasms occur less often because the suprapubic catheter does not irritate the trigone as does the urethral catheter.

Potential complications with chronic suprapubic catheterization are similar to those associated with indwelling urethral catheters, including leakage around the catheter, bladder stone formation, urinary tract infection, and catheter obstruction (Table 13.6).

Table 13.6 Complications of clean intermittent catheterization

Complication	Prevention
Bleeding—More frequently seen in new patients and prevalence is about one-third of patients	1. Ensure patient is using proper technique
	2. Encourage liberal lubrication
Urethritis—Prevalence varies widely but is below 8%	1. Ensure patient is using proper technique
	2. Change catheter material
Stricture—The incidence of stricture increases with longer follow-up with most events occurring 5 years after initiation. Prevalence is around 4%	1. Ensure gentle introduction of the catheter
	2. Use of hydrophilic catheters may benefit
Creation of a false passage—Trauma especially in men can create false passages; however incidence is rare	1. Ensure patient is using proper technique
	2. Gentle slow introduction of catheter
Epididymitis and prostatitis—Both are rare and can be related to recurrent UTI	1. Ensure patient is using proper technique
	2. Ensure adequate hydration
	3. Ensure bladder is being emptied frequently to maintain residuals less than 500 cc
	4. Treat only when symptomatic
UTI—Prevalence is between 12 and 88% secondary to definition used and patient populations	1. Ensure patient is using proper technique
	2. Ensure adequate hydration
	3. Ensure bladder is being emptied frequently to maintain residuals less than 500 cc
	4. Treat only when symptomatic
Bladder stone—Incidence is very rare and is usually related to introduction of a foreign body into the bladder such as a pubic hair, loss of catheter in the bladder, bladder perforation, or necrosis	1. Ensure patient is using proper technique
	2. Ensure adequate hydration

Intermittent Catheterization (IC)

IC is the insertion of a catheter several times daily to empty the bladder. Once the bladder is empty, the catheter is immediately removed. There is no evidence that recommends frequency of IC, other than to prevent overdistention of the bladder. According to the EAU guidelines on neurogenic lower urinary tract dysfunction, the gold standard for management is intermittent catheterization. The guidelines recommend using a 12–14 French catheter four to six times per day (Stohrer et al. 2009). CIC is also the preferred method of patients who have neurogenic bladder (Stohrer et al. 2009; Tubaro et al. 2012; Newman and Wilson 2011).

Newman and Wein (2009) stated that the advantages of CIC over indwelling included self-care and independence, reduced need for equipment, less barriers for intimacy and sexual activities, and potential for reduced lower urinary tract symptomology.

Sterile versus clean catheterization in this patient population remains a controversial topic; however, experts agree that clean intermittent catheterization (CIC) is appropriate for the majority of patients. Sterile catheterization is required for those with immunosuppression, those at risk for developing UTIs, and patients in acute or long-term care facilities (AUA 2014; Stohrer et al. 2009; Newman and Wein 2009).

The reuse of catheters remains controversial. The current standard of care is that catheters are for single use only. Several authors support this level of care (AUA 2014; Stohrer et al. 2009; Jamison et al. 2013).

Teaching patients CIC takes a knowledgeable practitioner and lots of patience. There are many patient handouts available; see resources for links on teaching patients.

Pharmacology

There are very few medications that are used to treat UAB. The main drug that is used is bethanechol (urecholine), a parasympathomimetic that provides direct stimulation of muscarinic receptors to allow a better detrusor contraction. Barendrecht and others (2007) did a systematic review and determined that the medication is not effective in the majority of patients studied. Bethanechol is currently the only approved medication for UAB. It must be titrated (5–10 mg per dose maximum dose 50 mg) individually and given 3–4 times daily. According to Chancellor et al. (2018) data via meta-analysis shows little benefit in the treatment of UAB.

Surgical Care

Sacral Nerve Stimulation

Sacral neuromodulation may be an effective minimally invasive intervention for some patients with underactive bladder. This is clinically indicated in some patients with nonobstructive urinary retention and incomplete bladder emptying. The therapy offers several potential benefits including avoidance of medications which could be associated with polypharmacy or drug–drug interactions. It may also be useful in those who either cannot perform or have not responded to other forms of behavioral therapy. At the writing of this book, MRI incompatibility is no longer an issue with SNS.

Although the exact mechanisms of sacral neuromodulation are not known, its principles are based on the fact that the S2–S4 nerve roots provide the primary autonomic and somatic innervation to the lower urinary tract, including the pelvic floor, urethra, and bladder. Neuromodulation works on the principle that activity in one neural pathway can influence activity in another neural pathway. Yoshimura and Chancellor (2011) have suggested that SNS causes somatic afferent inhibition of sensory processing in the spinal cord. The S2–S4 nerve roots provide the primary autonomic and somatic innervation to the bladder, urethra, and pelvic floor. Thus, sacral neuromodulation somehow helps in dysfunctional voiding of UAB by stimulating these nerve roots.

Botulinum Toxin

Botulinum toxin has been extensively used in the neurogenic population to prevent urgency and urge incontinence. The main concern with patients who have UAB is that the patient will almost always require ISC and must be taught before the procedure.

Normally, muscle contraction occurs after acetylcholine is released at the neuromuscular junction. Botulinum toxin blocks neurotransmission by binding to acceptor sites on motor or sympathetic nerve terminals, entering the nerve terminals and inhibiting the release of acetylcholine. Without acetylcholine release, the muscle is unable to contract (AHFS Drug Information 2009). This inhibition occurs as the neurotoxin cleaves a protein (SNAP-25) necessary to the docking and release of acetylcholine from the vesicles within nerve endings. As a result Botulinum toxin acts as a temporary biochemical neuromodulator, meaning that muscle contraction will resume after the effects of the medication have worn off (usually 3–6 months) (Chancellor 2009).

Preventing and Treating Infections

As a result of impaired storage and voiding function, UTIs occur frequently in UAB patients. UTI is the leading cause for septicemia in these patients which is associated with a significantly increased mortality (Pannek 2011). Symptomatic UTIs are often bothersome for the patients and are therefore related to a decreased quality of life. As UTIs are often recurrent and the bacterial strains are increasingly resistant to antibiotic treatment, UTIs are a clinical challenge for both patients and caregivers.

The EAU (Bok et al. 2018) and AUA white paper (2014) guidelines state that screening for and treatment of asymptomatic UTI in patients with UAB are not recommended (Bok et al. 2018). Patients should only be treated when there is

Table 13.7 Signs and symptoms associated with UTIs in the neurologically compromised patient

Signs and symptoms associated with a UTI include
1. New onset or worsening of fevers unexplained by other symptomatology
2. Rigors
3. Altered mental status changes unexplained by other pathology (i.e., dehydration)
4. Malaise or lethargy with no other identified cause
5. Flank pain
6. Costovertebral angle tenderness
7. Acute hematuria
8. Pelvic discomfort
9. In patients with spinal cord injury
(a) Increased spasticity
(b) Autonomic dysreflexia
Pyuria is not diagnostic of a UTI in catheterized patients; however the absence of pyuria in a symptomatic patient suggests a diagnosis other than UTI
The absence or presence of odorous urine or cloudy urine should not be used to diagnose a UTI

Table 13.8 Preventing UTIs in patients undergoing catheterization

1. Treat only symptomatic UTIs
2. Do not do routine urinalysis or culture
3. Maintain good hygiene
4. Maintain adequate hydration
5. Do not routinely irrigate
6. Ensure adequate emptying of the bladder
(a) In CIC catheterize to maintain 500 cc or less in the bladder
(b) In indwelling catheters secure to leg and ensure no kinking of dislodgement of tubing
7. Although controversial acidification of the urine with use of cranberry pills has shown to be useful in preventing UTI. Cranberry pills cannot be used on patients with anticoagulant therapy
8. Change patient catheter based on patient tolerance

symptomology, bacteriuria, and pyuria. Determining symptomology is based on infection in this population that can be challenging due to the overlap of symptoms (see Table 13.7). If treatment is determined to be necessary, see Chap. 10.

In this patient population, a urine culture should always be ordered if treatment is decided. The antibiotic ordered can then be changed or continued based on the susceptibility. Preventing infections in the UAB patient must be a part of the patient education. See Table 13.8 for suggestions.

Clinical Pearls

- There is no one magic number that can be used to declare the PVR volume to be abnormal in elderly patients; an elevated post-void residual volume alone should be handled with caution. Consider each patient individually: do they have bothersome symptoms and is their CR elevated? If the answer is no, consider watching the patient rather than intervening.

- Many patients respond well to conservative measures such as scheduled toileting, prompted voiding, or other treatments, particularly with the assistance of caregivers when needed. Double voiding, defined as urinating again after a brief delay from the initial void, can help to better empty the bladder in some patients.
- When a distended bladder is incidentally identified and reported by the radiologist, it is important to clarify with the patient whether he/she voided prior to the study. Also, a bladder scan should be performed post-void to confirm an elevated PVR.
- The impact of detrusor underactivity on older patients can range from minimal to severe. Bothersome nocturia may be improved by decreasing fluid intake several hours before retiring to bed.
- Patients with dependent edema in the lower extremities or an element of congestive heart failure may benefit from reclining with their legs elevated for a time before going to bed for the night. Timing of diuretic use is important, and these medications should be taken in the morning or early afternoon rather than closer to bedtime.
- The risk of urinary retention associated with pain medications appears to be higher with the longer-activating pain medication. Similarly, general anesthetics promote smooth muscle relaxation and can contribute to post-operative urinary retention. The risk is even higher in those patients treated with epidural pain management.
- Asymptomatic bacteria should not be treated ever in a patient with UAB. If there are no significant white blood cells in the urine, and the patient does not have symptoms, do not give an antibiotic.
- When doing a SP tube change it is helpful to measure the distance from the skin to the end of the catheter and use the same distance with the new catheter.

Resources for the Patient

Teaching CIC: http://www.cc.nih.gov/ccc/patient_education/pepubs/bladder/cisc-women5_22.pdf

https://www.suna.org/download/members/selfCatheterization.pdf

Bladder Diary: http://www.niddk.nih.gov/health-information/health-topics/urologic-disease/daily-bladder-diary/Pages/facts.aspx

Nerve Disease and Bladdder control: http://www.niddk.nih.gov/health-information/health-topics/urologic-disease/nerve-disease-and-bladder-control/Pages/facts. aspx

Sexual and Urological problems of Diabetes http://www.niddk.nih.gov/health-information/health-topics/Diabetes/sexual-urologic-problems-diabetes/Pages/index.aspx

Urinary retention: http://www.niddk.nih.gov/health-information/health-topics/urologic-disease/urinary-retention/Pages/facts.aspx

Resources for the Nurse Practitioner

http://www.auanet.org/common/pdf/education/clinical-guidance/Catheter-Associated-Urinary-Tract-Infections-WhitePaper.pdf

Managing and Treating Urinary Incontinence 2nd edition by Diane Newman and Alan Wein 2009 Health Professions Press

The Underactive Bladder Michael Chancellor and Ananias Diokno editors 2015 Springer

SUNA white paper on CAUTI: https://www.suna.org/resources/cautiWhitePaper.pdf

SUNA Practice Guidelines

Acute Urinary retention: https://www.suna.org/sites/default/files/download/indwellingCatheter.pdf

FemaleCatheterization:https://www.suna.org/sites/default/files/download/female-Catheterization.pdf

Male Catheterization: https://www.suna.org/sites/default/files/download/male-Catheterization.pdf

CAUTI: https://www.suna.org/sites/default/files/download/cautiGuideline.pdf

Supropubic cath change: https://www.suna.org/sites/default/files/download/suprapubic-Catheter.pdf

References

AHFS Drug Information (2009) BOTOX®. Retrieved 2 Sep 2009, from http://ashp.org/ahfs/index.cfm

Alimi Q, Hascoet J, Manunta A, Kammerer-Jacquet S, Verhoest G, Brochard C et al (2018) Reliability of urinary cytology and cystoscopy for the screening and diagnosis of bladder cancer in patients with neurogenic bladder: a systematic review. Neurourol Urodyn 37:916–925. https://doi.org/10.1002/nau.23395

American Urological Association (2014) White paper on catheter-associated urinary tract infections: definitions and significance in the urologic patient 2014. Downloaded from https://www.aua-net.org/common/pdf/education/clinical-guidance/Catheter-Associated-Urinary-Tract-Infections-WhitePaper.pdf. On 29 June 2015

American Urological Association (2016) White paper on Non-neurogenic chronic urinary retention: consensus definition, management strategies, and future opportunities.

Barendrecht MM, Oelke M, Laguna MP, Micheal MC (2007) Is the use of parasympathomimetics for treating an underactive bladder evidence based? BJU Int 99:749–752

Bok B, Pannek J, Castro-Diaz D, Del Popolo G, Groen J, Hamid R, Karesenty G, et al (2018) EAU guidelines on neuro-urology. Retrieved from http://www.uroweb.org/guideline/neurourology/

Chancellor M (2009) Ten years single surgeon experience with botulinum toxin in the urinary tract: clinical observations and research discovery. Int Urol Nephrol J 42(2):383–391

Chancellor M (2014) The overactive bladder progression to underactive bladder hypothesis. Int Urol Nephrol 46(Suppl 1):523–527

Chancellor M, Diokno AC (2014) CURE-UAB shedding light on the underactive bladder syndrome. Int Urol Nephrol 46(Suppl 1):S1

Chancellor MB, Bartolone SN, DeVries EM, Diokno AC, Gibbons M, Jankowski R et al (2018) New technology assessment and current and upcoming therapies for underactive bladder. Neurourol Urodyn 37:2932–2937

Chapple CR, Osman NI, Birder L, Dmochowski R, Drake MJ, van Koeveringe G, Abrams P et al (2018) Terminology report from the international continence society (ICS) working group on underactive bladder (UAB). Neurourol Urodyn 37:2928–2931

Dewulf K, Abrham N, Lamb LE, Griebling TL, Youshimura N, Tyagi P, Chancellor MB et al (2017). Addressing challanges in underactive bladder: recommendations and insights from the Congress on Underactive Bladder (CURE-UAB2). Int Urol Nephrol J 49(5):777–785

Diokno A (2015) Evaluation and diagnosis of underactive bladder in The Underactive Bladder. In: Chancellor M, Diokino A (Eds), pp 13–24

Diokno AC, Brock BM, Brown MB, Herzog AR (1986) Prevalence of urinary incontinence and other urological symptoms in the noninstitutionalized elderly. J Urol 136:1022–1025

Griebling T (2015) Geriatric urology and underactive bladder in The Underactive Bladder. In: Chancellor M, Diokno A (Eds). Springer, Basel, pp 177–188

Jamison J, Maquire S, Mcann J (2013) Catheter policies for management of long term voiding problems in adults with neurogenic bladder disorders (Review). Cochrane Libr 11:1–59

Lapides J, Diokno A, Silber S, Lowe B (1972) Clean intermittent self-catheterization in the treatment of urinary tract disease. J Urol 107(3):458–4613

McClurg D, Ashe RG, Marshall K, Lowe-Strong AS (2006) Comparison of pelvic floor muscle training, electromyography biofeedback and neuromuscular electrical stimulation for bladder dysfunction in people with multiple sclerosis: a randomized pilot study. Neurourol Urodyn 25:337–348

McClurg D, Ashe RG, Lowe-Strong AS (2008) Neuromuscular electrical stimulation and the treatment of lower urinary tract dysfunction in multiple sclerosis-a double blind, placebo controlled, randomised clinical trial. Neurourol Urodyn 27:231–237

Miyazato M, Yoshimura N, Chancellor M (2013) The other bladder syndrome: underactive bladder. Rev Urol 15(1):11–22

Musco S, Padilla-Fernández B, Del Popolo G, Bonifazi M, Blok M, Groen J et al (2018) Value of urodynamic findings in predicting upper urinary tract damage in neuro-urological patients: a systematic review. Neurourol Urodyn 37:1522–1540. https://doi.org/10.1002/nau.23501

Newman D, Wein A (2009) Managing and treating urinary incontinence, 2nd edn. Health Professions Press, Baltimore, pp 365–483

Newman D, Wilson M (2011) Review of intermittent catheterization and current best practices. Urol Nurs 31(1):12–28

Osman N et al (2014) Detrusor underactivity and the underactive bladder: a new clinical entity? A review of current terminology, definitions, epidemiology aetiology and diagnosis. Eur Urol 65(2):389–398

Pannek J (2011) Treatment of urinary tract infection in persons with spinal cord injury: guidelines, evidence, and clinical practice. A questionnaire based survey and review of the literature. J Spinal Cord Med 34(1):11–15

Patil NJ, Nagaratna R, Garner C, Raghurman NV (2012) Effect of integrated yoga on neurogenic bladder dysfunction in patients with multiple sclerosis—a prospective observational series. Compliment Ther Med 20:424–430

Prieto J, Murphy CL, Moore KN, Fader M (2014) Catheterisation for long term bladder management (Review). Cochrane Libr 9:1–97

Stohrer M, Blok B, Castro-Diaz D, Chartier-Kastler E, Del Popolo G, Kramer G, Pannek J, Piotr R, Wyandaele J (2009) EAU guidelines on neurogenic lower urinary tract dysfunction. Eur Urol 56:81–88

Taylor JA, Kuchel GA (2006) Detrusor underactivity: clinical freatures and pathogenisis of an underdiagnosed geriatric condition. J Am Geriatr Soc 54:(12)1920–1932

Tubaro A, Puccini F, De Nunzio C, Diggesu GA, Elneil S, Gobbi C, Khullar V (2012) The treatment of lower urinary tract symptoms in patients with multiple sclerosis: a systemic review. Curr Urol Rep 13:335–342

Valente S, Du Beau C, Chancellor D et al (2014) Epidemiology and demographics of the underactive bladder: a cross sectional survey. Int Urol Nephrol 46(Suppl):S7–S10

Weld K, Dmochowski R (2000) Effect of bladder management on urological complications in spinal cord injured patients. J Urol 163:768–772

Yoshimura N, Chancellor MB (2011) Physiology and pharmacology of the bladder and urethra. In: Wein AJ, Kavoussi LR, Novick AC, Partin AW, Peters CA (eds) Campbells urology, 10th edn. Elsevier, Philadelphia

Stress Incontinence

14

Natalie Gaines, John E. Lavin, and Jason P. Gilleran

Contents

Objectives
1. Discuss the incidence and definition of stress urinary incontinence (SUI).
2. Review and provide tips for the assessment of SUI.
3. Discuss management of SUI.

N. Gaines
Female Pelvic Medicine and Reconstructive Surgery, Department of Urology, Beaumont Health System, Royal Oak, MI, USA

J. E. Lavin
Department of Urology, Beaumont Health System, Royal Oak, MI, USA

J. P. Gilleran (✉)
Department of Urology, Oakland University William Beaumont School of Medicine, Royal Oak, MI, USA
e-mail: JGilleran@urologist.org

© Springer Nature Switzerland AG 2020
S. A. Quallich, M. J. Lajiness (eds.), *The Nurse Practitioner in Urology*,
https://doi.org/10.1007/978-3-030-45267-4_14

Introduction

Incidence

Stress urinary incontinence (SUI) is defined as involuntary urinary leakage with any activities that increase abdominal pressure, such as coughing, laughing, sneezing, or even moving from a seated to a standing position. SUI is a very common problem affecting 15–80% of women. In terms of financial burden, urinary incontinence of all types was estimated to cost over $19.5 billion dollars a year (Hu et al. 2004).

Unfortunately, incontinence has been considered by many as a normal, irreversible aspect of aging that is an indication of mental incompetence. It dramatically increases the risk that a patient will be institutionalized as the burden on the caregiver becomes too much to care for the patient at home. Because of the social stigma associated with its hygienic issues, incontinence is underreported by patients; other patients do not self-report and minimize their symptoms as they feel that incontinence is not a legitimate medical issue. Because of these barriers in societal perception, only 1/4–1/2 of patients with incontinence are adequately managed.

Pertinent Anatomy, Physiology

The female urethra is approximately 4 cm in length from the bladder neck to the urethral meatus. In order to maintain continence, the urethra must remain closed at rest and also during any activity that may increase in abdominal pressure, such as coughing, bearing down, or sneezing.

Three structures are required to permit urethral closure. First, the urethral mucosa and submucosa must have a good vascular supply to help form a watertight closure. This is under the influence of estrogens. The second structure is the striated urogenital sphincter, also called the rhabdosphincter, which surrounds the urethra and keeps it closed at rest. Third, muscular and fascial tissues form a supportive hammock for the upper and mid-urethra. The largest connective tissue component, the endopelvic fascia, has two important connections which form the pubourethral and urethropelvic ligaments, connecting the urethra to the pubic bone and other strong tissues in the pelvis. The levator ani is a group of skeletal muscles that act as a pelvic support structure, with the pubourethral muscle being one portion of the levator ani arranged in a "sling" configuration around the proximal urethra. The levator ani complex also includes the puborectalis and pubococcygeus; this pelvic floor musculature has a significant role in supporting not only the pelvic organs but also the weight of the abdominal contents. Within the midline of these muscles is an exit aperture called the urogenital hiatus, where the urethra and vagina exit the pelvis. The predominant innervation to these muscle groups is via the pudendal nerve.

Pathophysiology

Stress urinary incontinence can occur in women as a result of two primary mechanisms. The most common etiology is urethral hypermobility (UH), which causes 80–90% of cases. In normal anatomy, the endopelvic fascia and pelvic floor muscles (levator ani) stabilize the urethra within the pelvis. This support coapts the urethra against the vagina posteriorly, compressing the urethra during any increase in intra-abdominal pressure.

This "hammock theory" was proposed by DeLancey in 1994 (DeLancey 1994).

In a woman with urethral hypermobility, the support structures no longer maintain the urethra in its normal anatomic position during stress maneuvers, which permits movement of the bladder neck and proximal urethra. Consequently, abdominal pressure is not distributed equally to the urethra, and when the bladder pressure is greater than the closure pressure of the urethra, urinary leakage occurs.

Common causes for urethral hypermobility include childbirth, stretching of the portions of the fascia which support the urethra, and injury to the structures which support the uterus, causing the urethra to pull down and away from the pubic bone. These conditions worsen with age and hormonal changes.

Intrinsic sphincter deficiency (ISD) is a less common cause of stress urinary incontinence, occurring in 10–20% of SUI patients. In ISD, the urethral mucosa and submucosa coapt poorly despite adequate vaginal support. This can be caused by multiple previous surgeries, pudendal nerve injury (which causes decreased urethral resistance to leakage), radiation, or injury to the blood supply after pelvic or vaginal surgery. ISD is typically seen in the presence of urethral hypermobility, but can occur as an isolated finding, particularly in the geriatric population, or in women who have previously undergone a urethral support surgery.

History

Accurately recognizing the type of incontinence in a patient can be challenging and requires a detailed history. Pertinent points include when the leakage started, what situations or movements tend to exacerbate it, and the overall severity—is the patient leaking just a few drops or emptying her entire bladder? Leakage that occurs after cough, sneeze, standing up, or while straining to have a bowel movement is the hallmark of SUI, whereas leakage that occurs after the patient feels an intense need to urinate is characteristic of urge incontinence. However, patients may report leakage that occurs without awareness of the mechanism behind it, which is classified as unaware incontinence. In these situations, incontinence can be related to stress maneuvers with repeated small volume urine loss; similarly, older patients may no longer have the sensation of urgency that accompanies bladder overactivity. The Medical, Epidemiologic, and Social Aspects of Aging, or MESA, questionnaire can be used to help quantify symptoms and to determine if the patient is suffering from both stress and urge incontinence, called mixed urinary incontinence (See Fig. 14.1).

MESA URINARY INCONTINENCE QUESTIONNAIRE (UIQ)

NAME :_____DATE :_____
        LAST,   FIRST   MI

Please check (÷) the appropriate box.

1. Over the past 12 months, have you had urine loss beyond your control?
    _____ Yes   _____ No

2. How long ago did your urine loss start? _____ years   _____ months _____days

3. When does the urine loss usually occur?

    _____ Day time only

    _____ Night time only

    _____ Both day time and night time

4. Do you use anything for protection against leaked urine?

        _____ Yes (Go to the next question)   _____ No

5. On <u>average</u>, how many of each of these do you use for protection? (Please write the number used and check each day or week)

                                                            <u>Number
                                                            Used</u>

    Sanitary napkins   _____   ____each day or ____each week
    Pads like those placed on furniture (ex. Blue pads)   _____   ____each day or ____each week
    Adult wetness control garments (ex. Attends, Depends) _____   ____each day or ____each week
    Toilet paper or facial tissues   _____   ____each day or ____each week
    Something else (please list)   _____   ____each day or ____each week
    _____   ____each day or ____each week

    _____   ____each day or ____each week

6. While awake, when you are having urine loss problems, how much urine would you say you lose without control EACH TIME?

        _____ A few drops to less than ½ teaspoon
        _____ ½ teaspoon to less than 2 tablespoons
        _____ 2 tablespoons to ½ cup
        _____ ½ cup or more

7. When you lose urine, does it usually:

        _____ Just create some moisture
        _____ Wet your underwear
        _____ Trickle down you thigh
        _____ Wet the floor

8. Generally, how many times do you usually urinate from the time you wake up to the time before you go to

    bed? _____ times.

9. Generally, how many times do you usually urinate after you have gone to sleep at night? _____ times

Fig. 14.1 MESA Urinary Incontinence Questionnaire (Diokno et al. 2002)

Urge Incontinence Questions

1. Some people receive very little warning and suddenly find that they are losing, or about to lose urine beyond their control. How often does this happen to your?
   _____Often (3)   _____Sometimes (2)   _____Rarely (1)   _____Never (0)

2. If you can't find a toilet or find a toilet that is occupied and you have an urge to urinate, how often do you end up losing urine and wetting yourself?
   _____Often (3)   _____Sometimes (2)   _____Rarely (1)   _____Never (0)

3. Do you lose urine when you suddenly have the feeling that your bladder is full?
   _____Often (3)   _____Sometimes (2)   _____Rarely (1)   _____Never (0)

4. Does washing your hands cause you to lose urine?
   _____Often (3)   _____Sometimes (2)   _____Rarely (1)   _____Never (0)

5. Does cold weather cause you to lose urine?
   _____Often (3)   _____Sometimes (2)   _____Rarely (1)   _____Never(0)

6. Does drinking cold beverages cause you to lose urine?
   _____Often (3)   _____Sometimes (2)   _____Rarely (1)   _____Never (0)   TOTAL SCORE=____/18

URGE SYMPTOMS INDEX LOOK-UP TABLE				
1/18 = 6%	5/18 = 28%	9/18 = 50%	13/18 = 72%	17/18 = 94%
2/18 = 11%	6/18 = 33%	10/18 = 56%	14/18 = 78%	18/18 = 100%
3/18 = 17%	7/18 = 39%	11/18 = 61%	15/18 = 83%	
4/18 = 22%	8/18 = 44%	12/18 = 67%	16/18 = 89%	

Stress Incontinence Questions

1. Does coughing gently cause you to lose urine?

   _____Often (3)   _____Sometimes (2)   _____Rarely (1)   _____Never (0)

2. Does coughing hard cause you to lose urine?

   _____Often (3)   _____Sometimes (2)   _____Rarely (1)   _____Never (0)

3. Does sneezing cause you to lose urine?

   _____Often (3)   _____Sometimes (2)   _____Rarely (1)   _____Never (0)

4. Does lifting things cause you to lose urine?

   _____Often (3)   _____Sometimes (2)   _____Rarely (1)   _____Never (0)

5. Does bending over cause you to lose urine?
   _____Often (3)   _____Sometimes (2)   _____Rarely (1)   _____Never (0)

6. Does laughing cause you to lose urine?
   _____Often (3)   _____Sometimes (2)   _____Rarely (1)   _____Never (0)

Fig. 14.1 (continued)

7. Does walking briskly cause you to lose urine?
_____Often (3)   _____Sometimes (2)   _____Rarely (1)   _____Never (0)

8. Does straining, if you are constipated, cause you to lose urine?
_____Often (3)   _____Sometimes (2)   _____Rarely (1)   _____Never (0)

9. Does getting up from a sitting to a standing position cause you to lose urine?
_____Often (3)   _____Sometimes (2)   _____Rarely (1)   _____Never (0)   TOTAL SCORE=____/27

STRESS SYMPTOMS INDEX LOOK-UP TABLE						
1/27 = 4%	5/27 = 19%	9/27 = 33%	13/27 = 48%	17/27 = 63%	21/27 = 78%	25/27 = 93%
2/27 = 7%	6/27 = 22%	10/27 = 37%	14/27 = 52%	18/27 = 67%	22/27 – 81%	26/27 = 96%
3/27 = 11%	7/27 = 26%	11/27 = 41%	15/27 = 56%	19/27 = 70%	23/27 = 85%	27/27 = 100%
4/27 = 15%	8/27 = 30%	12/27 = 44%	16/27 = 59%	20/27 = 74%	24/27 = 89%	

Fig. 14.1 (continued)

One way of identifying SUI severity is to quantify the number of sanitary pads the patient uses daily, but the number and type of pad alone can be misleading. Thus, a clinician should ascertain not only whether the patient is using a thin liner versus a full diaper but also how wet they are when she changes them. Some patients change their pads after only a few drops of leakage, whereas others only change their pads when they are fully soaked. Additionally, one should inquire about a patient's overall voiding habits to evaluate for any concomitant voiding or bowel dysfunction. Does she also have daytime frequency and urgency, nighttime frequency or leakage while sleeping (nocturnal enuresis), any history of hematuria or dysuria, straining to void, or post-void micturition (dribbles of urine leaking out after she finishes urinating)? Constipation can frequently cause urinary leakage, so ensuring that a patient with leakage is having soft, formed bowel movements is very important. Hematuria or dysuria in a smoker could be an indication of a transitional cell cancer of the bladder or ureter and merit a full hematuria workup. A voiding diary can be helpful in the woman with frequency and nocturia, which can also provide insight on fluid intake, as polydipsia can exacerbate any type of urinary incontinence.

Incontinence can often accompany pelvic organ prolapse (POP), and the history should also include if the patient reports a sensation of a bulge coming out of her vagina. As laxity in the structural supports of the pelvis can cause UI, prolapse can occur in more severe cases. In a woman with a concomitant cystocele or rectocele, she may note the need to "splint," where she places a finger in the vagina to assist with emptying of the bladder and/or bowels. It is imperative to know that women with advanced POP often do not have SUI, as this can be "masked" by the bulge kinking off the urethra. In such cases, women may report having SUI in the past that spontaneously resolved, likely once their prolapse worsened.

Other pertinent aspects of the history include a complete medical history, with prior surgeries and current medications noted. Some medications can worsen SUI in patients, such as alpha-adrenergic antagonists, such as doxazosin (see Table 14.1). Current or prior tobacco use can lead to chronic cough, as can pulmonary conditions such as asthma or COPD. Chronic cough as a side effect of angiotensin-converting

Table 14.1 Medications that cause transient UI

Medication	Effect on urinary system
Alpha-adrenergic receptor antagonists	Smooth muscle relaxation of the bladder neck and urethral causing SUI (mainly women)
Tricyclic antidepressants Alpha-adrenergic agonists	Anticholinergic effect and alpha-adrenergic receptor agonist effect causing post-void dribbling, straining, and hesitancy in urine flow and even urinary retention
Psychotropics	May decrease afferent input resulting in decrease in bladder contractility. Can accumulate in the elderly causing confusion resulting in functional incontinence
Cholinesterase inhibitors	Increase bladder contractility and may cause incontinence
Narcotic analgesics, opioids	Decrease bladder contractility, decrease afferent input. Depress the central nervous system causing sedation, confusion, and immobility, leading to urinary retention and UI
Calcium channel blockers	Impair bladder contractility, causing UI
Diuretics	Overwhelm the bladder with rapidly produced urine for up to 6 h after ingestion
Methylxanthines	Polyuria, bladder irritation

Adapted from Ouslander (2004)

inhibitors is rare, but it should be noted in the patient's medication history. Obesity can also be a source of SUI, and weight loss of 10% can often correct the incontinence. Treatment of chronic cough can in and of itself relieve SUI and should be pursued either before or concomitantly with any treatments for SUI, as successful treatment is less likely if this symptom is not addressed adequately. Lastly, a full gynecologic history, including gravida/parity status, vaginal versus caesarean section deliveries, and any complications of pregnancies, should be noted. Menopausal status and the use of any type of hormone replacement are also important, although hormonal replacement therapy may only marginally help the woman with SUI.

Diagnostic Evaluation

Physical Exam

The goal of a proper physical examination is to reproduce the leakage that the patient reports while identifying anatomic abnormalities that could account for the incontinence. Examination with a full bladder is paramount in the evaluation of SUI. However, some patients may leak with an empty bladder evaluated with a supine empty bladder stress test (SEBST)—leakage from the urethral meatus during cough or Valsalva maneuver at the time of the pelvic examination. In 2010 Nager et al. reported that patients with a positive SEBST had increased pad weight and number of leaks per day compared to patients with a negative SEBST, that is, a positive supine empty bladder stress test is highly indicative of severe stress incontinence. Urethral hypermobility on exam is indicated by brisk, upward movement of the urethra of at least 30° with an increase in abdominal pressure. One method of measuring the degree of urethral mobility is via the "q-tip test," in which a soft lubricated applicator is passed through the urethra to the level of the bladder neck. The woman is asked to cough and/or Valsalva and the degree of rotation is measured, with >30° considered hypermobile. However, this test is not used as often clinically due to urethral discomfort.

A "stress test" is considered positive if one demonstrates urinary leakage; however, absence of urinary leakage does not mean the patient doesn't have SUI. Thirty-four percent of women with SUI have a negative stress test, which could be positional or due to inadequate filling of the bladder (Nager et al. 2010). If negative, reassess with the patient standing. Absence of urethral mobility, i.e., a "fixed" urethra, in the presence of stress leak is important since the most commonly used surgery for SUI, the mid-urethral sling, has a higher failure rate in these patients. This finding is more common in the elderly female, who may also have a finding of atrophic vaginitis.

Other findings to note on exam are whether there are signs of a urethral diverticulum, which can be identified as a fluid-filled sac along the urethra that expresses fluid through the meatus on palpation. These can also be quite tender, particularly if they are actively infected. Patients with a urethral diverticulum will often report the symptom of post-void dribbling, stress incontinence, or even continuous incontinence. The examination of the patient's pelvic floor while asking her to perform a Kegel maneuver—squeeze down around your finger and evaluate the strength of her pelvic floor musculature—can be very helpful. A woman with a weak pelvic floor and incontinence may significantly benefit from pelvic floor physical therapy.

A pelvic exam must also identify the presence of pelvic organ prolapse and its severity. This is especially important in a patient who reports previously having stress incontinence that spontaneously resolved as her vaginal bulge worsened. Some patients have such a large cystocele that it ultimately kinks off the urethra.

A rare cause of incontinence, particularly in the young nulliparous female, is the presence of an ectopic ureter, which can drain directly into the vagina. Usually, this is associated with a symptom of continuous, rather than activity-related, incontinence. Lastly, one should perform a general neurologic examination, evaluating for intact sensation and any deficits.

Diagnostic Tests

It is clinically indicated to obtain a urinalysis in every patient with SUI, looking for microscopic hematuria, which should prompt a workup according to the American Urological Association guidelines, or a urinary tract infection, which should be treated prior to additional workup.

Measuring post-void residual is also part of the basic evaluation for SUI, especially if there is planned surgical intervention. Incomplete emptying or urinary retention, the definition of which can vary but is generally accepted as a PVR >150 mL, identifies those who may have an issue with bladder emptying after surgery. An elevated PVR could be related to a neurologic deficit or a large cystocele that may need to be repaired simultaneously. These patients merit further workup, particularly in the absence of advanced-grade pelvic organ prolapse.

Urodynamic testing (UDT) is a routine outpatient diagnostic test designed to reproduce symptoms while assessing for other functional abnormalities of the lower urinary tract. In the woman with SUI alone, UDT is not routinely indicated. The Value of Urodynamic Evaluation, or VaLUE, study was a randomized trial comparing office evaluation only versus office evaluation and urodynamics prior to SUI surgery (Nager et al. 2012). This large multicenter study showed that in 97% of patients, urodynamics merely confirm the office evaluation; that is, in the vast majority of patients, urodynamic testing is not necessary to make a proper diagnosis. At 1-year follow-up, these patients had similar outcomes. The uncomplicated index patients included in the VaLUE study were defined as a woman with stress-predominant incontinence, a post-void residual of less than 150 mL, negative urinalysis or urine culture, and urethral hypermobility with a positive stress test on examination. Which patients should undergo urodynamic testing?

1. Any patient who reports SUI and in whom one cannot demonstrate it on exam with a full bladder in the standing position, prior to any surgical intervention.
2. Any patient with concern for, or a proven neurologic disease—leakage in this patient may be due to altered bladder compliance and neurogenic detrusor over-activity. Consider video urodynamics to look for vesicoureteral reflux at higher detrusor pressures—this can ultimately lead to deterioration of the upper tracts (kidneys).
3. Any patient who has previously undergone an anti-incontinence procedure and has persistent or recurrent incontinence. UDT can help evaluate if the prior surgery is causing urethral obstruction.
4. Patients with high-grade pelvic organ prolapse without stress incontinence may have occult stress incontinence, which can be "unmasked" during UDT.
5. Mixed incontinence patients who have both SUI and urgency, frequency, and urge urinary incontinence should undergo UDT to help the clinician decide which treatments should be initiated first.

The AUA and the Society for Urodynamics, Female Pelvic Medicine, and Urogenital Reconstruction (SUFU) published a set of guidelines in 2012 to assist clinicians in determining which patients may benefit from further urodynamic testing (Winters et al. 2012). For straightforward stress urinary incontinence, no routine imaging studies are indicated.

Management

Because SUI is a quality-of-life disease, the treatment is contingent upon the patient's bother. Remember, some patients are not severely bothered by what you may perceive as a severe symptomatology and choose not to pursue any treatment. Conservative first-line treatment consists of pelvic floor physical therapy and

Table 14.2 Behaviors to reduce stress incontinence

Behavior	Intervention
Fluid intake	Fluid intake should be 6–8 8 oz. glasses of fluid per day
Bowel function	Regulate bowel function to avoid straining and constipation
Smoking	Quit to relieve chronic cough associated with smoking
Obesity	Lose weight to decrease pressure on sphincter

Table 14.3 Kegel exercises

Kegel exercise instructions
1. Identify pelvic floor muscles
2. Squeeze and hold up to 10 s
3. Relax for 10 s after each contraction (relaxing is just as important as contracting)
4. Do not use the stomach, buttocks, or thighs
5. Do ten sets daily in each position, sitting, standing, and laying
6. Doing too many exercises can fatigue your muscles

behavioral changes (see Table 14.2). Teaching a client Kegel exercises (see Table 14.3) can be done in the office or with referral to physical therapist (PT) who specializes in pelvic floor therapy. When referring a patient to pelvic floor PT, the physical therapists use a number of modalities to target the levator muscle group, including intravaginal muscle strengthening exercises, biofeedback, and electrical stimulation. Behavioral therapy is helpful in patients who report excessive fluid intake (>100 oz. total daily) or who have incontinence due to delayed voiding, where leakage occurs due to overfilling. Addressing any causes of chronic cough or straining can resolve SUI in many women. Cough is a known side effect of angiotensin-converting enzyme (ACE) inhibitors, such as lisinopril, in some individuals. Appropriate referrals to otolaryngology for chronic cough or even discussion with their primary physician to adjust medications can be helpful.

For those patients with situational incontinence only (i.e., only occurring during certain sporting activities), one can use a urethral insert to "plug" the outlet and reduce leakage. The FemSoft is a soft, plastic insert that can be left in the urethra temporarily. Alternatively, a vaginal tampon has been reported to reduce leakage in younger women. In the most severe cases of sphincteric damage, or in the frail elderly individuals, catheter placement can be offered as a short- or even long-term option, but carries several risks, including urethral damage, hematuria, and urinary tract infections.

For patients who are not interested in or not candidates for physical therapy, or in those with incomplete symptom resolution after PT, the next option is surgery, as there are no Food and Drug Administration-approved pharmaceuticals for SUI. The most common procedure for SUI currently is the mid-urethral sling (MUS). The concept of an MUS, initially described as a tension-free vaginal tape, was first described by Ulmsten in 1996 (Ulmsten et al. 1996). A 17-year follow-up of 90 women published in 2013 reported an objective cure rate of over 90% (Nilsson et al.

2013). The surgical approach involves a small vaginal incision to permit passage of a thin strip of synthetic mesh using a trocar, or a thin metal carrier, through the obturator canal and exiting via the groin (the transobturator sling) or behind the pubic bone exiting via the suprapubic area (the retropubic sling). Once healed in position, the mesh rests underneath the middle of the urethra and, during any increase in intra-abdominal pressure, permits coaptation of the urethra to prevent urinary leakage.

The Trial of Mid-Urethral Slings (TOMUS) study evaluated for a difference in outcomes between the retropubic and the transobturator approach. At 24-month follow-up, both groups were found to have similarly high rates of satisfaction. The retropubic slings were found to have slightly better objective success rates, but also had higher rates of voiding dysfunction requiring surgery (3% vs. 0%, $p = 0.002$) and urinary tract infections (Nilsson et al. 2013). The transobturator slings, because they pass through the obturator fossa, can cause damage to the obturator nerve; thus, these patients had a higher rate of neurologic symptoms.

The most common complications of MUS include urinary obstruction, bladder or urethral injury, injury to bowel or vascular structures, and mesh erosion. Urinary obstruction may be reported by the patient and should be promptly managed within the first several weeks postoperatively. Many patients report a slower stream; however, any patient who is unable to void or requires catheterization needs prompt evaluation by the operating surgeon. Immediately after surgery, the mesh has not undergone maximal tissue ingrowth, and it is possible to perform a sling release, either in the operating room or the office. The vaginal incision is opened and the sling is grasped and pulled down to loosen. After about 3 weeks, the surrounding pelvic tissues have begun to grow into the mesh, and the patient may require a sling incision, where the sling must be cut in the operating room. If obstruction is not addressed, the bladder can be damaged due to high voiding pressures, which can ultimately cause myogenic failure (inability to contract normally) and/or bladder wall thickening, which can adversely affect bladder filling.

Bladder and urethral injuries are typically diagnosed via intraoperative cystoure-throscopy. Bladder perforation by a trocar has been reported in 3.5–6.6% of cases; management includes removal of the offending trocar and repassage as well as temporary catheterization, the duration of which is at the performing surgeon's discretion. In cases where the trocar has only passed through the bladder a single time, some surgeons feel comfortable leaving no catheter; in other cases, with multiple passages (as occasionally occurs in a patient with difficult anatomy), the catheter must remain in place for 1–7 days. If mesh erosion into the urethra or the bladder occurs as a late complication, the patient can present with gross hematuria, lower tract symptoms such as frequency or urgency, or recurrent urinary tract infections. Mesh that is eroded into the urinary tract must be removed completely. The choice to perform another sling at that time versus as a delayed approach is up to the surgeon's discretion, but the use of mesh in these revision cases may not be prudent.

Mesh erosion or exposure is a rare occurrence after MUS, but this condition can present as vaginal discharge or bleeding, especially after intercourse or partner discomfort. The patient herself may feel palpable mesh or other material in the vagina, but this is most often seen by the clinician during pelvic exam. If the exposure is minimal or the patient is asymptomatic, the erosion can be observed and the patient can use a topical estrogen cream. This is most commonly done in a woman who is not sexually active. If the patient is having symptoms, there are several management options, including excising the exposed portion, reapproximating vaginal epithelium over the exposure, or even removal of the entire mesh sling. Complete removal can lead to recurrence of the patient's incontinence. It should be noted that full-thickness exposure is not necessary for the sling to cause discomfort, and the finding of point tenderness over a portion of the sling that was not present preoperatively may warrant partial or total sling removal in select cases.

Bowel injuries are exceedingly rare but occur with passage of the trocar through the space of Retzius during retropubic sling placement. This occurs more commonly in women with a history of prior abdominal of pelvic surgery or with an abdominal hernia. Bowel injuries manifest after retropubic MUS with peritoneal signs—severe or persistent abdominal pain, guarding, rigidity, fever, or feculent drainage from the abdominal incision sites. Diagnosis may be solidified by a CT scan with oral contrast. This is a surgical emergency and requires prompt treatment.

A second procedure which dates to the early twentieth century but is still commonly used is the pubovaginal fascial sling. This procedure differs from the midurethral sling in several important ways. First, the anatomic location is more proximal than the MUS—the sling itself is placed at the bladder neck. These slings are historically intended to be at least partially obstructing and can be used in patients with intrinsic sphincter deficiency or in patients who have failed previous MUS. Instead of a piece of mesh, tissue is used—typically autologous tissue, taken from the patient's fascia lata on the thigh or from the rectus fascia on the abdominal wall. A vaginal incision is made, just like in the MUS, but the bladder neck is exposed and lateral dissection performed to enter the retropubic space. Next, an abdominal incision is made, typically a Pfannenstiel incision, and if using rectus fascia, this is harvested. The piece of tissue required to perform this procedure is typically 6–10 cm in length and 1–2 cm in width. Permanent suture is used to anchor the fascia on each end to tension it to the abdominal fascia. A ligature passer is passed on either side of the urethra down from the abdominal to the vaginal incision under fingertip guidance. The suture is grasped and brought up so that the fascia is lying flat against the urethra and then tensioned under direct visualization and palpation. This procedure takes longer, may have more blood loss, and typically requires an overnight stay, versus the MUS which permits same-day discharge. The complications are similar to those of the MUS and include injury to bowel, bladder, urethra, or vascular structures or urinary obstruction, but because the patient has no mesh placed and the tissue is her own, the exposure rate is quite low. However, because the fascial sling is much more obstructing than the MUS, many patients develop new-onset urgency, voiding dysfunction, and the need for catheterization. If the fascial sling is overly tensioned, it can be loosened, but this is always done in the operating room (not the office) and is more extensive than loosening a mesh sling.

The Burch colposuspension, which differs from slings as this procedure is performed via an abdominal incision, anchors the anterior vaginal wall at the level of the bladder neck to the iliopectineal line (Cooper's ligament) using 2–4 permanent sutures. This procedure is most commonly performed at the same time as an abdominal hysterectomy. In the Stress Incontinence Surgical Treatment Efficacy Trial, or SISTEr, the Burch colposuspension was compared to the previously discussed bladder neck sling (Albo et al. 2007). With 24-month follow-up, this multicenter trial showed that the fascial sling had higher overall success rates than the Burch procedure and that more patients who had undergone the Burch procedure needed a second surgery to correct their SUI. However, the success of the fascial sling was offset by its higher rate of complications, including UTI, urge incontinence, and the need for surgical treatment to permit voiding.

In patients with a fixed urethra, a fascial sling can be effective, but a less invasive, less obstructive approach is to use a bulking agent, such as calcium hydroxyapatite (Coaptite) or silicon elastomer (Macroplastique). Cross-linked collagen was commonly used in the past, but is no longer available on the market. Bulking agent injection is performed using a cystoscope through the wall of the mid-urethra to "bulk up" the urethral sphincter and allow the walls of the urethra to coapt together, reducing stress incontinence. Patients should be counseled that "cure" of the leakage with this technique is uncommon, but one can expect significant improvement with 1–2 injections. Risks are low and can include transient retention (1–3 days), urinary infection, and urethritis and dysuria in rare cases.

There is currently ongoing research regarding the use of autologous muscle cells injected into the urethra to "regenerate" the urethral sphincter. Muscle cells are harvested via biopsy of the thigh muscles, for example, and grown in an outside laboratory for several weeks before reinjection. Early studies are promising, but this treatment shows promise and may be commercially available in the near future.

Conclusion

SUI is a very correctable problem, and its management has evolved to a less invasive approach, with good long-term follow-up and several well-designed studies demonstrating efficacy of the MUS. Obtaining a thorough and appropriate history, performing a directed physical examination, and assessing urine and voiding function are critical to develop a therapeutic plan for each patient. Carefully assessing the patient's expectations and then providing appropriate counseling on nonsurgical and surgical options are requisites to ensure that each patient receives the outcome that she desires.

Clinical Pearls
- Conservative management is a preferred route in younger patients with mild stress incontinence or patients at high risk for surgical repair.
- Urodynamics are no longer indicated in the uncomplicated, "index" woman with stress urinary incontinence.
- Despite the FDA warnings and recent cessation of mesh "kits" for vaginal prolapse, the mid-urethral mesh sling is the most studied anti-incontinence

procedure to date and a safe, viable option in the appropriately selected woman with SUI.

- The treatment of intrinsic sphincter deficiency is still limited and can be challenging in the severe cases. For mild to moderate cases, bulking agents are an effective minimally invasive option with low morbidity, but patients must be counseled appropriately on expectations for improvement, rather than cure.

Resources for the Nurse Practitioner

http://www.auanet.org/education/guidelines/incontinence.cfm

Diane Newman and Alan Wein Urinary Incontinence 2nd edition Health Professionals Press 2009   https://www.auanet.org/guidelines/stress-urinary-incontinence-(sui)-guideline

Resources for the Patient

http://www.urologyhealth.org//Documents/Product%20Store/Surgical-VaginalMesh treat-SUI-PatientFactSheet.pdf

https://www.niddk.nih.gov/health-information/urologic-diseases/bladder-control-problems

https://urologyhealth.org/urologic-conditions/stress-urinary-incontinence-(sui)

https://sufuorg.com/about/news/message-about-fda-statement-on-mus.aspx

https://www.niddk.nih.gov/health-information/urologic-diseases/bladder-control-problems?dkrd=hispt0442

References

Albo ME, Richter HE, Brubaker L et al (2007) Burch colposuspension versus fascial sling to reduce urinary stress incontinence. N Engl J Med 356(21):2143–2155

DeLancey JO (1994) Structural support of the urethra as it relates to stress urinary incontinence: the hammock hypothesis. Am J Obstet Gynecol 170(6):1713–1720; discussion 1720–1713

Diokno AC, Catipay JR, Steinert BW (2002) Office assessment of patient outcome of pharmacologic therapy for urge incontinence. Int Urogynecol J Pelvic Floor Dysfunct 13(5):334–338

Hu TW, Wagner TH, Bentkover JD, Leblanc K, Zhou SZ, Hunt T (2004) Costs of urinary incontinence and overactive bladder in the United States: a comparative study. Urology 63(3):461–465

Nager CW, Kraus SR, Kenton K et al (2010) Urodynamics, the supine empty bladder stress test, and incontinence severity. Neurourol Urodyn 29(7):1306–1311

Nager CW, Brubaker L, Litman HJ et al (2012) A randomized trial of urodynamic testing before stress-incontinence surgery. N Engl J Med 366(21):1987–1997

Nilsson CG, Palva K, Aarnio R, Morcos E, Falconer C (2013) Seventeen years' follow-up of the tension-free vaginal tape procedure for female stress urinary incontinence. Int Urogynecol J 24(8):1265–1269

Ouslander JG (2004) Management of overactive bladder. New Engl J Med 350:786–799

Ulmsten U, Henriksson L, Johnson P, Varhos G (1996) An ambulatory surgical procedure under local anesthesia for treatment of female urinary incontinence. Int Urogynecol J Pelvic Floor Dysfunct 7(2):81–85; discussion 85–86

Winters JC, Dmochowski RR, Goldman HB et al (2012) Urodynamic studies in adults: AUA/SUFU guideline. J Urol 188(6 Suppl):2464–2472

Overactive Bladder

15

Jennifer L. Mosher and Leslie Saltzstein Wooldridge

Contents

Objectives

1. Discuss diagnosis, incidence, and assessment of overactive bladder.
2. Delineate treatments for OAB.
3. Describe the impact on quality of life for patients with overactive bladder.

J. L. Mosher (✉)
Mercy Health Physician Partners Pelvic Medicine and Urogynecology, Muskegon, MI, USA

L. S. Wooldridge
Mercy Health Bladder Clinic, Muskegon, MI, USA

© Springer Nature Switzerland AG 2020
S. A. Quallich, M. J. Lajiness (eds.), *The Nurse Practitioner in Urology*,
https://doi.org/10.1007/978-3-030-45267-4_15

This chapter on overactive bladder (OAB) is intended to guide the nurse practitioner in his/her practice through the proper linear treatment of patients. In doing so, the incidence and prevalence of OAB in North America will be stated. A review of pertinent history and a physical to determine the diagnosis of OAB will also be presented. Finally, treatment and therapies identified by the American Urologic Association (AUA) and Society for Urodynamics and Female Urology (SUFU) guidelines for treatment of OAB (Gormley et al. 2012-2015, Lightner et al. 2019) will be discussed.

Definitions

All definitions are determined by the International Continence Society (ICS) (Haylen et al. 2010).

Overactive bladder (*OAB*, Urgency) syndrome is defined as the presence of urinary urgency, usually accompanied by frequency and nocturia, with or without urgency urinary incontinence, in the absence of urinary tract infection (UTI) or other obvious pathology.

Daytime urinary frequency is defined by the number of voids by day (wakeful hours including last void before sleep and first void after waking and rising).

Twenty-four-hour frequency is the total number of daytime voids and episodes of nocturia during a specified 24-h period.

Increased daytime urinary frequency is the complaint that voiding occurs more frequently during waking hours than previously deemed normal. Traditionally seven episodes of voiding during waking hours has been deemed as the upper limit of normal, though it may be higher in some populations.

Nocturia is the complaint of interruption of sleep one or more times because of the need to void. Each void is preceded and followed by sleep.

Urgency is the complaint of a sudden, compelling desire to pass urine that is difficult to defer.

Urge urinary incontinence is the involuntary leakage of urine, associated with a sudden compelling desire to void.

OAB "wet" is OAB with urge urinary incontinence.

OAB "dry" is OAB without urge urinary incontinence.

Warning time is the time from the first sensation of the urgency to void.

Refractory OAB is present in the patient who has failed appropriate behavioral therapy of sufficient length and a trial of at least one antimuscarinic medication administered for 6–12 weeks (Gormley et al. 2012)

Incidence and Epidemiology

The prevalence of OAB has been difficult to define due to differing definitions and qualifications to obtain a specific diagnosis of overactive bladder. A review by

Powell et al. (2018) identified three key cross-sectional epidemiological studies of OAB in the United States. In 2003, the NOBLE (National Overactive Bladder Evaluation) study found the prevalence of OAB among noninstitutionalized adults to be 16.5% (33 million people). Prevalence increased to over 30% among those over 65 years old and was comparable in men and women. In 2007, the EpiLUTS (Epidemiology of Lower Urinary Tract Symptoms) study estimated the prevalence among adults 40 years and older to be 18.5% (42.2 million people). The most recent study in 2010, OAB-POLL (OAB on Physical and Occupational Limitations) estimates an even higher overall prevalence of 23.2% and found that approximately twice as many women as men are affected.

The estimated national total economic burden of OAB in the US has ranged from 12.6 billion (2000 USD) to 65.9 billion annually (2007 USD) (Durden et al. 2018). More recent research by Powell et al. (2018) has identified this burden of cost estimation to be much higher, over 100 billion annually. They found that the costs among individuals with OAB were 1.4 to more than twofold higher than those of the same age and sex-matched individuals without OAB.

In 2013 Coyne et al. identified higher prevalence of OAB among men and women aged 18–70 and significant differences by racial/ethnic group based on the results of the OAB-POLL. The prevalence of OAB was highest among African American men and women (20% and 33%). In men, this was followed by Hispanics (18%) and whites (15%), while in women the rates were comparable among Hispanic and white women (29%). African American and Hispanic men and women were significantly more likely to have OAB despite having a lower prevalence of self-reported co-morbidities and risk factors associated with OAB. McKellar et al. (2019) found that there is no apparent difference in use of medical therapy for OAB based on racial/ethnic differences.

Risk Factors

Overactive bladder can be idiopathic and develop over years. Aging is the most commonly found risk factor for both men and women. Age-related changes in both the bladder and pelvic floor tissues as well as changes in the nervous system result in higher prevalence of OAB in elderly women. As estrogen levels decrease with menopause, atrophy of the lower urinary tract and pelvic floor also may trigger urinary symptoms. In men 60 years or older, there is a higher prevalence of benign prostatic hyperplasia which can lead to bladder outlet obstruction and OAB symptoms.

Obesity is also shown to result in higher incidences of OAB. Elevated BMI leads to increased abdominal pressure as well as increased intravesical pressure, leading to stretching along the pudendal nerve and possible pelvic floor dysfunction. In men an increasing BMI has also been associated with larger prostate volumes increasing their risk of OAB due to bladder outlet obstruction.

Numerous studies have shown a higher incidence of OAB in relation to known bladder irritants, such as caffeine and carbonated beverages (Reisch et al. 2018). In regards to cigarette smoking and alcohol abuse, however, although both have significant burden of disease in general, they have not been shown to have a significant association with higher incidence of OAB (Zhu et al. 2019).

Guidelines for Treatment

The guidelines for treatment of OAB were designed and published (Gormley et al. 2012, 2015 and Lightner et al. 2019) to provide direction for all types of providers who evaluate and treat OAB. This project was conducted as part of the Agency for Healthcare Research and Quality (AHRQ) Evidence Report, Treatment of OAB in Women (2009). A literature search was conducted from 1966 to 2008, 2008 to 2011, 2014, and 2019. The first guidelines were initially presented May 2012 at the AUA annual meeting and continue to be updated as new information becomes available.

First-line therapy	Second-line therapy	Third-line therapy	Fourth-line therapy	Additional treatment
Behavioral management: Fluid management; Pelvic floor therapy; Toileting schedules. If partially effective, consider adding medications.	Medications: Anticholinergics Antimuscarinics Beta-3 adrenergic agents Combination therapy with an anticholinergic and beta-3 adrenergic agent If patient goals are not met consider further treatment.	Neuromodulation: Percutaneous tibial nerve stimulation (PTNS); Sacral nerve stimulation (SNS). OnabotulinumtoxinA (Botox)	Surgery: Augmentation cystoplasty; Urinary diversion	Indwelling catheters (including transurethral, suprapubic, etc.) are not recommended except as a last resort in selected patients.

History and Physical Examination

The history is one of the most important components of diagnosing OAB. Knowing the onset, duration, characteristics of complaints, and any previous pelvic surgery is very helpful. Included in the history is the patient's amount of urgency, frequency, and urge incontinence. In addition to their voiding history, it is equally important to assess their fluid intake, including both type and amount. The degree of bother from their bladder symptoms should also be assessed. If they are not bothered significantly by their symptoms, then you may not need to treat as aggressively. For example, if an individual was waking up twice per night to void due to fluid intake at

Before you begin, please read these Insructions carefully.
Keep a record for 3 days in a row, usIng a new form for each 24-hour period
Write down every time you urinate or lost urine, whether it was planned or accidental.
Musure urine. Or estimate total voiding amount.
Other points to remember:

- Use the column on the far left, which is not numbered, to mark the time that you get out of bed in the morning and the time you get into bed at night.
- **Column 1:** Each time you urinate on purpose, record the amount on the time that corresponds with the approximate time. If you go to the bathroom more than once an hour, write both amounts in the space, with a slash: 400/100 tcc. or M/S
- **Column 2:** Anytime you have accidental urine loss, make a check mark on the line that corresponds with the approximate time. If it happens twice in an hour, make 2 check marks.
- **Column 3:** Each time you make a check mark in column 2, estimate the amount of urine loss in column 3. Since you won't be able to measure urine leakage, use the number (1–4) that best describes what happened.
- **Column 4:** To provide more details about accidental urine loss, use the letter "S", "U", or "B" to diiscribe the episode
- **Column 5:** Write YES if the episode was bothersome to you, NO if it wasn't
- **Column 6:** Each time you drink fluids, enter the amount and the type of fluid-Boz (or 1 cup) of juice, coffee, or water, for example

Bring the 3 voiding diaries to your next visit-and remember not to empty your bladder just before you see the doctor.

In and out of bed	Time	Column 1 Internationa urination (quantity) S-M-L or Measured	Column 2 Accidental urine Loss (check)	Column 3 Quantity of urine loss S-M-L	Column 4 Activity at the time of urine loss	Column 5 Bothersome? YES/NO	Column 6 Type and amount of fluids
	Midnight						
	1 am						
	2 am						
	3 am						
	4 am						
	5 am						
	6 am						
	7 am						
	8 am						
	9 am						
	10 am						
	11 am						
	Noon						
	1 pm						
	2 pm						
	3 pm						
	4 pm						
	5 pm						
	6 pm						
	7 pm						
	8 pm						
	9 pm						
	10 pm						
	11 pm						
Totals							

Fig. 15.1 Voiding Diary (Adapted from the University of Michigan 2012)

bedtime, but they are not bothered by this, even though by definition this is nocturia, treatment may not be warranted. It is also important to determine if any particular event started or correlates with the bladder problem (Abrams 2010)?

The most objective form of documentation is the use of a bladder record (see Fig. 15.1). This document should tell you when and how often the patient voids and was there an urge and what was the severity of that urge. It is also important to note their perception of the need to void. Do they know when their bladder is full? Do they leak immediately after awareness? Do they leak 1–2 min after awareness? If there was a leaking episode, the time and activity at the time of the leak should also be noted. How many pads did they change in a 24 hour period? Also include everything the patient had to drink that day, time, type of fluid, and amount. All of these parameters can be correlated when developing a plan of care. More recently, electronic diaries have been introduced, although these are less commonly used in clinical trials than paper diaries. Abrams et al. (2016) found that electronic diaries seem to increase patient compliance and improve data quality. Based on this research, current recommendation for diaries would be 7-day electronic diaries to improve accuracy and reliability, with a 3-day diary minimum.

Rule out all transient causes of OAB including:

- Urinary tract infection.
- Atrophic vaginitis.
- Benign prostatic hypertrophy.
- Excessive flow (CHF, diabetes, diuretics).
- Restricted mobility.
- Medication review: determine any possible causes of OAB from new or current medications.
- Bladder cancer.

Other valuable components of the history include any previous treatment of OAB and the response to those treatments. Identify the comorbidities associated with OAB including neurologic diseases (i.e., stroke, multiple sclerosis, spinal cord injury), mobility deficits, medically complicated/uncontrolled diabetes, fecal motility disorders (fecal incontinence/constipation), chronic pelvic pain, history of recurrent urinary tract infections (UTIs), gross hematuria, prior pelvic/vaginal surgeries (incontinence/prolapse surgeries), or current significant prolapse, pelvic cancer (bladder, colon, cervix, uterus, prostate) and pelvic radiation (Gormley et al. 2012), etc. These problems most often have OAB components inherent in their physiology. It is also imperative to inquire about environmental considerations. Distance to the bathroom, mobility, and lifestyle contributions are all aspects that can exacerbate OAB.

Review all current medications, prescribed and over the counter. Look for medications that might contain alcohol or caffeine. Certain medications used to treat hypertension or peripheral edema including diuretics that are associated with polyuria can cause urgency, frequency, and incontinence.

A focused physical exam is important to rule out any physical abnormality and gives the clinician the opportunity to teach the patient Kegel exercises.

Female Examination

- Vaginal exam including inspection of the perineum, labia, vaginal tissues, urethra, and presence of prolapse. Also check for vaginal spasm, pain, or tenderness in the vagina and note the position. This is the time to teach proper technique for Kegel exercises and determine the strength of the pelvic floor. Rule out hypermobility of the bladder neck by doing the pad stress test or Q-tip test. Urethral hypermobility is defined as a maximum straining angle greater than or equal to 30° above the horizontal plane (Robinson et al. 2012).
- Rectal exam to rule out constipation, blood, or prolapse.

Male Examination

- Inspection of the genitals to rule out any abnormalities that may cause pain or urgency, condition of the foreskin, presence of urethral discharge, size of scrotum/testes, abnormal lesions, or masses.
- Rectal exam to identify any abnormalities of the prostate, presence or absence of pain or inflammation, constipation or blood or fissures, hemorrhoids, or stool.
- Teach Kegel exercises. Document strength of contraction and note rising of the tip of the penis, which indicates proper technique with contraction.

All Patients

- An abdominal exam should be performed to assess for scars, masses, hernias and areas of tenderness as well as for suprapubic distension that may indicate urinary retention.
- Urinalysis: rule out UTI, hematuria, glycosuria. A urine culture is not necessary unless indication of infection is found and is done based on the discretion of the clinician. If there is evidence of infection, a culture should be performed, the infection treated appropriately and the patient should then be reassessed in regard to their symptoms once the infection has cleared. If hematuria is noted in the absence of infection then workup should commence according to the AUA guidelines (Gormley et al. 2012).
- Check post-void residual to rule out overflow incontinence (>300 mL).
- Functional status: does the patient need assistance with walking that may inhibit their ability to get to the toilet? Wheelchair, walker, or cane? Can they manipulate their own clothing?
- Pain issues that may limit their desire to toilet.
- Note cognition: is the patient alert, oriented? Can he/she identify a toilet and/or urge to void, follow instructions? Consider issuing the Mini-Mental State Examination (MMSE) for those patients at risk for cognitive impairment.

- Check lower extremity nerve conduction. Use a tuning fork on the bony prominences of lower extremities to determine intact nerve pathways.
- Is there lower extremity edema that may increase nocturia?
- Perineal sensation (anal wink or bulbocavernosus reflex).
- Note abnormal lab values: elevated blood glucose or calcium.

Diagnostic Testing

Upon admission to the clinic, patients should have their post-void residuals (PVR) checked. A residual of 150 mL or greater can indicate incomplete bladder emptying and can cause constant urgency. Post-void residuals should be done within 10 min of voiding. Any perceived abnormal PVR requires confirmation before being considered significant.

Urodynamic testing can also determine the absence or presence of OAB in the form of detrusor overactivity, but cannot determine frequency. This test is not necessary for everyone but is helpful when the diagnosis is unclear because of a patient having difficulty expressing their symptoms or how they are leaking, or the physical exam is inconclusive differentiating between the presences of urge versus stress urinary incontinence. Urodynamics is not required to make the diagnosis of OAB and should not be used in the initial screening process (see Chap. 11).

Treatment for OAB: AUA Guidelines (Gormley et al. 2012)

First-Line Therapy: Behavioral Management

Elimination of bladder irritants is the first and foremost treatment for OAB. Common irritants are caffeine, artificial sweeteners, alcohol, grapefruit juice, tomatoes and spices, citrus, and excessive milk. When determining the amount of bladder irritants a patient can have, help them gradually decrease their intake to a minimum. You can also have them drink water simultaneously with their coffee or other drink or alternate their drink of preference with water to help dilute the irritant. Teach your patients to know their own body's tolerance for bladder irritants. Decrease the amount they eat or drink until their urgency, frequency, and incontinence are under control. A reduction in daily fluid intake of 25% is associated with a significant improvement in OAB symptoms (Gormley et al. 2012).

Fluid management can be a key issue in the presence or absence of OAB (Wyman et al. 2009). Patients need to know that drinking 6–8 glasses of fluid is normal intake. Half of total intake should be water. Water intake should be increased by at least a cup for every 30 min of strenuous exercise that is done. Intake should be creatively spaced throughout the day. Sip, do not gulp drinks. Patients should stop drinking fluids 2–3 hours prior to bedtime. If they become thirsty, sucking on one ice cube at a time can help. Caffeine should be eliminated after midafternoon to help with a good night's sleep.

Pelvic floor therapy is done several ways. Simple Kegel exercises, biofeedback, or pelvic floor stimulation are components of pelvic floor therapy.

Proper technique when performing Kegel exercises is to isolate the pelvic floor muscle, specifically the levator ani muscle. This is the muscle that helps control urinary leakage. Most women find this exercise difficult to master. However with proper instruction and practice it can be a good way to control detrusor contractions, increase pressure in the urethra, and control urinary leakage (Reisch 2020). Proper technique is very important in order to achieve positive results. Instruction is easily done with a vaginal exam when placing finger into the vagina, have the patient squeeze and pull the finger into her vagina without moving the rest of her body.

Kegel exercise instructions
1. Identify pelvic floor muscles
2. Squeeze and hold up to 10 seconds
3. Relax for 10 seconds after each contraction (relaxing is just as important as contracting)
4. Do not use stomach, buttocks, or thighs
5. Do ten sets daily in each position: sitting, standing, and laying
6. Doing too many exercises can fatigue your muscles

The pelvic floor muscles are a group of striated and skeletal muscle groups. There are two different types of muscle fibers in the pelvic floor: slow-twitch (Type 1) and fast-twitch (Type II) fibers. These fibers control strength and endurance. The levator ani is made up of mostly slow-twitch fibers that work to maintain normal resting and help with endurance. The fast-twitch muscle fibers (type II) aid in strong and forceful contractions. They can fatigue much faster. To improve these muscle fibers, doing a set of five quick flicks and resting 10 seconds in between can help strengthen these muscles and aid in recruitment of these muscles with a strong urge to urinate. Doing quick flicks can help reduce the urge to urinate. These too should be done daily, in sets of 2–3 in each position, sitting, standing, and laying.

In order to properly perform pelvic floor exercises, the patient should be cognitively intact. For those who are not, you can use a 6″ ball placed between the knees, while in a seated position with toes pointed inward and squeeze the ball, hold for 10 seconds and relax (Hulme 1998).

Biofeedback is a teaching technique with which you are taught to improve your pelvic floor muscle strength and learn to see these muscles work properly to help control urination, urgency, or relaxation. Special sensors or electrodes are placed near the pelvic muscles that help in controlling urination. There are two ways to provide "sensors". A vaginal probe, somewhat like a tampon, or a rectal probe can be used. Another method is the use of surface electrodes. Two electrodes are placed around the anus. Another electrode is placed on your thigh and yet another electrode is placed on your abdomen. These electrodes all have wires that are connected to a computer. The activity performed by these muscles can be seen on the computer in the form of lines. The information the patient receives from the signal can then be used to make adjustments in muscle activity. The job of the biofeedback therapist is to interpret the activity and coach the patient into improving the strength and endurance of the pelvic floor muscle. This is done through a variety of exercises that are performed, in the office, in front of the computer to see differences and changes. Practicing these exercises at home is essential in order to make progress and see changes in urinary leakage patterns, urgency, or relaxation. Through practice, patients become more aware of their pelvic muscles and eventually learn to use the muscles without having to depend on biofeedback.

Biofeedback is used in the treatments of stress or urge urinary incontinence (Voorham et al. 2017). It can also be used for other pelvic floor disorders, bladder control problems, or before and after surgery. There are no side effects or pain to this therapy. It is generally used in conjunction with behavioral therapies and sometimes medication. Treatment sessions vary but usually begin weekly. As symptoms improve, time in between sessions increases. There are computer programs available for biofeedback with programs specific to stress or urge incontinence or techniques in relaxation.

Electrical stimulation is the third type of pelvic floor therapy. It is a controlled delivery, via the vagina or rectum, of small amounts of stimulation to the nerves and muscles of the pelvic floor and bladder. Stimulation is generated through a vaginal or rectal probe that is placed in either the vagina or rectum, or surface electrodes. The purpose of this treatment is to relax the bladder muscle and reduce unwanted bladder contractions. The numbers of treatments that are needed are individualized to each patient and their problem.

Urge reduction techniques are ways in which to use your pelvic floor muscles to inhibit detrusor contractions to avoid leaking.

Urge reduction techniques
1. With the strong urge to urinate, stop what you are doing
2. Take a deep breath and do a couple of quick Kegel exercises
3. Distract yourself
4. If the urge goes away, slowly move toward the bathroom
5. Should the urge return, repeat the above
6. The key to controlling the urge is NOT to respond by rushing to the bathroom. This will almost always result in leaking urine

Toileting programs are highly effective with a motivated patient and/or caregiver.

Habit training	Bladder retraining	Prompted voiding
Voiding according to one's schedule Use bladder records as a guideline Can also be helpful for those with little or no sensation to void Prevention technique for those who forget to void	Use of Kegel exercises, urge reduction techniques, and timing to "teach" your bladder how to gradually hold more urine	Caregiver dependent; Specific behavioral protocol with opportunity to toilet at regular intervals Timing is based on results of bladder diaries
	Purpose is to resist the urge to void	Check the patient at designated times to prevent incontinence Opportunity (prompt) to toilet every 2 h
	Gradually lengthen time in between voiding by using relaxation and urge reduction techniques	Toileting assistance if requested If the patient is wet, change clothing and/or pads as needed and ask if the patient needs to use the toilet Social interaction and verbal feedback involved
Goal is to keep bladder pressure low and prevent leakage	Try to hold an additional 15 min to gradually increase voiding intervals	
	Successful outcomes can take up to 6–8 weeks to accomplish	*DO NOT SCOLD THE PATIENT!*
		Assist the patient as necessary Patience is key to success When approaching the patient be positive

Managing nocturia is important to help patients get a good night's sleep. Nocturia guidelines are hidden within the broader LUTS guidelines because it has historically been linked primarily to OAB, even though the main cause is nocturnal polyuria (Everaert et al. 2019). Five uninterrupted hours of sleep is normal for the elderly. Waking once to void at night is also normal for the elderly. However, these strategies can help with leakage:

- No fluids after supper. Suck on ice cubes if thirsty.
- Take evening medications no later than 7 pm unless sleep aids. May take sips of water with medications.
- Elevate legs 45° (higher than waist or 45–60 min in later afternoon). A simple strategy is to lay on the couch and elevate legs on 2–3 pillows.
- Alter time of diuretic administration to midafternoon (no later than 3 pm).
- Stay up as late as possible in order to sleep longer.
- Bedside commode/urinal for safety if necessary.
- Bladder and pelvic floor training.
- Weight loss if elevated BMI.
- Salt and protein restriction if appropriate.
- Practice good sleep hygiene.
- Evaluation for sleep apnea can also be useful.

Management of constipation with fluids, exercise, increasing natural fiber (artificial fiber can cause excess flatus), or medication is important to keep the bowels regular. A full colon has a tendency to push on the bladder causing urgency and/or leaking.

Pessaries are indicated for pelvic organ prolapse. Fitting a patient with a pessary may help with urgency caused by the pressure on the bladder from the prolapse. Pessaries should be fitted and cared for by a trained professional with experience with pessaries. There are multiple different types and sizes, each used for a unique problem.

When using *incontinent products* for urine containment, make sure they fit and the patient is using pads with appropriate levels of absorption for his/her problem. DO NOT use menstrual pads for urine containment. These products have coarse fibers that may cause irritation and skin breakdown. Also, do not use Kleenex, toilet paper, or paper towels for control of leakage as this too can cause skin breakdown. Only use incontinent products that are marketed as such.

Other strategies for decreasing bladder urgencies
1. Weight loss: obesity is associated with the risk of onset of OAB symptoms
2. Use diuretics judiciously and not before bedtime
3. Make toilet easier to get to: bedside commode and urinals. Condom catheters at bedtime
4. Think of the environment: cold and running water are triggers to void
5. Smoking cessation: nicotine is a bladder irritant

Second-Line Therapy: Medications

Currently there are two major classifications of drugs used for the treatment of OAB: antimuscarinics and beta-3 agonist. The antimuscarinics include oxybutynin, tolterodine, solifenacin, darifenacin, fesoterodine, and trospium. Their actions are similar. These drugs act during the filling/storage phases of the micturition cycle by inhibiting afferent (sensory) input from the bladder, as well as directly on the smooth muscle to decrease contractility (see the chart for detailed information regarding these drugs). These drugs are contraindicated in patients with slow gastric motility, narrow angled glaucoma, and severe renal or hepatic impairment. Major side effects include constipation, dry mouth, and blurred vision. These drugs are to be used with caution with the elderly (Fick et al. 2019).

The second major drug for treating OAB is mirabegron. It is an agonist of the human beta-3 adrenergic receptor. It relaxes the detrusor smooth muscle during the storage phase of the urinary bladder fill-void cycle by activation of beta-3 adrenergic receptor, which increases bladder capacity. The updated 2019 AUA guidelines now include combination therapy for the treatment of OAB, using both an antimuscarinics and a beta-3 adrenergic receptor agonist. Coadministration appears to not have a noticeable effect on pharmacokinetics. Studies have also shown improved efficacy with combination therapy without any significant effect on the safety profile when compared to monotherapy.

Vaginal estrogen cream has also been studied to have some effect on bladder urgency in postmenopausal women (Weber et al. 2015). Estrogenation of the vaginal tissues can be achieved with multiple different applications, including vaginal estrogen creams, rings, ovules, and tablets. Follow the dosing recommendation per product label.

General Comments Regarding Medications

- Do not administer these drugs to patients with narrow angled glaucoma, significant bladder outflow obstruction, GI obstructive disorders, or renal or hepatic dysfunction.
- All information provided is from package inserts or advertised company literature.
- Effectiveness similar in all drugs.
- None of these drugs should be chewed, divided, or crushed.
- Treatment discontinuation due to adverse effects of drugs is common.
- It is overall recommended for all drugs with anticholinergic properties that they be avoided in the elderly. Behavioral interventions should always be tried first.

Third-Line Therapy: Neuromodulation and Botox

Third-line therapies are indicated for patients with refractory OAB defined as the patient who has failed a trial of symptom-appropriate behavioral therapy of sufficient length to evaluate potential efficacy and who has failed a trial of at least one antimuscarinic medication administered for 6–12 weeks (AUA/SUFU guidelines 2013). See comparison list of third-line therapies.

Percutaneous tibial nerve stimulation (PTNS) is a minimally invasive therapy delivered in the office setting for 30 min. This is a treatment that can be delivered by a NP, PA, or RN under the direction of a physician. PTNS is a series of 12 treatments, typically once a week. It is a nonsurgical, nondrug therapy. This therapy has been approved for treatment of patients with urgency, frequency, and urge incontinence who do not want drugs, cannot tolerate drugs, failed conservative therapy including two OAB medications. PTNS is delivered through a device called Urgent PC or Medtronic NURO™ system along with a lead wire to the stimulator and a surface electrode. Stimulation occurs through a 34-gauge needle electrode inserted approximately 2 in. above the medial malleolus and one finger-width toward the back of the leg at a 60° angle. The patient is tested for proper response of the stimulation from the heel, foot, or toe vibration or flexion of the toes. Any or all of these responses are appropriate to note proper placement. If the patient complains about discomfort or "buzzing" immediately around the needle site, the needle may not be deep enough. If the stimulation is extremely uncomfortable, the needle may be too close to the tibial nerve (de Wall and Heesakkers 2017). The impulse travels up afferent fibers of the tibial nerve to the sacral nerve plexus. This treatment is designed to alter aberrant bladder signals. There are minimal side effects; they are mild and mainly related to needle insertion, bruising, discomfort, and slight bleeding (de Wall and Heesakkers 2017). PTNS is not intended for patients with pacemakers or implantable defibrillators, patients prone to excessive bleeding, patients with nerve damage that could impact either percutaneous tibial nerve or pelvic floor function, or on patients who are pregnant or planning pregnancy. Do not use if the skin in the area of use is compromised. Exercise caution for patients with heart problems (Medtronic 2018a, b, c). Patient response is generally seen after 5–6 treatments and sustained after the 12th treatment and ongoing maintenance therapy (MacDiarmid et al. 2010). There are new upcoming treatments options as well. The new implantable eCoin™ and BlueWind RENOVA™ devices stimulating the tibial nerve show reproducible and favorable clinical results when compared to standard PTNS systems. They are currently in ongoing FDA trials to evaluate the long-term efficacy (Yamashiro et al. 2019).

Sacral nerve stimulation (SNS) is an implantable system that stimulates the sacral nerves modulating the neural reflexes that influence the bladder, sphincter, and pelvic floor. SNS is indicated for treatment of urinary retention, fecal incontinence, and the symptoms of OAB including urgency, frequency, and urge incontinence after failure of first and second-line therapy with moderate to severe symptoms. SNS is also approved for fecal incontinence and urinary retention.

The theory of mechanism behind SNS is that the modulation enables more normal detrusor muscle behavior and helps reduce detrusor and pelvic floor muscle spasticity. It is a two-staged procedure. Test stimulation period allows informed choice for the patient and the doctor to proceed with implanting internal device based on effectiveness. Patients undergoing SNS must be cognitively intact in order to use the remote device to maximize treatment. Patients must also be aware that diagnostic MRIs are contraindicated from the neck down with Medtronic Interstim system, however the Axonics System is full-body MRI 1.5 T safe (Elterman 2018). Medtronic has filed a pre-market approval supplement with the FDA for approval of its InterStim Micro neurostimulator and the accompanying InterStim SureScan MRI leads (Medtronic 2019). The SNS may affect other implanted devices, such as a pacemaker or defibrillator, clinicians involved with both devices should discuss the possible interactions before surgery. To minimize or prevent detrimental effects, implant the devices on opposite sides of the body. Safety and effectiveness of this therapy has not been established however for pregnancy, pediatric use (under 18 years of age), those with progressive, systemic neurological diseases or with bilateral stimulation. (Medtronic 2018a, b, c).

Intravesical Onobotulinumtoxin-A is an acetylcholine release inhibitor and a neuromuscular blocking agent. It is FDA approved for treatment of urinary incontinence due to detrusor overactivity associated a neurologic condition, e.g., spinal cord injury or multiple sclerosis as well as treatment of idiopathic overactive bladder with symptoms of urge urinary incontinence, urgency, and frequency in patients who have failed first- and second-line therapy. The dosage is 100 units as 0.5 mL (5 units) injections across 20 sites into the detrusor muscle. Detrusor overactivity associated with a neurologic condition should not exceed 200 units. Treatments can be repeated after 12 weeks. Mean repeat time for OAB is 24 weeks, for neurogenic bladder, mean repeat time is 42–48 weeks. Adverse reactions include urinary tract infection, urinary retention, dysuria, and hematuria. (See comparison chart of all three treatments.)

When all third-line therapies fail, Dr Sandip Vasavada advocates OnabotulinumtoxinA (BOTOX) as most studies were done with patients who have moderate to severe urge incontinence. Dr Steven Siegel advocated for sacral neuromodulation after failed Botox after a 6–9 month waiting period after the last Botox injection to prevent false positive/negative testing. Dr Kenneth Peters went one step further to advocate the pudendal route. At this publication time, this route is not FDA approved. In Dr Peters' experience, he feels the location of the leads in a slightly different position can affect better outcomes as in his 10-year data, "80 % of patients felt their success was greater with PNM compared to SNM." Dr Stephen Krauss feels the data support a >75 % durable success for augmentation/diversion. However, these procedures are not often done due to their invasive nature (Freilich 2015).

Clinical Pearls
- First-line treatments for OAB have no risk and should be offered to all patients.
- Patient's goals for treatment outcomes should be realistic. OAB is a chronic syndrome and can be difficult to treat.
- Treating the cognitively impaired patient:
  - Treat all medical conditions or transient contributors to OAB.
  - Avoid change in environment.
  - Identify the bathroom.

- PATIENCE!!! Avoid blaming/scolding. It can trigger disruptive behavior.
- Watch for nonverbal cues that a person needs to toilet.
- Prompt to void. Use positive statements vs. questions: "Come with me. I will take you to the bathroom" is better than, "Do you have to go to the bathroom?" or, "Do you want to go to the bathroom?"
- Treating the patient with impaired mobility:
  - Pain control may be necessary in order for the patient to get to the bathroom on time. Think scheduled and break through pain management.
  - Safety first: make sure the patient is using assistive devices as needed.
  - Toileting assistive devices may be helpful, i.e., commodes, urinals, or condom catheters.
- Treating the geriatric patient:
  - Awareness of normal aging changes that affect the bladder and pelvic floor including the presence of:
  Decreased bladder contractility.
  Uninhibited contractions are present.
  Decreased bladder capacity.
  Increased nighttime production of urine.
  Atrophic vaginitis.
  Benign prostatic hypertrophy.
- Realization that OAB is a chronic syndrome without an ideal treatment and no treatment will "cure" the condition in most patients.
- Be prepared to manage the transitions between treatment levels appropriately.
- It is appropriate for patients to choose no treatment at all.
- Weigh benefit versus risk with all treatments.
  - Duration of potential adverse reactions.
  - Reversibility of adverse reactions.
- OAB may compromise quality of life but it does not affect survival.

Resources for the Nurse Practitioner

International Continence Society (ICS) www.ICS.org
  American Urogynecologic Society www.AUGS.org
  American Urologic Association: OAB guidelines http·//www.auanct.org/education/auaguidelines.cfm
  Society of Urologic Nurses and Associates (SUNA) www.suna.org
  OAB screening tools www.PfizerPatientReportedOutcomes.com
  NIH Bladder Diary

Resources for the Patient

National Association for Continence (NAFC) www.nafc.org
  Patient Pictures www.patientpictures.com

Simon Foundation www.simonfoundation.org
Patient Education Fact Sheets: www.SUNA.org
Third line of therapy options for overactive bladder

	PTNS	Botox	InterStim
Primary location of service	Clinic	Clinic or hospital	Clinic and hospital
Provider	Nurse	Physician	Nurse and physician
Indication	Urinary urgency, frequency, and urge incontinence	Urinary incontinence due to overactivity of bladder as well as urinary urgency and frequency in patients not responding to meds	Urinary urgency, frequency, urge incontinence, nonobstructive urinary retention, or urge fecal incontinence
Contraindications	Patients with defibrillators, pacemakers, pregnant or considering pregnancy, and bilateral lower extremity nerve damage	Urinary tract obstruction, history of frequent urinary tract infections Allergy to Botox	MRI, diathermy, implantable devices (pacemaker, defibrillator), pregnancy
Technique	Twelve treatments, 30 min each; No anesthesia	Local anesthesia to bladder and urethra. Sedative 45–60 prior to procedure; Twenty injections in the bladder wall through a cystoscope Treatments can be repeated after 12 weeks, generally repeats every 6–8 months	First-stage testing in office ~30 min procedure, local anesthesia, single wire stimulation through lower back Implant procedure in operating room under anesthesia
Complications	Rare, bleeding at site, painful sensation during stimulation that did not interfere with treatment	Urinary tract infection, inability to urinate, or empty bladder (need to catheterize self), bloody urine	Infection, pain at implantation site, lead movement, urinary and bowel problems, electric shock, need for revision
Posttreatment	No restrictions	The patient should void prior to leaving the clinic or hospital	Activity restricted 3–6 weeks post-op Battery change every 5–7 years based on usage
Improvement and cure rates	59–88%	50–70%	37–79%
References	MacDiarmid et al. (2010), MacDiarmid (2015)	Botox (2014)	Medtronic (2018a)

Medications for overactive bladder

Medication antimuscarinics	Dosages	Adverse events (>5%)	Drug/drug interactions	Half-life	Comments
Detrol LA (tolterodine)	2 or 4 mg daily Immediate release Also available, given BID	Dry mouth 23% Headache 6% Constipation 6%	NONE	8 h	No dosage adjustments needed for elderly residents Research available on elderly (Zinner et al. 2002) for safety, efficacy, and adverse events
Ditropan XL (oxybutynin)	5, 10, or 15 mg daily Available in tablet or syrup 5 mg/5 mL Available generic, immediate release (AE increased and given TID)	Dry mouth 29% Diarrhea 7% Constipation 7% Headache 6%	Studies not conducted	12 h	Likely to cross blood–brain barrier (Kay and Granville 2005) May have significant cognitive effects
Enablex b (darifenacin)	7.5 or 15 mg daily	Constipation 20.9% Dry mouth 18.7% Headache 6.7%	Digoxin, ketoconazole, itraconazole, ritonavir, nelfinavir, clarithromycin, and nefazodone (see package insert for details)	13–19 h	Highest % of constipation of all drugs in the class. Think of your patients with concomitant fecal in continence Data suggest safety in the elderly
Gelnique	10% sachet 3% pump	Dry mouth 7% UTI 7%	Studies not conducted		Do not take a bath, swim, shower, exercise, or get the application site wet for 1 h after you apply your dose

Medication antimuscarinics	Dosages	Adverse events (>5%)	Drug/drug interactions	Half-life	Comments
Oxytrol (oxybutynin)	3.9 mg patch Change twice weekly (q3–4 days)	Site pruritus 14% Site erythema 8.3%	Studies not conducted	7–8 h	Geriatric effectiveness no different than younger people 49% of patients in original study were >65 years old Likely to cross blood–brain barrier More convenient mode of delivery. Much fewer GI side effects
Sanctura (trospium chloride)	20 mg. BID 60 mg XR daily	Dry mouth 20.1% Constipation 9.6%	NONE	20 h	Needs to be taken on an empty stomach or 1 h before meals. In residents >75 years, dosage may need to be decreased to 20 mg. QD based on tolerability
Toviaz (fesoterodine fumarate)	4 and 8 mg extended release	Dry mouth 17% (4 mg) and 35% (8 mg) Constipation 4% (4 mg) and 6 % (8 mg)	Doses >4 mg not recommended in patients taking potent CYP3A4 inhibitors	7 h	Hot environment caution Better choice than trospium for patients with >2–3 episodes UI daily
Vesicare (solifenacin)	5 or 10 mg daily	Dry mouth 10.9% (5 mg) and 27.6% (10 mg) Constipation 5.4% (5 mg) and 13.4% (10 mg)	NONE	45–68 h	No CNS side effects Favorable tolerability profile Better choice than trospium for patients with >2–3 episodes UI daily

Medication antimuscarinics	Dosages	Adverse events (>5%)	Drug/drug interactions	Half-life	Comments
Beta-3 adrenergic receptor agonist Myrbetriq (mirabegron)	25–50 mg daily	Hypertension, nasopharyngitis, UTI, and headache <2% and > placebo	Monitoring needed with drugs metabolized by CYP2D6 (metoprolol and desipramine) and warfarin Digoxin: start at lowest dose of digoxin and monitor serum levels	50 h	Trial of 8 weeks is recommended to determine effectiveness No adjustment of dosage necessary for the elderly

General comments:

Do not administer these drugs to residents with controlled narrow angled glaucoma, significant bladder outflow obstruction, GI obstructive disorders, or renal or hepatic dysfunction
All information provided is from package inserts or advertised company literature
Effectiveness similar in all drugs
None of these drugs should be chewed, divided, or crushed
Treatment discontinuation due to adverse effects of drugs is common
It is overall recommended for all drugs with anticholinergic properties that they be avoided in the elderly. Behavioral interventions should always be tried first (Fick et al. 2019)

References

Abrams P, Andersson KE, Birder L et al (2010) Fourth international consultation on incontinence recommendations of the international scientific committee: evaluation and treatment of urinary incontinence, pelvic organ prolapse, and fecal incontinence. Neurourol Urodyn 29(1):213–240
Abrams P, Paty J, Martina R et al (2016) Electronic bladder diaries of differing durations versus a paper diary for data collection in overactive bladder. Neurourol Urodyn 35(6):743–749. https://doi.org/10.1002/nau.22800
BOTOX® (2014) Best practices for the treatment of overactive bladder patients. Allergan, Inc., Irvine
Coyne KS, Sexton CC, Bell JA et al (2013) The prevalence of lower urinary tract symptoms (LUTS) and overactive bladder (OAB) by racial/ethnic group and age: results from OAB-POLL. Neurourol Urodyn 32(3):230–237. https://doi.org/10.1002/nau.22295
de Wall LL, Heesakkers JP (2017) Effectiveness of percutaneous tibial nerve stimulation in the treatment of overactive bladder syndrome. Res Rep Urol 2017(9):145–157. https://doi.org/10.2147/RRU.S124981
Durden E, Walker D, Gray S et al (2018) The economic burden of overactive bladder (OAB) and its effects on the costs associated with other chronic, age-related comorbidities in the United States. Neurourol Urodyn 37:1641–1649. https://doi.org/10.1002/nau.23513

Elterman DS (2018) The novel Axonics® rechargeable sacral neuromodulation system: procedural and technical impressions from an initial North American experience. Neurourol Urodyn 37:S1–S8. https://doi.org/10.1002/nau.23482

Everaert K, Hervé F, Bosch R et al (2019) International Continence Society consensus on the diagnosis and treatment of nocturia. Neurourol Urodyn 38(2):478–498. https://doi.org/10.1002/nau.23939

Fick DM, Semla TP, Steinman M et al (2019) American Geriatrics Society 2019 updated AGS Beers Criteria for potentially inappropriate medication use in older adults. J Am Geriatr Soc 67(4):674–694. https://doi.org/10.1111/jgs.15767

Freilich D (2015) Panel: management of refractory overactive bladder: what to do when third line therapies fail—session highlights. Retrieved from www.UroToday.com

Gormley EA, Lightner DJ, Burgio KL, Chai TC, Clemens JQ, Culkin DJ, Das AK, Foster HE Jr, Scarpero HM, Tessier CD, Vasavada SP (2012) American Urological Association; Society of Urodynamics, Female Pelvic Medicine & Urogenital Reconstruction. Diagnosis and treatment of overactive bladder (non-neurogenic) in adults: AUA/SUFU guideline. J Urol 188(6 Suppl):2455–2463. https://doi.org/10.1016/j.juro.2012.09.079. Epub 2012 Oct 24

Gormley EA, Lightner DJ, Faraday M, Vasavada SP (2015) American Urological Association; Society of Urodynamics, Female Pelvic Medicine. Diagnosis and treatment of overactive bladder (non-neurogenic) in adults: AUA/SUFU guideline amendment. J Urol 193(5):1572–1580. https://doi.org/10.1016/j.juro.2015.01.087. Epub 2015 Jan 23. Review

Haylen BT, de Ridder D, Freeman RM et al (2010) An International Urogynecological Association (IUGA)/International Contienence Society (ICS) joint report on the terminology for female pelvic floor dysfunction. Neurourol Urodyn 29:4–20. https://doi.org/10.1002/nau

Hulme JA (1998) Beyond Kegels Book II: a clinician's guide to treatment algorithms and special populations. Phoenix Publishing, Missoula

Kay GG, Granville LJ (2005) Antimuscarinic agents: implications and concerns in the management of overactive bladder in the elderly. Clin Ther 27(1):127–138; quiz 139–40. Review

Lightner DJ, Gomelsky A, Souter L et al (2019) Diagnosis and treatment of overactive bladder (non-neurogenic) in adults: AUA/SUFU guideline amendment 2019. Neurourol Urodyn 202(3):558–563. https://doi.org/10.1097/JU.0000000000000309

MacDiarmid S (2015) PTNS for overactive bladder: patient selection and technique. Urol Times Feb 1, 2015. Available at http://urologytimes.modernmedicine.com/urology-times/news/ptns-overactive-bladder-patient-selection-and-technique

MacDiarmid SA, Peters KM, Shobeiri SA, Wooldridge LS, Rovner ES, Leong FC et al (2010) Long-term durability of percutaneous tibial nerve stimulation for the treatment of overactive bladder. J Urol 183(1):234–240

Mckellar K, Bellin E, Schoenbaum E et al (2019) Prevalence, risk factors, and treatment for overactive bladder in a racially diverse population. Urology 126:70–75. https://doi.org/10.1016/j.urology.2018.12.021

Medtronic (2018a) Information for prescribers Medtronic InterStim™ System. http://manuals.medtronic.com/content/dam/emanuals/neuro/M976705A_a_001_view.pdf. Accessed 20 Jan 2020

Medtronic (2018b) Indications insert Medtronic InterStim® Therapy. http://manuals.medtronic.com/content/dam/emanuals/neuro/CONTRIB_087797.pdf. Accessed 20 Jan 2020

Medtronic (2018c) PTNM guidebook. https://www.medtronic.com/content/dam/medtronic-com/us-en/patients/treatments-therapies/bladder/documents/ptnm-nuro-system-patient-guidebook.pdf. Accessed 20 Jan 2020

Medtronic (2019) Medtronic announces FDA submission for InterStim™ Micro Neurostimulator and SureScan™ MRI Leads. http://newsroom.medtronic.com/news-releases/news-release-details/medtronic-announces-fda-submission-interstimtm-micro. Accessed 20 Jan 2020

Powell LC, Szabo SM, Walker D et al (2018) The economic burden of overactive bladder in the United States: a systematic literature review. Neurourol Urodyn 37(4):1241–1249. https://doi.org/10.1002/nau.23477

Reisch R (2020) Interventions for overactive bladder: review of pelvic floor muscle training and urgency. J Womens Health Phys Therap 44(1):19–25. https://doi.org/10.1097/JWH.0000000000000148

Reisch R, Rutt R, Dockter M et al (2018) Overactive bladder symptoms in female health profession students: bladder diary characteristics and impact of symptoms on health-related quality of life. J Womens Health 27(2):156–161. https://doi.org/10.1089/jwh.2016.6181

Robinson BL, Geller EJ, Parnell BA et al (2012) Diagnostic accuracy of visual urethral mobility exam versus Q-Tip test: a randomized crossover trial. Am J Obstet Gynecol 206(6):528. e1–528.e6. https://doi.org/10.1016/j.ajog.2012.02.015

University of Michigan, A (2012) Voiding diary: what it's for, how to fill it out. J Fam Pract 61(9):547–548

Voorham JC, De Wachter S, Van den Bos TW et al (2017) The effect of EMG biofeedback assisted pelvic floor muscle therapy on symptoms of the overactive bladder syndrome in women: a randomized controlled trial. Neurourol Urodyn 36(7):1796–1803. https://doi.org/10.1002/nau.23180

Weber MA, Kleijn MH, Langendam M (2015) Local oestrogen for pelvic floor disorders: a systemic review. PLoS One 10(9):e0136265. https://doi.org/10.1371/journal.pone.0136265

Wyman JF, Burgio KL, Newman DK (2009) Practical aspects of lifestyle modifications and behavioral interventions in the treatment of overactive bladder and urgency urinary incontinence. Int J Clin Pract 63(8):1177–1191

Yamashiro J, de Riese W, de Riese C (2019) New implantable tibial nerve stimulation devices: review of published clinical results in comparison to established neuromodulation devices. Res Rep Urol 11:351–357

Zhu J, Hu X, Dong X et al (2019) Associations between risk factors and overactive bladder: a meta-analysis. Female Pelvic Med Reconstr Surg 25(3):238–246. https://doi.org/10.1097/SPV.0000000000000531

Zinner NR, Mattiasson A, Stanton SL (2002) Efficacy, safety, and tolerability of extended-release once-daily tolterodine treatment for overactive bladder in older versus younger patients. J Am Geriatr Soc 50(5):799–807

Problems in Female Urology: Interstitial Cystitis/Bladder Pain Syndrome, Pelvic Floor Disorders, and Pelvic Organ Prolapse

16

Giulia I. Lane and Lindsey Cox

Contents

G. I. Lane (✉)
Department of Urology, University of Michigan, Ann Arbor, MI, USA

L. Cox
Medical University of South Carolina, Charleston, SC, USA
e-mail: coxli@musc.edu

© Springer Nature Switzerland AG 2020
S. A. Quallich, M. J. Lajiness (eds.), *The Nurse Practitioner in Urology*,
https://doi.org/10.1007/978-3-030-45267-4_16

Objectives
1. Provide a resource for providers caring for female urology patients to aid in diagnosis and management of complex pelvic pain, including interstitial cystitis/ bladder pain syndrome (IC/BPS).
2. Review other female pelvic floor disorders (PFD) including pelvic organ prolapse (POP).
3. Differentiate among a broad range of differential diagnoses to exclude other causes of pelvic pain.
4. Recognize and manage IC/BPS according to the American Urological Association guidelines.
5. Outline the steps of evaluation and nonoperative as well as surgical management of pelvic floor disorders, e.g., pelvic organ prolapse.

Overview

The specialty of Urologic Surgery has traditionally had a strong focus on disorders of the male genitourinary tract. Urologists dedicated to treating disorders in women or "Female Urology" have recently joined with Urogynecologists in the formation of a new medical specialty called Female Pelvic Medicine and Reconstructive Surgery or FPMRS. Urologists trained in FPMRS treat a wide range of benign conditions in women and men, including urinary incontinence, overactive bladder, neurogenic bladder as well as the topics of this chapter, chronic pelvic pain or IC/BPS, and pelvic floor disorders. These topics are interrelated as patient presentation and symptoms can overlap, but each deserves discrete attention as management and therapy are distinctly different, and will be covered separately.

This chapter describes experimental and off-label uses of medications and devices for IC/BPS; the authors urge providers to follow all governmental and manufacturer protocols, precautions, warnings, indications, and contraindications.

IC/BPS

Definitions

Interstitial Cystitis/Bladder Pain Syndrome (IC/BPS) is a chronic condition that can be challenging both to diagnose and to treat. Various terms have been used to describe this condition, including Painful Bladder Syndrome (PBS), Chronic Pelvic Pain Syndrome (CPPS), and Interstitial Cystitis alone. IC/BPS and chronic prostatitis/CPPS (CP/CPPS) both fall within the broad category of urologic chronic pelvic pain syndromes (UCPPS) (Clemens et al. 2014; 2019). Men with CP/CPPS should be evaluated for IC/BPS (Hanno et al. 2015). This chapter will focus on female patients and will use IC/BPS for consistency with the American Urological

Association (AUA) and Society for Urodynamics, Female Pelvic Medicine & Urogenital Reconstruction (SUFU) Guidelines (Hanno et al. 2015).

The AUA/SUFU guidelines on IC/BPS use the 2009 SUFU definition of IC/BPS: "an unpleasant sensation (pain, pressure, discomfort) perceived to be related to the urinary bladder, associated with lower urinary tract symptoms of more than 6 weeks duration, in the absence of infection or other identifiable causes" (Hanno and Dmochowski 2009). As the definition implies, IC/BPS is a diagnosis of exclusion with symptoms consisting of chronic pain in the pelvis, pelvic floor, and/or genitalia that is often accompanied by lower urinary tract symptoms with symptoms consisting of chronic pain in the pelvis, pelvic floor, and/or genitalia. The condition is noninfectious, nonmalignant, and chronic in nature. Onset of symptoms range between 6 weeks and 6 months within research definitions and clinically, symptoms may fluctuate over time, but rarely resolve completely. Symptom flares are very common in IC/BPS (53% reporting >2 flares over 11 months) and female patients with worse baseline pelvic pain have worse pain intensity during symptom flares (Kessler 2019; Sutcliffe et al. 2019).

IC/BPS can be subcategorized based on the presence or absence of Hunner's lesions into Hunners Lesion (HL) or non-HL IC/BPS (Han et al. 2018). HL are identified on cystoscopy and consists of circumscribed, erythematous patches on the bladder mucosa with small vessels radiating toward a central scar (Han et al. 2018) (Fig. 16.1).

There is no well-defined pathologic etiology or specific definitive diagnostic testing for IC/BPS, despite much research on the topic; even epidemiologic studies with the goals of defining cases of IC/PBS for study were unable to find a single definition that was both sensitive and specific (Berry et al. 2010). At least seven guidelines exist for diagnosis and treatment of IC/BPS, with varying recommendations (Malde et al. 2018). Central to all guidelines is the premise that the diagnosis of IC/BPS relies primarily on patient reported symptoms and careful exclusion of other possible causes of pelvic pain. The National Institute of Diabetes and Digestive and Kidney Diseases (NIDDK) of the U.S. National Institutes of Health (NIH) are funding the Multidisciplinary Approach to the Study of Chronic Pelvic Pain (MAPP)

Fig. 16.1 Image of Hunners Lesion courtesy of Dr. Anne Cameron, University of Michigan

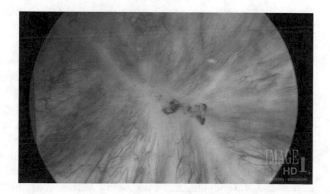

research network to study the spectrum of pelvic pain disorders including IC/PBS (Clemens et al. 2014).

In addition to diagnostic challenges, therapies for IC/BPS are not universally effective, and there are no curative medical therapies. Some studies have shown that patients with characteristic Hunner's lesions on cystoscopy have different symptoms and responses to therapy when compared to non-ulcerative patients; this may be due to different etiologies of HL versus non-HL IC/BPS (Chennamsetty et al. 2015; Han et al. 2018). HL IC arises from a primary bladder etiology while non-HL IC/BPS is representative of myofascial pain and pelvic floor dysfunction (Han et al. 2018).

The AUA guidelines for IC/BPS represent one of the current best practices guidelines for the diagnosis and treatment of patients with IC/BPS (Hanno et al. 2011, 2015; Malde et al. 2018). The algorithm presented allows for the provider to work from initial diagnosis through the care of patients with severe and refractory symptoms who have failed multiple treatment approaches.

These treatments will be discussed in detail under the section entitled *Management*. Patients may benefit from decision aids that include the AUA IC/BPS treatment algorithm to help explain the evidence-based approach to escalating therapy. Such decision aids are available for free download on the Urology Care Foundation website ("Educational Materials - Urology Care Foundation," n.d.).

Epidemiology

IC/BPS occurs in both men and women. Prior studies have shown a ratio of five females for every one male with IC/BPS, but recent evidence suggests that there may also be significant numbers of men who meet epidemiologic definitions, but are not diagnosed (Suskind et al. 2012). It is challenging to estimate the prevalence of IC/BPS because of the varying definitions over time. The most recent, survey based study, estimates that there are 3.3–7.9 million United States women 18 years old or older with IC/BPS, but only 9.7% of women surveyed had been clinically diagnosed (Berry et al. 2011).

Risk Factors

Research from the MAPP Network finds that lifetime stress (such as early adverse life events), poor coping, and psychosocial problems are associated with urologic chronic pelvic pain syndromes (UCPPS) including IC/BPS (Clemens et al. 2019; Naliboff et al. 2015). Specifically, those with IC/BPS have higher levels of anxiety, depression, negative affect, catastrophizing symptoms, neuroticism than healthy control subjects (Afari et al. 2019). Studies have revealed associations between IC/BPS and other non-bladder chronic conditions including fibromyalgia, chronic fatigue syndrome, irritable bowel syndrome, allergy, asthma, migraine, anxiety, depression, vulvodynia, and back pain (Warren et al. 2011). IC/BPS patients with associated conditions (specifically fibromyalgia, chronic fatigue syndrome, irritable bowel syndrome) have lower health-related quality of life scores than those without (Suskind et al. 2013).

New evidence from the MAPP Network suggests that IC/BPS is likely mediated by a centralized process (Clemens et al. 2019). Specifically, functional magnetic resonance imaging has found that there are brain-level disturbances in the sensory and motor signaling related to the bladder and pelvic floor that cause changes in brain structure and function in those with UCPPS (Asavasopon et al. 2014; Clemens et al. 2019; Rana et al. 2015). Quantitative sensory testing has revealed evidence of global hypersensitivity to unpleasant stimuli among those with IC/BPS, which also aligns with the theory that IC/BPS is a centrally mediated pain syndrome (Clemens et al. 2019).

Anatomy and Physiology

Familiarity with male and female pelvic anatomy (Fig. 16.2), inclusive of the external genitalia, is necessary for the diagnosis and management of IC/BPS. This chapter will focus on female pelvic anatomy, although it is essential to recognize that IC/BPS can occur in both men and women.

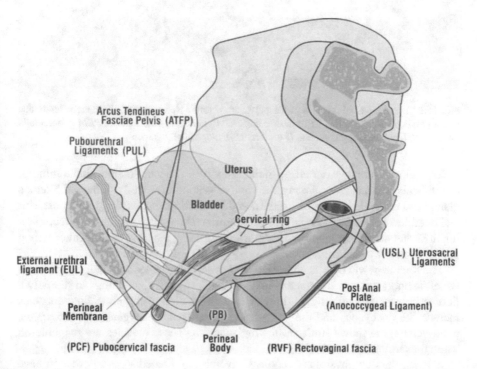

Fig. 16.2 Female pelvic anatomy and connective tissue. Connective tissue levels—This is a schematic 3D sagittal section of the main connective tissue structures of the pelvis, showing their relationship to the organs and pelvic bones

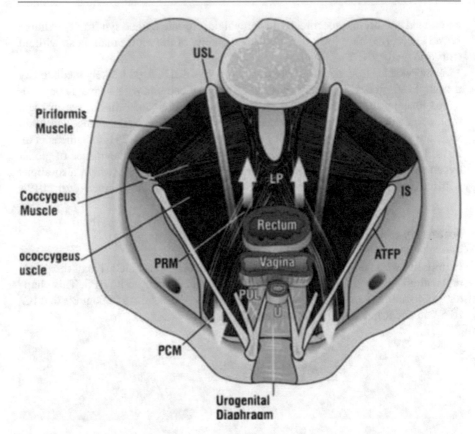

Fig. 16.3 Upper layer of muscles of the pelvic floor (after Netter 1989). *ATFP* arcus tendineus fascia pelvis, *IS* ischial spine, *LP* levator plate, *PCM* pubococcygeus muscle, *PRM* puborectalis muscle, *PUL* pubourethral ligament, *U* urethra, *USL* uterosacral ligament

The normal female external genitalia consist of the labia majora, labia minora, the clitoral hood and clitoral body, the vaginal vestibule, as well as bilateral Skene's glands and ducts (lateral to the urethra) and Bartholin's glands and ducts (posterior and lateral to the vaginal opening). The examiner should be familiar with recognizing the hymenal ring, which is a landmark for grading the level of descent of pelvic organs in pelvic organ prolapse.

The female pelvic floor is an interrelated group of muscles and their attachments which support the pelvic organs (Figs. 16.3 and 16.4). The openings in the pelvic floor accommodate voiding, childbirth, and defecation. The pelvic floor muscles include the coccygeus and the levator ani group (pubococcygeus, ileococcygeus, puborectalis), as shown in the following diagram. These muscles are palpable on vaginal examination.

Normal voiding physiology requires several coordinated steps in order to have comfortable and socially appropriate storage of urine, with voluntary voiding that is complete and efficient. The bladder muscle has multiple neurologic inputs and

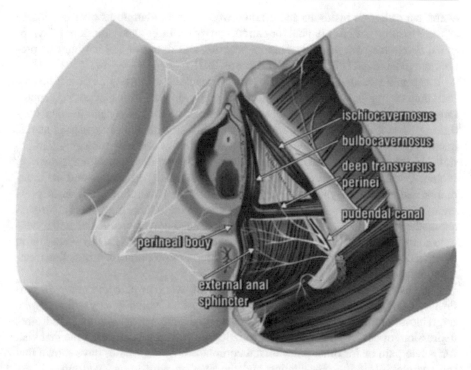

Fig. 16.4 Lower layer of muscles of the pelvic floor anchors the organs distally (after Netter 1989)

outputs that must be coordinated by higher centers. In the resting state, the bladder performs its storage function; signals to relax the detrusor muscle of the bladder are relayed through the autonomic nervous system. Both lack of parasympathetic input as well as sympathetic activity serve to relax the detrusor muscle of the bladder as the bladder fills. The urinary sphincters are contracted or closed during storage. When voluntary voiding is determined to be appropriate, the nervous system signals the pelvic floor and urethral sphincter to relax, the bladder neck opens, and the detrusor muscle contracts. This physiology can be altered in IC/BPS at several levels, including sensitivity to filling, overactivity during storage (possibly with involuntary bladder contractions that cause incontinence of urine), pain or difficulty with voiding and inefficient emptying. The cause (or causes) of these alterations in IC/BPS is not yet understood.

History

Commonly, patients with IC/BPS present with a chief complaint of pain. They can often describe an inciting event, or an event preceding the onset of symptoms. This event may be an episode of acute bacterial cystitis, or time when they were forced to hold urine for a prolonged period of time. Some patients describe no inciting event, but rather an insidious and gradual worsening of symptoms over the course of the condition, and it is typical for patients describe flares and remissions of symptoms. Flares may vary in presentation, severity, and duration and may not be predictable (Clemens et al. 2019; Sutcliffe et al. 2019).

Important considerations for history-taking include a thorough medical history including comprehensive history of other chronic pain conditions, neurologic, autoimmune or rheumatologic and endocrine conditions as well as general medical conditions. Thorough gynecologic and obstetrical history including menstrual status, detailed history of pregnancies and outcomes, history of sexually transmitted infections, history of sexual function, history of early adverse life events (death, divorce, violence, sexual abuse, illness), history of any abnormal pap smears and the treatments, history of any gynecologic or urologic disorders including urolithiasis, presence of any urologic or gynecologic cancers including treatments (surgery, chemotherapy, radiation) and current status of these conditions. A frequency-volume chart, or voiding diary, is also recommended (Hanno et al. 2011). A description of the patient's bowel habits can provide an intervention point for adjunctive treatment of dysfunctional elimination or constipation.

Patients may have characteristics or a diagnosis of other pain and non-pain syndromes including fibromyalgia, endometriosis, vulvodynia/vestibulodynia, migraines, chronic back pain, irritable bowel syndrome, chronic fatigue syndrome, depression, or anxiety. The visit to a urologic care provider is often not the first visit for pelvic pain or for other pain-related complaints. Some studies have shown that the complexity of the presentation and the overlap with other syndromes likely results in a delay in diagnosis for patients with IC/BPS (Chrysanthopoulou and Doumouchtsis 2013). It is imperative to detail prior evaluation, treatments and their effects, and the patients' level of insight into their pain. Listening to patients at this stage can help develop a broad differential diagnosis, avoid repeating prior testing and treatments, and allow the provider to gain a sense of the patients' psychosocial situation and preferences and values which can impact future shared decision-making. This is especially important if patients already have a diagnosis of IC/BPS, so as not to overlook potentially treatable conditions that could be present either concurrently with IC/BPS or alone.

In generating a differential diagnosis, some "red flags" for other conditions can be elicited on history. Patients with neurologic symptoms may need further workup to rule out multiple sclerosis, pudendal neuralgia, or spinal pathology such as cauda equina syndrome. Musculoskeletal symptoms could be the result of trauma or inflammation; gynecologic symptoms (vulvar pain, vaginal discharge, dysmenorrhea) may point to infectious causes or endometriosis. Urologic symptoms such as hematuria, colicky flank or groin pain can prompt investigations into conditions such as eosiniphilic cystitis, lupus cystitis, urothelial carcinoma in situ, atypical infections or urolithiasis.

Thorough characterization of pain is important in order to understand the aspects of the condition that are most bothersome and limiting to the patient, as well as to have insight into other (potentially undiagnosed) conditions. Symptom questionnaires for urinary symptoms as well as for pain should be administered at baseline and at subsequent visits to assess for response to treatment (Hanno et al. 2011).

In characterizing pain, it is important to elicit:

(a) Pain location: frequently pain can originate in the suprapubic area, however for some patients, the origin of pain is reported as urethral or vaginal. Pain can radiate throughout the pelvis, including the lower abdomen, flanks, and lower back, and/or pain can radiate toward the vagina or rectum. Patients will often describe a bothersome constant awareness of the bladder. Some patients use terms such as "pressure" or "discomfort" and will actually deny overt "pain."

(b) Timing of pain: in a given day, patients with IC/BPS may report pain is worse at nighttime, some patients can describe a correlation with pain flares and the menstrual cycle, and frequently pain flares can be correlated with times of psychosocial stress.

(c) Relationship of pain to urinary symptoms: often patients will report that pain is increased with filling and relieved by voiding, some patients will also report dysuria as a characteristic of pain flares, and for a small number this is the initial symptom of IC/BPS.

(d) Exacerbating and ameliorating factors—frequently patients recognize dietary triggers that can worsen pain due to IC/BPS, classically acidic or spicy foods. Patient position can have an effect on pelvic pain caused by pudendal neuralgia, which is often worse with prolonged sitting and improved by standing or by sitting on a toilet seat.

Physical Exam

Specific Maneuvers
The evaluation begins with a general examination noting patients' appearance and affect. Neurologic exam, extremity exam, abdominal exam, flank exam for CVA tenderness, and a detailed pelvic exam are also recommended. Patients may have had severe pain with pelvic examination and/or negative experiences with examination, therefore it is important to emphasize to patients that the exam will be fully explained to them and completed at their pace. Having a chaperone available that can facilitate the provider's ability to perform the exam expeditiously and at the same time provide support to the patient while the exam is being completed is also helpful.

Abnormal Findings
A limited neurologic examination should include any abnormalities in mental status, gait and balance, sensation and muscle tone of the perineum and pelvic floor. Musculoskeletal and/or abdominal exam may reveal tender points, and a useful eponymous test is performing an evaluation for Carnett's sign. The patient is asked to raise the head and shoulders, or to raise both legs with straight knees. The

examiner will find a positive Carnett's sign if the abdominal pain worsens with tensing the abdominal wall, indicating that the source of the pain is less likely originating from an intra-abdominal source. Positive Carnett's sign could indicate possible nerve entrapment (especially from prior surgery), myofascial pain, or trigger points.

The pelvic exam begins with inspection for skin abnormalities including skin lesions consistent with herpes simplex or other infections, including yeast. The examiner should also be familiar with other chronic vulvar skin conditions like lichen sclerosus and lichen planus. The vulva and vaginal vestibule can be examined with a cotton-tipped swab to map light touch sensation, numbness, or areas of tenderness. The vaginal vestibule and introitus should be examined carefully and notation made of the quality of the vaginal epithelium—signs of atrophy, signs of yeast, signs of contact dermatitis, friable tissue, inflammation, as well as vaginal discharge. Abnormalities such as Bartholin's and Skene's gland/duct cysts should also be noted.

Examining the urethra begins with the urethral meatus. Note should be made of urethral meatal stenosis, urethral prolapse, urethral caruncle or signs of urethral diverticulum, including any mass along the anterior vaginal wall. Any surgical scars should be noted, and the presence of any visible or palpable mesh or sutures should be reported. Tenderness, spasm or increased tone of the pelvic floor muscles should be assessed, and voluntary control of both the ability to perform contraction and relaxation of the pelvic floor should be evaluated.

A speculum/ "split" speculum should be used to visualize the cervix or vaginal cuff scar; the vaginal epithelium should be interrogated for signs of fistula, granulation tissue or other lesions, cervical tenderness should also be assessed. Bimanual examination may reveal vaginal wall masses, adnexal tenderness or mass, abnormal uterine size or lie, or one of the hallmark findings for patients with IC/BPS: bladder tenderness to palpation both transvaginally and suprapubically. Attempts to correlate findings on exam to the patient's pain description are extremely helpful.

Pelvic organ prolapse should also be reported and patients should be examined at full valsalva to determine if prolapse is present. Full evaluation of pelvic organ prolapse will be discussed later in the chapter. If the bladder is relatively full, the examiner can also assess for stress urinary incontinence on cough and valsalva. If the patient has complaints of feeling of incomplete emptying, weak stream or straining to void, the examiner may elect to perform straight catheterization to determine post-void residual; or to document sterile urine if infectious causes haven't been thoroughly ruled by obtaining a catheterized urine sample to send for further testing.

Diagnostic Tests

Laboratory Evaluation

The initial laboratory evaluation should include a urinalysis and urine culture. These should be evaluated to rule out infection and to screen for other abnormalities. Urinalysis with microscopy should be ordered as a follow-up for any abnormalities on urinalysis, and guidelines for microscopic hematuria workup should be followed.

The less common finding of sterile pyuria should be worked up as well. Urine can also be sent for special testing for atypical organisms that can cause urethritis, namely *Ureaplasma urealyticum* and *U.* parvum as well as *Mycoplasma genitalium* and *M. hominis* (Crescenze et al. 2018). Patients who test positive for *M. genitalium* should be informed that this is a sexually transmitted infection (STI), they should be screened for other STIs and they (and their partners) should be given information about the prevention and treatment of the infection (Jensen et al. 2016).

If the patient reports associated vulvar and vaginal symptoms, or if the examination is concerning for a yeast infection, it is reasonable to send a swab for yeast culture, as there are strains of yeast that are resistant to commonly used over the counter and prescription treatments. Other sexually transmitted infections (gonorrhea, chlamydia and trichomonas, *M. genitalium*) as well as bacterial vaginosis should be ruled out in the setting of vaginal discharge. Urinary biomarkers have been extensively studied as adjuncts to the diagnosis of IC/BPS; these are not typically used outside of the research setting, and there are no clinically available tests for urine markers that are recommended in the AUA guidelines for IC/BPS.

Imaging Studies

There are no imaging studies that are recommended as part of the basic diagnostic algorithm for IC/BPS. Imaging studies may be considered if other conditions are suspected. A CT urogram should be ordered for confirmed microscopic hematuria, gross hematuria or concern for congential abnormalities such as an ectopic ureter. History of urolithiasis, colicky pain, especially that which radiates to the groin or flank can also prompt CT evaluation for a distal ureteral stone.

Pelvic ultrasound is useful for evaluating findings on abnormal pelvic exam, especially adnexal mass. Transvaginal ultrasound can show the presence and location of mesh in patients with prior pelvic surgery, although it is not required. Concern for urethral diverticulum or unclear examination findings on the anterior vaginal wall can prompt a pelvic MRI.

Procedures

Testing for post-void residual volume by ultrasound or catheterization is recommended for all patients as part of the basic evaluation (Hanno et al. 2011). If catheterization is undertaken and suspicion for IC/BPS is high, a one-time bladder instillation of 40 cc of 2% lidocaine at the time of examination can help determine if instillation therapy is a viable treatment option for future management.

Cystoscopy can aid in diagnosis for complex presentations, when diagnosis is unclear, such as when there is concern for bladder cancer congenital abnormalities or iatrogenic cause for the patients' symptoms (Hanno et al. 2015). However, some advocate early cystoscopy, even in uncomplicated cases, in order to identify Hunner's lesions and guide a HL IC/BPS focused treatment algorithm (Han et al. 2018). Vaginoscopy can be added to evaluate for vaginal scarring, septa, fistula, or other unexplained findings on physical examination.

Urodynamic studies can also be considered, including a simple uroflometry to screen for functional or structural obstruction or detrusor underactivity, or more sophisticated cystometrogram and pressure flow studies to evaluate complex incontinence or voiding dysfunction.

Management

Behavioral, Conservative, Complementary, and Alternative Medicine

The AUA guidelines recommend that all patients should be educated on behavioral modifications, fluid management, dietary changes, exercise, and stress reduction that can help them cope with their IC/PBS diagnosis and symptoms (Hanno et al. 2015). Specific dietary educational materials on excluding bladder irritants using the elimination diet are available for patients on the Interstitial Cystitis Association website (http://www.ichelp.org). Dietary changes, fiber supplements and stool softeners can help avoid constipation, which may exacerbate IC/BPS. Providers should not underestimate the contribution of education, self-care, stress management and behavioral modification in the therapy of IC/BPS.

Complementary and alternative oral therapies for IC/BPS that have some evidence include the urinary alkalizing agent, calcium glycerophosphate (Prelief®), and the multi-agent supplement, CystoProtek® (Atchley et al. 2015). Calcium glycerophosphate supplementation (Prelief®; AkPharma, Pleasantville, NJ, USA) can be used prior to ingesting trigger foods (Atchley et al. 2015). CystoProtek® (chondroitin sulfate (150 mg), quercetin (150 mg), rutin (20 mg), glucosamine sulfate (120 mg), hyaluronate sodium (10 mg), olive kernal extract (45%); Tischon Corporation, Westbury, NY for Alaven Pharmaceutical, LLC, Marietta, GA, USA) is thought to help by providing support to rebuild the bladder surface glycosaminoglycans. Over the counter phenazopyridine and aloe vera supplements can also help provide symptom control during flares, specifically for dysuria associated with IC/BPS.

Patients with IC/PBS may benefit from additional multidisciplinary referrals. Patients who have pain outside of the pelvis or pain that is difficult to manage can be referred to an anesthesiologist or physical medicine and rehabilitation provider who specializes in pain management. If patients feel they have a significant psychological impact of their pain/symptoms, they can be offered a referral to counseling with a pain psychologist. Patients with impact on sexual function can be referred for sexual health counseling. Referral to gastroenterology for refractory bowel symptoms, including constipation is often warranted, and referral to gynecology for a discussion of treatment of endometriosis, dysmenorrhea, or oral contraceptives/hormonal manipulation for patients with hormone sensitive IC/BPS symptoms can also be worthwhile.

Pelvic floor physical therapy (PFPT) is an important tool for the treatment of patients with pelvic floor muscle tenderness and IC/BPS. PFPT is a second-line therapy for IC/BPS based on strong evidence (Hanno et al. 2015). A recent randomized clinical trial showed that 10 sessions of 60 min of myofascial physical therapy resulted in significantly more patients (59%) reporting they were moderately or markedly improved compared to those undergoing therapeutic massage (26%) (Fitzgerald et al. 2012).

Pharmacotherapy

Oral IC/BPS Medications

Several oral medications are options for second line treatment per the AUA guidelines (Hanno et al. 2015). They are listed here in alphabetical order, as they are listed in the guideline.

1. Amitriptyline is a tricyclic antidepressant that is used off-label for several chronic pain conditions. Amitriptyline has a high rate of side effects, most commonly sedation/drowsiness and nausea; the sedation can be taken advantage of for patients who have difficulty with sleep due to symptoms, and the anticholinergic effects can help relax the bladder. It is typically started at 25 mg daily and increased to 100 mg daily; lower doses can be used to start the titration if the medication is not tolerated due to side effects. The medication can be titrated up over a period of weeks, studies have shown that patients who reach the 50 mg daily dose show significant improvement in symptom scores or global response to symptom improvement compared to placebo (Van Ophoven et al. 2004; Foster et al. 2010). These doses are lower than those typically used for antidepressant effects.
2. Cimetidine is a histamine H2-receptor blocker that is not FDA approved for IC/BPS, but has been shown to be effective with few side effects in small studies. The dosage used in studies varies from 200 mg three times daily, 300 mg twice daily to 400 mg twice daily (Hanno et al. 2011).
3. Hydroxyzine (pamoate or hydrochloride salt) is a first generation antihistamine that is also used in certain conditions for its anxiolytic effects. Side effects are typically limited, and include sedation with initial use. Doses used in studies range from 10 mg titrated to 50 mg daily to 25 mg titrated to 75 mg daily over a period of weeks. The evidence for general use in IC/BPS is unclear, however experts postulate that hydroxyzine may be beneficial for the subset of IC/BPS patients with systemic allergies (Sant et al. 2003).
4. Pentosan Polysulfate is the only oral medication that is FDA approved for use in IC/BPS. The polysaccharide drug is proposed to improve the glycosaminoglycan layer that protects the lining of the bladder. There have been conflicting reports on the performance of pentosan polysulfate in randomized, placebo-controlled trials, but a pooled analysis. Dimitrakov et al. (2007)) shows that it likely has a modest benefit for patient reported symptom improvement, and the expert consensus of the AUA guideline panel recommend pentosan polysulfate as a second-line treatment. The most common adverse effects are diarrhea, abdominal pain, and rectal bleeding. In 2018, Pearce et al reported on six patients who developed a nonreversible pigmentary maculopathy associated with long-term Pentosan Sulfate use (median cumulative exposure was 2263 g and duration of use was 186 months) (Pearce et al. 2018). Caution should be used when prescribing pentosan polysulfate in patients with macular disease and those with current or prior pentosan polysulfate use with vision changes are recommended referral for ophthalmologic exams (Ferguson et al. 2019).

Oral immunomodulation with cyclosporine A is a fifth-line treatment in the AUA algorithm. Several studies demonstrate efficacy in small groups of patients with refractory IC/BPS symptoms. It appears that cyclosporine A may be most effective in patients with ulcerative IC/BPS. The most common adverse events are rising serum creatinine and hypertension, and therefore patients must be monitored very closely (Hanno et al. 2011, 2015; Forrest et al. 2012).

Oral medications previously used as anticonvulsants that are widely used as treatments for neuropathic pain (pregabalin and gabapentin) have been used in small trials and case reports for both chronic prostatitis/pelvic pain in men and in women with IC/BPS (Vas et al. 2014; Pontari et al. 2010), but the effectiveness of these medications is unclear.

Lower urinary tract symptoms (LUTS) can also be treated per usual pathways, with the caveat that patients may not experience the responses expected in patients with LUTS without IC/PBS. Patients with significant hesitancy can be trialed on alpha blockers, those with frequency and urgency can be trialed on antimuscarinics and or mirabegron.

The AUA guidelines specifically recommend against long-term antibiotic use as well as systemic glucocorticoid use. The use of opioids for IC/BPS is controversial; patient surveys report high efficacy of opioids however experts in IC/BPS feel that long-term narcotics are not beneficial (Gupta et al. 2015; Lusty et al. 2018) Within the AUA guidelines, narcotics are described as a part of multimodal therapy that should be used with caution (Hanno et al. 2015).

Topical ointments containing various drugs can be useful for patients with concomitant vulvar pain or vulvodynia; the most commonly used is lidocaine 5% ointment. These ointments are variable in the vehicle base, as well as in active ingredient concentration and combination; many compounding pharmacies can add neuropathic agents, tricyclic antidepressants, antispasmodics as well as other anesthetics (Haefner et al. 2005). Patients with pelvic floor muscle involvement, although the evidence for its use is sparse and contradictory, can also be given a trial of vaginal valium, either 5 or 10 mg tablets or compounded as a suppository (Carrico and Peters 2011; Crisp et al. 2013).

Intravesical Instillations

Using a urethral catheter to directly instill medications into the bladder in a retrograde fashion is a commonly used treatment for patients with IC/BPS, and is usually referred to as bladder instillation or intravesical instillation therapy. Patients can be somewhat reluctant to undergo catheterization due to concerns of the catheterization itself being painful; counseling and a knowledgeable nursing staff familiar with IC/BPS patients can help facilitate treatments. A review of the evidence for the various instillations medications summarizes them well (Colaco and Evans 2013). A Cochrane review also exists that predates the AUA guidelines, which found no conclusive evidence for any therapy other than resiniferatoxin, which was not shown to be effective (Dawson and Jamison 2007). The intravesical treatments are recommended as second-line treatments by the AUA, and are again listed in alphabetical order.

1. Dimethyl sulfoxide (DMSO) is an organosulfur compound that has been used as an intravesical treatment for IC/BPS for decades, with two randomized crossover trials showing efficacy. There is some variability in the amount, dwell time, and interval of instillations, however the guideline reports protocols of successful trials of DMSO alone as using 50 cc of 50% DMSO for a dwell time of 15 min in weekly or every 2 week intervals for a course of 4–6 treatments (Hanno et al. 2011). Notably, DMSO is absorbed by the bladder and can be painful if left to dwell too long. Adverse events are noted to be variable, including garlic taste, bladder irritation, and headache, but overall are not serious.

2. Heparin is well known for its use as an anticoagulant, however, structurally it is a glycosaminoglycan, and because of the theory that the glycosaminoglycan layer is inadequate or disrupted in IC/BPS, it has also been widely used as an intravesical treatment for IC/BPS. It is used in preparations ranging from 10,000 to 40,000 IU in 3–10 cc of sterile or distilled water, given one to three times per week with dwell times up to 1 h. Heparin's efficacy has been shown in observational studies, and in more recent studies it has been combined with alkalinized lidocaine (to take advantage of the shorter term effectiveness of lidocaine) with good results (Hanno et al. 2011).

3. Lidocaine is a local anesthetic that has been shown to have short-term efficacy in reducing symptoms of IC/BPS in several studies, which are mostly observational (Hanno et al. 2011). In the study protocols 8–20 cc of 1–2% lidocaine is often mixed with bicarbonate to alkalinize and potentially increase penetration of the medication, with a dwell time of up to 1 h for daily to weekly instillations. A pretzel-shaped intravesical device that releases lidocaine into the bladder continuously called LiRIS (Lidocaine Releasing Intravesical System, Allergan) was being tested in clinical trials (NCT02395042) and showed promising results (Nickel et al. 2012) However, recent reports find that development of this therapy has ceased (Osborne 2019).

The use of other medications in combination with the above or alone has been described in the literature. In clinical practice, various compounds are added to "cocktails" that are provider-specific, including bupivacaine, gentamicin, pentosan polysulfate, other glycosaminoglycans (hyaluronic acid and chondroitin sulfate), and various glucocorticoids (triamcinolone or hydrocortisone). Because DMSO is absorbed by the bladder and may affect the absorption of other agents, caution is advised when using DMSO as part of a cocktail. The AUA recommends *against* using intravesical BCG, a commonly used treatment for bladder cancer.

After a patient is determined to have a significant response to bladder instillations, the provider can continue to arrange for office visits for the administration of the treatments, or the patient and family can be taught self-catheterization and prescribed medications and supplies to perform instillations at home. This strategy demands a motivated patient, as well as advanced coordination of care to overcome hurdles with insurance coverage, prescriptions that may require a compounding pharmacy, and the lack of shelf-stable cocktails, but can help patients be independent in their symptom management.

Neuromodulation

Sacral neuromodulation (SNM) is considered a fourth-line treatment for IC/BPS, although it is not FDA approved for this use. SNM is approved for use in patients with urinary frequency and urgency, which often overlap with IC/BPS symptoms. Patients are given a trial of neurostimulation which begins with implantation of a sacral stimulator lead, and then an implanted device is surgically inserted if the patient reports successful alleviation of symptoms and/or improvement on voiding diary. A similar technique that targets the pudendal nerve for stimulation has also been studied in a small cohort and found to be effective for pain and voiding symptom relief (Peters et al. 2007) Patients with implanted neurostimulators should be aware of battery life limitations (around 5 years) and restrictions on undergoing spinal MRI with the device in place.

Percutaneous tibial nerve stimulation (PTNS) is another type of neuromodulation that is approved for use for relief of urinary symptoms secondary to overactive bladder syndrome. In this treatment, a fine needle, the size of those used in acupuncture, is placed along the course of the tibial nerve on the medial aspect of the ankle. The needle is then attached to a device that provides electrical stimulation temporarily, with no permanent implants. Very small studies in patients with IC/BPS have shown a decrease in pain intensity with PTNS, although larger and longer-term studies are needed (Gokyildiz et al. 2012).

Intradetrusor Botulinum Toxin

Cystoscopy with injection of botulinum toxin into the bladder detrusor muscle is an FDA approved therapy for neurogenic (200 U) and non-neurogenic (100 U) detrusor overactivity. It has been studied in refractory IC/BPS since 2004. The AUA guidelines initially recommended its use as a fifth-line treatment, partly due to adverse events and the potential for the need to catheterize if unable to void after injection at the 200U dose. The 2014 guideline amendment moved botulinum toxin injection to a fourth-line treatment (Hanno et al. 2015). The guideline panel notes that most of the evidence, even the newer studies, is observational, not placebo controlled, and have arms that combine botulinum toxin with hydrodistention, making the overall effect of botulinum toxin injection in IC/BPS difficult to pinpoint. A recent review of the evidence for botulinum toxin use in IC/BPS showed a trend toward using the 100 U dose and repeat injection protocols (Jhang et al. 2014). Patients have to be willing to catheterize if botulinum toxin injection causes the inability to empty the bladder well, those who are unable to tolerate catheterization are not candidates for this treatment.

Other Pain Injections

Some providers who treat complex pelvic pain also provide trigger point injections and/or pudendal nerve blocks based on clinical evaluations (Gupta et al. 2015; Han et al. 2018). These are performed in a series of three injections (one injection every 6–8 weeks) via a transvaginal approach using a combination of ropivicaine, lidocaine, and triamcinolone (Han et al. 2018). Caudal epidural injections and other more sophisticated locoregional pain procedures can be performed as part of multi-disciplinary teams that include pain management specialists.

Hyperbaric Oxygen

Hyperbaric oxygen therapy is another investigational treatment that has been shown in very small studies to have a potential role in treating IC/BPS due to its use in other forms of cystitis, but it is not currently an approved or commonly used therapy (Tanaka et al. 2011; Van Ophoven et al. 2006).

Surgical

The most common surgical procedures for IC/PBS are cystoscopy with hydrodistention of the bladder, and cystoscopy with treatment for Hunner's ulcers (biopsy, fulguration, triamcinolone injection) (Gupta et al. 2015; Han et al. 2018).

Criteria for Surgery

Patients who have failed conservative management can choose to undergo cystoscopy and hydrodistention as a diagnostic aid as well as for therapeutic benefit. This is a third-line treatment in the AUA algorithm (Hanno et al. 2015). If characteristic findings are present (petechiae, glomerulations, Hunner's lesion) these can add to the evidence for a diagnosis of IC/BPS, provide an avenue for treatment (Hunner's lesion), and determination of anesthetized bladder capacity can identify patients with severe forms of IC/BPS. Some patients will not have these findings, but will still have the characteristic flare of symptoms followed by weeks to months of symptom improvement. This pattern of response to hydrodistention also helps support a diagnosis of IC/BPS if the diagnosis is unclear. The long-term efficacy for symptom relief varies, but typically declines over a period of months in observational studies. There are no sham/placebo-controlled studies to determine how effective hydrodistention will be, and no category of patients that are particularly likely to have benefit from the treatment.

Very few patients will meet criteria for major surgical intervention for IC/BPS. Patients with intractable pain and very small, contracted bladder have been treated with open surgical techniques, including augmentation cystoplasty, substitution cystoplasty, continent and incontinent urinary diversion with and without simple cystectomy. The patients must be counseled that these are major surgeries which are irreversible, have significant morbidity, and are not guaranteed to alleviate all pain (Andersen et al. 2012; Rössberger et al. 2007; Peters et al. 2013).

Preoperative Considerations and Additional Tests That May Be Appropriate Prior to Surgery

Preoperative considerations would be similar to any minor endoscopic procedure; guidelines for workup of any patient undergoing general anesthesia should be followed, with the inclusion of a urine culture with treatment to sterilize the urine prior to instrumentation.

Medications

Typically the procedure is done with general anesthesia, but because of the high levels of preoperative pain, patients are also medicated intraoperatively with urethral 2% lidocaine jelly, and an instillation of 40 mL of 2% lidocaine at the conclusion of the hydrodistension. While anesthetized, a belladonna and opium suppository can also be administered to prevent bladder spasms in the postoperative period, and patients are given prescriptions to manage the pain flare that typically occurs after and medication pain control after. Triamcinolone, a corticosteroid, is injected into Hunner's ulcers, with the guideline specifying 10 mL of triamcinolone acetonide, 40 mg/mL, injected in 0.5 mL aliquots into the submucosal space of the center and periphery of ulcers using an endoscopic needle, with 60 mg maximum dose (Hanno et al. 2011).

Teaching Points

Reports from cystoscopy and hydrodistention will typically characterize the bladder capacity under anesthesia, as well as the appearance of the bladder mucosa both before and after filling the bladder to capacity. Hydrodistention can cause findings consistent with IC/BPS including terminal hematuria on draining the bladder, petechiae or glomerulations. There may be no abnormal findings, and a normal cystoscopy does not rule out IC/BPS. Hunner's Ulcers are typically erythematous ulcers that can appear anywhere on the bladder mucosa and are present even before hydrodistentions. Suspicious lesions should be biopsied prior to any treatment of the lesion with fulguration or injection.

Postoperative Management and Short-Term Complications

Patients should be counseled that the first few days to 1 week after their hydrodistention, their IC/BPS symptoms may flare before they improve. Managing expectations perioperatively is critical, patients should be advised that they may experience dysuria and difficulty voiding postoperatively. Postoperative pain should be managed in escalating fashion starting with scheduled Tylenol and ibuprofen, phenazopyridine, and if needed short opioid courses (less than 3 days of short acting narcotics) (Dowell et al. 2016). Patients should receive instructions to help identify signs and symptoms of urinary retention and urinary tract infection and should notify their provider if these occur.

Bladder perforation is an extremely rare but serious intraoperative complication of any cystoscopic procedure, including hydrodistention, with or without treatment of Hunner's lesions. The bladder can tear or crack during bladder stretching, which may require prolonged catheterization, or in extreme circumstances, intraoperative open surgical repair. The AUA guidelines state that high-pressure, long-duration hydrodistention should not be offered.

Long-Term Complications

Long-term complications from hydrodistention are also unusual. Repeated fulgurations could lead to scarring of the bladder and decreased capacity, but only if extensive.

Pelvic Organ Prolapse and Pelvic Floor Disorders

Definitions

Pelvic organ prolapse is a term that describes the overall condition of female pelvic organs descending from their normal position into or through the vagina. The International Urogynecological Association/International Continence Society (IUGA/ICS) terminology committee defines POP as "The descent of one or more of the anterior vaginal wall, posterior vaginal wall, the uterus (cervix), or the apex of the vagina (vaginal vault or cuff scar after hysterectomy)"(Haylen et al. 2010). The American Urogynecologic Society developed a best practice statement for the evaluation and counseling of women with POP in 2017 (Carberry et al. 2017).

The description of pelvic organ prolapse has also been standardized, and is described by the portion of the vagina that is observed to be prolapsing. The term "cystocele" is often applied to an observed anterior vaginal wall prolapse, as a bulge in the anterior vaginal wall most commonly occurs with bladder protrusion into the vagina, but may also contain small bowel (enterocele) or the uterus, making the term "anterior vaginal wall prolapse" more appropriate. Uterine or cervical prolapse occurs when the uterus or cervix descends into the vaginal canal. Enterocele can occur in the anterior vaginal wall, posterior vaginal wall or at the vaginal apex. Vaginal vault or vaginal cuff prolapse describes the prolapse of the upper vagina after hysterectomy, uterine prolapse, and vaginal vault prolapse also be described as apical compartment prolapse. A bulge in the posterior vaginal wall, adjacent to the rectum, is termed a "rectocele." This should not be confused with "rectal prolapse," which is reserved for prolapse of the rectal mucosa through the anal opening. A perineocele is a bulge caused by a defect in the perineal body causing perineal descent.

Epidemiology

There is an 11% risk of undergoing an operation for POP or urinary incontinence by the age of 80 (Fialkow et al. 2008) and it is projected that there will be as many as 9.2 million women in the United States with POP by 2050 (Wu et al. 2009) (Fig. 16.5). Pelvic organ prolapse is known to have a significant impact on women's quality of life, sexual health, and body image (Lowder et al. 2011).

Anatomy and Physiology

The structure and function of the female pelvis is described above. The pelvic floor must support the genitourinary and gastrointestinal organs, and at the same time, allow them to perform the functions of voiding, childbirth and defecation. The normal support of the pelvic organs itself is complex, and dysfunction of the muscles, "ligaments," and "fascia" that keep these organs within the pelvis are not fully

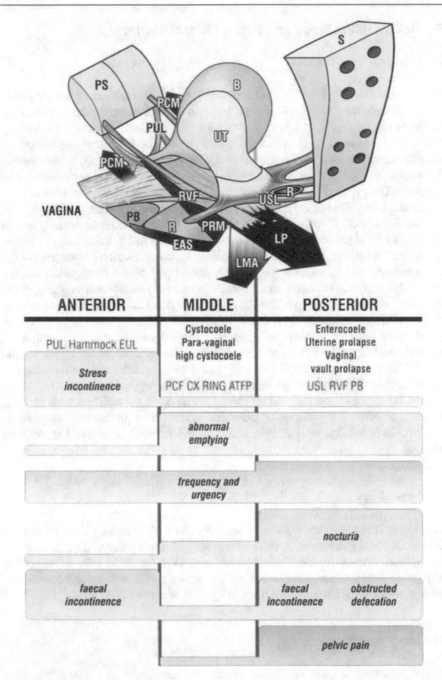

Fig. 16.5 The pictorial diagnostic algorithm. This algorithm summarizes the relationships between structural damage (prolapse) in the three zones and functions (symptoms). The size of the bar gives an approximate indication of the prevalence (probability) of the symptom. Laxities (red lettering) which can be repaired: pubourethral ligament (PUL); external urethral ligament (EUL); pubocervical fascia (PCF); CX ring/cardinal ligament; arcus tendineus fascia pelvis (ATFP); utero-sacral ligament (USL); rectovaginal fascia (RVF); perineal body (PB)

understood. Advanced computer modeling is currently being employed to understand the dynamic forces involved in the development of POP (Chen et al. 2013; Jing et al. 2012).

History

The symptom of a bothersome vaginal bulge is the most specific for POP (Carberry et al. 2017). The patient can describe this as pain but also as "pulling", or "heaviness" in the pelvis or vagina (Haylen et al. 2010). Patients will often describe the sensation that they are sitting on a small ball or other object.

It may be that an asymptomatic patient arrives at the appointment with a history of being told by another provider that they have prolapse, a cystocele, or that one of their pelvic organs has "dropped." It is especially important to reassure these patients that prolapse itself is not a dangerous or life-threatening condition and that sexual activity will not cause them harm. Patients should also be counseled that asymptomatic prolapse does not require treatment and can be managed expectantly or conservatively (Carberry et al. 2017).

Similar history-taking considerations exist for female patients with pelvic floor dysfunction as with IC/BPS, including a detailed sexual, gynecologic, and obstetric history, including complications and details of delivery. Due to differences in surgical options for treatment of POP and the fact that POP can adversely impact sexual health, it is important to ask patients whether they are sexually active or desire to have penetrative vaginal intercourse in the future and whether their POP symptoms interfere with sexual function (Carberry et al. 2017).

A thorough evaluation of symptoms of prolapse as well as bowel and bladder function should be reported and assessed with validated questionnaires. Anterior wall prolapse (cystocele) can cause increased resistance at the bladder outlet and lead to urinary hesitancy, incomplete voiding and also mask stress urinary incontinence. Therefore patients should be specifically asked whether stress urinary incontinence symptoms were present prior to developing prolapse—whether they have hesitancy, feeling of incomplete bladder emptying, position-dependent voiding and straining. Patients may report using their hand to reduce the prolapse in the vagina or on the perineum, termed "splinting," in order to facilitate bladder emptying or defecation. Fecal incontinence, flatal incontinence, straining to defecate, feeling of incomplete defecation, constipation, and other associated symptoms of anorectal dysfunction should be investigated. Symptoms of sexual dysfunction include pain during intercourse (dyspareunia), obstructed intercourse and vaginal laxity (Haylen et al. 2010).

The examiner should also elicit a detailed surgical history, with review of records if possible. It can be difficult for patients to recall remote surgeries, or concomitant procedures performed at the time of hysterectomy. It is useful to determine if a patient has had oophorectomy, and some patients may not know this information, and efforts should be made to confirm the status. Additionally, if pelvic surgeries were performed in recent years, it is also helpful to know what materials were used for any anti-incontinence or reconstructive surgeries in the event that reoperation is necessary.

The biggest risk factor for POP is vaginal childbirth causing trauma to the levator ani musculature (DeLancey et al. 2007; Morgan et al. 2011). Recent studies also find associations between POP and heavy occupational lifting, obesity, defecatory dysfunction (Dumoulin et al. 2016).

Physical Exam

Specific Maneuvers

Prior to the pelvic examination, it is useful to get an idea of the size of the prolapse by asking the patient how the bulge looks/feels when it is at its largest. This will help the examiner know if they are seeing the full extent of the prolapse during examination. Often patients will require specific instructions to achieve the full extent of prolapse (Fig. 16.6). One helpful maneuver is to ask the patient to take a deep breath and hold it, and while not allowing exhale, to bear down, causing a full valsalva. When the prolapse reaches its full extent, the vaginal rugae will smooth out. The patient should be able to demonstrate the control of the pelvic floor and the force of a pelvic floor contraction should be noted.

The pelvic exam follows the same format as described in the IC/BPS section above, but should also include prolapse assessment using the pelvic organ prolapse quantification scale (POP-Q; Table 16.1). POP-Q is a system of measurements that describe pelvic organ prolapse based on a fixed point of reference (the hymenal

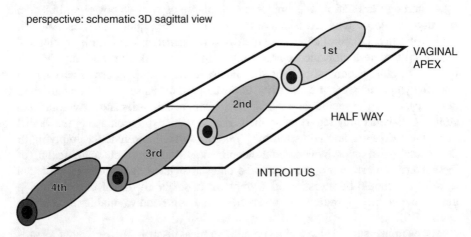

Fig. 16.6 Grading prolapse. Halfway Classification System. Perspective: schematic 3D sagittal view. The Halfway Classification System is used for prolapse from grades 1 to 4. Prolapse assessment is best performed under gentle traction (preferably in the operating room): First degree = prolapse to the halfway point; second degree = prolapse between the halfway point and introitus, but not beyond; third degree = prolapse beyond introitus; fourth degree = total eversion of either uterus or vaginal vault with traction

Table 16.1 Pelvic Organ Prolapse Quantification (POP-Q)

Enter POP-Q values here:	
Aa	Anterior wall 3 cm from external urethral meatus _____ cm (−3 to +3)
Bb	Most dependent part of anterior wall _____ cm (−3 to +TVL)
C	Cervix or vaginal cuff _____cm (±TVL)
D	Posterior fornix (if no prior hysterectomy) _____ cm (±TVL)
Ap	Posterior wall 3 cm from hymen _____cm (−3 to +3)
Bp	Most dependent part of posterior wall _____ cm (−3 to +TVL)
GH	Genital hiatus _____cm
PB	Perineal body _____cm
TVL	Total vaginal length _____cm

Staging pelvic organ prolapse using the POP-Q measurement

STAGE 0	STAGE I	STAGE II	STAGE III	STAGE IV
Aa = −3 cm	Aa = −2 cm	Aa = −1 to +1	Aa = +2 to +3	Aa = +3 or more
Ba = −3 cm	Ba = −2 cm	Ba = −1 to +1	Ba = +2 but <(+TVL-2)	Ba = +3 or more
Ap = −3 cm	Ap = −2 cm	Ap = −1 to +1	Ap = +2 to +3	Ap = +total TVL
Bp = −3 cm	Bp = −2 cm	Bp = −1 to +1	Bp = +2 but <(+TVL-2)	Bp = +TVL-1 or -2
C = −(≤TVL-2)	C = −2 to −(TVL-3)	C = −1 to +1	C = +2 but <(+TVL-2)	C = +total TVL
D = −(≤TVL-2)	D = −2 to −(TVL-3)	D = −1 to +1	D = +2 but <(+TVL-2)	D = +TVL-1 or -2

Note. Stage is assigned to the most severe prolapsing organ. Measurement is rounded to the nearest centimeter. TVL means the total measured vaginal length
Courtesy of Ananias Diokno, MD. Used with permission

Table 16.2 The Pelvic Organ Prolapse Quantification staging system

Stage	Description
0	No prolapse
I	Most distal portion of prolapse is >1 cm above the level of the hymen
II	Most distal portion of the prolapse is <1 cm proximal or distal to the hymen
III	Most distal portion of prolapse protrudes more than 1 cm below the hymen but no farther than 2 cm less than the total vaginal length (not all of the vagina has prolapsed)
IV	Complete procidentia or vaginal eversion; the most distal portion is at least total vaginal length of 2 cm

remnant) (Table 16.2). This system was developed to help both researchers and clinicians to standardize the description of prolapse in individual patients which allows for staging of prolapse with comparison of patients. The POP-Q is well described in the literature (Haylen et al. 2010) and is best learned from an experienced practitioner.

The position of the anus should be evaluated and a rectal exam should be undertaken in the evaluation of bowel symptoms, noting the sphincter tone, ability to contract and to attempt to expel an examining digit, and a rectovaginal exam can reveal the quality of the tissues and the extent of rectocele, and hard stool in the rectal vault can indicate functional bowel problems.

Abnormal Findings

As described above, thorough pelvic examination should be undertaken with notation of the tissue quality, any skin abnormalities, and any areas of tenderness or pain. Other abnormalities on pelvic exam that may be associated with previous surgeries should be well documented. These would include the presence of mesh or sutures and the presence of scars or banding.

Additionally, patients with prior surgery, medical conditions that would make one prone to fistulas, or complicated childbirth should incite a high index of suspicion for vesicovaginal, rectovaginal, urethrovaginal, peritoneovaginal, or ureterovaginal fistulas. The anus should be examined for asymmetry, indicating muscle injury or weakness. Rectal prolapse should be described and any concerns for fistulas or chronic or poorly healed obstetrical lacerations should be noted.

Diagnostic Tests

There are no required diagnostic tests in the evaluation of POP. Diagnostic testing, therefore, should be ordered based on patients' symptoms or clinical suspicion in order to rule out alternative diagnoses or support the diagnosis of POP (Carberry et al. 2017).

Laboratory Evaluation

In women with lower urinary tract symptoms (LUTS), a urinalysis and urine culture should be obtained (Carberry et al. 2017). These studies are also recommended for patients who are scheduled for surgical intervention with expected urinary tract instrumentation.

Imaging Studies

Dynamic magnetic resonance imaging, 3D ultrasound and other complex imaging modalities are often used for research in POP, but are not recommended as part of the standard evaluation. Imaging can be indicated for abnormal findings on pelvic exam, such as concern for fistula or urethral diverticulum, or for dysfunction of the urinary tract (fluoro urodynamics) or the gastrointestinal tract (defecography) (Carberry et al. 2017).

Procedures

A post-void residual urine volume can be obtained by ultrasound bladder scan or by catheterization. A full bladder stress test where the patient is examined with a full bladder (either by natural filling or by retrograde bladder filling with a catheter) can be useful to document the presence or absence of stress incontinence. If the patient is considering prolapse repair, the full bladder stress test can also be performed with the prolapse reduced, either with a pessary or a speculum in the vagina, to demonstrate stress incontinence that may occur with the prolapse reduced (occult stress urinary incontinence). More complex voiding dysfunction can be evaluated with a simple cystometric examination, or with urodynamics. Defecatory dysfunction can be evaluated with defecography or anorectal manometry (Carberry et al. 2017).

Management

It is important to elicit the patients' preferences, values and goals of care when discussing the management of pelvic organ prolapse. Fact sheets and decision aids for pelvic organ prolapse are available online and can help guide discussions about treatment options (Loss of Bladder Control - Bladder Prolapse - Urology Care Foundation n.d., Patient Fact Sheets - Healthcare Providers I AUGS n.d.)

Behavioral, Conservative, Complementary and Alternative Medicine

Patients should be counseled regarding concerns about safety, sexual functioning and body image (Lowder et al. 2011). For many patients, expectant management along with education about their condition and reassurance that POP is not dangerous is a reasonable treatment option.

One physical intervention that is often recommended for patients with prolapse is pelvic floor physical therapy. Pelvic floor physical therapy for patients with POP is focused on pelvic floor muscle training and strengthening, rather than muscle relaxation in patients with IC/BPS. Individualized one on one pelvic floor physical therapy has been shown in a randomized controlled trial to improve patient reported symptoms of POP (Hagen et al. 2014). This type of therapy can be offered to patients as a low risk intervention (Hagen and Stark 2011).

Vaginal pessaries have been used as a mechanical intervention for pelvic organ prolapse for centuries. Contemporary vaginal pessaries are devices made of medical-grade silicone of various shapes and sizes and are designed to treat any size or type of prolapse. Pessary fitting entails choosing the right size and shape of pessary to comfortably reduce a women's prolapse. During a pessary fitting, a trial of valsalva and voiding in the office can help ensure that the pessary is properly sized (pessaries that are too small may be expelled with these maneuvers and pessaries that are too large may feel uncomfortable). Pessary treatment is described as having a moderate dropout rate, but a review of the evidence shows that studies report 50–80% continuation at 1 year, with a high patient satisfaction in the medium term (Lamers et al. 2011). Pessary maintenance is performed by the patient and/or the provider to varying degrees depending on the patient's abilities. Ideally, patients can be taught and clean the pessaries themselves at home. These patients can be monitored with a yearly speculum exam to ensure that there is no damage to the vaginal tissues. Other patients do not have the ability to remove and clean the pessary and therefore require periodic removal and cleaning by a provider. There is no strict time interval between visits for these visits for pessary removal and cleaning, but experts recommend an initial vaginal exam at 2–4 weeks after placement and then removal and cleaning by a provider about every 3 months thereafter (Carberry et al. 2017). The most common side effects of pessary use are vaginal discharge, odor, bleeding pain and constipation (Lamers et al. 2011). Retained pessaries after loss to follow up or neglect can cause serious complications, but these are exceedingly rare.

Medical

There are essentially no pharmacologic treatments for POP. Topical estrogen cream can help improve the vaginal tissues and some of the associated irritative voiding symptoms and dyspareunia associated with atrophy, and will possibly make pessary use more comfortable, but will not improve prolapse.

Surgical

Surgical treatment for POP can be divided in to obliterative versus reconstructive approaches (Carberry et al. 2017). Obliterative surgery should only be considered among women who are sure that they will not desire vaginal intercourse in the future (Carberry et al. 2017). Colpocleisis, an obliterative surgery, is a transvaginal surgery which shortens and narrows the vagina to reduce the prolapsed organs and, in layman's terms, "closes" the vaginal canal. Colpocleisis is usually performed with concomitant perineorraphy to decrease the size of the genital hiatus (Abbasy and Kenton 2010). Colpocleisis can be performed with the uterus intact, termed LeFort Colpocleisis, or in patients with prior or hysterectomy (Carberry et al. 2017). When performed without hysterectomy, colpocleisis is a safe and fairly low morbidity operation that can be performed under regional anesthesia (spinal) (Carberry et al. 2017). Patient satisfaction and anatomic success are very high in the literature, with a recent large case series of one type of colpocleisis reporting over 92% satisfaction in 310 elderly women, with 15.2% complication rate and 1.3% mortality rate (Zebede et al. 2013).

Reconstructive surgery can consist of a single or multiple procedures designed to restore the anatomy and function of the prolapsed organs. These procedures are typically described by the compartment that they address and the route by which the procedures are performed.

Uterine prolapse, apical compartment prolapse, vaginal vault prolapse can be repaired transabdominally or transvaginally; both approaches resuspend the vagina by attaching it to a structure within the pelvis for support. Abdominal sacrocolpopexy involves attaching the vaginal apex via a reinforcing graft (often synthetic polypropylene mesh) to the sacral anterior longitudinal ligament (Nygaard et al. 2013). This can be performed as an open, laparoscopic or robotic surgery either post-hysterectomy or at the same time as total or supracervical hysterectomy. Transvaginal native tissue repairs for apical prolapse suspend the vaginal apex by attaching it with sutures to the sacrospinous ligament or to the uterosacral ligaments, often with concomitant hysterectomy but uterine sparing approaches (hysteropexy) have been described (Bradley et al. 2018). Vaginal mesh repairs for apical prolapse use mesh that is placed transvaginally to re-suspend the vaginal apex, typically by attachment to the sacrospinous ligament. However, there are currently no vaginal pelvic organ prolapse mesh products marketed in the United States (see details below). Choice of apical prolapse repair is often surgeon dependent and the risks and benefits of the planned repair should be discussed on an individualized basis.

Reconstructive surgery for anterior vaginal wall defects, often called "anterior colporraphy" or "anterior repair" can be colloquially described by patients as "bladder lift," "bladder sling," "bladder suspension," making it imperative to obtain operative reports in patients who have had prior surgery. Anterior compartment repairs are most often transvaginal surgeries and consist of native tissue repairs where the cystocele is reduced using plicating sutures (anterior colporraphy), or transvaginal mesh repairs where polypropylene mesh is used as a graft to reinforce the vaginal wall. In April 2019, the United States Food and Drug Administration (FDA) "ordered all manufacturers of surgical mesh intended for transvaginal repair of anterior compartment prolapse [the only transvaginal mesh available on the market] to stop selling and distributing their products immediately" (Center for Devices & Radiological Health 2019). This decision was made after determination that the manufacturers had not demonstrated "reasonable assurance of safety and effectiveness for these devices" (Center for Devices & Radiological Health 2019). It is important to note that this order does not apply to mesh used for mid urethral sling surgeries nor does it apply to transabdominal mesh for POP such as in sacrocolpopexy.

Surgical repairs for posterior wall defects include rectocele repair ("posterior colporraphy" or "posterior repair") and perineorraphy. These are most typically completed transvaginally without any graft material as there is no current evidence that grafting of any type improves outcomes in the posterior compartment (Gomelsky et al. 2011).

Criteria for Surgery
The most important preoperative consideration for patients considering prolapse repair is that surgeries for POP are elective surgeries. Patients should be counseled extensively on the risks and benefits, the durability and the success rates of the procedures, as well as the alternatives to surgery. This counseling has been shown to play an important role as patient's preparedness for surgery is associated with their satisfaction with the outcome of the procedure (Kenton et al. 2007). Patients must meet criteria for general anesthesia, with the exception of colpocleisis, which can be performed under spinal anesthetic.

Preoperative Considerations and Additional Tests That May Be Appropriate Prior to Surgery
Patients with POP are frequently middle-aged or older, and may have significant comorbidities. Guidelines should be followed for preoperative workup for any patient undergoing general anesthesia. Patients should also have preoperative urine cultures if there is concern for UTI, or the urinary tract is going to be extensively

instrumented. For patients considering surgical intervention, the American College of Surgeons National Surgery Quality Improvement Program surgical risk calculator is helpful in estimating perioperative morbidity and mortality (ACS Risk Calculator - Patient Information n.d.; Carberry et al. 2017).

Medications
Guidelines for perioperative surgical prophylactic antibiotics should be followed. Multimodal, preoperative pain medication administration can be considered as part of an enhanced recovery after surgery pathway (Carter-Brooks et al. 2018). Phenazopyridine can be administered preoperatively to aid with ureteral efflux identification. Medications used during surgery include vasopressin or local anesthetic with epinephrine for hydrodissection. Methylene blue or indigo carmine can also aid in confirmation of ureteral efflux during cystoscopy, however due to side effects and shortages, these are less commonly used in recent years. The use of vaginal packing (with or without soaking in medications) is surgeon dependent and varies greatly.

Teaching Points
Prolapse repair is a dynamic field of surgery and an active area of research in the specialty of FPMRS. Anatomic success is not the only factor that is important when judging the success of an operation for prolapse, as the absence of symptoms (vaginal bulge) is strongly related to how much overall improvement patients subjectively report after surgery (Barber et al. 2009). Failure rates determined by varying definitions of success show a wide range in the literature, however most studies show that there is a reasonable chance that a patient may undergo a second surgical prolapse repair, which makes complex reoperative surgery not uncommon for the pelvic surgeon, and patients must be counseled on risks for repeat surgical repair.

Intraoperatively, the surgeon must recognize that patients under anesthesia have relaxation of the pelvic floor musculature, and that these muscles will regain normal tone. Surgical planning should take into account the patients' preoperative exam, symptoms, personalized goals and examination under anesthesia.

Postoperative Management
Postoperatively, patients undergoing POP repairs can be discharged on the same day or observed for a 23 h stay, depending on their clinical course (Carter-Brooks et al. 2018). Patients are frequently catheterized during surgery and will undergo catheter removal with void trial prior to discharge from the hospital. If a vaginal pack is placed, the packing will need to be removed prior to trial of voiding. If patients are unable to void, they can be taught how to perform intermittent catheterization after each void in order to facilitate transition back to normal voiding. Spontaneous voiding typically returns within a few days to a few weeks after surgery. If the patient is unable to self-catheterize, she can be sent home for a short time (usually about 5–7 days) with an indwelling Foley catheter.

Postoperative pain control begins in the preoperative area with patient counseling on pain expectations and administration of multimodal preoperative pain medications (Carter-Brooks et al. 2018). Scheduled, non-narcotic medications, such as acetaminophen and NSAIDs are recommended in the postoperative period. Short courses of postoperative narcotic pain medication can be prescribed with adherence to recent guidelines, for similar pelvic surgeries (vaginal hysterectomy) a recommendation of between 0 and 15 5 mg tablets of oxycodone has been recommended (Dowell et al. 2016; Prescribing Recommendations n.d.). Provider and patient resources and best practices statements on postoperative pain optimization can be found via the Michigan Opioid Prescribing Engagement Network (Michigan OPEN) (Home n.d.).

Short-Term Complications

Short-term complications of POP surgery parallel those seen with any surgical intervention. Small risks of abdominal wound infections, port site complications, or complications from vascular, genitourinary or gastrointestinal injuries during minimally invasive or open intra-abdominal surgery exist. A meta-analysis of sacrocolpopexy complication rates showed a rate of wound infection of 2.4% and a rate of cystotomy of 2.8% (Hudson et al. 2014). Patients are positioned in lithotomy for POP surgeries, this positioning has risk of peroneal, obturator, lateral femoral cutaneous and sciatic nerve injury from compression of these nerves against the table, lithotomy stirrups or hyper-extension or flexion (Warner et al. 2000) and careful intraoperative positioning is critical.

Transvaginal surgery also carries a risk of postoperative bleeding, both vaginal, paravaginal, and intra-abdominal, and special consideration should be given to bleeding into the retroperitoneum after sacrospinous ligament suspension suture placement. Intra-abdominal bleeding or bowel complications can occur (obstruction or injury) during vaginal hysterectomy or enterocele repair where the peritoneum is entered or with passage of mesh kit trocars (although these are no longer marketed). A series of 438 consecutive transvaginal native tissue repairs also showed a very low rate of complications, with a cystotomy rate of 0.2% and a reoperation rate for hemorrhage of 0.9%, without differences in serious complications for patients undergoing sacrospinous ligament suspension or hysterectomy (Mothes et al. 2014) There are risks of bladder or ureteral injury during hysterectomy regardless of route, as well as in anterior and apical prolapse repairs and passage of mesh kit trocars (although these are no longer marketed), and a high index of suspicion is warranted and routine cystoscopy is recommended

Infection of the vaginal incisions are rare, vaginal wounds can more commonly develop bleeding or dehiscence. Granulation tissue can form within the vagina at the site of vaginal incisions, which can often be treated in the office, or as a short outpatient procedure. Urinary tract infection can occur regardless of type of surgery, and patients should be counseled on the signs and symptoms of this relatively common occurrence.

Long-Term Complications

Long-term complications of prolapse repair can include small bowel obstruction (if peritoneum is entered), dyspareunia, lower urinary tract dysfunction, mesh complications (exposure, erosion, pain), and failure of the repair or recurrent prolapse. Following prolapse surgery, around 12% of women develop de novo urinary frequency and urgency, and 9% develop voiding dysfunction (Maher et al. 2013) Follow-up of mesh grafts used in prolapse show an exposure rate around 7.3–18% for transvaginal mesh (Gomelsky et al. 2011; Maher et al. 2013) (although these are no longer marketed). A long-term study of abdominal sacrocolpopexy showed that 10.5% of patients would be expected to have a mesh or suture erosion at 7 years of follow-up (Nygaard et al. 2013). In all studies, mesh exposures in the vagina were often managed conservatively.

Clinical Pearls
- Be mindful of cultural/religious considerations, relative to members of the opposite sex performing these examinations and procedures.
- Management of constipation is key to management of both prolapse and IC/BPS.
- Current guidelines recommend against long-term antibiotic and systemic glucocorticoid use for IC/BPS.
- Patients who are unwilling to perform ISC, or lack the manual dexterity for ISC, are not candidates for botulinum toxin bladder injections.
- Education, self-care, and behavioral modifications are key to successful management of IC/BPS.
- Always consider preoperative urine cultures in this population, if the GU tract will be extensively instrumented.

Resources

Resources for the Nurse Practitioner

1. AUA Guideline: Diagnosis and Treatment of Interstitial Cystitis/Bladder Pain Syndrome http://www.auanet.org/education/guidelines/ic-bladder-pain-syndrome.cfm
2. American Urogynecologic Society www.augs.org
3. Interactive POP-Q http://www.bardmedical.com/products/pelvic-health/pop-q/
4. Michigan Opioid Prescribing Engagement Network https://michigan-open.org

Resources for the Patient

1. Urology Care Foundation Patient Information http://www.urologyhealth.org/urology/index.cfm?article=67
2. Interstitial Cystitis Association http://www.ichelp.org
3. American Urogynecologic Society www.augs.org
4. Voices for Pelvic Floor Dysfunction http://www.voicesforpfd.org/p/cm/ld/fid=5

References

Abbasy S, Kenton K (2010) Obliterative procedures for pelvic organ prolapse. Clin Obstet Gynecol 53(1):86–98. https://doi.org/10.1097/GRF.0b013e3181cd4252

ACS Risk Calculator - Patient Information (n.d.) Retrieved December 2, 2019, from http://riskcalculator.facs.org/RiskCalculator/PatientInfo.jsp

Afari N, Buchwald D, Clauw D, Hong B, Hou X, Krieger JN et al (2019) A MAPP network case-control study of urologic chronic pelvic pain compared with non-urologic pain conditions. Clin J Pain 36(1):8–15. https://doi.org/10.1097/AJP.0000000000000769

Andersen AV, Granlund P, Schultz A, Talseth T, Hedlund H, Frich L (2012) Long-term experience with surgical treatment of selected patients with bladder pain syndrome/interstitial cystitis. Scand J Urol Nephrol 46:284–289. https://doi.org/10.3109/00365599.2012.669789

Asavasopon S, Rana M, Kirages DJ, Yani MS, Fisher BE, Hwang DH et al (2014) Cortical activation associated with muscle synergies of the human male pelvic floor. J Neurosci 34(41):13811–13818. https://doi.org/10.1523/JNEUROSCI.2073-14.2014

Atchley MD, Shah NM, Whitmore KE (2015) Complementary and alternative medical therapies for interstitial cystitis: an update from the United States. Transl Androl Urol 4(6):662–667. https://doi.org/10.3978/j.issn.2223-4683.2015.08.08

Barber MD, Brubaker L, Nygaard I et al (2009) Defining success after surgery for pelvic organ prolapse. Obstet Gynecol 114(3):600–609. https://doi.org/10.1097/AOG.0b013e3181b2b1ae

Berry SH, Bogart LM, Pham C et al (2010) Development, validation and testing of an epidemiological case definition of interstitial cystitis/painful bladder syndrome. J Urol 183(5):1848–1852. https://doi.org/10.1016/j.juro.2009.12.103

Berry SH, Elliott MN, Suttorp M et al (2011) Prevalence of symptoms of bladder pain syndrome/interstitial cystitis among adult females in the United States. J Urol 186(2):540–544. https://doi.org/10.1016/j.juro.2011.03.132

Bradley S, Gutman RE, Richter LA (2018) Hysteropexy: an option for the repair of pelvic organ prolapse. Curr Urol Rep 19(2):15. https://doi.org/10.1007/s11934-018-0765-4

Carberry CL, Tulikangas PK, Ridgeway BM, Collins SA, Adam ARA (2017) American Urogynecologic Society best practice statement: evaluation and counseling of patients with pelvic organ prolapse. Female Pelvic Med Reconstr Surg 23(5):281–287. https://doi.org/10.1097/SPV.0000000000000424

Carrico DJ, Peters KM (2011) Vaginal diazepam use with urogenital pain/pelvic floor dysfunction: serum diazepam levels and efficacy data. Urol Nurs 31(5):279–284, 299. http://www.ncbi.nlm.nih.gov/pubmed/22073898

Carter-Brooks CM, Du AL, Ruppert KM, Romanova AL, Zyczynski HM (2018) Implementation of a urogynecology-specific enhanced recovery after surgery (ERAS) pathway. Am J Obstet Gynecol 219(5):495.e1–495.e10. https://doi.org/10.1016/j.ajog.2018.06.009

Center for Devices, & Radiological Health (2019) Urogynecologic surgical mesh implants. Retrieved December 2, 2019, from U.S. Food and Drug Administration website: http://www.fda.gov/medical-devices/implants-and-prosthetics/urogynecologic-surgical-mesh-implants

Chen L, Ramanah R, Hsu Y, Ashton-Miller JA, Delancey JOL (2013) Cardinal and deep uterosacral ligament lines of action: MRI based 3D technique development and preliminary findings in normal women. Int Urogynecol J Pelvic Floor Dysfunct 24:37–45. https://doi.org/10.1007/s00192-012-1801-4

Chennamsetty A, Ehlert MJ, Peters KM, Killinger KA (2015) Advances in diagnosis and treatment of interstitial cystitis/painful bladder syndrome. Curr Infect Dis Rep 17(1):454. https://doi.org/10.1007/s11908-014-0454-5

Chrysanthopoulou EL, Doumouchtsis SK (2013) Challenges and current evidence on the management of bladder pain syndrome. Neurourol Urodyn 30:169–173. https://doi.org/10.1002/nau.22475

Clemens JQ, Mullins C, Kusek JW, Kirkali Z, Mayer EA, Rodríguez LV et al (2014) The MAPP research network: a novel study of urologic chronic pelvic pain syndromes. BMC Urol 14:57. https://doi.org/10.1186/1471-2490-14-57

Clemens JQ, Mullins C, Ackerman AL, Bavendam T, van Bokhoven A, Ellingson BM et al (2019) Urologic chronic pelvic pain syndrome: insights from the MAPP Research Network. Nat Rev Urol 16(3):187–200. https://doi.org/10.1038/s41585-018-0135-5

Colaco MA, Evans RJ (2013) Current recommendations for bladder instillation therapy in the treatment of interstitial cystitis/bladder pain syndrome. Curr Urol Rep 14(5):442–447. https://doi.org/10.1007/s11934-013-0369-y

Crescenze I, Shah P, Adams G, Cameron AP, Stoffel J, Romo PB et al (2018) MP15-05 Treatment Outcomes Of Ureaplasma And Mycoplasma Species Isolated From Patients With Pain And Lower Urinary Tract SympTOMS. J Urol 199(4S):e190. Retrieved from https://www.auajournals.org/doi/abs/10.1016/j.juro.2018.02.518

Crisp CC, Vaccaro CM, Estanol MV et al (2013) Intra-vaginal diazepam for high-tone pelvic floor dysfunction: a randomized placebo-controlled trial. Int Urogynecol J Pelvic Floor Dysfunct 24:1915–1923. https://doi.org/10.1007/s00192-013-2108-9

Dawson TE, Jamison J (2007) Intravesical treatments for painful bladder syndrome/interstitial cystitis. Cochrane Database Syst Rev 4:2007–2009. https://doi.org/10.1002/14651858.CD006113.pub2

DeLancey JOL, Morgan DM, Fenner DE et al (2007) Comparison of levator ani muscle defects and function in women with and without pelvic organ prolapse. Obstet Gynecol 109:295–302. https://doi.org/10.1097/01.AOG.0000250901.57095.ba

Dimitrakov J, Kroenke K, Steers WD et al (2007) Pharmacologic management of painful bladder syndrome/interstitial cystitis: a systematic review. Arch Intern Med 167(18):1922–1929. https://doi.org/10.1001/archinte.167.22.2452

Dowell D, Haegerich TM, Chou R (2016) CDC guideline for prescribing opioids for chronic pain - United States, 2016. MMWR Recomm Rep 65(1):1–49. https://doi.org/10.15585/mmwr.rr6501e1

Dumoulin C, Hunter KF, Moore K, Bradley CS, Burgio KL, Hagen S et al (2016) Conservative management for female urinary incontinence and pelvic organ prolapse review 2013: summary of the 5th international consultation on incontinence. Neurourol Urodyn 35(1):15–20. https://doi.org/10.1002/nau.22677

Educational Materials - Urology Care Foundation (n.d.) Retrieved November 29, 2019, from https://www.urologyhealth.org/Documents/Product%20Store/IC_PatientGuide.pdf

Ferguson TJ, Geraets RL, Barker MA (2019) Review of Chronic use of pentosan polysulfate sodium associated with risk of vision-threatening disease. Int Urogynecol J 30(3):337–338. https://doi.org/10.1007/s00192-018-3850-9

Fialkow MF, Newton KM, Lentz GM, Weiss NS (2008) Lifetime risk of surgical management for pelvic organ prolapse or urinary incontinence. Int Urogynecol J Pelvic Floor Dysfunct 19:437–440. https://doi.org/10.1007/s00192-007-0459-9

Fitzgerald MP, Payne CK, Lukacz ES et al (2012) Randomized multicenter clinical trial of myofascial physical therapy in women with interstitial cystitis/painful bladder syndrome and pelvic floor tenderness. J Urol 187(6):2113–2118. https://doi.org/10.1016/j.juro.2012.01.123

Forrest JB, Payne CK, Erickson DR (2012) Cyclosporine A for refractory interstitial cystitis/bladder pain syndrome: experience of 3 tertiary centers. J Urol 188:1186–1191. https://doi.org/10.1016/j.juro.2012.06.023

Foster HE, Hanno PM, Nickel JC et al (2010) Effect of amitriptyline on symptoms in treatment naïve patients with interstitial cystitis/painful bladder syndrome. J Urol 183(5):1853–1858. https://doi.org/10.1016/j.juro.2009.12.106

Gokyildiz S, Kizilkaya Beji N, Yalcin O, Istek A (2012) Effects of percutaneous tibial nerve stimulation therapy on chronic pelvic pain. Gynecol Obstet Invest 73:99–105. https://doi.org/10.1159/000328447

Gomelsky A, Penson DF, Dmochowski RR (2011) Pelvic organ prolapse (POP) surgery: the evidence for the repairs. Br J Urol 107(11):1704–1719. https://doi.org/10.1111/j.1464-410X.2011.10123.x

Gupta P, Gaines N, Sirls LT, Peters KM (2015) A multidisciplinary approach to the evaluation and management of interstitial cystitis/bladder pain syndrome: an ideal model of care. Transl Androl Urol 4(6):611–619. https://doi.org/10.3978/j.issn.2223-4683.2015.10.10

Haefner HK, Collins ME, Davis GD et al (2005) The vulvodynia guideline. J Low Genit Tract Dis 9:40–51. https://doi.org/10.1097/00128360-200501000-00009

Hagen S, Stark D (2011) Conservative prevention and management of pelvic organ prolapse in women. Cochrane Database Syst Rev 12:CD003882. https://doi.org/10.1002/14651858. CD003882.pub4.Copyright

Hagen S, Stark D, Glazener C et al (2014) Individualised pelvic floor muscle training in women with pelvic organ prolapse (POPPY): a multicentre randomised controlled trial. Lancet 383:796–806. https://doi.org/10.1016/S0140-6736(13)61977-7

Han E, Nguyen L, Sirls L, Peters K (2018) Current best practice management of interstitial cystitis/bladder pain syndrome. Ther Adv Urol 10(7):197–211. https://doi.org/10.1177/1756287218761574

Hanno P, Dmochowski R (2009) Status of international consensus on interstitial cystitis/bladder pain syndrome/painful bladder syndrome: 2008 snapshot. Neurourol Urodyn 28(4):274–286. https://doi.org/10.1002/nau.20687

Hanno PM, Burks DA, Clemens JQ, Dmochowski RR, Erickson D, Fitzgerald MP et al (2011) AUA guideline for the diagnosis and treatment of interstitial cystitis/bladder pain syndrome. J Urol 185(6):2162–2170. https://doi.org/10.1016/j.juro.2011.03.064

Hanno PM, Erickson D, Moldwin R, Faraday MM, American Urological Association (2015) Diagnosis and treatment of interstitial cystitis/bladder pain syndrome: AUA guideline amendment. J Urol 193(5):1545–1553. https://doi.org/10.1016/j.juro.2015.01.086

Haylen BT, De Ridder D, Freeman RM et al (2010) An International Urogynecological Association (IUGA)/International Continence Society (ICS) joint report on the terminology for Female Pelvic Floor Dysfunction. Neurourol Urodyn 29:4–20. https://doi.org/10.1002/nau.20798

Home (n.d.) Retrieved December 2, 2019, from Michigan OPEN website: https://michigan-open.org/

Hudson CO, Northington GM, Lyles RH, Karp DR (2014) Outcomes of robotic sacrocolpopexy: a systematic review and meta-analysis. Female Pelvic Med Reconstr 20:252–260. http://journals. lww.com/jpelvicsurgery/Abstract/2011/11000/Bladder_Pain_Syndrome__A_Review.4.aspx

Jensen JS, Cusini M, Gomberg M, Moi H (2016) 2016 European guideline on Mycoplasma genitalium infections. J Eur Acad Dermatol Venereol 30(10):1650–1656. https://doi.org/10.1111/jdv.13849

Jhang J-F, Jiang Y-H, Kuo H-C (2014) Potential therapeutic effect of intravesical botulinum toxin type A on bladder pain syndrome/interstitial cystitis. Int J Urol 21(Suppl 1):49–55. https://doi.org/10.1111/iju.12317

Jing D, Ashton-Miller JA, DeLancey JOL (2012) A subject-specific anisotropic visco-hyperelastic finite element model of female pelvic floor stress and strain during the second stage of labor. J Biomech 45:455–460. https://doi.org/10.1016/j.jbiomech.2011.12.002

Kenton K, Pham T, Mueller E, Brubaker L (2007) Patient preparedness: an important predictor of surgical outcome. Am J Obstet Gynecol 197(6):654.e1–654.e6. https://doi.org/10.1016/j.ajog.2007.08.059

Kessler TM (2019) Flares of chronic pelvic pain syndrome: lessons learned from the MAPP Research Network. BJU Int 124(3):360–361. https://doi.org/10.1111/bju.14843

Lamers BHC, Broekman BMW, Milani AL (2011) Pessary treatment for pelvic organ prolapse and health-related quality of life: a review. Int Urogynecol J 22:637–644. https://doi.org/10.1007/s00192-011-1390-7

Loss of Bladder Control - Bladder Prolapse - Urology Care Foundation (n.d.) Retrieved December 2, 2019, from https://www.urologyhealth.org/educational-materials/loss-of-bladder-control-bladder-prolapse

Lowder JL, Ghetti C, Nikolajski C, Oliphant SS, Zyczynski HM (2011) Body image perceptions in women with pelvic organ prolapse: a qualitative study. Am J Obstet Gynecol 204(5):441. e1–441.e5. https://doi.org/10.1016/j.ajog.2010.12.024

Lusty A, Kavaler E, Zakariasen K, Tolls V, Nickel JC (2018) Treatment effectiveness in interstitial cystitis/bladder pain syndrome: Do patient perceptions align with efficacy-based guidelines? Can Urol Assoc J 12(1):E1–E5. https://doi.org/10.5489/cuaj.4505

Maher C, Feiner B, Baessler K, Schmid C (2013) Surgical management of pelvic organ prolapse in women. Cochrane Database Syst Rev 4:CD004014. https://doi.org/10.1002/14651858. CD004014.pub5

Malde S, Palmisani S, Al-Kaisy A, Sahai A (2018) Guideline of guidelines: bladder pain syndrome. BJU Int 122(5):729–743. https://doi.org/10.1111/bju.14399

Morgan DM, Larson K, Lewicky-Gaupp C, Fenner DE, DeLancey JOL (2011) Vaginal support as determined by levator ani defect status 6 weeks after primary surgery for pelvic organ prolapse. Int J Gynaecol Obstet 114(2):141–144. https://doi.org/10.1016/j.ijgo.2011.02.020

Mothes AR, Mothes HK, Radosa MP, Runnebaum IB (2014) Systematic assessment of surgical complications in 438 cases of vaginal native tissue repair for pelvic organ prolapse adopting Clavien– Dindo classification. Arch Gynecol Obstet 291(6):1297–1301. https://doi.org/10.1007/s00404-014-3549-1

Naliboff BD, Stephens AJ, Afari N, Lai H, Krieger JN, Hong B et al (2015) Widespread psychosocial difficulties in men and women with urologic chronic pelvic pain syndromes: case-control findings from the multidisciplinary approach to the study of chronic pelvic pain research network. Urology 85(6):1319–1327. https://doi.org/10.1016/j.urology.2015.02.047

Netter FH, Colacino S. Atlas of human anatomy. Elsevier-health sciences division; 1989. 01–01.

Nickel JC, Jain P, Shore N, Anderson J, Giesing D, Lee H et al (2012) Continuous intravesical lidocaine treatment for interstitial cystitis/bladder pain syndrome: safety and efficacy of a new drug delivery device. Sci Transl Med. 4(143):143ra100. https://doi.org/10.1126/scitranslmed.3003804

Nygaard I, Brubaker L, Zyczynski HM et al (2013) Long-term outcomes following abdominal sacrocolpopexy for pelvic organ prolapse. JAMA 309(19):2016–2024. https://doi.org/10.1001/jama.2013.4919

Osborne J (2019) LiRIS device for interstitial cystitis & Hunner's lesions DEPRIORITIZED by Allergan - Interstitial Cystitis Network. Retrieved December 1, 2019, from Interstitial Cystitis Network website: https://www.ic-network.com/liris-device-for-interstitial-cystitis-hunners-lesions-deprioritized-by-allergan/

Patient Fact Sheets - Healthcare Providers I AUGS (n.d.) Retrieved December 2, 2019, from https://www.augs.org/patient-fact-sheets/

Pearce WA, Chen R, Jain N (2018) Pigmentary maculopathy associated with chronic exposure to pentosan polysulfate sodium. Ophthalmology 125(11):1793–1802. https://doi.org/10.1016/j.ophtha.2018.04.026

Peters KM, Feber KM, Bennett RC (2007) A prospective, single-blind, randomized crossover trial of sacral vs pudendal nerve stimulation for interstitial cystitis. BJU Int 100:835–839. https://doi.org/10.1111/j.1464-410X.2007.07082.x

Peters KM, Jaeger C, Killinger KA, Rosenberg B, Boura JA (2013) Cystectomy for ulcerative interstitial cystitis: sequelae and patients' perceptions of improvement. Urology 82(4):829–833. https://doi.org/10.1016/j.urology.2013.06.043

Pontari MA, Krieger JN, Litwin MS et al (2010) Pregabalin for the treatment of men with chronic prostatitis/chronic pelvic pain syndrome: a randomized controlled trial. Arch Intern Med 170:1586–1593. https://doi.org/10.1001/archinternmed.2010.319

Prescribing Recommendations (n.d.) Retrieved December 2, 2019, from Michigan OPEN website: https://michigan-open.org/prescribing-recommendations/

Rana M, Yani MS, Asavasopon S, Fisher BE, Kutch JJ (2015) Brain connectivity associated with muscle synergies in humans. J Neurosci 35(44):14708–14716. https://doi.org/10.1523/JNEUROSCI.1971-15.2015

Rössberger J, Fall M, Jonsson O, Peeker R (2007) Long-term results of reconstructive surgery in patients with bladder pain syndrome/interstitial cystitis: subtyping is imperative. Urology 70:638–642. https://doi.org/10.1016/j.urology.2007.05.028

Sant GR, Propert KJ, Hanno PM et al (2003) A pilot clinical trial of oral pentosan polysulfate and oral hydroxyzine in patients with interstitial cystitis. J Urol 170(3):810–815. https://doi.org/10.1097/01.ju.0000083020.06212.3d

Suskind AM, Berry SH, Ewing BA, Elliott MN, Suttorp MJ, Clemens JQ (2012) The prevalence of interstitial cystitis/bladder pain syndrome (Ic/Bps) and chronic prostatitis/chronic pelvic pain syndrome (Cp/Cpps) in men; results of the rand interstitial cystitis epidemiology (Rice) male study. J Urol 187:e29–e30. https://doi.org/10.1016/j.juro.2012.02.115

Suskind AM, Berry SH, Suttorp MJ et al (2013) Health-related quality of life in patients with interstitial cystitis/bladder pain syndrome and frequently associated comorbidities. Qual Life Res 22:1537–1541. https://doi.org/10.1007/s11136-012-0285-5

Sutcliffe S, Gallop R, Henry Lai HH, Andriole GL, Bradley CS, Chelimsky G et al (2019) A longitudinal analysis of urological chronic pelvic pain syndrome flares in the Multidisciplinary Approach to the Study of Chronic Pelvic Pain (MAPP) Research Network. BJU Int 124(3):522–531. https://doi.org/10.1111/bju.14783

Tanaka T, Nitta Y, Morimoto K et al (2011) Hyperbaric oxygen therapy for painful bladder syndrome/interstitial cystitis resistant to conventional treatments: long-term results of a case series in Japan. BMC Urol 11:11. https://doi.org/10.1186/1471-2490-11-11

Van Ophoven A, Pokupic S, Heinecke A, Hertle L (2004) A prospective, randomized, placebo controlled, double-blind study of amitriptyline for the treatment of interstitial cystitis. J Urol 172(2):533–536. https://doi.org/10.1097/01.ju.0000132388.54703.4d

Van Ophoven A, Rossbach G, Pajonk F, Hertle L (2006) Safety and efficacy of hyperbaric oxygen therapy for the treatment of interstitial cystitis: a randomized, sham controlled, double-blind trial. J Urol 176:1442–1446. https://doi.org/10.1016/j.juro.2006.06.065

Vas L, Pattanik M, Titarmore V (2014) Treatment of interstitial cystitis/painful bladder syndrome as a neuropathic pain condition. Indian J Urol 30(3):350–353. https://doi.org/10.4103/0970-1591.128513

Warner MA, Warner DO, Harper CM, Schroeder DR, Maxson PM (2000) Lower extremity neuropathies associated with lithotomy positions. Anesthesiology 93(4):938–942. https://doi.org/10.1097/00000542-200010000-00010

Warren JW, Van De Merwe JP, Nickel JC (2011) Interstitial cystitis/bladder pain syndrome and nonbladder syndromes: facts and hypotheses. Urology 78:727–732. https://doi.org/10.1016/j.urology.2011.06.014

Wu JM, Hundley AF, Fulton RG, Myers ER (2009) Forecasting the prevalence of pelvic floor disorders in U.S. Women: 2010 to 2050. Obstet Gynecol 114(6):1278–1283. https://doi.org/10.1097/AOG.0b013e3181c2ce96

Zebede S, Smith AL, Plowright LN, Hegde A, Aguilar VC, Davila GW (2013) Obliterative LeFort colpocleisis in a large group of elderly women. Obstet Gynecol 121(2):279–284. https://doi.org/10.1097/AOG.0b013e31827d8fdb

Updated Citations

Altman D, Väyrynen T, Engh ME, Axelsen S, Falconer C (2011) Anterior colporrhaphy versus transvaginal mesh for pelvic-organ prolapse. N Engl J Med 364(19):1826–1836. https://doi.org/10.1056/NEJMoa1009521

Maher C, Baessler K, Glazener CMA, Adams EJ, Hagen S (2008) Surgical management of pelvic organ prolapse in women: a short version Cochrane review. Neurourol Urodyn 27(1):3–12. https://doi.org/10.1002/nau.20542

Menchen LC, Wein AJ, Smith AL (2012) An appraisal of the food and drug administration warning on urogynecologic surgical mesh. Curr Urol Rep 13(3):231–239. https://doi.org/10.1007/s11934-012-0244-2

Winters JC, Togami JM, Chermansky CJ (2012) Vaginal and abdominal reconstructive surgery for pelvic organ prolapse. In: Wein AJ, Kavoussi LR, Novick AC, Partin AW, Peters CA (eds) Campbell-Walsh urology, 10th edn. Elsevier, Philadelphia

Diagnosis and Management of Localized Prostate Cancer

17

Brett Watson, Pamela Jones, and Jason Hafron

Contents

Objectives
1. Discuss the diagnosis and incidence of localized prostate cancer.
2. Review screening and staging of prostate cancer.
3. Discuss treatment options in localized prostate cancer.

B. Watson · J. Hafron (✉)
Department of Urology, Beaumont Health, Royal Oak, MI, USA
e-mail: Jason.Hafron@beaumont.edu

P. Jones
Advanced Prostate Cancer Clinic, Michigan Institute of Urology, St Clair Shores, MI, USA
e-mail: JonesP@michiganurology.com

© Springer Nature Switzerland AG 2020
S. A. Quallich, M. J. Lajiness (eds.), *The Nurse Practitioner in Urology*,
https://doi.org/10.1007/978-3-030-45267-4_17

Definitions

The prostate gland is a small, smooth exocrine gland that surrounds the urethra. It is located inferior to the bladder and anterior to the rectum. The purpose of the prostate is to secrete seminal fluid to protect the sperm from the acidity of the vaginal tract during reproduction.

The prostate-specific antigen (PSA) test is a serum test used for screening for prostate cancer and other prostate abnormalities. PSA is a protein enzyme produced by the prostate gland to liquefy semen. PSA levels are low in men with healthy prostates.

The Gleason score (GS) is the standard grading system for prostate cancer based on pathologic tissue evaluation obtained from a prostate biopsy or prostate surgery. The tissue is graded based on the glandular structure or pattern as it appears under the microscope. The two most common patterns (the predominant one is primary) are added to obtain the Gleason score (sum).

Incidence and Epidemiology

Prostate cancer is the most common noncutaneous cancer in American men (Cooperberg et al. 2013). Approximately 1 out of 9 men will be diagnosed with prostate cancer in their lifetime. The American Cancer Society (ACS) projects that an additional 192,000 men will be diagnosed with prostate cancer each year. Second to only lung cancer, prostate cancer is a leading cause of cancer-related death in American men, with over 33,000 deaths expected in 2020. Despite its high prevalence, only 1 in 41 men die of prostate cancer (ACS 2020). The number of prostate cancer diagnoses far exceeds the mortality rate due to numerous factors including increased screening, earlier diagnosis, improvements in treatment, and the indolent nature of many prostate cancers. The risk of prostate cancer diagnosis increases with age to about 60% in men 65 and older.

The anatomy of the prostate gland is divided into three distinct zones: the peripheral, central, and transition. The peripheral zone contains 70% of the glandular tissue and is the most common site of prostate cancer. It is the region palpated during a digital rectal examination (DRE). The central zone contains the ejaculatory ducts and contributes about 25% of the glandular tissue. It is an uncommon site for prostate cancer. The transition zone contains the remaining 5% of the glandular tissue, but accounts for about 15% of prostate cancers. The transition zone is the area of the prostate from which benign prostatic hyperplasia (BPH) typically develops (Kampel 2013). Most prostate cancers are multifocal and involve multiple zones of the prostate.

Prostate cancer develops when the rates of cell division and cell death are no longer equal, leading to uncontrolled tumor growth. Following the initial transformation event, further mutations in a multitude of genes, including the tumor suppressors PTEN and p53, as well as the androgen receptor, can lead to tumor progression and metastasis. Most prostate cancers (95%) are adenocarcinomas.

History/Presentation

The majority of early prostate cancers are identified in patients who are asymptomatic, as result of the prevalent use of PSA screening and digital rectal exams. Genitourinary symptoms such as frequency, urgency, nocturia, incomplete emptying, and hesitancy are more commonly related to BPH, prostatitis, and other benign conditions; these symptoms are rarely caused by a prostate cancer with local tumor growth into the urethra or bladder. It is also common for both BPH and prostate cancer to occur simultaneously. Until otherwise proven, for older men who present with urinary symptoms, prostate cancer remains in the differential for diagnosis.

PSA screening was developed in the 1980s with use of the test increasing throughout the 1990s before declining in the past decade. PSA testing is controversial because while it is helps detect a large amount of patients with prostate cancer, many of these cancers are clinically insignificant. There is uncertainty if widespread screening and treatment of these low-grade cancers actually improves mortality rates. Various organizations have published guidelines for the use of PSA screening in prostate cancer screening. These guidelines are constantly evolving and will be discussed later in this chapter. Other biomarkers have been developed, but none are superior to PSA for the detection of prostate cancer and PSA remains a mainstay of screening for now.

Risk Factors

The cause of prostate cancer is not clearly understood. However, there are multiple risk factors associated with it. The leading risk factors are age, race, and family history. Dietary, environmental, genetic, and hormonal factors are also reported to increase the risk of prostate cancer, with varying levels of reported evidence. Age is a significant risk factor for development of prostate cancer. Autopsy studies have revealed a high prevalence of premalignant (high-grade prostatic intraepithelial neoplasia [HGPIN]) and malignant disease (mostly low grade) starting in the third and fourth decade of life and increasing steadily thereafter (Sakr and Partin 2001). Prostate adenocarcinoma prevalence significantly increases from the fifth decade onward, with a 1-in-3 chance of carrying incidental cancer in the 60- to 69-year-old age group and with 46% of 70- to 81-year-old men harboring prostate cancer (Yin et al. 2008).

The prevalence rates of prostate cancer remain significantly higher in African-American men than in white men, while the prevalence in Hispanic men is similar to that of white men. The prevalence in men of Asian origin is lower than that of whites. Although mortality rates are continuing to decline among white and African-American men, mortality rates in African-American men remain more than twice as high as in any other racial group. There are possible etiologies for the noted disparity in prostate cancer mortality. Some data reveals that African-American men tend to present with prostate cancer at a younger age, higher prostate cancer grade and more advanced in stage. Therefore, the higher mortality rate could potentially be due to more advanced disease at the time of diagnosis, i.e., stage migration (Zagars et al. 1998). The explanation for racial stage migration includes disparities in socioeconomic status leading to less access to health care and PSA screening, as well as racial differences in tumor biology, possibly attributable to dissimilarity in dietary, hormonal, or molecular factors leading to more aggressive tumors (Morton 1994; Powell 1998).

A family history of prostate cancer presents as a hereditary risk factor for this disease. Men with a family history of prostate cancer in one or more first-degree relatives have a higher risk of developing prostate cancer and are also likely to present 6–7 years earlier. Genetic studies suggest that a strong familial predisposition may be responsible for as many as 5–10% of prostate cancer cases. Several reports have suggested a shared familial risk (inherited or environmental) for prostate cancer. BRCA-2 mutations increase the risk for a more aggressive prostate cancer that develops at a younger age (ACS 2020; Taylor et al. 2019).

Physical Exam

A complete history and physical examination with a digital rectal exam (DRE) are essential in the assessment of a potential prostate cancer patient. When a DRE is performed, the technique used and the comfort of the patient are important for yielding optimal results from the exam.

In preparation of the exam, the patient should be allowed to urinate, and then properly positioned. The patient should be positioned bent over at the waist with elbows/forearms on the examining table, with the feet shoulder-width apart. The lateral decubitus position on the examining table is also a commonly used position for a DRE. The practitioner should be prepared with a pair of gloves, lubricant, and tissue for cleanup.

DRE Technique

- Lubricate examining index finger of dominant hand.
- Spread the buttocks apart to take a visual inspection of the gluteal folds, anus, and perineum.
- Tell patient to anticipate touch as gentle pressure is applied to opening of anus.
- Slowly advance finger through sphincter into the rectum.
- Begin the palpation of the prostate at the apex toward the base while including the lateral sulci with finger sweeping from side to side to examine the entire prostate.
- Upon removal of examining finger, make note of any blood.

The physical exam reveals the health status and abnormal findings that may indicate a need for further evaluation. Abnormal DRE findings, such as a firm/hard and very enlarged prostate, induration, and nodularity, are possible indications of prostate cancer (Ball et al. 2019). The findings above, in addition to DRE abnormalities that include pain, tenderness on exam, enlargement, a boggy prostate, or abnormal findings in the rectum, warrant further evaluation (see Chap. 20). Consideration and appropriate referral should also be given to discovery of swelling, enlarged lymph nodes, back pain, palpable bone pain, weakness, fatigue, or decreased appetite during the history or physical exam. These signs and symptoms could also suggest locally advanced prostate cancer or other malignancies.

Diagnostic Testing

Laboratory Studies

The recommendations for PSA screening for prostate cancer vary between organizations and have changed significantly since the test was approved by the FDA in 1986. The controversy surrounding the test stems from the fact that while the test can help detect a large amount of prostate cancers, the majority of these cancers are low risk and not clinically significant, potentially leading to overdiagnosis and overtreatment. Despite past disagreements in screening recommendations, two major organizations, the American Urologic Association (AUA) and the United States Preventative Services Task Force (USPSTF) now have very similar guidelines (AUA 2018; USPSTF 2019).

In men aged 55–69, the decision to undergo PSA testing should be an individual one, based on shared decision-making between the patient and health care provider. This discussion should include known risk factors, a discussion of the risks and benefits of screening, and the patient's own preferences. The AUA provides a shared decision making tool to help providers fulfill this standard (see Resources).

Routine screening is not recommended for men between 40 and 55 years who are at average risk. However, men at elevated risk due to race or a strong family history of lethal or metastatic cancers, can consider screening after a thorough discussion with their healthcare provider.

Screening in men younger than 40, men 70 and older, as well as men with a life expectancy of less than 10 years, is not recommended.

A PSA test may be ordered as a diagnostic tool to further evaluated urinary complaints or abnormal clinical findings on DRE. A normal PSA result should not negative further evaluation if prostate cancer is suspected. A PSA result of 2.5 ng/mL or less is considered normal, however the range of PSA levels is a continuum of risk, and prostate cancer can be present at low or normal PSA levels. In addition, younger men tend to have lower PSA levels than older men. The positive predictive value (PPV) for prostate cancer of a PSA 4–10 ng/mL is about 20–30%, and PSA >10 ng/mL has a PPV or 74% (Kampel 2013). Essentially, the higher the PSA, the higher the risk of prostate cancer.

In addition to PSA testing, there are a number of products which help to identify patients at higher risk for clinically significant prostate cancer. Select MDx and ExoDx are urine-based tests which analyze specific gene products and provide a score which indicates the risk of clinically significant prostate cancer. 4K score is a blood-based test which analyzes subtypes of PSA molecule, hk2 biomarkers, and clinical factors to provide a risk score.

Imaging Studies

Multiple imaging studies may be utilized to assist in visualizing the prostate and determining the stage of prostate cancer. The information obtained from these studies is useful when determining treatment options. Imaging studies may also be used to determine an extraprostatic spread of cancer and to evaluate clinical symptoms. The specific imaging tests and rationale for their use will be briefly discussed here.

Transrectal Ultrasound (TRUS) A type of ultrasonography commonly used in guiding prostate biopsies. The prostate is easily visualized on the TRUS and can guide placement of the biopsy needle into each region of the prostate. TRUS is also used to determine the size and volume of the prostate gland. If it is able to detect non-palpable lesions, the visualization may be helpful in the staging and diagnosis of prostate cancer.

Computed Tomography (CT) Scan The cross-sectional imaging of a CT scan may be helpful in revealing organ, bone, and soft tissue details of the abdomen and pelvis. More specifically, the CT scan can identify large or bulky diseases of the prostate, involvement of the bladder, or nodal involvement. Unless contraindicated for a specific patient, the CT scan is performed with IV contrast for enhancement of tissues and lesion detection. Typically, in patients with localized prostate cancer, CT imaging is reserved for high-risk cases (PSA >20 and/or Gleason score >8 and/or

T3 disease on DRE) to rule out metastatic disease. The CT scan may also be used for treatment planning, if a patient elects to undergo radiation therapy treatment.

Magnetic Resonance Imaging (MRI) The MRI images are produced using a magnetic field with radio frequency. An MRI is superior to a CT scan when imaging soft tissue, the prostate capsule, and the lymph nodes. Multiparametric MRI has been increasingly used to detect lesions within the prostate gland itself. Using a system called the Prostate Imaging-Reporting and Data System (PI-RADS), lesions within the prostate are able to be stratified based on risk of clinically significant cancer. The scoring ranges from PI-RADS 1 (Very low risk of clinically significant cancer) to PI-RADS 5 (Very high risk of clinically significant cancer) (Weinreb et al. 2016). A technology called MRI-fusion allows for the overlay of MRI images with live TRUS images during biopsy. This technique allows for suspicious lesions seen on MRI to be precisely targeted during biopsy.

Bone Scan This nuclear medicine imaging is used to identify disease that has spread to the bone. When prostate cancer metastasizes, the most common site of the spread is to the bone (Box 17.1). Typically, in patients with localized prostate cancer, bone scan imaging is reserved for high-risk (PSA >20 and/or Gleason score >8 and/or T3 disease on DRE) or locally advanced prostate cancer to rule out metastatic disease. Bone scans may also be ordered when a patient develops pain unrelated to the prostate gland itself.

Positron Emission Tomography (PET) PET scans use radioactive tracers to show areas of increased metabolic activity within the body. Depending on the specific tracer used, PET scans can be used to detect and localize areas of cancer cells. Several tracers are available that are targeted at detecting recurrent prostate cancer in men who previously underwent treatment. F-18 Fluciclovine (Axumin) and Gallium 68/F-18 prostate-specific membrane antigen (PSMA) are two of the more commonly used tracers (Li et al. 2018).

Box 17.1 Common Sites of Prostate Cancer Metastasis (Kampel) Sites of Spread
- Bones
- Lymph nodes
- Lung
- Liver
- CNS (Brain)

Procedures

A prostate needle biopsy is required to confirm the diagnosis of prostate cancer. It is most commonly performed with TRUS guidance and a local anesthetic in the outpatient setting, either an office or surgery center. Prior to the biopsy, enema is usually recommended. After the ultrasound probe is inserted into the rectum, the

Table 17.1 Side effects/complications of a prostate biopsy

Pain or discomfort	UTI, small risk
Hematuria	Rectal bleeding, small risk
Hematospermia	Fainting immediately following procedure (vasovagal reaction)
Urinary retention	Sepsis (rare)
Fever	

prostate is able to be visualized and a systematic biopsy, typically 12 samples, is obtained. The biopsy needle travels through the rectal wall and into the prostate. Recently, the adoption of multiparametric MRI has led to a new technique called MRI-Fusion biopsy. In this technique, computer software overlays the MRI images on the live TRUS images. This allows for the surgeon to precisely sample any suspicious lesions seen on MRI.

In 2016, Liss et al., reviewed the complications and risks related to prostate biopsy. It is important to educate patients on the side effects and the potential complications of this procedure (Table 17.1). Patients should discontinue anticoagulant therapy and nonsteroidal anti-inflammatory medications prior to the biopsy. Antibiotic therapy is required before and after the biopsy procedure. AUA recommends a fluoroquinolone or cephalosporin for prophylaxis. However, the protocol of local practices and flora should guide the choice of antibiotic therapy (Liss et al. 2016; AUA 2019). Patients should also be aware of potential complications (Table 17.1).

An alternate method of prostate biopsy, the transperineal approach, is becoming more widely adopted. The ultrasound probe is still inserted via the rectum for visualization of the prostate, but the biopsy needles are placed via the perineum. This avoids puncture of the rectal wall. Studies have shown decreased rates of sepsis with this technique (Borghesi et al. 2017).

Procedure

When the results of the biopsy are positive for prostate cancer, this pathology and histology along with the PSA, DRE, and imaging results are used to determine the grade and stage of the cancer. This information is necessary in identifying the risk of spread/metastasis. As mentioned earlier in this chapter, most prostate cancers are of adenocarcinoma histology, more specifically acinar-type adenocarcinoma.

Prostate cancer is graded by using the Gleason score or sum (GS). It is graded on a system ranging one, meaning well differentiated, up to five, meaning poorly differentiated. The higher the score, the more likely the tumor will spread. The GS correlates well with the prognosis, stage for stage, however the patient is managed (Albala et al. 2011).

The staging for prostate cancer is identified by using the American Joint Committee on Cancer (AJCC) TNM system. The T (primary tumor), N (nodes), and M (metastatic disease) are determined by clinical and/or pathologic findings. Staging helps

AJCC Prostate Cancer Prognostic Stage Groups
(8th edition, 2017)

When T is...	And N is...	And M is...	And PSA is...	And Grade Group is...	Then the stage group is...
cT1a-c, cT2a	N0	M0	<10	1	I
pT2	N0	M0	<10	1	I
cT1a-c, cT2a	N0	M0	≥10 <20	1	IIA
cT2b-c	N0	M0	<20	1	IIA
T1-2	N0	M0	<20	2	IIB
T1-2	N0	M0	<20	3	IIC
T1-2	N0	M0	<20	4	IIC
T1-2	N0	M0	≥20	1-4	IIIA
T3-4	N0	M0	Any	1-4	IIIB
Any T	N0	M0	Any	5	IIIC
Any T	N1	M0	Any	Any	IVA
Any T	Any N	M1	Any	Any	IVB

NOTE: When either PSA or Grade Group is not available, grouping should be determined by T category and/or either PSA or Grade Group as available.

Fig. 17.1 Prostate cancer staging

identify if the cancer localized, locally advanced, or spread to other areas of the body. TNM staging does not include tumor grade or PSA level.

Gleason grade group is another, simpler, way to risk stratify the patients. Based on the Gleason scores, patients are assigned a Gleason Grade Group (GG). A gleason score of 6 corresponds to GG 1. Gleason score of $3 + 4 = 7$ corresponds to GG 2. Gleason score $4 + 3 = 7$ corresponds to GG3. Gleason score 8 prostate cancer is assigned GG4. And any gleason score 9 or 10 prostate cancers are assigned GG5.

May need to add Fig. 17.1 with the Gleason scores and grade groups side by side

---

Management of Localized Prostate Cancer

Multiple management options are available for newly diagnosed patients with localized prostate cancer. Clinical and pathological characteristics at presentation are important prognostic factors that must be considered when deciding management and treatment options. These characteristics are utilized to determine the relative risk of disease progression for an individual patient upon deciding treatment. Multiple risk instruments are used for prostate cancer. For the purpose of this chapter, the D'Amico risk classification groups (1998), commonly used in the management of prostate cancer, will be illustrated here:

- Low risk: PSA ≤10 ng/mL, Gleason ≤6, and stage T1 or T2a
- Intermediate risk: PSA 10–20 ng/mL, Gleason 7, or clinical stage T2b
- High risk: PSA >20 ng/mL, Gleason 8–10, or clinical stage T2c or T3a

Management options for localized prostate cancer range from conservative to aggressive. The best treatment options should be clearly presented to each prostate cancer patient. This will require consultation with other clinical specialists, including radiation oncologists and medical oncologists. In certain cases, management of prostate cancer may involve multiple modalities of treatment.

Watchful waiting is an option in which the decision is made to forgo definitive prostate cancer treatment at the time of diagnosis. This is the most conservative option. Patients with severe health risks due to comorbidities and/or limited life expectancy are cases when this option is a consideration. This option may be without routine follow-up.

Active surveillance is another option where definitive treatment is not received at the time of diagnosis. This option is usually considered for certain low- and intermediate-risk prostate cancer patients. These patients are "actively" and carefully followed with PSA level tests, DREs, and biopsies according to clinical guidelines and protocols. These patients are treated accordingly when there are signs of progression. Although between 20 and 41% of the patients on this regimen may require treatment at 3–5 years following the diagnosis, for most patients, treatment at progression appears to be as effective as it would have been if delivered at the time of diagnosis (Cooperberg et al. 2013).

For patients considering active surveillance, or already on active surveillance protocols, there are several molecular tests that can help guide treatment decisions. Oncotype Dx, Prolaris, and Decipher are genetic tests that are performed on the prostate cancer tissue after biopsy. These tests can help determine the aggressiveness of the cancer and how likely it is to progress or metastasize. Depending on the results, patients may choose more or less aggressive treatment options.

Radiation therapy (RT) is an outpatient option for definitive treatment for prostate cancer. Like surgery, radiation therapy has multiple techniques and has advanced over the years. Radiotherapy is a commonly used modality for localized prostate cancer. Each radiation modality has a clinical indication for use. Complications and side effects are a result of the toxic effects of radiation on normal tissue within the treatment field. Acute toxic effects of radiation typically occur after 2–3 weeks of starting the treatment course, but can occur even sooner. Late effects of radiation occur at least 3 months after treatment is completed. These delayed effects can presents years or even decades after the treatment course.

External beam radiotherapy (EBRT) is the least invasive form of radiation for prostate cancer treatment. It is indicated for low-, intermediate-, and high-risk groups (Hansen and Roach 2007). EBRT is delivered via X-rays using photon and more recently proton energies. Improved treatment planning and imaging involves three-dimensional conformal radiotherapy (3DCRT) and intensity-modulated radiation therapy. These techniques have allowed for improvement in targeting and shaping volumes, which permits higher doses to be delivered to the prostate, while sparing the surrounding tissues, with the goal of decreasing acute and late toxicity. Hyperfractionation is delivered in more fractions (treatments) with a lower dose per fraction. Hypofractionation is delivered in fewer fractions with a higher dose per fraction. EBRT usually begins 1 week after an hour planning session (simulation). It is delivered in daily fractions 5 days per week up to approximately 9 weeks depending on the prescribed dose or whether it is hyperfractionated versus hypofractionated.

Brachytherapy is an interstitial radiation therapy technique where radioactive seeds are implanted directly into the prostate, with TRUS guidance. The radioactive seeds are deposited into the tissues using a mechanical device preloaded with tiny catheters/tubes. Patients are not radioactive at completion of brachytherapy treatment. There are low-dose-rate (LDR) and high-dose-rate (HDR) brachytherapy techniques. The HDR technique will be the focus in this section. This is a minimally invasive treatment requiring spinal anesthesia and a potential overnight stay in the hospital. HDR brachytherapy alone (monotherapy) or in combination with EBRT are the two forms of brachytherapy commonly used. HDR alone is indicated for low- and intermediate-risk groups. It can be delivered in two implants a week apart with two fractions/treatments each or as one implant with two fractions. Single-fraction HDR brachytherapy is being studied currently.

Combined HDR/EBRT is indicated for intermediate- and high-risk groups. The HDR dose per fraction is less than in monotherapy. Patients receiving this modality undergo two implants 1 week apart, each with two HDR treatments, along with a 4–5 week course of EBRT (Table 17.2).

Table 17.2 Radiation therapy modalities with acute/late toxicities

Modality	Acute toxicities	Late toxicities
EBRT	Frequency, nocturia, urgency, dysuria, frequency BMs, diarrhea, rectal urgency and irritation, urinary retention (rare), fatigue	Dysuria, frequency, urgency, hematuria d/t RT cystitis, urethral stricture, diarrhea, rectal urgency, rectal bleeding, d/t proctitis, gradual ED (>30%) at 5 years
Brachytherapy/ HDR	Frequency, urgency, dysuria, urinary retention, diarrhea, rectal frequency, urgency, and spasms; perineal hematoma	Urethral stricture, retention, incontinence, cystitis, proctitis, ED (40%) 5 years
Combined EBRT/HDR	No significant changes as toxicities are similar to those of single modality	No significant changes as toxicities are similar to those of single modality

Surgery

Surgery for prostate cancer involves the removal of the entire prostate gland and the seminal vesicles. The pelvic lymph nodes will only be removed if the preoperative risk of lymphatic spread is high enough to warrant surgical resection. Preoperative risk is based on preoperative nomograms or published risk tables. The goals of surgical resection are to removal all of the prostate cancer while limiting damage to the urethral sphincter (preserves urinary continence) and the cavernous nerves (preserves erectile function). The decision for surgery is based on the patient's overall life expectancy, comorbidities, prostate cancer risk, and previous surgical history. Generally, surgery is reserved for men under 70 years of age and in overall good health. The current techniques to remove the prostate include open radical retropubic prostatectomy, laparoscopic radical prostatectomy, robotic-assisted laparoscopic radical prostatectomy, and radical perineal prostatectomy. The decision to utilize any of these techniques is based on the patients' body habitus, surgical history, and the surgeons' experience.

Open radical retropubic prostatectomy is the traditional method for removal of the prostate gland. The procedure is performed through a mid-line infraumbilical incision under general or spinal anesthesia. The procedure commonly takes 3–4 h and requires 1–2 day hospitalization. Patients will have a Foley catheter in their bladders for 7–14 days. Common side effects of the procedure include urinary incontinence, erectile dysfunction, and bleeding.

Robotic-assisted laparoscopic radical prostatectomy is a minimally invasive approach performed through small incisions, with the surgeon in the room controlling arms on a surgical robot to perform the procedure. Robotic surgery affords the surgeon outstanding surgical vision and more precise movements within the body. Patients have less abdominal trauma due to smaller incisions and most will have less pain compared with open surgery. Additionally, blood loss is less with robotic surgery. Patients require general anesthesia and the surgery typically takes 3–4 h. Most remain in the hospital for one night and require a Foley catheter for approximately 1 week. The vast majority of prostatectomies in the US are performed with this technique. Side effects may include urinary incontinence, erectile dysfunction, and urethral strictures.

Laparoscopic radical prostatectomy is a minimally invasive technique that preceded the robotic-assisted prostatectomy. The approach and surgical steps are essentially the same, but without the robotic interface between the patient and surgeon. This surgery has largely been replaced by the robotic prostatectomy, and is not commonly performed in the US. The outcomes and side effects are similar to the robotic-assisted laparoscopic radical prostatectomy.

Radical perineal prostatectomy involves removal of the prostate through an incision made through the perineum. The recovery time after this surgery may be shorter than with the open radical retropubic approach. Outcomes and side effects are similar to other approaches, with the exception of preservation of erectile function. The maintenance of erectile function following perineal prostatectomy is limited.

Cryosurgery involves the freezing of the entire prostate gland (or sometimes just the focal areas) to temperatures which are lethal to cancer cells. The procedure is typically performed using small probes that are placed under transrectal ultrasound guidance through the perineum into the prostate. During treatment, the surgeon can monitor the ice ball to ensure it encompasses the entire prostate. Common side effects include urinary symptoms, hematuria, erectile dysfunction, and (rarely) rectal injuries.

High-Intensity Focused Ultrasound (HIFU) is another technique for treatment of localized prostate cancer. HIFU utilizes a rectal ultrasound probe to generate high frequency ultrasound waves, which induce destruction of cancer cells while sparing the surrounding structures (Chaussy 2017). It should be noted that neither cryosurgery or HIFU are currently considered standard care options by the AUA.

Follow-up for all procedures requires scheduled PSA testing generally every 6 months. Following surgery it is expected for the PSA to return to zero. If the PSA does not return to zero or rises above zero, unresected or recurrent prostate cancer should be suspected. However, following radiation or cryosurgery, the PSA will reach a nadir that is above zero. In these patients, significant rises from the PSA nadir indicate recurrent prostate cancer. Usually, the urologist will obtain imaging with a bone scan, CT scan, or PET scan, as well as consider a prostate biopsy to determine the location of the recurrent prostate cancer.

Additionally, the patients return of erectile function and continence is closely monitored following any treatment. If a patient was potent prior to surgery and underwent a nerve-sparing surgical procedure, penile rehabilitation programs are helpful. Typically, these programs encourage sexual activity with the use of pharmacotherapy and therapeutic devices. Frequently, patients will be placed on a scheduled dose of phosphodiesterase inhibitor. Lastly, patients are encouraged to perform Kegel exercises and often are referred for pelvic floor physical therapy if available to help restore urinary continence. Patient support and encouragement are critical, especially during the early stages of recovery. If potency and continence fail to return after an adequate trial of the techniques listed above, there are surgical procedures that can be offered.

Clinical Pearls
1. The use of an antibiotic prior to removal of a catheter following prostatectomy maybe helpful.
2. Handouts on what to expect during and after the surgery help alleviate anxiety. Include
   (a) Length of surgery
   (b) Length of hospitalization
   (c) Catheter removal date
   (d) Follow-up date
   (e) Medications that will be prescribed routinely post-op (pd5 inhibitors)
   (f) Kegel exercises how and when to do

Resources for the Nurse Practitioner

Clinically Localized Prostate Cancer: AUA/ASTRO/SUO Guideline (2017) https://
www.auanet.org/guidelines/prostate-cancer-clinically-localized-guideline
    http://urologyhealth.org//Documents/Product%20Store/Prostate-Cancer-
Screening-Checklist-Foundation-English.pdf
    Memorial Sloan Kettering Prostate Cancer Nomograms https://www.mskcc.org/
nomograms/prostate

Resources for the Patient

ustoo.org. A nonprofit organization established in 1990 that serves as a resource of
volunteers, with peer-to-peer support and educational materials to help men and
their families/caregivers make informed decisions about prostate cancer detection,
treatment options, and related side effects.
    cancer.org. The official website of the American Cancer Society. The website
contains information and resources for patients and families with prostate cancer.
    http://www.urologyhealth.org/Documents/Product%20Store/Localized-
Prostate-Cancer.pdf
    Shared Decision Making Tool: https://www.urologyhealth.org/educational-
materials/is-prostate-cancer-screening-right-for-me

References

Albala DM, Morey AF, Gomella LG, Stein JP (2011) Oxford American handbook of urology.
    Oxford University Press, New York, pp 190–221. Print
American Cancer Society (2020) Cancer facts & figures for prostate cancer. American Cancer
    Society, Atlanta. Web
American Urological Association (2018) Clinical guideline on early detection of prostate cancer.
    American Urological Association Education and Research, Linthicum
American Urological Association (2019) Best practice statement. Urologic procedures and anti-
    microbial prophylaxis. American Urological Association Education and Research, Linthicum
Ball JW et al (2019) Seidel's guide to physical examination: an interprofessional approach, 9th
    edn. Elsevier, St Louis, pp 507–522. Print
Borghesi et al (2017) Complications after systematic, random, and image-guided prostate biopsy.
    Eur Urol 71(3):353–365
Chaussy CG (2017) High-intensity focused ultrasound for the treatment of prostate cancer: a
    review. J Endourol 31(S1):S30–S37
Cooperberg MR et al (2013) Neoplasms of the prostate gland. In: McAninch JW, Lue TF (eds)
    Smith & Tanagho's general urology, 18th edn. McGraw-Hill Co., New York, pp 357–370
D'Amico AV et al (1998) Biochemical outcome after radical prostatectomy, external beam radia-
    tion therapy, or interstitial radiation therapy for clinically localized prostate cancer. JAMA
    280(1998):969–974. Web
Hansen EK, Roach M (2007) Handbook of evidence-based radiation oncology. Springer,
    New York, pp 293–311. Print

Kampel LJ (2013) Dx/Rx: prostate cancer, 2nd edn. Jones & Bartlett Learning, Burlington, pp 3–134. Print

Li R, Ravizzini GC, Gorin MA et al (2018) The use of PET/CT in prostate cancer. Prostate Cancer Prostatic Dis 21:4–21

Liss MA et al (2016) AUA white paper. The prevention and treatment of the more common complications related to prostate biopsy update. American Urological Association, Linthicum

Morton RA (1994) Racial differences in adenocarcinoma of the prostate in North American men. Urology 44:637–645. Print

Powell IJ (1998) Prostate cancer in the African American: is this a different disease? Semin Urol Oncol 16:221–226. Print

Sakr W, Partin AW (2001) Histological markers of risk and the role of high-grade prostatic intraepithelial neoplasia. Urology 57(1):115–120. Print

Taylor RA, Fraser M, Rebello RJ et al (2019) The influence of BRCA2 mutation on localized prostate cancer. Nat Rev Urol 16:281–290. Web

USPSTF (2019) Final update summary: prostate cancer: screening. U.S. Preventive Services Task Force, Rockvile. web

Weinreb JC, Barentsz JO, Choyke PL et al (2016) PI-RADS prostate imaging—reporting and data system: 2015, version 2. Eur Urol 69(1):16–40

Yin MI, Bastacky S, Chandran U, Becich MJ, Dhir R (2008) Prevalence of incidental prostate cancer in the general population: a study of healthy organ donors. J Urol 179(3):892–895. Web

Zagars GK, Pollack A, Pettaway CA (1998) Prostate cancer in African-American men: outcome following radiation therapy with or without adjuvant androgen ablation. Int J Radiat Oncol Biol Phys 42(5):17–523. Print

Bladder and Urothelial Cancer

18

Anne Lizardi-Calvaresi, Staci Mitchell, and Julie Derossett

Contents

A. Lizardi-Calvaresi (✉)
Department of Urology, Thomas Jefferson University, Philadelphia, PA, USA
e-mail: Anne.Calvaresi@jefferson.edu

S. Mitchell
Department of Urology, University of Michigan Health System, Ann Arbor, MI, USA
e-mail: stacilin@med.umich.edu

J. Derossett
Division of Cancer Center Urology, Department of Urology, University of Michigan Health System, Ann Arbor, MI, USA

Objectives

1. Explain the diagnosis, assessment, and management of urothelial carcinoma.
2. Identify the incidence, risk factors, and signs and symptoms associated with cancer of the bladder, ureters, and urethra
3. Discuss the pathology, staging, diagnostic evaluation of urothelial carcinoma
4. Review management of urothelial carcinoma

Overview

Urothelial Carcinoma is defined as the abnormal division of cells within the layers of tissue or urothelium of the renal pelvis, bladder, ureters, and the urethra. Cancer of the bladder, ureters, and urethra most commonly are missed diagnosed as urinary tract infections or nephrolithiasis. Patients are given multiple courses of antibiotics and/or pain medication without resolution of their symptoms. Diagnosis and management of the disease is delayed, with risk of disease progression.

Incidence

Bladder Cancer

In 2019, there were approximately 80,000 new cases of bladder cancer and an estimated 17,600 people who died from this disease (Surveillance, Epidemiology, and End Results [SEER] 2020). Bladder cancer represents 4.5% of all new cases in the United Sates. In 2016, there were an estimated 699,450 people living with bladder cancer in the United States. It is the second most common urologic cancer and has the highest recurrence rate of any cancer. With advancing age, bladder cancer is more common and is more common in men than women with a median age at diagnosis of before 73. Bladder cancer is most frequently diagnosed among people aged 75–84, with the highest mortality among this group as well.

When comparing race, more Caucasian Americans are diagnosed with bladder cancer than African Americans, and more Asian Americans than American Indians and Hispanic Americans. There are a higher percentage of caucasian men (38.5%) than African American men (19.7%) diagnosed with bladder cancer in the United States. There is a higher incidence of bladder cancer in caucasian women (9.5%) than in African American women (6.6%).

Bladder cancer is the sixth leading cause of cancer death in the United States. There are 3.2% deaths in people ranging in age from 45 to 54, 11.4% in people aged 55–64, 21.9% in people aged 65–74, 31.9% in people between the ages of 75–84, and 31.0% in people over the age of 80 (SEER 2020). The median age at death is 79. The percentage of people diagnosed with bladder cancer surviving 5 years in 2016 was 78.3%. This 5-year relative survival rate has increased over the last 30 years. In 1975, the percentage of people diagnosed with bladder cancer surviving 5 years was 71.5% compared to 80.6% in 2006. The 5-year survival rate also depends upon the cancer stage or extent of disease at the time of diagnosis. The highest 5-year survival rates are those diagnosed with cancer in the originating layer of cells of the bladder or in situ (95.8%) as compared to localized bladder cancer, confined to the primary site (69.5%). When bladder cancer spreads outside of the bladder to the regional lymph nodes, the 5-year survival rate decreases to 36.3% and dramatically decreases to 4.6% when the cancer is staged at distant or has metastasized to other organs.

Upper Tract Urothelial Cancer

The incidence of cancer within the upper tracts (renal pelvis and ureter) is much lower, is more common in people older than 65, and accounts for less than 5% of all cancers of the kidney and upper urinary tract. According to cancer surveillance reports published from the American Cancer Society (Cancer Statistics 2019), there were an estimated 3000 people diagnosed with ureteral cancer in 2019 in the United States, and 2600 were male compared to 1300 female (Cancer Statistics 2019).

The most common type of cancer that originates within the kidney in adults is renal cell carcinoma (RCC) (85%). Upper tract urothelial carcinoma (UTUC) is the most common type of cancer of the renal pelvis and ureter. The prognosis of upper tract cancer is directly related to the stage at diagnosis. The recurrence of bladder cancer after treatment for renal pelvis or ureteral cancer occurs in 15–50% of cases (Azemar et al. 2011).

Urethral Cancer

Primary urethral cancer is extremely rare, with fewer than 2000 cases reported, and less than 1% of the total incidence of malignancies. (Guidos 2018). At the time of diagnosis, the disease is usually advanced, making it difficult to distinguish between primary urethral cancer and locally advanced urothelial carcinoma of the bladder.

African Americans are twice as likely than Caucasians to develop primary urethral carcinoma. The SEER database reports that the majority of primary urethral cancers (55–77.6%) are urothelial carcinoma. Other histology types reported include squamous cell carcinoma (11.9–21.5%), adenocarcinoma (5–16.4%), and rare cases of melanoma. The incidence of urethral cancer increases with age, with the majority of cases diagnosed at age 75 or older. (Swartz et al. 2006).

Pertinent Anatomy and Physiology

The wall of the bladder has four main layers. The innermost lining is comprised of cells called urothelial or transitional cells, known as urothelium or transitional epithelium. Beneath the urothelium is a thin layer of connective tissue, blood vessels, and nerves, the lamina propria. The next layer is the muscle of the bladder, the muscularis propria. Outside of this muscle is a layer of fatty connective tissue that separates the bladder from other organs.

The types of bladder cancer are identified by the layers, or cells, in which the cancer originates and the depth of invasion. Urothelial carcinoma (UC) is the most common type of bladder cancer and originates in the innermost lining of the bladder. UC has the appearance of urothelial cells that line the inside of the bladder; urothelial cells also line the renal pelvis, ureters and urethra, meaning UC can occur at any site along the ureter or renal pelvis. Urothelial cell carcinoma is classified further based on depth of invasion and subtype (Table 18.1).

Table 18.1 Classification of bladder cancer

Type	Description	
Urothelial carcinoma (UC)	Most common type of bladder cancer Originates in the innermost lining of bladder; urothelial cells line the renal pelvis, ureters, and urethra; UC can also occur in these organs.	*Noninvasive:* remained in the inner lining (transitional epithelium). *Invasive:* grown into lamina propria, or into muscularis propria *Superficial or nonmuscle-invasive*: describe noninvasive tumors as well as invasive tumors that have grown into the lamina propria but not the muscularis propria. *Papillary carcinoma*: grow in stalk-like formations toward center of the bladder. Appear to resemble stalks of cauliflower, but do not extend into the deeper layers. Called noninvasive papillary carcinoma. *Papillary urothelial neoplasm of low malignant potential (PUNLUMP)*: very low grade and noninvasive; appear at lateral posterior wall of the bladder and ureteric orifices. Rarely associated with invasion or metastasis and have a good prognosis. *Flat Carcinomas:* do not grow toward the center of bladder and remain in the inner layer. Also called noninvasive flat carcinoma or flat carcinoma in situ (CIS).
Squamous cell carcinoma (SCC)	1–2% of bladder cancers are squamous cell carcinoma and nearly all are invasive Associated with squamous metaplasia May occur at multiple areas of the bladder; most commonly found at lateral wall and trigone On cystoscopy, the tumor appears nodular and has a plaque like, irregular surface Most of the tumors are large, exophytic, and necrotic and bulge into the bladder cavity Having bladder diverticula may increase likelihood of developing SCC	

Table 18.1 (continued)

Type	Description
Adenocarcinoma	Rare Accounts for 0.5–2% of all bladder cancers Higher rate of extravesical disease as compared to urothelial carcinoma Tumor often appears as a solitary lesion, has a tendency for local invasion, and the symptoms appear late
Small cell carcinoma	Aggressive, poorly differentiated neuroendocrine neoplasm similar to small cell carcinoma of the lung Rare, accounting for <500 new cases annually Can involve any area of the bladder; most common sites are lateral wall and bladder dome
Sarcoma	Malignant mesenchymal tumor that is rare 50% of bladder sarcomas are leiomyosarcomas, and ~20% are rhabdomyosarcomas May be present in any region of the bladder, but most commonly identified in the trigone or fundus
Carcinosarcoma and sarcomatoid carcinoma	Rare and highly aggressive Sarcomatoid cracinomas of the bladder are primarily spindle cell tumors with epithelial differentiation, most commonly urothelial
Lymphoepithelioma-like carcinoma	Rare epithelial tumor characterized by lymphoid infiltrate suggestive of lymphoma Typically muscle-invasive at time of diagnosis Appears to have a better prognosis than other primary bladder cancers

Nonurothelial bladder cancers are rare and more aggressive than UC. Presenting symptoms of nonurothelial bladder cancer appear late, and tend to indicate an invasive and more advanced diagnosis, with a poor prognosis. Nonurothelial bladder cancers are further classified as epithelial or nonepithelial. According to Hayes and Gilligan (2014), approximately 90% of these cancers are epithelial in origin, including squamous cell carcinomas (SCCs), adenocarcinomas, and small cell (neuroendocrine) tumors. Nonepithelial cancers are rare and include sarcomas, carcinosarcomas, sarcomatoid cancers, paragangliomas, pheochromocytomas, primary bladder melanomas, and lymphomas. Melanoma and lymphoma are the most common cancers that metastasize to the bladder. Cancer from the colon, rectum, prostate, or uterus can extend directly into the bladder.

Risk Factors

Urothelial carcinoma is associated with several risk factors: smoking, environmental/chemical exposures, and chronic urinary tract infections. Smoking is the primary risk factor, and former smokers are twice as likely to develop bladder cancer as those who never smoked, while current smokers are four times more likely to develop transitional cell kidney and ureter cancer as nonsmokers (National Institutes of Health [NIH] 2014).

Workplace exposure is associated with an increased risk as well. Industrial chemicals such as aromatic amines, benzidine, and beta-naphthylamine along with rubber, leather, textiles, and paint products have been linked to urothelial carcinoma. Hairdressers, painters, machinists, printers, truck drivers (diesel fumes), and firefighters (chemical/foam fire retardants) are at risk due to exposure to chemicals on the job. Urothelial carcinoma is also commonly identified in populations living near factories, chemical plants, and highly industrialized areas. Chronic overuse of analgesic medications (analgesic nephropathy) has also been associated with upper tract urothelial carcinoma.

Chronic urinary tract irritants such as bacterial infections, foreign bodies (recurrent bladder calculi, catheters), and chronic outlet obstruction have been associated with a higher incidence of developing urothelial carcinoma. Use of chronic indwelling catheters in patients with spinal cord injury has been associated with urothelial malignancies. A population-based retrospective analysis of spinal cord injured patients conducted by West et al. (1999) concluded that squamous cell carcinoma was more common in spinal cord injured patients with indwelling urethral catheters and suprapubic catheters (42%) than those using clean intermittent catheterization, condom catheterization, or spontaneous voiding (19%).

Additional studies have cited other etiologies specifically identified for cancer of the urethra. Wiener et al. (1992) demonstrated HPV DNA in 4 (29%) of 14 cases of primary urethral cancer. Kaplan et al. (1967) found that 37% of males with urethral cancer had some history of venereal disease.

Specific Risk Factors to Assess:
- Smoking: assess type of tobacco used: cigarette, cigar, E-cigarettes, chewing tobacco, snuff, number of years smoked, number of packs per day, and date of cessation for former smokers.
- Chemicals in the workplace: assess for environmental exposures of current and former places of residence; people that live in highly industrialized areas have a higher risk.
- People who have had bladder cancer have a greater risk for getting the disease again.
- Family history of lynch syndrome
- Bladder cancer is more common in people aged 55 and older.
- Bladder cancer is more common in men than women.
- Life-long bladder irritation and infections: people who have had multiple bladder infections are at greater risk for bladder cancer. This includes a history of urinary retention requiring an indwelling catheter or the need for intermittent self-catheterization.
- Low fluid intake may add to the risk.
- Arsenic is a poison that raises the risk of bladder cancer. In some parts of the world, arsenic may be found at high levels in drinking water; the chance of exposure in the US depends on location and whether water is from a well or a sanitation system.

History

A complete and thorough history is crucial in the diagnosis of urothelial carcinoma. Identifying risk factors and assessment of signs and symptoms will be helpful in guiding diagnostic evaluation and the evaluation of differential diagnosis.

Medical History: A complete medical history is necessary to evaluate for prescribing medications, diagnostic testing, and treatment planning. Especially important to note, is any previous radiation to the abdomen and pelvis.

Surgical History: A history of previous procedures and/or surgeries, especially of the urinary system and to the abdomen and pelvis will help in treatment planning.

Medication History: A thorough medication history is necessary to evaluate for drug interactions and contributes to a differential diagnosis. Note use of anticoagulation medications, nicotine gum/patch, testosterone replacement in men, and previous antibiotic use.

Allergies: Especially important is noting allergies to antibiotics and IV contrast.

Social History: A complete social history should include: alcohol use (amount and type), illicit drug use (amount and type), support system, and home environment. Baseline sexual function is also important to note.

Clinical Presentation: The assessment of each symptom should include: duration, frequency, severity, intermittent or chronic, and treatments utilized. Urothelial carcinoma can mimic other conditions (Table 18.2).

Table 18.2 Symptom assessment

Signs and symptoms that can be associated with urothelial carcinoma	Signs and symptoms that can be associated with urothelial carcinoma *of the urethra*	Symptoms of advanced (metastatic) disease

• Fever, chills, sweats, nausea/vomiting
• Gross hematuria (visible blood in the urine): most common sign; usually painless and should never be ignored
• Clots and/or tissue within the urine.
• Microscopic hematuria
• Lower urinary tract symptoms (LUTS): frequency, urgency, nocturia, and dysuria (pain or burning)
• Incomplete emptying of the bladder.
• Urinary Incontinence
• Back/flank pain (upper tract carcinoma)
• Abdominal/pelvic pain
• Urethral discharge
	• Diminished stream, straining to void
	• Frequency, nocturia, itching, dysuria (most commonly reported with carcinoma in situ)
	• Urinary retention from progressive urethral stricture disease
	• Hematuria, urethral or vaginal spotting
	• Purulent, foul-smelling, or watery discharge
	• Hematospermia
	• Perineal, suprapubic, or urethral pain
	• Dyspareunia
	• Swelling
	• Tenesmus
	• Priapism
	• No symptoms except for findings on physical exam including hard nodule in the perineum, labia, or along the shaft of the penis.
		• Unexplained weight loss
		• Loss of appetite
		• Fatigue
		• New skeletal pain
		  – Chest pain/shortness of breath
		  – Cachexia

Box 18.1 Clues on physical examination

Abnormal physical exam findings that may be associated with bladder cancer and/or metastatic disease:

Unintentional weight loss, especially over a short period of time. Changes of cognition, mood, affect. Palpable enlarged cervical, supraclavicular lymph nodes, and/or inguinal lymph nodes. Pain with direct palpation of vertebral bodies, bilateral ribs, pelvis, bilateral hips, and thighs. Palpable abdominal mass.	Palpable pelvic/rectal fullness/mass Palpable urethral mass: men and women Lower extremity edema: Can be an indicator of deep vein thrombosis (DVT). Unilateral edema can be an indicator of metastatic disease. Declining performance status, especially a rapid decline. *Men:* palpable prostatic nodules (possible prostate cancer), scrotal/testis mass.

Physical Examination

A complete head to toe physical examination should be performed. Abdominal exam should focus on any potential enlargement of spleen or liver, masses and tenderness with direct palpation, and/or suprapubic pain. Females need a pelvic and rectal exam to assess for mass and fullness. Males need a complete genitourinary exam including penis, meatus, scrotum, testis, epididymis, and rectal exam including prostate to assess for nodules and mass/fullness of rectal wall. Both men and women should have palpation for lateral inguinal lymph nodes and direct palpation of sites of skeletal pain.

Baseline performance status may also be assessed, with a tool such as the Eastern Cooperative Oncology Group (ECOG) performance status measure (Oken et al. 1982). These will help to assess how a patient's disease progression, assess how the disease affects the daily living abilities of the patient, and determine appropriate treatment and prognosis (Box 18.1).

Diagnosis

There are alternative diagnoses that can mimic bladder cancer (Box 18.2). Gross or microscopic hematuria are often treated like a urinary tract infection or nephrolithiasis; multiple courses of antibiotics or pain medications may have been prescribed without a full evaluation for urothelial carcinoma. Never assume hematuria is a urinary tract infection.

Urothelial Carcinoma of the Upper Tracts: Urothelial carcinoma of the renal pelvis and ureters is the most common type of cancer that affects the upper tracts.

Box 18.2 Diagnoses that can mimic urothelial carcinoma

Urinary tract infection (UTI)
Nephrolithiasis
Hemorrhagic cystitis: noninfectious (history of radiation to the pelvis)
Renal cell carcinoma
Overactive bladder
Benign stricture disease (bladder outlet obstruction, overflow incontinence)
Benign prostatic hypertrophy (BPH) in men
Gynecologic causes in women
Urethral trauma
Anticoagulation medication

Approximately 10% are squamous cell carcinomas. A primary tumor within the bladder can involve the ureteral orifice and extend into the ureter.

After definitive treatment of carcinoma within the bladder, there is a high recurrence rate of urothelial carcinoma within the upper tracts. About 30–50% of patients with cancer of the upper tracts have or will have bladder cancer.

Urothelial Carcinoma of the Urethra: Urethral carcinoma is characterized by unique anatomic and histologic differences between males and females. The average male urethra is 21 cm and divided into anterior and posterior components. The shorter female urethra is approximately 4 cm with less complex anatomy. In both men and women, the histologic pattern of the urethral mucosa progresses from transitional epithelium to squamous epithelium as it continues distally. The mucosal cells of the urethra are replaced at a rapid rate which can lead to dysplasia and neoplasia; these mucosal cells histologically classify urethral cancer as TCC or adenocarcinoma secondary to metaplasia (Guidos et al. 2018). Inflammation, infection, and irritation may also impede the natural DNA repair mechanisms of the urethral mucosal cells (Guidos et al. 2018).

The most common sites of tumor invasion in females are the labia, vagina, and bladder neck. In males, the most common sites of extension are the vascular spaces of the corpora and periurethral tissues, deep tissues of the perineum, urogenital diaphragm, prostate, and the penile and scrotal skin, where it can cause abscesses and fistula (Guidos et al. 2018). Urethral tumors usually invade locally and extend into adjacent soft tissues. At time of diagnosis, the tumors are often locally advanced and are associated with a poor prognosis.

Staging of Urothelial Carcinoma

Management of Urothelial Carcinoma is dependent upon the stage and grade of the cancer. Staging is based on the 2016 American Joint Committee on Cancer (AJCC) TNM guidelines. The "T" stage refers to clinical staging only, based on the results of diagnostic testing. The "p" stage is determined by the pathologic examination of the tissues *after* the removal of the bladder, ureter, or urethra. For example: Ta is the clinical stage of noninvasive papillary carcinoma and pTa is the pathologic stage of noninvasive papillary carcinoma.

Diagnostic Testing

Laboratory Evaluation

Comprehensive blood panel: Assesses for electrolyte imbalances, liver function, and most important baseline renal function: creatinine, BUN, and glomerular filtration rate (GFR). Evaluating baseline renal function is necessary to determine if it is appropriate for the patient to receive intravenous contrast with imaging. Patients should *not* receive IV contrast with CT scans if creatinine is 2.0 mg/dL or higher.

Complete blood count with platelets and differential: Assesses for an elevated white blood cell count (WBC) to evaluate for possible infection, baseline hemoglobin, and hematocrit.

Coagulation studies (PT, PTT, INR): Assesses the potential for bleeding disorders, baseline INR (especially if on anticoagulation medications).

Urinalysis: Always send a urine specimen to the lab for a macroscopic and a microscopic analysis. A macroscopic urinalysis will identify the presence of bacteria and red blood cells (RBC). Never rely on an office urinalysis; this can only give preliminary data on the presence of nitrates and/or blood, while a complete laboratory evaluation is important to evaluate for differential diagnosis.

Urine culture and sensitivity: Sending the urine for a culture and sensitivity despite the results of the macro and microscopic urinalysis is a prudent choice, especially if the patient is symptomatic. The culture will identify the type of bacteria present, and sensitivities will identify the appropriate antibiotic to treat the bacteria present in the sample.

Urine cytology: A urine cytology is the most valuable and reliable urine test to detect bladder cancer. A voided urine sample is sent for a laboratory evaluation to determine the presence of cancer cells. The results can be negative, positive, or atypical; atypical urine cytology does not necessarily confirm or deny the presence of cancer cells. Further evaluation based on risk factors and signs and symptoms is recommended. Urine cytology is most helpful in diagnosing high-grade tumors and carcinoma in situ (CIS). Low-grade noninvasive tumors may be missed by routine cytologic analysis. Urine cytology is also used for surveillance after the initial treatment of bladder cancer to detect a recurrence.

FISH (UroVysion Fluorescence in situ hybridization): This is a urine-based genetic test for the diagnosis and surveillance of bladder cancer. This method detects genetic alterations of the urothelial cells found in the urine, using fluorescent DNA probes binding to the regions of chromosomes 3, 7, and 17 as well as on the 9p21. (Riesz et al. 2007). A positive test result will identify the amount of positive cells present in the sample.

Diagnostic Studies

Because the presentation of UC is extremely variable and staging plays a vital part in planning treatment, a wide variety of diagnostics may be used (Table 18.3). An ultrasound post-void residual (PVR) is a noninvasive and time-efficient test that can be completed in the office. Immediately after a voluntary void, the patient's bladder is scanned with a portable ultrasound bladder scanner. The amount of residual urine left in the bladder is measured.

Hydronephrosis or incomplete emptying of the kidneys, can be identified on CT scan, MRI or renal US, and is an indicator of obstructed urine flow from the kidneys through the ureters to the bladder. This is a significant finding and can indicate tumors within the ureters, at either of the ureteral orifice, excessive tumor burden within the bladder, and/or metastatic disease.

Table 18.3 Imaging studies to evaluate UC

Study	Discussion
Ultrasound	Abdominal or renal ultrasound is an appropriate initial test to evaluate abdominal/flank pain, nausea/vomiting, and hematuria.
Chest Imaging (X-ray and chest CT)	Baseline chest X-ray including anterior, posterior, and lateral views, is helpful in evaluating for pulmonary and cardiac disease, and nodules or mass.
	Pulmonary nodule protocol chest CT may be considered to further evaluate areas of concern present on X-ray and/or concern for metastatic disease.
Computerized Tomography (CT) Urogram	***Should always be considered in cases of hematuria***
	Evaluate for any allergies to IV contrast.
	Specialized CT scan that fully evaluates the upper urinary tracts (kidneys and ureters) and the bladder; typically includes abdomen and pelvis.
	Helps to identify tumors present within the urinary system, other organs, and within the abdomen and pelvis.
	Lymphadenopathy (size, location, and number of enlarged lymph nodes) is also assessed.
	Bladder wall thickness can also be identified and measured; this is associated with the presence of a bladder wall tumor.
Stone protocol CT scan	Evaluates renal calculi as a potential source of pain/hematuria
	Usually done without contrast.
Intravenous Pyelogram (IVP)	X-ray test that provides pictures of the kidneys, bladder, ureters, and urethra.
	Evaluate for any allergies to IV contrast.
	Shows size, shape, and position of the urinary tract, and collecting system within the kidneys.
	Intravenous contrast is injected, and a series of X-ray pictures are taken at timed intervals.
	Identifies diseases of the urinary tract, such as kidney stones, tumors, or infection.
	Identifies congenital urinary tract defects.

(continued)

Table 18.3 (continued)

Study	Discussion
Retrograde Pyelogram	Type of X-ray that allows visualization of the bladder, ureters, and renal pelvis.
	A catheter is inserted through the urethra and up into the bladder and/or ureters; contrast is injected through the catheter to opacify the lining of the urinary system.
	Identifies filling defects (e.g., stones or tumors).
	Option when an intravenous excretory study (IVP or contrast CT scan) cannot be done because of renal disease or allergy to intravenous contrast.
	Relative contraindications include the presence of infected urine, pregnancy, and contrast allergy.
MRI (Magnetic Resonance Imaging)	Sensitive test to detect the presence of metastatic disease.
	MRI urogram is similar to a CT urogram: fully evaluates upper tracts and the bladder.
	May not be appropriate for patients with metal implants, pacemakers/defibrillators, and significant claustrophobia.
Bone Scan (whole body)	Crucial diagnostic test to evaluate for concerns of metastatic disease to the skeletal system.
Diuretic Renal Scan (DRS)	Further evaluates appearance, function, and presence of obstruction (hydronephrosis) of the kidneys.
	Renal function is described by the T ½ times before and after Lasix administration of each kidney, estimated contribution of each kidney to effective renal plasma flow, and split renal function of each kidney.
	Clarifies degree of obstruction and loss of function for each kidney.
	Also known as a Lasix renal scan or renogram.

Cystoscopy is the gold standard of care in evaluating the bladder and urethra for cancer. It is typically completed in the outpatient clinic, but can be done in the operating room when bladder biopsies are needed. In the outpatient setting, the patient is prepped using a topical anesthetic, often xylocaine gel. The cystoscope is gently advanced through the urethra into the bladder. Attached to the cystoscope is a port for the administration of normal saline into the bladder to improve visualization of the bladder wall and the bilateral ureteral orifice. This also aides in the collection of urine samples. The lining of the urethra is also visualized and assessed for an area of abnormality. Visualization can be reduced by bleeding, or debris, and flat urothelial lesions such as CIS may be difficult to distinguish from normal bladder tissue. If cystoscopy findings are negative in the setting of a positive urine cytology, further evaluation of the upper tracts is indicated.

Bladder biopsies are tissues samples taken from the bladder lining using the cystoscope. The tissue samples are sent to pathology for examination, and are essential for obtaining a tissue diagnosis. These samples provide the histology, grade, and the depth of invasion. After bladder biopsies, the patient may experience gross hematuria, passing clots, dysuria, urgency and frequency, symptoms that are typically self-limiting and resolve within 2–3 days. During this time, a short course of phenazopyridine (Pyridium) can help to alleviate the symptoms.

Ureteroscopy with biopsy is an upper tract endoscopy completed in the operating room under anesthesia, and is performed by a urologist. A ureteroscope is inserted through the urethra and advanced into the right and/or left ureter. The lining of the ureter and the ureteral orifice are inspected, and biopsies of any visually abnormal areas may be taken.

Urethroscopy: A urethroscopy is an endoscopy of the lining of the urethra, and is completed at the time of a cystoscopy. If abnormalities are seen on outpatient cystoscopy, then the patient is taken to the operating room for biopsy.

Lymph node biopsy: A biopsy of enlarged lymph nodes can be completed by either a fine needle aspiration (FNA) or under CT guidance to identify and confirm metastatic disease.

Management of Urothelial Carcinoma

Treatment for Urothelial Carcinoma can be quite challenging for patients. Review of important behavioral modifications before treatment can improve patient outcomes during and after treatment.

- **Smoking Cessation:** The number one most important task is to quit tobacco use; many patients cannot accept that smoking has a direct correlation to the diagnosis of urothelial carcinoma. Tobacco consultation teams, support groups, cognitive therapy, and medication management programs can be extremely helpful.
- **Chemical and Environmental Exposures:** Reducing exposures to chemicals will minimize risks even further, and remind patients to follow all safety guidelines when handling chemicals.
- **Physical Wellness:** Encouraging daily activity such as walking, gentle strengthening exercises (if appropriate for the patient), biking, and swimming before starting treatment, will help to improve strength and endurance. This will help facilitate recovery and improve patient outcomes.
- **Nutrition:** Maintaining proper nutrition is essential during and after treatment. Side effects from systemic chemotherapy can alter a patient's appetite and ability to eat. It is common for patients to lose 15–20 lb after a radical surgical resection. Referral for nutrition counseling will help to outline an appropriate meal plan for each patient.
- **Hydration:** Maintaining good hydration will maintain urinary tract health. Dehydration can cause electrolyte imbalance and impair renal function; instruct patients to avoid bladder irritants such as alcohol, caffeine, and soda.
- **Psychosocial Support:** Providing continued support through treatment, recovery, and surveillance will improve patient outcomes and decrease distress. Referral to a Psychology Oncology program or social work can assist with anxiety and depression, not only for the patient, but for the caregiver as well. Social work can also assist the caregiver and patient with financial concerns, transportation, meals, and household chores.

- **Optimize Medical Comorbidities:** Optimizing medical comorbidities prior to treatment will improve outcomes; well-controlled diabetes, hypertension, and chronic obstructive pulmonary disease (COPD) will maximize recovery. Consultation with primary care providers and specialty providers is necessary coordination of care.

Management of Urothelial Carcinoma of the Bladder

Intravesical Immunotherapy and Chemotherapy

Intravesical therapy is an important treatment modality in the management of nonmuscle-invasive (Ta) or minimally invasive bladder cancers. This treats persistent microscopic tumors persistence and prevents tumor reimplantation, new tumor formation, and possible tumor grade and stage progression. Intravesical therapy is given directly into the bladder through the urethra with a catheter, and typically begins 2–4 weeks after a transurethral resection (TURBT). An initial induction course is once per week for 6 consecutive weeks, followed by cystoscopy and/or bladder biopsies in 4–6 weeks. Depending upon response, the patient may go on to maintenance intravesical therapy in the form of immunotherapy or chemotherapy. Immunotherapy is the instillation of agents that work by triggering the body's immune response to destroy cancer cells that may be present in the bladder after a transurethral resection. Intravesical chemotherapy is the instillation of chemotherapeutic agents that inhibit or slow cancer cell production.

Intravesical Immunotherapy
Bacillus Calmette–Guerin (BCG) is a live attenuated strain of *Mycobacterium bovis*, first indicated as a tuberculosis vaccine, and has been used in intravesical immunotherapy since the 1970s. The mechanism of action is a T-helper type I immune response, and is considered first line treatment for nonmuscle-invasive bladder cancer.

Interferon is an immunotherapeutic agent that may be used as monotherapy or in combination with BCG. The mechanism of action is lymphocyte activation and potentiates a T-helper type I immune response.

Intravesical Chemotherapy
Mitomycin C (MMC) is the most common intravesical chemotherapeutic agent used for nonmuscle-invasive bladder cancer. It is an antibiotic and inhibits DNA synthesis; it can be used for induction and maintenance therapy. MMC can also be used in a perioperative fashion at the time of a transurethral resection (TURBT). The rationale for perioperative dosing is the destruction of residual microscopic tumor at the site of TURBT and of circulating cells, thereby preventing reimplantation at the time of TURBT.

Gemcitabine is an intravesical chemotherapeutic agent that has been used to treat nonmuscle-invasive bladder cancer. This agent may be used in intermediate-risk patients as an alternative to MMC, and in high-risk, BCG refractory patients, and may be active in reducing tumor recurrence.

Docetaxel is an intravesical chemotherapeutic agent that has been used to treat nonmuscle-invasive bladder cancer. This agent may be used in intermediate-risk patients in combination with gemcitabine, as an alternative to MMC, and in high-risk, BCG refractory patients, and may be active in reducing tumor recurrence (Thomas et al. 2019).

Valrubicin is an intravesical chemotherapeutic agent that has been used to treat nonmuscle-invasive bladder cancer. This agent may be used in BCG refractory patients, and may be active in reducing tumor recurrence (Cookson et al. 2014).

BCG Shortage Recommendations: BCG shortages have led to recommended alterations in treatment agents and courses. Recommendations include the following:

- Do not use BCG for low-risk nonmuscle-invasive bladder cancer (NMIBC) patients. Use intravesical chemotherapy such as mitomycin
- Consider alternative intravesical agents for second-line therapy (BCG refractory)
- High-risk NMIBC including high-grade T1 and CIS should be prioritized for full strength BCG. If not available, consider ½ or 1/3 dose
- For maintenance BCG use 1/3 dose with limitation of the treatment course to 1 year
- Prioritize BCG-naïve patients
- If BCG is not available, consider alternative agents including mitomycin, gemcitabine (with or without sequential docetaxel or mitomycin), or valrubicin
- Patients with high-risk features who are good surgical candidates should be offered radical cystectomy (BCG Shortage Information 2019)

Side Effects of Intravesical Therapy: Intravesical therapy produces a local reaction to the bladder urothelium which can cause significant symptoms during treatment. The most common side effects are irritative voiding symptoms (dysuria, frequency, urgency), pain in the bladder, gross hematuria, low-grade fever and malaise. These usually occur in the first 24–48 h after treatment. If symptoms persist, a urine culture should be completed to rule out a bacterial urinary tract infection. If the urine culture is negative, then medications such as anticholinergics, topical antispasmodics (phenazopyridine), analgesics, and NSAIDS can be used to alleviate symptoms.

If the urine culture is positive, intravesical therapy is held, and the patient is treated with the appropriate antibiotic determined by the culture sensitivities. A follow-up urine culture 2–3 days post-antibiotic therapy is completed to confirm resolution of the infection prior to the continuation of treatment. If the patient has difficulty voiding, small frequent voids, weakening urinary stream, they should be evaluated with an ultrasound prior to resuming treatments.

Side effects can become increasingly severe over time with long-term intravesical therapy, and doses may by half or one-third. In some cases, patients are not able to tolerate subsequent treatments and the therapy is discontinued. In some patients, severe chemical cystitis can occur, especially with MMC and can be managed with intravesical dimethyl sulfoxide (DMSO: includes methylprednisone, dimethyl sulf-oxide, lidocaine HCL 2%, sodium bicarbonate) given once per week for 6 weeks. Antihistamines, long-acting anticholinergics and oral prednisone can also be used.

Surgical Management

Transurethral Resection of the Bladder Tumor (TURBT) is both diagnostic and therapeutic, and can be used in the initial management of nonmuscle-invasive (Ta) disease and recurrent Ta disease. The configuration (flat, sessile, or papillary), loca-tion (trigone, base, dome, or lateral walls), size (centimeters), and number of tumors are noted during a TURBT. These characteristics provide critical staging information imperative for treatment recommendations. If there is tumor present at the bladder neck or within the prostatic urethra, biopsy or resection of the prostatic urethra is included at the time of the TURBT. A single dose of MMC given immediately follow-ing a TURBT in patients with both low- and high-risk nonmuscle-invasive urothelial carcinoma reduces the risk of recurrence. Potential complications include irritative lower urinary tract symptoms, bleeding, bladder perforation, urethral stricturing, and scarring of the ureteral orifices that could potentially lead to renal obstruction.

Radical Cystectomy is the standard of care for invasive urothelial carcinoma, and is indicated when there is infiltrating muscle-invasive bladder cancer without evidence of metastasis or with low volume regional metastasis (stage T2-T3b), extensive disease not amenable to cystoscopic resection, invasive prostatic urethral involvement, or low-grade disease that has been refractory to intravesical immuno-therapy or chemotherapy. Conditions that can influence cystectomy include bleed-ing diathesis, evidence of gross, unresectable metastatic disease (unless performed for palliation), and medical comorbidities that preclude operative intervention such as advanced heart disease, and poor pulmonary function. Five-year survival rate for radical cystectomy plus pelvic lymph node dissection and negative nodes is 85–100% for T2a disease but 10–30% for node positive disease.

Consideration for neoadjuvant chemotherapy should be made for patients with muscle-invasive bladder cancer who are scheduled to undergo cystectomy. Sufficient evidence exists to show improved reduced tumor burden, decreased micrometastatic disease, and improved survival cancer following cystectomy with a cisplatin-based neoadjuvant chemotherapy course (Patel and Campbell 2009). Even with improved survival, the use of neoadjuvant chemotherapy remains severely underutilized with less than 20% patients who undergo radical cystectomy receiving neoadjuvant che-motherapy (Porter et al. 2011). Non-cisplatin-based chemotherapy regimens have not shown improved outcomes in this patient population (Advanced Bladder Cancer Meta-analysis Collaboration 2003). Newer data suggests improved outcomes in patients who are not cisplatin eligible, and who received neoadjuvant anti-programmed cell death (PD)-1/ligand I (PD-L1) agents. These are referred to as checkpoint inhibitors. Studies to date have examined the use of pembrolizumab and atezolizumab. Both have shown high pathologic response rates with larger studies currently underway (Necchi et al. 2018).

For men, a cystoprostatectomy is performed, involving bilateral lymphadenectomy, removal of the bladder, peritoneal covering, perivesical fat, distal ureters, prostate, seminal vesicles, and vas deferens. Men without tumors at the bladder base or prostate may be considered for a nerve-sparing procedure. For women, an anterior exenteration is completed (bilateral pelvic lymphadenectomy, cystectomy, hysterectomy, salpingo-oophorectomy, partial anterior vaginectomy).

Several types of urinary diversions can be completed with a cystectomy. When considering a urinary diversion, it is crucial to discuss with the patient his/her preference, along with the surgical criteria for each diversion. For an ileal conduit, the patient must be willing to have a stoma that continuously drains urine into an external appliance. With a continent cutaneous urinary diversion, the patient must be willing and able to catheterize the pouch through and external stoma at least every 3 h. With an orthotopic neobladder, the patient must understand that initially it is labor intensive to train the neobladder. He/she must also be willing and physically able to perform intermittent straight catheterization if needed; neobladder patients must also understand they may experience urinary incontinence or retention.

Management of Urothelial Carcinoma of the Renal Pelvis and Ureter

The treatment for localized upper tract transitional cell carcinoma is surgery and medical management. Nephroureterectomy is the standard of care for upper tract disease, and is indicated in patients with renal pelvis UC, regionally extensive disease, and high-grade or high-stage lesions. A neprhoureterectomy can be performed by an open or a laparoscopic approach. The kidney, ureter, and bladder cuff is removed. If the upper tract disease is confined to the distal segment of the ureter, a distal nephrourectomy with reimplantation of the proximal ureter can be completed. The 5-year survival by stage after a total nephroureterectomy is 91% for stage Tis, Ta, T1, and 0% for stage N3/M1.

Like patients with bladder cancer, consideration for neoadjuvant chemotherapy should be made for patients with UTUC who are scheduled to undergo a nephroureterectomy. Preliminary evidence exists to show improved survival and less residual cancer with a cisplatin-based neoadjuvant chemotherapy course. This has been extrapolated from evidence showing improved outcomes in patients who received neoadjuvant chemotherapy prior to cystectomy. Furthermore, as cisplatin-based chemotherapy requires intact renal function, it is ideal to administer before surgical removal of the kidney. Despite this, objective evidence supporting its use preoperatively is still limited. (Grossman et al. 2003).

Medical management of upper tract urothelial tumors involves the instillation of chemotherapeutic agents Mitomycin C, or immunotherapy BCG. These agents can be administered either percutaneously, through a ureteral catheter (percutaneous nephrostomy tube) or intravesically in patients with vesicoureteral reflux. This approach is most appropriate for patients with multiple superficial disease or carcinoma in situ.

Management of Urothelial Carcinoma of the Urethra

Management of urothelial carcinoma of the urethra varies with stage and location of the lesion. Tumors of the distal urethra are usually discovered earlier and at a lower stage. Tumors of the proximal urethra usually present at a more clinically advanced stage. Surgical management of small superficial tumors includes: laser resection, transurethral resection, fulguration, and Mohs surgery. Large tumors or tumors that invade other structures or tissues require a radical resection. Indications for urethrectomy include: tumor in the anterior urethra; prostatic stromal invasion that is noncontiguous with the primary site; positive urethral margin during radical cystectomy; or diffuse CIS of bladder, prostatic ducts, or prostatic urethra.

The management of distal urethral tumors is different for men and women. For superficial tumors in women treatment may include transurethral resection, electroresection and fulguration, laser surgery, or brachytherapy with or without external beam radiation. For invasive tumors in women, treatment may include an anterior exenteration with or without lymphadenectomy. The management of superficial tumors in men may include transurethral resection, electroresection and fulguration, or laser surgery. Tumors that are located near the tip of the penis may include a partial penectomy with or without lymphadenectomy. For tumors in the distal urethra (but not at the tip of the penis) that are noninvasive, a partial urethrectomy with or without lymphadenectomy may be performed. Invasive urethral tumors in men may require a radical penectomy with or without lymphadenectomy; treatment modalities may include radiation therapy with or without chemotherapy and chemotherapy given together with radiation.

The management of cancer that involves the proximal urethra is also different for men and women. In women with small tumors, radiation therapy and/or surgery (anterior exenteration with lymph node dissection and urinary diversion) may be performed. In men, management may include, radiation therapy, or radiation therapy and chemotherapy, followed by surgery (cystoprostatectomy, penectomy, lymph node dissection, and urinary diversion).

Preoperative Education Prior to Surgery for Urothelial Carcinoma

Prior to surgery the patient will meet with an enterostomal therapist for education and marking for stoma placement. Education will include strategies for living a full life with an ostomy, resources for obtaining ostomy supplies, peristomal skin care, and proper fit of the appliance. Patients may consider a family member or a friend that may be available to assist with ostomy care. The goal for patients is to become confident and independent with care of their stoma and application of their appliance.

Neobladder training will include strategies to promote optimal functional capacity of the neobladder. These include, voiding utilizing the crede' maneuver, timed voiding with gradually increasing the voiding interval, intermittent self-catheterization and irrigation, and pelvic floor therapy.

Patients with a urinary diversion should obtain a medical ID bracelet/necklace to identify the presence and type of their diversion.

Postoperative Management: In the immediate postoperative period, there are several complications that can occur after cystectomy. The most common complication that may require readmission to the hospital is failure to thrive. The patient has difficulty recovering at home, are unable to maintain proper nutrition and hydration, resulting in causing weakness and electrolyte imbalance. Intermittent outpatient IV hydration and monitoring of labs including a comprehensive and a CBC with platelets and differential may be considered. If condition continues to decline, readmission to the hospital is considered for supportive care.

A wound infection, and/or dehiscence may also occur after cystectomy. Erythema, redness, drainage or pain at the abdominal incision may occur. Oral antibiotics, such as Keflex on an outpatient basis may be considered. If condition progresses to fever, chills, foul odor, elevated white blood cell count, the patient may require readmission for IV antibiotics, and/or a possible surgical wound irrigation and debridement followed by dressing changes. After cystectomy, patients are discharged with an abdominal binder to help support the abdominal incision. A wound with intact underlying fascia may be managed with wet to dry dressing changes on an outpatient basis. This will require patient and caregiver education of wound management and signs/symptoms of infection. If the underlying fascia becomes compromised, then a surgical repair may be considered.

Alteration of the intestinal tract can lead to bowel complications after surgery, including development of a postoperative ileus or hypomotility of the GI tract. Symptoms of an ileus may include moderate, diffuse abdominal discomfort, constipation, abdominal distention, nausea and vomiting, vomiting bile, lack of bowel movement and/or flatulence, and excessive belching. This condition may require readmission for hydration and bowel rest.

A urinary tract infection or pyelonephritis can also occur after surgery. If a UTI is suspected, a urine specimen should be sent for culture and sensitivity. Most uncomplicated UTI can be treated on an outpatient basis with oral antibiotics and increased fluid intake. On occasion, a UTI can progress to pyelonephritis requiring readmission and IV antibiotics and hydration. In severe cases pyelonephritis can lead to sepsis with aggressive management in the intensive care unit.

Surveillance Recommendations for Urothelial Carcinoma

Nonmuscle-invasive urothelial carcinoma: The frequency for local recurrence and the potential for stage progression, especially in those with high-risk disease, require vigilant surveillance lifelong. The clinical follow-up includes an appropriate patient history including voiding symptoms and hematuria, urinalysis, cystoscopy and urine cytology according to the NCCN (2014) guidelines. This includes cystoscopy at 3–6 month intervals and urine cytology for the first 2 years and at increasing intervals as clinically indicated thereafter. Upper tract imaging should be considered every 1–2 years for high-grade tumors.

Muscle-invasive urothelial carcinoma following cystectomy and urinary diversion: The NCCN (version 2.2014) guidelines for surveillance after cystectomy include imaging of the chest, upper tracts, abdomen, and pelvis every 3–6 months for 2 years based on risk of recurrence and then as clinically indicated. A urine cytology and comprehensive blood panel should be completed every 3–6 months for 2 years then as clinically indicated. Also, a vitamin B12 and Folic acid should be completed annually. In addition, a urethral wash is recommended every 6–12 months. A urethral wash is completed primarily in male post cystectomy ileal conduit patients to detect abnormal cells within the urethra.

Clinical Pearls
- Tobacco use is the leading risk factor for urothelial carcinoma.
- A complete evaluation of symptoms is essential, as urothelial carcinoma can mimic other conditions such as UTI and renal calculus. Never assume hematuria is a urinary tract infection.
- Always complete an US post-void residual (PVR) to evaluate for urinary retention
- Never ignore blood in the urine. All hematuria must be further evaluated with urinalysis (microscopic and macroscopic), urine culture and sensitivity, urine cytology, CT urogram, and cystoscopy.
- The presence of hydronephrosis on imaging is a significant finding that must be further evaluated and treated.
- A CT urogram is an essential diagnostic tool to fully evaluate the bladder and upper tracts.
- Side effects from intravesical therapy usually occur within the first 24–48 h after treatment.
- Side effects from intravesical therapy can become increasingly severe with each subsequent treatment.
- An Enterostomal Therapy consultation and follow-up is essential for patients with an ileal conduit urinary diversion.
- Maintaining good voiding habits is essential in maintaining neobladder health.
- The frequency for local recurrence and the potential for stage progression of patients with urothelial carcinoma require lifelong surveillance.
- There is increasing evidence to show improved outcomes with the use of neoadjuvant systemic chemotherapy and immunotherapy in this patient population.

Resources

The following is a list of resources available for the patient and for the provider:

- American Bladder Cancer Support www.bladdercancersupport.org
- American Cancer Society www.cancer.org
- American Society for Clinical Oncology www.cancer.net

- American Urological Association Foundation www.auafoundation.org
- Bladder Cancer Advocacy Network (BCAN) www.bcan.org
- Bladder Cancer Webcafe www.blcwebcafe.org
- CancerCare www.cancercare.org
- Lance Armstrong Foundation www.livestrong.org
- National Cancer Institute www.cancer.gov
- National Comprehensive Cancer Network (NCCN) www.nccn.org
- United Ostomy Associations of America, Inc. www.uoaa.org
- The Wellness Community www.thewellnesscommunity.org
- The Wound, Ostomy and Continence Nurses Society™ (WOCN®) www. wocn.org

References

Advanced Bladder Cancer Meta-analysis Collaboration (2003) Neoadjuvant chemotherapy in invasive bladder cancer: a systemic review and meta-analysis. Lancet 361(9373): 1927–1934

Azemar MD, Comperat E, Richard F, Cussenot O, Roupret M (2011) Bladder recurrence after surgery for upper urinary tract urothelial cell carcinoma; frequency, risk factors, and surveillance. Urol Oncol 29(2):130–136

BCG Shortage Information (2019) American Urological Association. https://www.auanet.org/about-us/bcg-shortage-info

Cancer Statistics (2019) American Cancer Society. https://acsjournals.onlinelibrary.wiley.com/doi/full/10.3322/caac.21551. Accessed 23 Jan 2020

Cookson MS, Chang SS, Lihou C, Li T, Harper SQ, Lang Z, Tutrone RF (2014) Use of intravesical valrubicin in clinical practice for treatment of nonmuscle-invasive bladder cancer, including carcinoma in situ of the bladder. Ther Adv Urol 6(5):181–191

Grossman HB, Natale RB, Tangen CM (2003) Neoadjuvant chemotherapy plus cystectomy compared with cystectomy alone for locally advanced bladder cancer. N Engl J Med 349(9):859–866. [Medline]

Guidos J, Powell C, Donohoe J, et al (2018) Urethral cancer. Medscape. https://emedicine.medscape.com/article/451496-overview

Hayes J, Gilligan T (2014) Nonurothelial bladder cancer. UpToDate. http://www.uptodate.com/contents/nonurothelial-bladder-cancer

Kaplan GW, Bulkey GJ, Grayhack JT (1967) Carcinoma of the male urethra. J Urol 98(3):365–371. [Medline]

National Comprehensive Cancer Network (2014) NCCN clinical practice guidelines in oncology (NCCN guidelines). Bladder Cancer (Version 2). http://www.tri-kobe.org/nccn/guideline/urological/english/bladder.pdf

National Institutes of Health (2014) Smoking and Bladder Cancer. http://www.nih.gov/research-matters/august2011/08292011cancer.htm

Necchi A, Anichini A, Raggi D, Briganti A, Massa S, Luciano R (2018) Pembrolizumab as neoadjuvant therapy before radical cystectomy in patients with muscle-invasive urothelial bladder carcinoma (PURE-01): an open-label, single-arm, phase II study. J Clin Oncol 36(34):3353–3360

Oken MM, Creech RH, Tormey DC, Horton J, Davis TE, McFadden ET, Carbone PP (1982) Toxicity and response criteria of the Eastern Cooperative Oncology Group. Am J Clin Oncol 5:649–655. Eastern Cooperative Oncology Group, Robert Comis M.D., Group Chair The ECOG Performance Status is in the public domain therefore available for public use

Patel A, Campbell S (2009) Current trends in the management of bladder cancer. J Wound Ostomy Continence Nurs 31(3):91–93

Porter MP, Kerrigan MC, Donato BM, Ramsey SD (2011) Patterns of use of systemic chemotherapy for Medicare beneficiaries with urothelial bladder cancer. Urol Oncol 29(3):252–258

Riesz P, Lotz G, Páska C, Szendrôi A, Majoros A, Németh Z, Törzsök P, Szarvas T, Kovalszky I, Schaff Z, Romics I, Kiss A (2007) Detection of bladder cancer from the urine using fluorescence in situ hybridization technique. Pathol Oncol Res 13(3):187–194. Epub 2007 Oct 7

SEER Cancer Statistics Factsheets: Bladder Cancer (2020) SEER survival monograph: cancer survival among adults: US SEER program, 1988-2001, patient and tumor characteristics. SEER program. NIH Pub. No. 07-6215. National Cancer Institute, Bethesda. http://seer.cancer.gov/statfacts/html/urinb.html. Accessed 23 Jan 2020

Swartz MA, Porter MP, Lin DW, Weiss NS (2006) Incidence of primary urethral carcinoma in the United States. Urology 68(6):1164–1168

Thomas L, Steinberg R, Gerard Nepple K, O'Donnell MA (2019) Sequential intravesical gemcitabine and docetaxel in the treatment of BCG-naïve patients with non-muscle invasive bladder cancer. J Clin Oncol 37(7):469

Valerio M, Lhermitte B, Bauer J, Jichlinski P (2011) Metastatic primary adenocarcinoma of the bladder in a twenty-five years old woman. Rare Tumors 3(1):e9

West DA, Cummings JM, Longo WE, Virgo KS, Johnson FE, Parra RO (1999) Role of chronic catheterization in the development of bladder cancer in patients with spinal cord injury. Urology 53(2):292–297

Wiener JS, Liu ET, Walther PJ (1992) Oncogenic human papillomavirus type 16 is associated with squamous cell cancer of the male urethra. Cancer Res 52(18):5018–5023

Kidney Cancer

19

Brian Odom, Luke Edwards, and Jason Hafron

Contents

B. Odom · L. Edwards · J. Hafron (✉)
Department of Urology, Beaumont Health System, Royal Oak, MI, USA
e-mail: Jason.Hafron@beaumont.edu

© Springer Nature Switzerland AG 2020
S. A. Quallich, M. J. Lajiness (eds.), *The Nurse Practitioner in Urology*,
https://doi.org/10.1007/978-3-030-45267-4_19

Objectives
1. Provide a basic foundation of knowledge for providers regarding renal tumors, particularly renal cell carcinoma.
2. Discuss cystic renal lesions which are a frequent cause for urologic consultation.
3. Review commonly encountered benign renal tumors.
4. Focus on diagnosis, workup, and management of malignant renal masses.

Overview

The purpose of this chapter is to provide a basic foundation of knowledge for clinicians specializing in urologic care regarding renal tumors, particularly renal cell carcinoma. Cystic lesions which are a frequent cause for urologic consultation will be discussed as well as some of the more commonly encountered benign renal tumors. This chapter will focus mostly on diagnosis, workup, and the management of malignant renal masses. Management must be tailored to each individual patient based on renal function and comorbidities, as well as characteristics of the mass itself.

Definitions

Clear Cell Carcinoma The most common type of renal cell carcinoma (RCC).
Papillary Carcinoma The second most common type of RCC, further characterized as type I (less aggressive) and type II (more aggressive).
Chromophobe Carcinoma The third most common type of RCC, generally less aggressive than other subtypes.
Fuhrman Grade A grading system to predict tumor behavior based on nuclear characteristics. It is used for clear cell and papillary RCC but not the other less common subtypes.
Percutaneous Renal Biopsy A needle core biopsy obtained through the skin to obtain renal tissue in order to obtain a histological diagnosis. Performed with either ultrasound or CT guidance.
Paraneoplastic Syndromes Constellation of both systemic symptoms and laboratory abnormalities which can be associated with RCC and may remit with tumor resection.
Bosniak Criteria A classification system to risk stratify cystic renal lesions based on CT or MRI characteristics.

Incidence

Renal cell carcinoma (RCC) is the most common malignant renal cancer with an incidence of 73,820 new cases per year in the United States and accounts for roughly

13,000 cancer deaths per year (Siegel et al. 2019). RCC is most commonly diagnosed in the sixth and seventh decade of life. A male predominance does exist with the disease (Siegel et al. 2019). The incidence of RCC is increasing over the last 30 years and many attribute this to the increased utilization of cross-sectional imaging (Hock et al. 2002).

Anatomy and Pathology

Most RCCs are thought to originate from the epithelium of the proximal convoluted tubules. While beginning in the renal cortex, these masses often grow out bulging into perinephric fat aiding in their visualization on imaging studies. Additionally they demonstrate a propensity to involve the renal vein either by direct invasion or tumor thrombus. Historically nearly 30% of patients have metastatic disease at presentation, with the most common sites being lung, followed by bone, and regional lymph nodes. Metastases occur via both hematologic and lymphatic spread. The prevalence of metastatic disease correlates with tumor size at presentation in nonlinear sigmoidal relationship (Nguyen and Gill 2009) as demonstrated in Table 19.1.

Not all RCCs behave the same and there is a spectrum of behavior in terms of metastatic risk and recurrence. Grading is based on Fuhrman nuclear grade which takes into account both nuclear size, contour, and nucleoli and ranges from grade I to grade IV. Higher grades connote a higher degree of aggression and portend a worse prognosis.

There are various subtypes of RCC, and a few bear mentioning. The most common type of RCC by far is clear cell RCC, the name given due to the abundance of clear cytoplasm seen on histologic examination of tumor specimen. Clear cell accounts for 70–80% of all RCC. The second most common subtype is papillary RCC. This is seen more commonly in patients with end-stage renal disease. There are two subtypes of papillary RCC, type I and type II. The distinction is important with regards to prognosis and recurrence as papillary type II has been shown to be more aggressive, whereas type I is considered more indolent. The third most common subtype of RCC is chromophobe, which, like type I papillary, demonstrates less aggressive behavior.

Table 19.1 The prevalence of metastatic disease based on tumor size

Primary tumor size (cm)	Risk of mets at diagnosis (%)
≤3	<4
3–4	7
4–7	16
7–10	30
>10	43

Benign Renal Masses

The two most common benign renal tumors are oncocytoma and angiomyolipomas (AML). An estimated 3–5% of solid renal masses are oncocytomas (Romis et al. 2004). There is no imaging modality which can reliably differentiate oncocytoma from malignant masses and thus tissue is required for diagnosis, obtained either by percutaneous biopsy or surgical excision.

AMLs are benign tumors that are characterized by three major histologic components: fat cells, smooth muscle, and blood vessels. Unlike oncocytoma, AMLs can be diagnosed reliably with imaging alone. The presence of macroscopic fat on CT imaging is considered diagnostic. While AMLs are benign, they carry the risk of spontaneous life-threatening hemorrhage, and this risk increases with larger tumors. For tumors >4 cm in diameter treatment is preferred given this potentially serious adverse event. Selective renal arterial embolization (SAE) is a safe alternative to surgical intervention with a 94.1% freedom from surgery at 10 years of follow-up (Anis et al. 2020). Although it has a high freedom from surgery and renal preservation, re-embolization rates can be as high as 41% (Anis et al. 2020). Smaller AMLs can be managed with serial imaging on a surveillance protocol.

Cystic Renal Lesions

Often times a patient may be referred to a urology clinic based on renal ultrasound findings which demonstrate a cystic mass. These lesions, with the exception of simple cysts which can be reliably diagnosed by ultrasound, should undergo further imaging usually in the form of CT to better elucidate their nature. A useful classification system for cystic masses has been developed and is commonly used in clinical decision-making, namely, Bosniak classification, which is further described in Table 19.2. This classification is particularly helpful in that the different classes have widely varying risks of being malignant (Israel and Bosniak 2005) and thus have important differences in clinical management. Briefly, classes I and II are considered benign and do not require further imaging. Class IIF are lesions that in all

Table 19.2 Bosniak classification system of renal cysts

Bosniak class	Features	Risk of malignancy	Management
I	Water density, homogenous, no septa, calcifications, or enhancement	None	Reassurance
II	Thin septa, fine calcifications, no enhancement	Negligible	Reassurance
IIF	Hyperdense, multiple thin septa, may have thick calcifications but no enhancement	3–5%	Periodic surveillance
III	Thickened walls or septa in which enhancement is present	50%	Surgical excision
IV	Same as III with additional clearly enhancing soft tissue components	75–90%	Surgical excision

likelihood are benign, but consideration should be given to periodic imaging as a form of surveillance. Class III and IV are considered likely malignant and are the only classes characterized by enhancement, which is absent from the others. Accordingly, class III and IV lesions are managed with surgical intervention. This classification has recently had a proposed update to incorporate MRI, establish definitions for vague radiographic terms, and reduce over treatment of renal cystic lesions however it has yet to be validated (Silverman et al. 2019).

History and Presentation

Flank pain, a palpable mass, and hematuria has historically been described as the classic triad of RCC, however given the increased use of cross-sectional imaging, this triad is rarely seen in today's practice. Additional symptoms with which patients may present include hypertension, hypercalcemia, in addition to constitutional symptoms such as fevers, night sweats, malaise, and weight loss. This constellation of symptoms should prompt body imaging.

RCC is notorious for paraneoplastic syndromes which can occur in the setting of localized disease. These include hypercalcemia, hypertension, anemia or polycythemia, and liver dysfunction which is termed Stauffer's syndrome when seen in the absence of metastatic disease. Paraneoplastic syndromes can be observed in 10–40% of RCC cases and often remit after the tumor is removed. The persistence of these abnormalities after surgical excision may suggest undetected metastatic disease and portends a worse prognosis (Hanash 1982).

Fortunately many patients seen in practice today are asymptomatic with masses noted on imaging obtained for other reasons, with greater than half of all RCC cases now detected incidentally (Pantuck et al. 2000). Studies suggest that patients with incidentally detected masses as opposed to symptomatic presentation may have improved survival although it is difficult to fully account for lead and length time bias (Gudbjartsson et al. 2005). Review of Surveillance, Epidemiology, and End Results (SEER) data from 2016 demonstrates 65% of patients diagnosed during that time period had localized disease (SEER Database).

Risk Factors

The cause of renal cell carcinoma is unclear and most cases are sporadic. Smoking has been demonstrated to be a moderate risk factor with some studies suggesting a roughly doubled relative risk in these patients. Interestingly obesity has more recently been identified as an independent risk factor for development of RCC, relative risk being increased by as much as 2.3 by the sixth decade of life for patients in the highest quartile of BMI (Chiu et al. 2006). This may partly explain the high incidence noted in North America compared to other parts of the globe.

There are many hereditary forms of RCC; however, these syndromes only represent 2–3% of all RCC diagnosed today. Von Hippel–Lindau warrants mention given its nature as an autosomal dominant disorder which results in an RCC incidence of 50% in patients affected. RCC in these patients is often multifocal and bilateral and these patients are at higher risk for recurrence. As such, renal sparing intervention is particularly important. Of note, these patients are at risk for nonrenal cancers as well such as cerebellar hemangioblastomas, retinal angiomas, and pheochromocytomas, among others. These patients when identified should be referred for genetic counseling.

Physical Exam

A physical exam can provide additional information about the signs and symptoms associated with RCC. A physical exam in a patient with suspected malignancy or a known mass demonstrated on imaging should always include a blood pressure measurement as well as a thorough lymph node examination. An abdominal examination should be performed to determine if the kidney mass is palpable. Rarely large masses will be palpable on abdominal or flank examination. Additionally in males the presence of a nonreducing varicocele, particularly right sided, may indicate the presence of a retroperitoneal mass. Unilateral lower extremity edema may be a result of venous compression, but like most physical findings caused by renal masses, denotes advanced disease. The presence or absence of spinal tenderness should be documented as the spine is most frequently involved by bony metastases. Hypertension may be secondary to increased renin secretion and can improve with surgical excision of tumors.

Diagnostic Tests

Laboratory Evaluation

The purpose of laboratory testing is to rule out paraneoplastic syndromes, identify other potential sites of metastases, and determine the overall health of the patient. Laboratory analysis in patients with a renal mass should include renal function as measured by BUN and Cr, a serum calcium level, CBC, liver function panel, alkaline phosphatase, and urinalysis.

Imaging Studies

The minimum standard imaging in all cases of renal masses suspicious for malignancy should include abdominal and pelvic imaging in the form of either CT or MRI with intravenous contrast and a chest X-ray.

Ultrasonography (US) Ultrasound is a useful imaging modality which utilizes a transducer that both creates and receives high frequency sound waves to create grayscale images. It has the advantage of being a radiation-free modality and is adequate for diagnosis of benign simple cysts. Additional benefits include patient tolerance, wide clinical availability, and low cost. Clinically it is often used to follow mildly complex cysts, such as Bosniak IIF lesions, to assess for interval growth or changes in complexity. It is important to remember however that complex or echogenic cysts detected by ultrasound must be further investigated with either CT or MRI imaging modalities.

Computed Tomography (CT) A thin-slice CT scan collects data based on how much various tissues attenuate radiation and generates an axial image based on this data. For evaluation of a renal mass, CT is obtained with and without IV contrast to evaluate for enhancement. Enhancement is defined as an increase in Hounsfield units (a measure of attenuation) of 15 or more after administration of contrast. Enhancing renal masses are considered RCC until proven otherwise.

Magnetic Resonance (MRI) MRI generates cross-sectional imaging based on both hydrogen ion density in various tissues as well as the response of these ions to the presence of a strong magnetic field. It has the distinct advantage of higher sensitivity for tumor thrombus and venous involvement, making it the study of choice when either of these entities is suggested by CT. Along the same lines it provides greater clarity of soft tissue planes helping delineate potentially locally invasive disease. MRI is additionally radiation-free. The studies do however take longer to perform, during which time patients must remain still to ensure image quality. Not all patients can undergo MRI imaging as they may have magnetic material in their body in the form of pacemakers or neurostimulators, among other medical devices.

Positron Emission Tomography (PET) This imaging modality involves injection of a radiotracer intravenously and subsequent imaging to determine areas of increased molecular uptake and activity. Currently with regard to RCC, it is best used as an adjunct when traditional imaging is equivocal for the presence of metastatic disease, in patients for whom the diagnosis of metastatic disease would influence further management.

Bone Scan Additionally, laboratory abnormalities such as elevated calcium or alkaline phosphatase should raise suspicion for metastatic disease and may prompt a bone scan.

Chest X-Ray A chest X-ray is a mandatory study in the initial evaluation of these patients. If the chest X-ray is abnormal or if pulmonary symptoms such as new onset cough or hemoptysis are present, this should prompt a CT of the chest, however CT chest is not required in all patients.

Intravenous Pyelogram (IVP) It is worth noting that axial imaging in the form of CT or MRI has essentially entirely replaced IVP as an imaging modality for renal masses. Nonetheless it is of historical significance. A scout plain X-ray film is obtained followed by administration of intravenous iodinated contrast and serial radiographs at timed intervals provide an image of the renal unit as the kidney takes up and ultimately excretes the contrast.

Percutaneous Biopsy

Historically renal mass biopsy has been avoided in most cases of enhancing renal masses due to previously reported high false negative rates as well as concern for cancerous seeding of the biopsy tract and other complications such as bleeding (Abel et al. 2012). More recently however percutaneous biopsy has been enjoying a renaissance of sorts. Roughly 20% of T1a masses (<4 cm) are actually benign, and an accurate biopsy can spare these patients the morbidity of surgical intervention. It has been reported that greater than 90% of needle core biopsies are sufficient to render a diagnosis (Wang et al. 2009; Millet et al. 2012). More importantly, in biopsies which have sufficient tissue for diagnosis several studies have reported near or up to 100% accuracy (Wang et al. 2009; Menogue et al. 2013), which has alleviated the historical concern of false negative and potentially not intervening in the case of a missed cancerous tumor. Complication rates are satisfactorily low and as more biopsies are performed, tract seeding has been shown to be exceedingly rare. It is now generally recommended by the American Urological Association (AUA) that renal biopsy be offered to patients who are surgical candidates for whom a diagnosis has the potential to change management, with the understanding that some patients when faced with a renal mass will consider even low levels of diagnostic uncertainty unacceptable.

Management

Management of suspected malignant renal masses is directed by numerous variables such as tumor size, stage, patient comorbidities, life expectancy, and biopsy results, among others. A discussion of management requires a basic understanding of tumor, node, and metastasis (TNM) staging which is presented for review in Table 19.3.

Surveillance of Renal Masses

With the frequency of body imaging an increasing number of small, incidental renal masses have been discovered in elderly patients who are poor surgical candidates and this has granted insight into the natural history of such masses in the absence of intervention. It has been demonstrated that these tumors have relatively slow growth rates and low risks for metastases, with only 1.1% progression to metastatic disease for lesions <4 cm in size at 28 months follow-up and a growth rate of roughly 0.1 cm/year (Jewett et al. 2011). As such, the AUA 2017 guidelines state active

Table 19.3 TNM staging of kidney cancer as published by American Joint Committee on Cancer (AJCC)

Primary tumor (T)	
Tx	Primary tumor cannot be assessed
T0	No evidence of primary tumor
T1	Tumor ≤7 cm confined to kidney
• T1a	Tumor ≤4 cm confined to kidney
• T1b	Tumor 4–7 cm confined to kidney
T2	Tumor >7 cm confined to kidney
• T2a	Tumor 7–10 cm confined to kidney
• T2b	Tumor >10 cm confined to kidney
T3	Tumor extends into major veins or perinephric tissue but not ipsilateral adrenal gland and not beyond Gerota's fascia
• T3a	Tumor grossly extends into renal vein or its segmental branches or invades perirenal fat, or invades the pelvicalyceal system, or invades perirenal and/or renal sinus fat (Not beyond Gerota's fascia)
• T3b	Tumor extends into vena cava below diaphragm
• T3c	Tumor extends into vena cava above diaphragm or invades wall of vena cava
T4	Tumor invades beyond Gerota's fascia or into ipsilateral adrenal
Regional lymph nodes (N)	
NX	Regional nodes cannot be assessed
N0	No regional lymph node metastasis
N1	Metastasis present in regional lymph nodes
Distant metastasis (M)	
M0	No distant metastasis
M1	Distant metastasis

surveillance should be recommended initial management of "small solid of Bosniak 3/4 complex cystic renal masses, especially those <2 cm." In addition per the guidelines it should be offered to patients with limited life expectancy or for those unfit for or do not desire intervention.

Surgical Intervention

There have been novel treatments introduced, some of which will be discussed, however surgical excision remains a mainstay in the management of localized renal tumors.

Radical Nephrectomy

Radical nephrectomy (RN) has been a long-standing gold standard surgical procedure for localized RCC. This involves removing the entire kidney and all of the contents within Gerota's fascia. Traditionally this included removal of the adrenal but it has been demonstrated more recently for the majority of kidney tumors the ipsilateral adrenal can be spared during radical nephrectomy. RN is often performed laparoscopically or robotically at many institutions and offers excellent oncologic outcomes with shortened hospital stays while avoiding the morbidity of open surgery.

Partial Nephrectomy

Recently more attention has been paid to the health consequences of CKD, specifically increased cardiovascular morbidity, and subsequent mortality (Go et al. 2004). Not surprisingly, radical nephrectomy leads to CKD in a higher number of patients than partial nephrectomy. PN entails clamping of the renal vessels and excision of the tumor with removal of a rim of normal renal parenchyma. When performed via an open surgical approach, cold ischemia in the form of ice on the kidney is used, but laparoscopically this is not as feasible and is usually done without cold ischemia. Given our understanding of the potential for CKD and its sequelae, for patients with T1 tumors and a normal contralateral kidney, there has been a push in recent years to perform partial nephrectomy given that the mass is amenable to this approach. This decision is based largely on feasibility as determined by the individual surgeon. Partial nephrectomy (PN) can be performed via open, laparoscopic, or robotic-assisted approaches and management will vary based on surgeon expertise. It has been demonstrated that PN does carry with it an increased morbidity in terms of potential for bleeding and urinary leak which are complications not seen as often after RN; however, with the benefit of better preserved renal function.

Important preoperative considerations for both radical and partial nephrectomy are those common to most surgical interventions. All patients should receive preoperative medical clearance from either an internist or cardiologist, and further preoperative risk stratification and testing will be obtained at their discretion. Coordination of care across specialties is an important principle of preoperative surgical care.

Thermal Ablation

Thermal ablation for renal masses encompasses a variety of minimally invasive procedures done either percutaneously with CT guidance or laparoscopically including cryotherapy, radiofrequency ablation, among others. The literature regarding these is limited by short-term follow-up and the absence of standardized methodology; however it suggests roughly equivalent cancer-specific survival when compared to traditional surgical management, albeit with shorter follow-up. Recurrence-free survival, while high, does not match the rates noted with surgical management. It is important to note that these studies have been performed mostly on elderly patients who are considered high surgical risk and on small renal masses generally <3 cm in size. As such, the AUA guidelines in 2017 suggest that thermal ablation "should be considered an alternative approach for the management of T1a renal masses <3 cm in size." Renal mass biopsy should be performed prior to thermal ablation. In addition, when counseling patients about thermal ablation it is important to "include information regarding an increased likelihood of tumor persistence or local recurrence" after thermal ablation compared to surgical removal. Decision making regarding these alternative options is complex and the urologist should play an integral role in patient counseling.

Follow-Up

After surgical excision of RCC, continued follow-up is essential given the estimation that 20–30% of patients will experience relapse. Patients are at various risks of relapse depending on stage, grade, and size of tumor at resection, and thus there is no standard follow-up protocol which can be applied to all patients. NCCN guidelines vary depending on stage or treatment modality. Please see Table 19.4 for more details in regards to follow-up schedules. Additionally patients with solitary kidneys or those with risk factors for renal insufficiency should be screened annually with 24 h urine protein measurements, as proteinuria is often the first sign of progressing renal disease. When detected a nephrology referral is appropriate.

With regard to imaging the lung is the most common site of distant recurrence, and as such, a chest imaging is an integral component of follow-up. The frequency of abdominal CT scans will vary based on T-stage and grade of the primary tumor. A concise review of post-treatment follow-up based on NCCN guidelines is located in Table 19.4. In regards to stage T4 tumors and their subsequent follow-up, frequency of lab work and imaging is determined on a case-by-case basis. Greater detail on follow-up recommendations can be found both at the NCCN and AUA links provided in the resources section.

Table 19.4 Kidney cancer follow-up based off T-stage as published by the National Comprehensive Cancer Network (NCCN)

Stage T1 following partial or radical nephrectomy
• H&P annually ± labs
• Abdominal CT or MRI within the first year, then annually for at least 3 years
• Chest X-ray or CT annually for 5 years
Stage T1 following thermal ablation
• Annual H&P ± labs
• Abdominal CT or MRI within 3–6 months, annually for 5 years or longer
• If signs of recurrence consider more frequent imaging, renal mass biopsy or further treatment
• Chest X-ray or CT annually for 5 years
Stage T2-3
• H&P every 3–6 months for 3 years, annually up to 5 years
• Comprehensive metabolic panel every 6 months for 2 years, then annually up to 5 years
• Abdominal (CT or MRI) and chest imaging (CT preferred) obtained every 3–6 months for at least 3 years, then annually up to 5 years

Clinical Pearls

- Many renal tumors are found incidentally during evaluation for other issues; the classic triad (flank mass, hematuria, pain) is now rare.
- Angiomyolipoma is the only solid renal mass which can reliably be diagnosed as benign on imaging alone; this is determined by the presence of macroscopic fat.
- Renal US is adequate to diagnose simple renal cysts for which reassurance is appropriate, but more complex renal cysts require CT or MRI to further evaluate.
- Biopsy is not necessary before excision of primary solid renal mass.
- 20–30% of patients may demonstrate paraneoplastic syndrome (elevated erythrocyte sedimentation rate, cachexia, fever, anemia, hypertension, elevated serum calcium and alkaline phosphatase, polycythemia).

Resources for the Nurse Practitioner

http://www.auanet.org/education/clinical-practice-guidelines.cfm
　　https://www.nccn.org/professionals/physician_gls/PDF/kidney.pdf

Resources for the Patient

http://www.urologyhealth.org/urologic-conditions/kidney-cancer
　　http://www.nccn.org/patients/default.aspx

References

Abel EJ et al (2012) Limitations of preoperative biopsy in patients with metastatic renal cell carcinoma: comparison to surgical pathology in 405 cases. BJU Int 110(11):1742–1746

Anis O, Rimon U, Ramon J et al (2020) Selective arterial embolization for large or symptomatic renal angiomyolipoma: 10 years of follow-up. Urology 135:82

Chiu BC et al (2006) Body mass index, physical activity, and risk of renal cell carcinoma. Int J Obes 30(6):940–947

Go AS et al (2004) Chronic kidney disease and the risks of death, cardiovascular events, and hospitalization. N Engl J Med 351:1296

Gudbjartsson T, Thoroddsen A, Petursdottir V et al (2005) Effect of incidental detection for survival of patients with renal cell carcinoma: results of population-based study of 701 patients. Urology 66:1186

Hanash KA (1982) The nonmetastatic hepatic dysfunction syndrome associated with renal cell carcinoma (hypernephroma): Stauffer's syndrome. Prog Clin Biol Res 100:301

Hock LM et al (2002) Increasing incidence of all stages of kidney cancer in the last 2 decades in the United States: an analysis of surveillance, epidemiology and end results program data. J Urol 16:57

Israel GM, Bosniak MA (2005) An update of the Bosniak Renal Cyst Classification system. Urology 66:484

Jewett MA et al (2011) Active surveillance of small renal masses: progression patterns of early stage kidney cancer. Eur Urol 60(1):39–44

Menogue SR et al (2013) Percutaneous core biopsy of small renal mass lesions: a diagnostic tool to better stratify patients for surgical intervention. BJU Int 111(4 Pt B):E146–E151

Millet I et al (2012) Can renal biopsy accurately predict histological subtype and Fuhrman grade of renal cell carcinoma? J Urol 188(5):1690–1694

Nguyen MM, Gill IS (2009) Effect of renal cancer size on the prevalence of metastasis at diagnosis and mortality. J Urol 181(3):1020–1027

Pantuck AJ et al (2000) Incidental renal tumors. Urology 56(2):190–196

Romis L et al (2004) Frequency, clinical presentation and evolution of renal oncocytomas: multicentric experience from a European database. Eur Urol 45:53

SEER Stat Fact Sheet (n.d.) Kidney and renal pelvis. http://seer.cancer.gov/statfacts/html/kidrp.html

Siegel RL et al (2019) Cancer statistics, 2019. CA Cancer J Clin 69(1):7–34

Silverman SG, Pedrosa I, Ellis JH et al (2019) Bosniak classification of cystic renal masses, version 2019: an update proposal and needs assessment. Radiology 292(2):475–488

Wang R et al (2009) Accuracy of percutaneous core biopsy in management of small renal masses. Urology 73(3):586–590

Neoplasms of the Penile and Testis

20

Sara Drummer, Hillary B. Durstein,
and Susanne A. Quallich

Contents

S. Drummer (✉)
AdventHealth Medical Group Urology, Altamonte Springs, FL, USA

H. B. Durstein
Las Vegas Urology, Las Vegas, NV, USA
e-mail: hdurstein@lasvegasurology.com

S. A. Quallich
Division of Andrology and Urologic Health, Department of Urology, Michigan Medicine,
University of Michigan, Ann Arbor, MI, USA
e-mail: quallich@umich.edu

© Springer Nature Switzerland AG 2020
S. A. Quallich, M. J. Lajiness (eds.), *The Nurse Practitioner in Urology*,
https://doi.org/10.1007/978-3-030-45267-4_20

Objectives
1. Describe penile and testicular neoplasms.
2. Identify populations that benefit from screening for penile and testicular neoplasms.
3. Appropriately order imaging studies and relevant labs to make the diagnosis of penile or testicle testicular neoplasm.
4. Discuss surveillance issues unique to these malignancies.

Penile Neoplasms

Neoplasms of the penis arise from the squamous epithelium of the glans and penile shaft. These cancers are rare in the United States, with an expected 2200 cases for 2020 (American Cancer Society [ACS]). Although other cell types may occur, the most prominent subtype is squamous cell carcinoma, and these lesions develop from the mucosal surface of the penis in the prepuce making the primary risk for this condition in the presence of the foreskin. This tends to be a particularly aggressive type of neoplasm with lesions that arise typically to the glans, prepuce, and penile shaft and infiltrate through lymphatic dissemination. Treatment for penile cancer commonly involves surgery, radiation, and chemotherapy.

Epidemiology and Risk Factors

The greatest risk for penile cancer is seen in men between the ages of 50 and 70. Industrialized nations have a much lower rate of penile cancer; among nonindustrialized countries, prevalence rates are up to five to ten times higher than that seen in the United States. It is an uncommon disease in children and young men, with exceptions seen among men who have human immunodeficiency virus and human papilloma virus (HPV).

Several distinct risk factors have been associated with penile cancer including phimosis, lack of circumcision, HPV infection, lower socioeconomic status, chronic inflammatory conditions such as balanitis, smoking, and overall poor genital hygiene. Uncircumcised men continue to have the highest risk, as a group, for penile cancer. Circumcision as an infant can prevent almost all penile cancer from developing. A lack of circumcision can contribute to chronic inflammatory states such as phimosis and balanitis, with these conditions present in 45–85% of men with penile cancers. This is compounded by poor hygiene, tobacco use, and other chronic inflammatory states. HPV infection has also gained recognition as a causative factor for penile cancer, with serotypes 16 and 18 remaining the most common influences on the malignant conversion of cells.

Clinical Diagnosis and Staging

Most penile cancers are superficial and low grade. Previous nomenclature for penile cancers have included terms such as carcinoma in situ (CIS), Bowen's disease, and erythroplasia of Queyrat, but have been more recently termed penile intraepithelial neoplasia (PeIN). Further subdivision is based upon morphologic and microscopic characteristics. When the penile cancer is diagnosed, it can be termed superficial spreading, described by vertical growth, and can be described as verruciform, multicenter, and mixed. Squamous cell carcinoma remains the most common type of penile cancer and is seen up to two-thirds of cases. The most important predictors for metastatic spread and survival remain as diagnosed tumor grade, depth of invasion, and presence or absence of perineural invasion. Clinical staging is assigned using the 2010 AJCC TMN staging for penile cancer (Table 20.1).

Table 20.1 TMN staging of penile cancer

TX	Primary tumor cannot be assessed
T0	No evidence of primary tumor
Tis	Carcinoma in situ
Ta	Noninvasive verrucous carcinoma
T1a	Invasion into subepithelial connective tissue, no lymph vascular invasion; *not* poorly differentiated
T1b	Invasion into subepithelial connective tissue, with lymph vascular invasion, or *is* poorly differentiated
T2	Invasion into corpus spongiosum or cavernosum
T3	Invasion into the urethra
T4	Invasion to other adjacent structures
Regional lymph nodes (N) *clinical stage definition*	
cNX	Regional lymph nodes cannot be assessed
cN0	No palpable or visibly enlarged inguinal lymph nodes
cN1	Palpable mobile unilateral inguinal lymph node
cN2	Palpable mobile multiple or bilateral inguinal lymph nodes
cN3	Palpable fixed inguinal nodal mass or pelvic lymphadenopathy unilateral or bilateral
Regional lymph nodes (N) *pathologic stage definition*	
X	Regional lymph nodes cannot be assessed
pN0	No regional lymph node metastasis
pN1	Metastasis in a single inguinal lymph node
pN2	Metastases in multiple or bilateral inguinal lymph nodes
pN3	Extranodal extension of lymph node metastasis or pelvic lymph node(s) unilateral or bilateral
Distant metastasis (M)	
0	No distant metastasis
M1	Distant metastasis

Adapted from AJCC (2010)

Metastasis occurs in a predictable stepwise fashion; it spreads from the penis to the sentinel node, the superficial inguinal nodes, to deep inguinal nodes, to pelvic nodes, and then to distant metastasis sites. This stepwise progression is because the lymphatics of the penis do not drain directly to the pelvic lymph nodes.

History and Physical Examination

The focused history includes age at circumcision (if relevant), history of balanitis or other chronic inflammatory conditions, history of prior penile trauma, and history of sexually transmitted infections (especially HPV), along with questions about tobacco use and personal hygiene habits. An individual's history should also be reviewed for previous treatment for dermatologic conditions such as lichen sclerosis or balanitis xerotica obliterans (BXO). A delay in seeking treatment is common, and men may present with paraneoplastic syndromes such as hypercalcemia.

Physical examination involves careful inspection of the penis, penile shaft, and bilateral inguinal regions. The foreskin should be retracted when possible. Each lesion must be assessed by including the diameter, whether it is fixed or mobile, location relative to the phallus and other anatomical structures, and obvious morphological features (keratinization, ulceration, nodular). Inguinal lymph nodes should be characterized as well, e.g., mobile versus fixed; the most common site of metastasis is the inguinal lymph nodes. Note should be made of potential underlying infection. Excisional biopsy or punch biopsy may be performed in clinic to confirm diagnosis.

Other conditions can present with lesions to the male genitals. A Buschke–Lowenstein tumor (giant condyloma) is a large exophytic mass that can occur in the genital, inguinal, or anorectal region. It is benign but can be locally invasive, and surgical excision may be quite extensive. Bowenoid papulosis presents as red-brown papules to the glans or shaft and is similar in appearance to carcinoma in situ. It is commonly treated with topical medications or laser ablation. Zoon's balanitis is a well-circumscribed, red, flat lesion, and it contains darker red spots. It looks similar to carcinoma in situ and is diagnosed by biopsy. It is also treated with topical preparations or laser ablation.

Lichen sclerosis (LS) results from a chronic infection, trauma, or inflammation to the male genitals. Two percent to 9% of men diagnosed with lichen sclerosis progress to penile cancer. LS presents as flat white patches on the glans and prepuce. It may feel fibrotic and is usually asymptomatic, although men may complain of burning and itching, and painful erections.

Diagnostic Tests

Initial evaluation will include a biopsy of the primary lesion. If the patient is appropriate for organ-sparing (penis-sparing) therapy, a penile ultrasound or MRI with contrast may help determine the extent of any tissue invasion. A biopsy of the sentinel lymph node may also be helpful. Patients at risk for cancer in the regional lymph nodes should also undergo a chest X-ray, CT scan of the abdomen and pelvis, and routine blood tests including serum chemistries including calcium and liver function tests. If the patient has bone pain, elevated calcium or alkaline phosphatase, a bone scan is indicated.

Management

The suitability of an individual patient for various therapies is determined by the clinical stage of his lesion(s). The American Urological Association offers guidelines for managing primary penile tumors (see Appendix). Tis and Ta primary tumors can be managed with topical treatments (5% imiquimod, 5-fluorouracil) with or without local resection. Men with higher-stage penile tumors should be offered wide local excision, penile-preserving surgery with skin grafts, and/or possibly laser ablation surgery. Penile-sparing surgery is heavily dependent on the grade, stage, and location of the primary tumor, but has a higher local recurrence rate. Surgery may take the form of penectomy or glansectomy; penectomy is considered when a penile stump of >2 cm cannot be preserved. A regional lymph node dissection may also be indicated, and emphasis on negative margins is paramount.

Chemotherapy is indicated when the primary tumor or inguinal node metastasis are unresectable. Regimens usually include 5-FU and cisplatin.

Perioperative Management

All team members caring for patients with penile cancer must be sensitive to the fact that this treatment can have significant psychosocial and sexual implications for men, independent of the stage of their tumor. Men may benefit from psychosocial counseling and possibly counseling with a specialized sex therapist as well.

Ongoing management involves intensive follow-up over the first 2 years, although there is a paucity of scientific literature supporting rigid follow-up guidelines. Men should be taught self-examination of the penis and inguinal lymph nodes. Men should be examined by clinician every 3–6 months over the first 2 years. If they undergo a lymph node dissection, men will need serial chest imaging (every 6 months) and abdominal/pelvic CT or MRI (every 3 months for the first year, every 6 months for the second year). Prognosis depends on surgical staging; men with invasion of the corpus spongiosis appear to have a better prognosis. Relative survival rate for cancers combined to the penis is 85% at 5 years.

Metastatic disease at time of diagnosis is treated with a multimodal approach than can include chemotherapy with consolidative surgery (preferably), radiotherapy, or chemoradiation, but prognosis is poor.

Long-Term Follow-Up

Men who have undergone penile-sparing surgery will be seen closely for the first 2 years (every 3 months), while those who have undergone partial/total penectomy will be seen every 6 months for the first 2 years (Clark et al. 2013). If there were bulky lymph nodes, men will need a physical examination and abdominal/pelvic imaging (CT or MRI) every 3 months for the first year and then every 6 months during year 2; chest X-ray is added according to this same imaging schedule. If there were negative lymph nodes, men will need a physical examination every 3–6 months for 2 years and then every 6–12 months for another 3 years. Imaging will target men whose examination is challenging (e.g., obesity). Management of local recurrences is poorly explored, but can include surgical resection, external beam radiotherapy, and/or systemic chemotherapy.

Testis Neoplasms

Neoplasms of the testes are relatively uncommon and are rare in the United States with an expected 9560 cases in 2019. Over 95% are germ cell tumors, with the remaining types split among germ cell tumors. These germ cell tumors are also classified as seminoma or non-seminoma germ cell tumors (NSGCT) and are the most common malignancy seen in men between the ages of 20–40. Only 10–30% of men present with metastatic disease; most men present with a localized testicular seminoma.

Epidemiology and Risk Factors

The well-recognized risk factors for testicular cancer include cryptorchidism, family or personal history of testicular cancer, or intratubular germ cell neoplasia (ITGCN). For men with a history of cryptorchidism, a higher risk for testicular cancer is associated with a higher location of the testes, meaning highest risk occurs in men with a history of intra-abdominal testis. Relative risk in men with cryptorchidism remains at 4–6 when compared with a matched cohort (Albers et al. 2011). Other conditions also increase risk for testis cancer including HIV infection, gonadal dysgenesis, male infertility, Klinefelter's syndrome, and testicular feminization after 30 years of age. The incidence of testicular cancer is highest among non-Hispanic whites and lowest among African Americans. Men ages 50 or greater are more likely to have a spermatocytic seminoma.

Anatomy

Testicular neoplasms are more common on the right, because cryptorchidism is more common on the right. Retroperitoneal lymph nodes are the most common site of metastasis; lymphatic spread occurs in a stepwise pattern. Within normal lymphatics, right testis tumors spread to interaortocaval retroperitoneal nodes, while left testis tumors are to be para-aortic retroperitoneal nodes. Distant metastasis, in the order of most common to least common, includes lung, and liver, brain, bone, kidney, adrenal, gastrointestinal, and spleen.

Clinical Diagnosis and Staging

The most common presentation is painless mass or swelling in the testis, usually found incidentally by the patient or his partner. Physical examination will reveal a firm, tender, or nontender testis mass. About 5–10% of men may present with a hydrocele which can obscure examination of any potential tumor (Ghoreifi and Djaladat, 2019). Other presenting symptoms can include clues to metastatic disease such as abdominal mass, supraclavicular mass, shortness of breath, or hemoptysis. Back pain can occur with bulky retroperitoneal metastasis and is more commonly seen with non-seminomas. Clinical staging is assigned using the 2010 AJCC TMN staging for testis cancer (Table 20.2).

History and Physical Examination

A key point in the history of men presenting with a testis mass is their personal history of cryptorchidism: where the testicle was located and at what age they underwent orchiopexy. There can be a typical delay in seeking treatment from 3 to 6 months after a nodule is noticed by the individual; length of delay correlates with the risk for metastasis. A history of acute testicular pain may be an indication of intratesticular hemorrhage or infarction.

Physical examination includes careful examination of the genitals, lymph nodes, abdomen, and breast tissue. A mass may be readily noted on examination of the testis; if the mass is sizable enough, there may also be erythema and pain associated with the examination due to distention of the scrotal skin. Transillumination of the scrotum will yield no evidence of light passing through scrotum. The patient abdomen may reveal bulky retroperitoneal disease, if the patient is thin enough. Gynecomastia may also be present.

Diagnostic Tests

A scrotal ultrasound is mandatory when physical exam reveals any testicular mass. If the scrotal ultrasound confirms a mass, tumor markers (Table 20.3) should be ordered along with liver function tests, creatinine, and CBC. Testosterone, FSH, and LH may be added if the patient is particularly interested in his fertility status pre- and posttreatment. If scrotal ultrasound is inconclusive then an MRI of the pelvis/scrotum may be obtained. An MRI of the testis is quite sensitive in diagnosing

Table 20.2 TMN staging of testicular tumors

Primary tumor (T)	
pTx	Primary tumor cannot be assessed
pT0	No evidence of primary tumor
pTis	Intratubular germ cell neoplasia
pT1	Tumor limited to the testis and epididymis without lymphovascular invasion; may invade the tunica albuginea but not the tunica vaginalis
pT2	Tumor limited to the testis and epididymis with lymphovascular invasion or tumor involving the tunica vaginalis
pT3	Invasion into spermatic cord with or without lymphovascular invasion
pT4	Invasion of scrotum with or without lymphovascular invasion
Regional lymph nodes (clinical) (N)	
Nx	Regional lymph nodes cannot be assessed
N0	No regional lymph node metastasis
N1	Metastasis within one or more lymph nodes <2 cm in size
N2	Metastasis within one or more lymph nodes >2 cm but <5 cm in size
N3	Metastasis within one or more lymph nodes >5 cm in size
Regional lymph nodes (pathologic) (N)	
Nx	Regional lymph nodes cannot be assessed
N0	No regional lymph node metastasis
N1	Metastasis within 1–5 lymph nodes; all node masses <2 cm in size
N2	Metastasis within a lymph node >2 cm but not >5 cm in size, or >5 lymph nodes involved, none >5 cm; none demonstrating extranodal extension
N3	Metastasis within one or more lymph nodes >5 cm in size
Distant metastasis (M)	
Mx	Distant metastasis cannot be assessed
M0	No distant metastasis
M1	Distant metastasis
M1a	Nonregional nodal or pulmonary metastasis
M1b	Distant metastasis at site other than nonregional lymph nodes or the lung
Serum tumor markers (S)	
Sx	Tumor markers not available or performed
S0	Tumor markers within normal limits
S1	LDH <1.5× normal, hCG <5000 IU/L, AFP <1000 ng/mL
S2	LDH 1.5–10× normal, hCG 5000–50,000 IU/L, AFP 1000–10,000 ng/mL
S3	LDH >10× normal, hCG >50,000 IU/L, AFP >10,000 ng/mL

Adapted from AJCC Cancer Staging Manual (2010) (National Comprehensive Cancer Network Clinical Practice Guidelines, 2018)

malignant versus benign testicular masses, yet is not considered to be a cost effective option. It is not recommended to be performed on a regular basis and is only suggested in the rare case that the scrotal ultrasound does not confirm the diagnosis (Thomas, et al. 2019; Mathur and Spektor, 2019). Chest X-ray should also be ordered; if the clinician's suspicion is high for a testicular neoplasm, a CT scan of the abdomen and pelvis with contrast can be ordered, anticipating the need for staging studies. It is important to note that abdominal CT scan has a 30% false negative rate—some men will have tumor in the retroperitoneal nodes. Additional workup is performed after a radical inguinal orchiectomy and confirmation of tumor pathology.

Table 20.3 Discussion of testicular cancer tumor markers

Marker	Non-seminoma germ cell tumors (NSGCT)	Yolk sac tumor	Seminoma	Embryonal carcinoma	Choriocarcinoma
Alphafetoprotein (AFP)	Elevated in 50–80%	Produced	Not produced	Not produced	Not produced
β-Human chorionic gonadotropin (bHCG)	Elevated in 20–60%	Never produced	Elevated in 15%	Produced	High levels
Lactate dehydrogenase (LDH)	Elevated but nonspecific	Nonspecific but produced	Nonspecific but produced	Nonspecific but produced	Nonspecific but produced

Table 20.4 Recommendations for a stage I seminoma surveillance

Year	1	2	3	4	5
History and physical exam	Every 3–6 months	Every 6–12 months	Every 6–12 months	Every 12 months	Every 12 months
Beta-HCG, AFP, and LDH	Optional	Optional	Optional	Optional	
Abdominal/pelvic CT	At 3, 6, 12 months	Every 6–12 months	Every 6–12 months	Every 12–24 months	Every 12–24 months
Chest X-ray	As clinically indicated				

Management

Radical inguinal orchiectomy is the standard of treatment when a primary testis cancer is suspected. This involves complete removal of the testicle and spermatic cord to the level of the internal inguinal ring, through inguinal incision. Management and surveillance are based on type of and stage of the tumor and can involve surveillance (Table 20.4), radiation therapy, or chemotherapy. Platinum is the most effective chemotherapeutic agents against germ cell tumors, but can result in long-term arrest of spermatogenesis.

Some men may need retroperitoneal lymph node dissection (RPLND) for bulky disease; this eliminates possible relapse and a simpler regimen for follow up. Some centers may offer this option laparoscopically. In many men RPLND leads to ejaculatory dysfunction.

Perioperative Management
All men preparing to be treated for a testicular mass should be offered the opportunity for sperm cryopreservation. Many men with a diagnosis of testicular neoplasm suffer from pretreatment subfertility, meaning that their sperm production has been

in some way adversely affected by the presence of the testicular neoplasm. In the majority of patients, their sperm production will rebound; however, if they are treated with radiation or chemotherapy, this rebound can be unpredictable and may occur over 5 years.

All team members caring for patients with testicular cancer must be sensitive to the fact that this treatment can have significant psychosocial and sexual implications for men, independent of their age and independent of the stage of their tumor. Men may benefit from psychosocial counseling and possibly counseling with a specialized sex therapist as well. Emphasis should be placed on the curability of testicular neoplasms, regardless of stage. Men may be offered information about a testicular prosthesis, although there may be issues relative to insurance coverage of these devices.

Long-Term Management
Specific long-term follow-up is dependent on the biology of the tumor, in conjunction with the tumor markers and their changes after removal of the testicle. The highest risk for recurrence is generally in the first 2 years after initial treatment. For germ cell tumors, follow-up involves regular tumor markers, imaging, and physical examinations. Men should be taught self-examination of the remaining testis. Any evidence of recurrence on imaging studies will require surgical resection.

Because of the success of treatment for testicular neoplasms, there can be issues of survivorship for these men, especially relative to the late effect of treatments. This can include monitoring for risk of cardiovascular disease, secondary malignancies such as leukemia, ongoing sub- or infertility, kidney dysfunction, lung toxicity, anxiety, or depression.

Cultural Considerations with Penile and Testicular Neoplasms

Because of the private nature and reproductive and sexual functions inherent to the genitals, all team members caring for these men should be sensitive to the potential for cultural, religious, and social implications involved with treatment. Penile cancer is very rare in Jewish men where circumcision is an accepted ritual and higher in Muslim populations where circumcision at puberty is a ritual. These factors may influence their comfort level with providers of the opposite gender and influence an individual's choice to seek treatment. Survivorship for men with testicular cancer is vital, as the disease is curable at almost every stage of presentation.

Clinical Pearls
- All testicular masses should be considered tumors until proven otherwise.
- A scrotal ultrasound is mandatory for any suspected testicular mass.
- Penile cancer is strongly linked to HPV strains, especially HPV-16.
- *Clinical* staging for testicular cancers is very important.
- Men undergoing surgery for penile or testicular cancer may benefit from psychosocial support, due to the disfiguring nature of the surgery.

Resources for the Nurse Practitioner

American Cancer Society: www.cancer.org

NCCN Clinical Practice Guidelines in Oncology (NCCN Guidelines®) www.nccn.org

Testicular prosthesis: http://www.coloplast.us/torosa-en-us.aspx

RESOLVE: The National Infertility Association: www.resolve.org

American Society for Reproductive Medicine: http://www.reproductivefacts.org

Resources for the Patient

American Cancer Society: www.cancer.org

The Urology Care Foundation: www.urologyhealth.org/urologic-conditions/penile-cancer

Testicular Cancer Foundation: www.testicularcancer.org

RESOLVE: The National Infertility Association: www.resolve.org

American Society for Reproductive Medicine: http://www.reproductivefacts.org

References

Albers P, Albrecht W, Algaba F, European Association of Urology et al (2011) EAU guidelines on testicular cancer: 2011 update. Eur Urol 60:304–319

American Joint Committee on Cancer (2010) Penis. In: Edge SB, Byrd DR, Compton CC et al (eds) AJCC cancer staging manual, 7th edn. Springer, New York, NY, pp 447–455

Clark PE, Spiess PE, Agarwal N, Biogioli MC, Eisenberger M, Greenberg RE, Herr HW, Inman BA, Kuban DA, Kuzel TM, Lele SM, Michalski J, Pagliaro L, Pal SK, Patterson A, Plimack ER, Pohar KS, Porter MP, Richie JP, Sexton WJ, Shipley WU, Small EJ, Trump DL, Wile G, Wilson TG, Dwyer M, Ho M (2013) Penile cancer: clinical practice guidelines in oncology. J Natl Compr Cancer Netw 11(5):594–615

Ghoreifi A, Djaladat H (2019) Management of primary testicular tumor. Urol Clin N Am 46:333–339

Mathur M, Spektor M (2019) MR imaging of the testicular and extratesticular tumors; when do we need? Magn Reson Imaging Clin N Am 27:151–171

Thomas L, Brooks M, Stephenson A (2019) The role of imaging in the diagnosis, staging, response to treatment, and surveillance of patients with germ cell tumors of the testis. Urol Clin N Am 46:315–331

Radiology in Urologic Patients

Ahmed El-Zawahry

Contents

A. El-Zawahry (✉)
Division of Urology, Southern Illinois University School of Medicine, Springfield, IL, USA
e-mail: Ahmed.ElZawahry@UToledo.Edu

© Springer Nature Switzerland AG 2020
S. A. Quallich, M. J. Lajiness (eds.), *The Nurse Practitioner in Urology*,
https://doi.org/10.1007/978-3-030-45267-4_21

Objectives
1. Explain common radiologic procedures and their indications in urology.
2. Review appropriate indications and patient preparation [as appropriate] for these studies.
3. Discuss benefits/risks associated with radiation exposure.
4. Determine appropriate radiation modality based on clinical concern, and specific advantages and limitations of each study.

Imaging in radiology is an important and integral part of urologic patient evaluation. Most urologic diseases will need confirmation by an appropriate radiology test. However, one should be alert to possible risks associated with radiation exposure. Radiation safety knowledge is important to balance risks/benefits associated with radiation exposure.

This chapter will act as a guide to choosing the correct diagnostic test modalities. Different imaging techniques are available and in this chapter, various modalities will be explored.

Plain Abdominal X-ray (KUB)

A simple plain film of the abdomen is a quick tool to help to visualize radiopaque calculi in the urinary tract. Currently, plain films are replaced by digital imaging in most of the locations. Radiation exposure is low and is about 0.53–0.7 millisieverts (mSv) (ACR 2020). Radiation exposure is less with fluoroscopy when compared to conventional plain film.

Indications

1. Assess the presence of radiopaque calculi. Small or faint calculi may not be visualized especially if patient is constipated.
2. Visualize kidney shadow and other soft tissue shadows.
3. Assess bone for any abnormalities.
4. Assess patients with constipation and voiding dysfunction related to constipation.

Patient Preparation

1. No special preparation is needed in most patients.
2. Bowel preparation may be needed in patients with constipation.

Contraindications

1. Pregnancy

Basic Equipment and Techniques

- X-ray machine has several components. A high voltage power supply, an X-ray tube, a collimating device, an X-ray detector or film. In addition, an electronic image intensifier and an image display system for fluoroscopic machines. Most of the images are stored and displayed digitally.
- **Image Recording:** Conventional recording of an X-ray image uses film and intensifying screens. The image intensifier and camera can be used to capture dynamic and static images. Real-time images are now typically recorded using conventional or digital video. Conventional spot or cine images may be acquired on X-ray film or digitally recorded.

Intravenous Urogram (IVU)

Also known as excretory urography or intravenous pyelogram (IVP), IVU is used to evaluate the upper urinary tract for abnormalities. IVU is rarely used these days if CT scans or MRI are available since more information can be obtained. However, it can be used in certain circumstances especially if the information needed is not obtained from the CT scan. In some instances, it can be done in conjunction with a CT scan evaluation to help to obtain more information.

This study includes:

- A preliminary plain film of the abdomen,
- This is followed by IV contrast based on the body weight,
- Subsequent films at different time intervals to obtain a good image of the kidneys at the nephrogram phase followed by a good film at excretory phase. It requires about 4–6 films. This can be tailored to patient condition, preference, and clinical diagnosis. Radiation exposure is about 2.0–2.5 mSv.

Indications

IVU is widely replaced by other more sensitive cross imaging studies (CT or MRI) in most indications. They are rarely used except when the other images are not available (Ramchandani 2014).

1. Hematuria: It helps to evaluate both the renal parenchyma, the pelvicalyceal system, the ureters, and the urinary bladder.
2. Urinary calculi: IVU can help to identify the location of the stones and assess the urinary tract. It helps to assess the kidneys and help to diagnose obstruction.
3. Urothelial cancer: IVU can be used for surveillance in patients with urothelial cancer.
4. Recurrent urinary tract infections.
5. Evaluation of kidney lesions.
6. Urgent evaluation of renal trauma. In cases of renal trauma or intraoperative questions about urinary tract, an IV bolus of contrast material could be used. This will help to visualize kidneys and ureters as well as bladder. The proper dosing would be 2 mL/kg with a maximum of 150 mL. The film can be taken in 2–10 min after injection.

Proper Preparation Includes

- Exclude patients at risk of contrast allergies.
- Bowel cleansing is helpful but not mandatory.
- Proper hydration is important to avoid contrast material adverse events. Some advocate limiting fluid intake before the study to have a proper concentration of contrast material. If this technique is adopted, it should be used cautiously in patients with possible kidney diseases or chronic renal insufficiency.

Contraindications

- Pregnancy
- Allergy to contrast material. It is usually contraindicated to use contrast materials if there is history of adverse reaction to contrast material. This will be discussed separately. It is better to use other cross-sectional modalities if available.

Complications

- Allergic reactions
- Contrast material complication.

Retrograde Urogram (Retrograde Pyelogram, RP)

Retrograde urography is a minimally invasive procedure that is performed under sterile conditions where cystoscopy and fluoroscopy are needed.

Retrograde urograms may be necessary if excretory urograms or CT urogram (CTU) are unsatisfactory, if the patient has a history of adverse reaction to intravenous contrast media, or if other methods of imaging are unavailable or inappropriate.

This study includes:

- Cystoscopy for evaluation of the bladder and identifying the ureteric orifice.
- A radiopaque contrast medium is used at the proper concentration.
- A ureteral catheter (open tip or other types) is used to enable injection of the contrast into the ureter and the collecting system.
- Fluoroscopy machine.
- Form of anesthesia (general anesthesia or monitored anesthesia).

Indications

- Visualize the pelvicalyceal system and the ureters if they were not properly visualized on cross-sectional imaging.
- Allergy or contraindications to IV contrast material.
- Evaluate the level of urinary tract obstruction if CT scan or MRI is not informative/available.
- Evaluation of patients with hematuria if CT scan or MRI is contraindicated or more evaluation is needed.

Patient Preparation

- Obtain urine culture before the intervention to rule out the presence of active UTI.
- Caution should be exercised in patients with contrast allergy but it is not a contraindication to proceed.
- Proper assessment for general anesthesia.

Contraindications

- Active urinary tract infections
- Pregnancy

Complications

- Urinary tract infections and possible sepsis especially in patients with untreated active infections.
- Ureteral injury: can range from minor mucosal tear or ureteral perforation.
- Ureteral damage or avulsion: complete ureteral damage is a serious problem but extremely rare when all the ureter is damaged.
- Contrast extravasation which has no consequences but if extensive may require prolonged stent placement (usually 7–10 days).
- Allergic reaction although it is not a contraindication to the procedure but exercise caution during the procedure. Patients with contrast allergy may need to be premedicated reaction may occur if extensive contrast extravasation occurs during the procedure.

Antegrade Pyelography

It is a study where the pelvicalyceal system and ureter are visualized by injecting contrast material in an antegrade fashion through percutaneous access of the kidney.
  This study includes:

- Accessing the kidney percutaneously using a percutaneous needle to inject the contrast material or using a preexisting renal tube (nephrostomy tube).
- Injecting contrast material through the needle or the nephrostomy tube.
- Using fluoroscopy.
- Taking pictures as needed.

Patient Preparation

- Obtain urine culture before intervention to rule out the presence of active UTI.
- Caution should be exercised in patients with contrast allergy but it is not a contraindication to proceed.
- Proper assessment for general anesthesia if needed.
- Hold anticoagulation therapy prior to attempt to access the kidney (discuss with PCP or cardiologist time frame).

Indications

- Visualize the upper tract when other images are not satisfactory.
- Evaluate the level of obstruction of the urinary tract if the whole ureter or portion of the ureter is not visualized through retrograde ureterogram.
- As a part of other surgeries.

Contraindications

- Active urinary tract infection.
- Uncontrolled coagulopathy.

Complications

- Injury to neighboring organs or structures during access.
- Bleeding.
- Sepsis in patients with active urinary tract infections.
- Urinary tract infections.
- Contrast extravasation which is not serious except in patients with contrast material allergy.

Voiding Cystourethrogram (VCUG)

The aim of this study is to visualize the anatomy of the urinary bladder and the urethra during voiding. This will allow the visualization of the bladder and the urethra and identify anatomical and some functional abnormalities in the lower urinary tract.
   This study includes:

- Inserting a urethral catheter into the bladder.
- A radiopaque contrast medium instilled into the bladder.
- Amount of dye should be about 300 cc or until the patient feels the urge to void.
- Fluoroscopy machine.
- Usually, no anesthesia is required.
- The patient is allowed to void while taking different pictures with fluoroscopy.

Indications

- Evaluation of possible anatomic abnormalities especially in pediatric population. Examples: Posterior urethral valve, vesicoureteral reflux especially in children with fever and recurrent urinary tract infections.
- Evaluation of possible causes of voiding dysfunction especially in patients with neurogenic bladder.
- Evaluation of some patients with urethral stricture.

Patient Preparation

- Obtain urine culture prior to intervention to rule out the presence of active UTI
- Caution should be exercised in patients with contrast allergy but it not a contraindication to proceed.

Contraindications

- Active urinary tract infections.
- Recent bladder surgery is a relative contraindication.

Complications

- Urinary tract infection.
- Dysuria.
- Minimal bleeding may occur after the procedure.

Retrograde Urethrogram (RUG)

The aim of this study is to visualize the anatomy of the urethra in male patients. This usually helps to visualize the anterior urethra since the posterior urethra is usually difficult to visualize because of the competent external urethral sphincter.

This study includes:

- Inserting a urethral catheter into the tip of the urethra and inflate the balloon with about 2 mL of water. This will allow the balloon to settle in the fossa navicularis.
- A radiopaque contrast medium injected into the urethra. A high-pressure injection should be avoided to avoid extravasation of contrast.
- Fluoroscopy machine to take appropriate pictures. Films should be done in anteroposterior and oblique views.
- Usually, no anesthesia is required.

Indications

- Assessment of the urethra in case of suspected urethral trauma. Consider in patients who present with blood drop at the urethral meatus after trauma.
- Evaluation of patients with known or suspected urethral stricture disease.
- Visualization of the urethra in case of suspected urethral disease such as urethra diverticula or fistula.

Patient Preparation

- Obtain urine culture prior to intervention to rule out the presence of active UTI.
- Caution should be exercised in patients with contrast allergy but it is not a contraindication to proceed.

Contraindications

- Active urinary tract infection.
- Caution should be adopted in patients with contrast allergy. Consider premedication.

Complications

- Urinary tract infection.
- Dysuria.
- Minimal bleeding may occur after the procedure.

Renal Nuclear Scan (Radionuclide Imaging)

The aim of this study is to assess kidney function, perfusion and/or obstruction using nuclear scans (Ramchandani 2014).

This study includes:

- A specific radioactive isotope tracer, injected IV.
- Gamma camera to capture the tracer.
- Many images are obtained depending on the type of information needed.
- A diuretic such as furosemide may be given at certain time to help with assessment of renal obstruction.

Indications

- Assessment of glomerular filtration rate (GFR). This will help to obtain information about split renal function.
- Evaluation of kidney obstruction.
- Evaluation of patients with kidney transplant to rule out the presence of obstruction, lack of perfusion from renal artery stenosis, presence of renal tubular necrosis or rejection.
- May be used to follow up of patients with vesicoureteral reflux (VUR).
- Evaluation of patients with acute scrotum. It helps to rule out testicular hypoperfusion secondary to torsion.
- In PET scans.

Patient Preparation

- No specific patient preparation is needed.
- Patients should have an empty bladder. A Foley catheter may be inserted in some patients during the study to ensure empty bladder.

Contraindications

- Active urinary tract infection.

Complications

1. Urinary tract infection.
2. Dysuria.
3. Minimal bleeding may occur after the procedure.

Angiography

It is the study where the contrast material is injected to visualize the arterial and venous system. This may be requested in urology patients in certain conditions.

Indications (Bishoff and Art 2016)

- Renal artery stenosis if suspected from clinical history. However, this is largely replaced by CT angiography or MR angiography.
- Preoperative evaluation for patients who may have arterial anomalies.
- Renal trauma, when vascular lesions are suspected.
- Postoperative bleeding if arterial injury or arteriovenous fistula are suspected?
- Adrenal gland tumors if adrenal vein sampling is desired.
- Varicocele: Patients with varicocele who would prefer embolization for treatment.

Complications

Complications after these procedures are rare and include but not limited to:

- Pain at the site of the puncture.
- Bleeding.
- Bruises at the site of the puncture.
- If embolization is used, it may lead to loss of the organ (very rare).
- Infection.

Contraindication

- Allergy to contrast material.
- Active infection at the site of injection.

Ultrasonography (US)

The most commonly utilized imaging modalities for urologic patients' evaluation. It has the advantages of being noninvasive with no radiation exposure and real-time evaluation. Gray-scale imaging allows for the evaluation of the anatomy and architecture structure of the organs while Doppler imaging allows to assess the vascularity and direction of blood flow in the organs and masses. Three-dimensional imaging allows for better quality evaluation. Different transducers are used based on the organs needed to be examined (Bishoff and Art 2016; Ramchandani 2014; Wieder 2014).

There are different probes that are used for the ultrasound examinations. It depends on the organ to be evaluated. There are also different frequencies of the probe. The lower the frequency of the probe, the deeper penetration of the tissues. For this reason, low-frequency probes such as 3–5 MHz are used for the kidneys. The high-frequency probes 6–7.5 MHz are usually used for the transvaginal or the transrectal ultrasound examinations. While higher frequency probes 7.5–10 MHz are usually used for more superficial tissues such as penile and scrotal evaluation (Wieder 2014).

Patient Preparation

1- There is not specific preparation needed.
2- It is possible to consider treatment of constipation prior to evaluation with US.
3- Good hydration may be helpful but not required.

Indications

Ultrasound has different utilization based on the organs needed to be evaluated. Different probes are used based on the organ and depth of penetration.

Kidneys

1. Kidney architecture and rule out obstruction.
2. Evaluation and surveillance of suspected kidney lesion or mass.
3. Assessment of kidney architecture in case of impaired renal function.
4. Evaluation of renal cysts.
5. Evaluation of rental transplant using Gray-scale and color Doppler.
6. Evaluation of perinephric collection.
7. Renal access for biopsy and procedures.
8. Intraoperative to help identifying kidney lesions during partial nephrectomy or ablation of lesions.
9. Antenatal kidney evaluation for hydronephrosis.
10. Evaluation of kidneys with unresolved infection to rule out the presence of renal abscess.
11. Monitoring renal abscess for improvement with treatment.

Urinary Bladder

1. Evaluation of the bladder for abnormalities such as stones, diverticula, or masses.
2. Measurement of residual urine.
3. Assess for the presence of urine efflux based on visualization of ureteral jets to rule out kidney obstruction (Wieder 2014).
4. Bladder access for procedure.

Prostate

1. Evaluation of the prostate and seminal vesicles.
2. Transrectal Ultrasound for evaluation of the prostate and other pelvic organs.
3. Transrectal US guided biopsy or aspiration of cysts.
4. Part of MRI fusion biopsy.

Scrotum (Ramchandani 2014)

1. Evaluation of scrotal and scrotal contents.
2. Evaluation of acute scrotum using color Doppler.
3. Undescended testis.
4. Assessment of cord lesions or varicocele.

Genital Evaluation

1. Evaluation of patients with erectile dysfunction using color Doppler.
2. Localizing plaques in patient with Peyronie disease.
3. Evaluation of patients with suspected penile fracture.
4. Pelvic or translabial US in women may help to identify anatomy and location or urethral diverticula and slings or mesh used for pelvic floor construction.

Complications

No complications.

Contraindications

There are no contraindications to using ultrasounds. It is a safe modality to use and it is good to consider for evaluation of pregnant women. However, it should be noted that interpretation of the US is operator dependents. Some difficulty may be encountered with patients who experience obesity or abnormal body habitus. Renal ultrasound will not visualize a stone in the ureters.

Computed Tomography (CT) Scan

A collimated X-ray beam that is taken in cross-sectional slices with variable thickness. Thickness can vary according to the indication for the study from 3 mm to 1 cm. It can be used with or without contrast depending on the organ and pathology under evaluation. It is the most versatile and most common used modalities for evaluation of urologic disease (Ramchandani 2014). It is more informative and more accurate than IVU in diagnosis of upper urinary tract abnormalities.

Radiation exposure is higher than KUB. It is estimated to be approximately 4–14 mSv per study. This could increase with increasing CT scan studies by obtaining series. If a CT scan without contrast and then a CT scan with contrast are obtained then that exposure increases.

Patient Preparation

1. Proper hydration when the contrast material is used.
2. Caution should be exercised in patients with contrast allergy but it is not a contraindication to proceed.
3. Pregnancy test in sexually active women of child bearing age.

Indications

1. Evaluation and assessment of patients with urolithiasis.
2. Evaluation and staging of renal mass.
3. Surveillance of renal mass postoperatively.
4. Assessment of renal cyst.
5. Evaluation for urinary obstruction and causes of obstruction

Complications

1. Radiation exposure for a CT scan abdomen and pelvis is about 10 mSv while it is more with CT urogram. It is usually >1.5 times of the radiation exposure of IVU.
2. These related to contrast material.

Magnetic Resonance Imaging (MRI)

MRI is a valuable cross-sectional imaging for the evaluation of soft tissues. It has less radiation exposure and is a good alternative option in patients who are allergic to contrast materials. MRI can be used with or without contrast. Gadolinium is the contrast used.

Patient Preparation

1. Ensure that the patient does not have any metal implants in the body.
2. Patients who are known to have claustrophobia may not be candidates for this study and may require additional preparation.

Indications (Ramchandani 2014)

1. Evaluation of soft tissue mass.
2. Characterization of renal mass or cyst especially if other modalities are not conclusive.
3. The image of choice for visualization of venous thrombus associated with renal cancer.
4. Staging of cancer, especially if more information about soft tissue invasion is needed.
5. May help with the evaluation of urinary obstruction, however, it is not good for stones visualization.
6. Diagnosis of Pheochromocytoma which will appear bright on MRI.
7. Dynamic MRI may be helpful for evaluation of pelvic organ prolapse.
8. Multiparametric MRI is currently used for providing anatomic details about prostate cancer. It is used in conjunction with MRI fusion technology for prostate biopsy in selected patients.
9. It is the image of choice for evaluation of pelvic lesions such as urethral diverticulum.

Contraindications

- Patients with metal implants.
- Patients who have chronic renal insufficiency that may be predisposed to contrast reaction.

Complications

- Nephrogenic systemic sclerosis associated with using gadolinium contrast.

Contrast Materials

Contrast media is very important to understand. Often used frequently to visualize the urinary tract system, contrast media help to improve resolution and differentiation between different organs and structures. The extracellular distribution of these agents results in improved contrast resolution and conspicuity of various structures. It also may help in the differential diagnosis of pathologies in organs. It can help to differentiate between benign renal lesions and malignant lesions. It can help to identify different types of cysts.

Made of water-soluble iodinated compounds, contrast media when excreted form a radiopaque image. Primarily used in IVU, different interventional radiology procedures, and CT scans.

The contrast material can be injected directly intravenous (IV) in case of IVU and CT scans. It also could be instilled directly into the urinary tract. In interventional radiology procedures, the contrast material can be used in different ways. Direct instillation to the collecting system or bladders uses similar media diluted to 15–45% concentration. This technique can avoid the risks of intravenous contrast material. When instilled into the bladder (cystography or cystogram) helps to visualize the bladder and identify bladder pathology if done correctly. The collecting system and ureters could be visualized by directly injecting contrast material into the collecting system. It can be performed in an antegrade fashion through a nephrostomy tube or retrograde fashion using cystoscopy and ureteric catheters.

The contrast materials used in CT scan are of low osmolarity or iso-osmolarity which are better tolerated and have a less frequent adverse reaction when compared to high osmolarity contrast material. The regular dose of iodine is about 2 mL/kg bodyweight with a maximum of 150 mL.

Contraindications

- Chronic kidney insufficiency: Injecting contrast materials in patients with known renal insufficiency may add risks of deterioration of kidney function.
- Allergic reaction to contrast materials.
- Congestive heart failure (CHF): contrast material may add to the workload due to added osmotic load in patients with severe or uncontrolled CHF.
- Metformin: patients should stop the medication 24–48 h before the study and resume when kidney function is back to baseline about 48 h after contrast use. These patients rarely at risk of developing fatal lactic acidosis.

Complications

Contrast-Induced Nephrotoxicity
- Acute renal insufficiency in predisposed patients. In this situation, acute renal insufficiency may ensue and then return to its baseline within 14 days [3].
- To avoid this problem:
  - Patients should be well hydrated.
  - Avoid any nephrotoxic agents such as NSAID, ACE inhibitors, and diuretics within 24 h before the scan.
  - Consider using none–ionic low osmolality contrast material.

Adverse Reactions to Contrast Material
- **Predisposing conditions to contrast adverse reaction:**
  - Iodine allergy.
  - Renal insufficiency: This is the most important risk factor that should be looked for. It is associated with a higher risk of developing contrast-induced nephrotoxicity.

- History of asthma or diabetes.
- Severe cardiac disease and heart failure.
- Dehydration.
- Sickle cell anemia
- Hyperthyroidism.
- Adrenal pheochromocytoma.
- **Types of adverse reactions:**
  - These reactions are more common with high osmolar contrast materials and less common with low-osmolar or iso-osmolar contrast materials.
  - Anaphylaxis (idiosyncratic, anaphylactoid) (ACR 2020): This is a severe reaction that can occur without expectation. It is associated with severe anaphylaxis and could be fatal (Spring et al. 1997). These reactions are not dose dependent.
  - Non-idiosyncratic reactions: These are dose-dependent and are related to the osmolality, concentration, volume, and injection rate of contrast material (ACR 2020).
  - Symptoms of non-idiosyncratic reactions include (ACR 2020) Sever:
  - Mild reactions:

    Nausea, vomiting, cough, warmth, headache, dizziness, altered taste, itching, flushing, chills, sweats, rash and hives, nasal stiffness, swelling of the eyes, and increased anxiety.

    Treatment for this reaction usually requires reassurance and observation. Antiallergic H1 receptor blocker (diphenhydramine orally, intramuscular or IV 1–2 mg/kg up to 50 mg) may be used.
  - Moderate reactions:

    Tachycardia or bradycardia, dyspnea, pulmonary edema, hypertension or hypotension, bronchospasm, and laryngeal edema.

    Treatment and monitoring are necessary. Treatment depends on the symptoms and should consider hydrocortisone 100–500 mg IV or IM and B-agonist inhalation for bronchospasms.
  - Severe reactions:

    Severe laryngeal spasms, cardiopulmonary arrest, unresponsiveness, hypotension, convulsions, and arrhythmias.

    This is an emergency that requires prompt treatment with attention to proper management of cardiovascular and respiratory symptoms. Epinephrine, IV fluid, and oxygen are the treatment for this situation. Patients will need close monitoring.

Preparation of Patients with Contrast Allergy (Bishoff and Art 2016)

1. Antihistaminics (H1 or H2 blockers).
2. Steroids
3. Epinephrine

- Patients with high risk to contrast media severe adverse reactions should be premedicated. This premedication will not eliminate the risk of this reaction however it will help to control them.

- Strategies used include:
  - Using nonionic contrast media will help to reduce the risks, and
  - 50 mg p.o. at 13, 7, and 1 h before contrast media injection plus diphenhydramine 50 mg IV, IM or p.o. 1 h before contrast injection, OR
  - Methylprednisone (Medrol) 32 mg p.o. 12 and 2 h before contrast media injection plus diphenhydramine 50 mg IV, IM or p.o. 1 h before contrast injection.

Cautions in Using Contrast Material Should Be Exercised in These Patients

- Extra precautions should be considered in
  - Patients taking metformin as there is a risk of developing lactic acidosis. This may be fatal in 50% of patients with renal insufficiency.
  - Patients with chronic renal disease, DM and dehydration status as these may predispose to kidney damage secondary to contrast-induced nephropathy:

Gadolinium is a contrast material that is used with the MRI scan.

- **Nephrogenic systemic sclerosis**
  - When renal function (GFR) is less than 30 mL/min.
  - Fibrosis of the skin, subcutaneous tissues, lungs, esophagus, heart, and skeletal muscles.
  - Initial symptoms can occur between 2 and 90 days.
  - Starts by swelling of the distal extremities and then induration of the skin.
  - Death may result in some patients.

Radiation Safety

Radiation safety protocols should be followed to limit the hazards as much as possible (Table 21.1). Aim of radiation safety is to keep radiation exposure "as low as reasonably achievable (ALARA)."

How to reduce radiation exposure?

These are important considerations to remember:

Table 21.1 Radiation exposure to different modalities

Diagnostic modality	Expected radiation exposure dose (mSv)
Chest X-ray (PA film)	0.02
Lumbar spine	1.5
I.V. urogram	3
Upper G.I. exam	6
CT head	2
CT chest	7
CT abdomen	8
Coronary CT angiogram	16

Adapted from McCollough CH, Bushberg JT, Fletcher JG, Eckel LJ (2015) Answers to Common Questions About the Use and Safety of CT Scans. Mayo Clin Proc 90 (10):1380–1392. https://doi.org/10.1016/j.mayocp.2015.07.011

1. Distance: increased distance decreases radiation exposure. Radiation exposure is inversely related to square distance.
2. Time: limiting the time of exposure as much as possible is important.
3. Shielding: Using proper shields to minimize radiation exposure is crucial.
4. Exposure to body parts should be limited.
5. Risks include the development of cataract and radiation-induced cancer.

"Radiation dose during fluoroscopy is directly proportional to the **time of exposure** and to the **number of exposures.**"

One should not underestimate the effect of radiation exposure. The Food and Drug Administration (FDA) reported: "A CT examination with an effective dose of 10 mSv may be associated with an increase in the possibility of fatal cancer of approximately 1 chance in 2000." This issue raises concerns about the excessive use of CT scans. Some studies showed that a low dose (<3.5 mSv) and ultra-low dose CT scan (<1 mSv) may be helpful in the diagnosis of stones in patients in emergency department to reduce radiation exposure (Moore et al. 2016; Rodger et al. 2018) and avoid radiation exposure.

Clinical Pearls
- Confirm that list of patient allergies is current, to avoid contrast media reactions.
- When ordering imaging studies, consider the probable need for insurance prior authorization.
- Most GU imaging does not require patient preparation.
- For patients that have an extensive history of imaging or radiation used for treatment (e.g., stone or trauma patients) consider total radiation dose and consider a non-radiation test when appropriate.
- Always evaluate renal function prior to any exam that involves contrast media.
- Several factors impact an individual's risk from radiation exposure: age, gender, genetic factors, type of study, and the fractionation and protraction of the radiation.

References

(ACR) ACoR (2020) ACR Committee on Drugs and Contrast Media. https://www.acr.org/-/media/ACR/Files/Clinical-Resources/Contrast_Media.pdf. Accessed 2 Mar 2020

Bishoff JTR, Art R (2016) Urinary tract imaging: basic principles of computed tomography, magnetic resonance imaging, and a plain film. In: Wein AJ, Kavoussi L, Partin AW, Peters CA (eds) Campbell-Walsh urology, vol 1, 11th edn. Elsevier, Philadelphia, PA, pp 26–62e23. 19103-2899

McCollough CH, Bushberg JT, Fletcher JG, Eckel LJ (2015) Answers to common questions about the use and safety of CT scans. Mayo Clin Proc 90(10):1380–1392. https://doi.org/10.1016/j.mayocp.2015.07.011

Moore CL, Daniels B, Singh D, Luty S, Gunabushanam G, Ghita M, Molinaro A, Gross CP (2016) Ureteral stones: implementation of a reduced-dose CT protocol in patients in the emergency department with moderate to high likelihood of calculi on the basis of STONE score. Radiology 280(3):743–751. https://doi.org/10.1148/radiol.2016151691

Ramchandani P (2014) Diagnostic and interventional radiology. In: Hanno TJG PM, Malkowicz SB, Wien AJ (eds) Penn clinical manual of urology, 2nd edn. Saunders, Elsevier, Philadelphia, PA

Rodger F, Roditi G, Aboumarzouk OM (2018) Diagnostic accuracy of low and ultra-low dose CT for identification of urinary tract stones: a systematic review. Urol Int 100(4):375–385. https://doi.org/10.1159/000488062

Spring DB, Bettmann MA, Barkan HE (1997) Deaths related to iodinated contrast media reported spontaneously to the U.S. Food and Drug Administration, 1978-1994: effect of the availability of low-osmolality contrast media. Radiology 204(2):333–337. https://doi.org/10.1148/radiology.204.2.9240516

Wieder J (2014) Imaging and radiology. In: Pocket guide to urology, 5th edn. J-Wieder-Medical, Oakland, CA

Procedures for the Nurse Practitioner in Urology

22

Heather Schultz and Sarah R. Stanley

Contents

H. Schultz (✉) · S. R. Stanley
Department of Urology, University of North Carolina at Chapel Hill, Chapel Hill, NC, USA
e-mail: hschultz@med.unc.edu

© Springer Nature Switzerland AG 2020
S. A. Quallich, M. J. Lajiness (eds.), *The Nurse Practitioner in Urology*,
https://doi.org/10.1007/978-3-030-45267-4_22

Objectives
1. Describe indications for specific outpatient office-based procedures appropriate to the urology patient.
2. Review both provider and patient preparation.
3. Discuss necessary post-procedure monitoring and follow-up.

Introduction

Physician shortages have opened the doors for advanced practice nurses and physician assistants to enter into the field of urology. As a surgical subspecialty, urology provides opportunities for providers to perform procedures in both the OR and office. This chapter on clinic-based urologic procedures is not meant to be instructive on how to perform the procedures themselves. Rather, this chapter is meant to be a discussion of indications, follow-up, potential insurance issues, and resources for the advanced practice provider (APP). This chapter will act as a guide for the APP to begin their journey in learning procedures.

The procedures that are reviewed in this chapter are certainly not exhaustive, and there are many other procedures that APPs are performing that are not included. According to the 2010 AUA survey sent to the APRN/PA/allied health membership database with 205 respondents (included APNs, PAs, RNs, and other allied health members) and a 30% response rate, APRN/PAs were found to be performing urodynamics, stent removal, urethral dilation, vasectomy, injection treatment for priaprism, and bladder biopsy (prostate biopsy and cystoscopy were not reported). Quallich reported in a survey from 2011 (53 surveys and 46.7% response rate) that ANPs were performing a wide variety of procedures, some at very advanced levels. The primary cultural and religious considerations relative to these procedures relate to providers of the opposite sex performing procedures and need to be addressed as the situation requires.

It was found through Medicare claims of procedures performed by APPs that there has been a dramatic increase between 1994 and 2012. Cystoscopy was found to have a 7.483% increase, from annual frequency of 25 to 2635 procedures per year. Transrectal prostate biopsy was found to have a 4.806% increase, from annual frequency of 17 to 834 procedures per year (Langston et al. 2017a, b; Erickson et al. 2017). A national workforce study from 2015 found that of the 296 responders, 63% were performing procedures of moderate to high complexity. Furthermore, it was found that 81% of the APPs reported performing procedures in urology (Langston

2017a). In the same 2015 survey, as percentages related to this chapter, the following were reported as being performed:

- 8% diagnostic cystoscopy
- 2% cystoscopy with bladder biopsy
- 12% cystoscopy for difficult catheter placement
- 18% cystoscopy for stent removal
- 6% transrectal ultrasound guided prostate biopsy
- 4% penile Doppler
- 18% implant insertion (Testopel and Vantas)
- 3% XIAFLEX injection

For the purposes of this chapter, the following procedures will be the focus: cystoscopy (diagnostic and stent removal), prostate biopsy, Testopel®, Vantas®, urethral dilation, penile block, reduction of paraphimosis, and penile injection for Peyronie's disease.

This chapter should not act as the only consideration of reference for a procedure. Rather this chapter should act as a guide that will supplement the hands on training that you may get from national organization meetings and, most importantly, the training that you will get from your supervising/collaborating physician. Every practice will have their own intricacies/protocols for performance. Every state and institution will have their own laws/rules of the APP performing procedures. This would need to be researched through your local board, credentialing committee, hospital committee, supervising/collaborating physician, and/or practice manager.

The American Urological Association (AUA) consensus statement on utilization of APPs in urologic practice (http://www.auanet.org/advocacy/advanced-practice-providers.cfm) may also be referenced when thinking of how the APP role can be utilized.

Questions to Keep in Mind When Considering Learning Procedures
1. Is this part of my practice agreement with my supervising/collaborating physician?
2. Does the state and practice I work in allow me to perform the procedures?
3. If I am allowed, is there any training/tracking of progress that is required by either my state or practice?
4. Do I work in a supportive environment that will be willing to teach the skill?
5. How would I incorporate this skill into my practice and is there a need?

Two other important articles/statements that should be kept in mind that support the role of APPs in practice:

1. Institute of Medicine (2010)
2. Fairman et al. (2010)

Objectives

1. The learner will be able to identify three resources for beginning their didactic training.
2. The learner will be able to identify three pre-procedure considerations.
3. The learner will be able to name three post-procedure instructions.

Urethral Dilation

Define Procedure

Dilation of urethral strictures on awake patient with the goal of draining the bladder and temporarilly treating stricture until a more formal surgical repair can be performed. These techniques may include the use of filiforms/followers, flexible cystoscopy, and glide wires.

Indications

The most common reason for the need for catheter placement is the need for bladder emptying. The most common reasons for difficult urinary catheter placement are enlarged prostate, urethral stricture(s), bladder neck contracture, or false passage.

Prep Required

1. Ensure that patient does not have an active urinary tract infection (UTI), and, if suspicious, treat.
2. Antibiotic prophylaxis according to institution policy.

Pre-procedure Considerations

1. Urethral dilation in setting of infection can lead to sepsis.
2. Urethral dilation in setting of anticoagulation can lead to bleeding.
3. Urethral dilation is a painful procedure for awake patients.
4. Urethral dilation can cause rectal perforation in some patients, for example, post prostatectomy and pelvic radiation patients.
5. If the patient is an uncircumcised male, replace foreskin in the reduced position to prevent paraphimosis.
6. Trauma to the urethra can occur with use of Heyman or filiforms and followers.
7. Consider not performing dilation in unstable patients.
8. Consider not performing dilation in patients with pelvic fracture.
9. Vagal response can occur and can present with orbital numbness, hypotension, tachycardia, diaphoresis, syncope, and weakness.

Post-procedure Instructions to Call Clinic

1. Fever >101°F.
2. Foley blockage.
3. Severe abdominal pain or rectal pain/drainage.

Follow-up

1. Urethral stricture may be assessed with Uroflow, international prostatic symptom score.

Discussion

The trend is that urethral dilation on the awake patient is a temporary option until formal surgery can be achieved. With that said, the provider placing the catheter or perhaps in performance of diagnostic cystoscopy may run into the stricture etiology, such as a urethral stricture. Then the provider would have to decide how to proceed.

Referral Suggestions

1. Formal surgical repair can be considered after urethral dilation of either urethroplasty or bladder neck contracture repair and should be performed by a urethral surgeon.
2. Urethral dilation may make formal surgical repair more difficult.
3. Urethral surgeon may want imaging in the form of:
    (a) Retrograde urethrogram.
    (b) Voiding cystogram.

Insurance Issues

Reimbursement for urethral dilation has been low. So low that urologist will at times look for alternatives for a difficult urinary catheter placement. There are Foley catheter teams that have been put in place at some institutions to help meet this need by trained nurses or APPs. There has been a report that with the use of APPs, the quality of life of the urologist can be better. Urethral dilation can be seen as emergent at times, and preauthorization is typically not required in such cases.

1. Reimbursement has been reported to be low.
2. Can be an emergent procedure: prior authorization is not indicated.

Guidelines

1. No current guidelines exist for urethral dilation.

Option for Difficult Urinary Catheterization

1. http://www.percuvision.com/index.html for Direct vision® that is meant for nurses to have a visual guide for difficult urethral catheterization (DUC) in patients that have a history of DUC to help prevent the need for use of guide wires in the case of false passages.

Resources for Learning

AUA Core Curriculum Available at Auanet.org with Membership

1. Anatomy and physiology of the lower urinary tract

CME Review Article

1. AUA update series paid subscription. 2011 Urethral Dilation: Tricks of the trade Carlos Villanueva, M.D. and George P. Hemstreet III, M.D., Ph.D. vol 30 lesson 5.
   (a) Blitz technique is reviewed here for placement of glide wire through Foley

National and Local Meeting Courses

1. UAPA and SUNA National Meetings: Cystoscopy Course
   (a) Check specific details of course for urethral dilation or if just for performing cystoscopy depending on learning needs.

Book Chapters

1. Mendez-Probst et al.
2. Duffey and Monga
3. Chung et al.
4. Fulgham and Bishoff
5. Gerald and McCammon

General Urethral Stricture Management

1. Blitz (1995)
2. Mendez-Probst et al. (2012)
3. Villanueva and Hemstreet (2008)
4. Athanassopoulos et al. (2005)
5. Beaghler et al. (1994)
6. Chelladurai et al. (2008)
7. Krikler (1989)
8. Villanueva and Hemstreet (2010)
9. Freid and Smith (1996)

Journal Articles on Local Anesthetic Use
1. Tzortzis et al. (2009)
2. Ho et al. (2003)
3. Patel et al. (2008)

Cystoscopy

Define the Procedure

Cyctoscopy is performed with the goal of identifying lower urinary tract pathology by directly visualizing the anterior urethra, posterior urethra, and the bladder.

Indications

- Gross and microscopic hematuria
- Recurrent UTIs
- Trauma
- Obstructive voiding symptoms
- Irritative voiding symptoms
- Dysuria
- Atypical cytologies
- Bladder abnormalities on imaging studies
- Obstruction after transurethral resection of the prostate (TURP)
- Interstitial cystitis (or chronic pelvic pain syndrome)
- Known history of bladder cancer
- Incontinence
- Urethral stricture disease
- Hematospermia
- Pelvic mass
- Bladder stones
- Removal of foreign bodies
- Facilitate catheter insertion
- Suprapubic tube, Foley, or clean intermittent catheterization >5 to 10 years

Prep Required

1. Rule out active UTI.
2. Counsel patient regarding indications for procedure/informed consent.
3. Sterilely prep and drape.
4. Supine position for flexible cystourethroscopy (with a slight frog-leg position for females).
5. 5 to 10 mL of lubricant-anesthetic jelly should be instilled into the urethra before the procedure.

Pre-procedure Considerations

1. Stability of patient.
2. Active bleeding (may require irrigation).
3. Will urine for cytology be collected (if for diagnostic cystoscopy)?
4. Will antibiotics be given based on patient risk or facility policy?
   (a) High risk: Anatomic anomalies of the urinary tract, poor nutritional status, smoking, chronic corticosteroid use, immunodeficiency, externalized catheters, colonized endogenous/exogenous material, distant coexistent infection, and prolonged hospitalization (Wolf et al. 2008) otherwise can be avoided. If patient is not high risk but there is need for fulguration, biopsy, or catheterization, antibiotic should be used (Wolf et al. 2008).

Discussion/Pearls of Cystoscopy

1. Preventing procedural discomfort: Most studies will state that lubrication does not make a difference (Patel et al. 2008). Male patients may report more of a benefit, while female may not (Patel et al. 2008; Taghizadeh et al. 2006). Viewing the monitor and talking may benefit the patient through relieving anxiety and helping him/her feel more in control of the situation. This is most helpful for men when reaching the membranous urethra and prostate and encouraging relaxation (Taghizadeh et al. 2006).
   (a) Water-soluble lubricant-anesthetic.
   (b) Male: urethral clamp—30 mL of lubricant.
   (c) Position video tower in patient view.
   (d) Explain procedure in real time.
   (e) During entrance into membranous urethra, have patient relax pelvic floor muscles and wiggle toes.
2. Technique: Finding the female urethral meatus is the challenging aspect for the female patient. Obesity, estrogen-deficient tissue, and anatomic anomalies can make this a challenge. For the male patient, ensure penile stretch throughout the procedure for maximum visibility of the fossa navicularis, penile urethra, and bulbar urethra (Duffey and Monga)
   (a) Obese female may need assistance with positioning and visualization of the meatus.
   (b) Penile stretch: of 90° angle to the abdominal wall.
   (c) Penile stretch: The glans is held by the third and fourth digits, and the thumb and forefinger will remain free for guiding scope into the meatus.
   (d) Turn irrigation on once the tip is in the meatus.
   (e) With flexible scope: more anterior angulation aid in passage over the bladder neck in men.
   (f) You can drain the bladder for comfort once inspection is complete.
3. Special considerations:
   (a) Suprapubic tubes:
      • You may be able to navigate through the urethra, but, when not able, you may be able to navigate through the mature suprapubic tract.

- Guide wire through the suprapubic tract to aid the endoscope in difficult cases (Duffey and Monga).
  (b) Continent urinary diversions:
    - Understanding of construction:
      - Type and location of ureteroenteric anastomosis
      - Presence or absence of an afferent limb
      - Continence mechanism employed (Duffey and Monga)
    - Mucus, debris, bowel peristalsis, and mucosal folding may inhibit visualization.
4. Stent removal:
  (a) The process is similar to diagnostic cystoscopy.

Post-procedure Instructions/Red Flags

1. Fever over 101°F
2. Profuse urethral bleeding
3. Inability to void
4. Significant dysuria or abdominal pain

Referral Suggestions

1. For any findings that would require general anesthesia
2. For any finding that the APP is not trained in performing, e.g., urethral dilation and removal of small stone in the bladder

Resources for Learning and Suggested Reading

Joint AUA/SUNA White Paper on the reprocessing of flexible cystoscopes 2013: https://www.auanet.org/education/other-aua-clinical-guidance-documents.cfm or https://www.suna.org/resource/clinical-practice?page=1
Quallich et al (2020). Standardized Office Cystoscopy for Advanced Practice Providers in Urology. Urology Practice (7):228–233.

National and Local Meeting Courses
1. UAPA and SUNA national meetings: cystoscopy course.
  (a) Check specific details of course for stent removal or if just for performing cystoscopy depending on your learning needs.

Guidelines
1. No current US guidelines exist for cystoscopy.
2. UK guidelines: http://www.baus.org.uk/Updates/publications-new/flexi-cystoscopy.

AUA Core Curriculum Available at Auanet.org with Membership
1. Anatomy and physiology of the lower urinary tract

Book Chapters
1. Mendez-Probst et al.
2. Duffey and Monga
3. Chung et al.
4. Gerald and McCammon

Local Anesthetic Use and Discomfort
1. Tzortzis et al. (2009)
2. Ho et al. (2003)
3. Patel et al. (2008)
4. Patel et al. (2008)
5. Taghizadeh et al. (2006)

Antibiotic Prophylaxis
1. Herr (2014)
2. Jiménez-Pacheco et al. (2012)
3. Wilson et al. (2005)
4. Latthe et al. (2008)
5. Wolf et al. (2008)

Role of APP in Cystoscopy
1. Kleier (2009)
2. Quallich (2011)
3. Schultz (2011)
4. Chatterton (2010)
5. Fagerberg and Nostell (2005)
6. Gidlow et al. (2000)
7. Radhakrishnan et al. (2006)

Artificial Urinary Drainage and Surveillance
1. Subramonian et al. (2004)
2. Hess et al. (2003)

Complications
1. Sung et al. (2005)

Testopel® (Testosterone Pellets)

Define the Procedure

In-office procedure on awake patients using local anesthetic for insertion of pellets (each pellet 75 mg) of dissolvable testosterone into the subcutaneous tissue of the gluteal area.

Indications

Testosterone replacement therapy in adult males for conditions associated with low or absent testosterone from either primary hypogonadism (congenital or acquired) or hypogonadotrophic hypogonadism (congenital or acquired).

Contraindications

1. Men with known breast cancer and/or known or suspected prostate cancer
2. Pregnant women (not approved for use in women)

Warnings/May Cause

- Gynecomastia
- DVT/PE
- Edema
- BPH
- Prostate cancer
- With high doses for long periods of time, may cause peliosis hepatitis or hepatocellular carcinoma
- Hirsutism
- Male pattern baldness
- Abnormal liver function studies
- Polycythemia
- Prolonged erection
- Acne
- Increase or decrease in libido
- Depression and/or anxiety
- Generalized paresthesia
- Breast discomfort
- Decreased sperm count
- Rarely anaphylaxis
- Decreased size in testicles
- Decrease insulin dosage need

Site Reactions

1. Pain at insertion site
2. Scar development (site rotation decreases risk)
3. Infection
4. Bleeding
5. Expulsion of pellets

Patient Prep

1. Pre-labs as indicated: hematocrit/hemoglobin, PSA, total and free testosterone, liver function studies, and cholesterol.
2. Physical male GU exam as indicated.
3. Assess the skin for scar.
4. Informed consent.
5. Sterile prep of the skin.
6. Each pellet is supplied in a glass ampule. Careful inspection should be made of each ampule. When opening, care should be taken to open away from the sterile field to prevent small shards of glass from dropping on pellet tray.

Post-procedure Instructions/Red Flags

1. No soaking in water for 72 h.
2. No vigorous exercise for 72 h.
3. Bruising is typical.
4. Discomfort for the first couple of days may occur.
5. Leave bandage on for 24 to 48 h.
6. Steri-Strips will fall off in about 4 to 5 days.
7. No showering for 24 h.
8. Ice for about 15 min to help decrease swelling/pain.
9. Patient should report bleeding that is continuous, hematoma, expulsion of pellets from the site, fluid discharge from the site, exquisite tenderness to the site or discomfort that persists for more than 5 days, and erythema to the site that lasts longer than 5 days.

Discussion

The use of subcutaneous testosterone can be a great way to reduce risk of testosterone exposure to others and can eliminate the need for biweekly injection or daily application. Typical training is onsite at the facility, with instruction from a seasoned provider.

Dose adjustment is less flexible with Testopel® than with other products; if treatment needs to be discontinued, surgical removal of the pellets may be necessary. If patient is testosterone replacement naïve, consideration should be made for shorter-acting modalities, such as topical gels, that can be discontinued without the need for an invasive procedure. Starting with another product will also help establish a beginning dose for Testopel®. Dose adjustment can vary from patient to patient, based on sensitivity to medication and absorption rates. Starting doses can vary, but between 10 and 12 pellets is common (McCullough 2014; Mechlin et al. 2014; Pastuszak et al. 2012), with the higher end of dosing at 6 pellets. The maximum treatment number of pellets can be debated, and when considering dose adjustment, there should be continued communication with the provider-mentor in Testopel® management. There are no formalized guidelines on starting dose or dose adjustment; it is up to the patient/provider and joint decision-making. There is certainly an "art" to finding the therapeutic dose for each individual patient. Counseling the patient that there may be a "trial and error" period of dose adjustment is helpful to set expectations when initially starting Testopel®.

Expulsion of pellets is rare and can be avoided with proper technique in depth of pellet placement and use of proper aseptic technique (Kelleher et al. 1999). Stitches are not required; typically Steri-Strips are applied, but one suture can be used. If at any point there are side effects, they may be reported at www.fda.gov/medwatch.

Referral

1. Polycythemia: hematology
2. Surgical removal of pellets if discontinuation is needed
3. Maximum pellet allowance with suboptimal objective or subjective outcome

Insurance

1. Prior authorization recommended https://www.testopel.com/reimbursement for prior authorization forms and letter of medical necessity/appeals
2. Testopel® reimbursement hotline: 1–800–897–9006
3. Claim form: http://www.auanet.org/advnews/hpbrief/view.cfm?i=364&a=873

Billing Codes

CPT1 (procedure) code	*11, 980*	*Subcutaneous hormone pellet implantation (implantation of testosterone pellets beneath the skin)*
HCPCS code (private insurance)	S0189	Testosterone pellet, 75 mg
HCPCS code (Medicare)	J3490	Unclassified drugs
NDC (for Medicare claims except CA and NV)	66, 887–004–20	100-count box. Use in Box 19 of CMS 1500 form
NDC (for Medicare claims, CA and NV)	66, 887–004–10	10-count box. Use in Box 19 of CMS 1500 form

Retrieved from https://www.testopel.com/reimbursement

1. Coding hotline: AUA's coding hotline at 866-746-4282, option 2, or e-mail at codinghotline@AUAnet.org

Resources

Training Videos
1. Cartoon video: https://www.youtube.com/watch?v=KeS395ePpX4
2. Patient video: https://www.youtube.com/watch?v=O3kOY46ZakE
3. Other multiple videos available with search of Testopel® video

Guidelines: Currently no guidelines exist for management or placement of Testopel®.

Seminars
1. SUNA, UAPA, and AUA (regional and national) meetings with search of "Hands on Course"

Patient Satisfaction
1. Kovac et al. (2014)
2. Smith et al. (2013)

Dosing
1. McCullough et al. (2012)
2. McCullough (2014)
3. Mechlin et al. (2014)
4. Pastuszak et al. (2012)
5. Kelleher et al. (2004)

Complications
1. Kelleher et al. (1999)

Book Chapters
1. Morales
2. Paul

Vantas® (Histrelin Acetate)

Define the Procedure

In-office procedure using a local anesthetic for subcutaneous placement of long-term LHRH agonist (histrelin acetate) into the upper inner aspect of the nondominant arm. It requires removal and replacement yearly.

Indications

Metastatic prostate cancer with treatment of Vantas®, intended to help alleviate symptoms, but not cure.

Contraindications

1. Hypersensitivity to gonadotropin-releasing hormone
2. Pregnant women

Warnings/May Cause

- Hot flashes/night sweats
- Osteoporosis
- Decreased size of testicles
- If disease to the bone/spine, may cause increase in pain
- Gynecomastia
- Erectile dysfunction/decreased libido
- Fatigue
- Voiding complaints
- Constipation
- Increase in blood sugar
- Implant site reactions
- Convulsions
- Pituitary apoplexy
- Drug-induced liver injury
- Decrease in cognitive function
- Anemia
- Change in body habitus

Patient Prep

1. Pre-labs as indicated
2. Physical male GU exam as indicated
3. Assess the skin for scar
4. Informed consent
5. Sterile prep of the skin

Post-procedure Instructions/Red Flags

1. No soaking in water for 72 h.
2. No vigorous exercise for 72 h.
3. Bruising can occur.
4. Discomfort for the first couple of days may occur.
5. Leave bandage on for 24 to 48 h.
6. Steri-Strips will come off in about 4 to 5 days. Suture: follow-up based on type used.
7. No showering for 24 h.

8. Ice for about 15 min to help decrease swelling/pain.
9. Patient should report bleeding that is continuous, hematoma, expulsion of pellets from the site, fluid discharge from the site, exquisite tenderness to the site or discomfort that persists for more than 5 days, and erythema to the site that lasts longer than 5 days.

Insurance/Coding

Endo Pharmaceuticals Reimbursement Services: 1-800-462-ENDO NDC #: 67, 979-500-01, J code: J9225.
Administration (CPT Codes):

- 11981 insertion, nonbiodegradable drug delivery implant
- 11982 removal, nonbiodegradable drug delivery implant
- 11983 removal, with reinsertion, nonbiodegradable drug delivery implant

ICD-9-CM Code: 185 Prostate Cancer.

Discussion

The use of year long Vantas can help in those who do not want surgical castration, compliance, decreased visits, and decreased injections (Shore et al. 2012). It has been found that histrelin can be efficacious for several years for PSA suppression (Chertin et al. 2000), but one would need to consider cost-effectiveness. In one study that included 97 men who were on a LHRH agonist for a 10 year or longer period, there was a greater than 3.2 to 10.7 times the cost compared to that of bilateral orchiectomy (Mariani et al. 2001). It has been found that orchiectomy and the use of a LHRH agonist are both simillarily efficacious in the treatment for prostate cancer (Mariani et al. 2001). In the setting of the prostate cancer patient that only has a few months to live, the use of a LHRH agonist compared to bilateral orchiectomy is more cost-effective (Mariani et al. 2001). There are many reasons for patient decision for chemical versus surgical castration with the most common psychological implications of orchiectomy perhaps with the permanence of and body image issues (Nelson 2013).

Other considerations should be made with initiation of a LHRH agonist in the setting of metastatic disease to the spine and bones (in symptomatic patients) and the LH flare (Weckermann and Harzmann 2004). With this there may need to be consideration of complete androgen blockage with the use of antiandrogens prior to the use of a LHRH agonist to decrease risks associated with flare in particular pain (Labrie et al. 1987; Kuhn et al. 1989).

With regard to technique, anecdotally, if there is difficulty with removal of previous implant, transverse incision versus traditional horizontal incision may aid in the removal. With the obese patient, it may be difficult to palpate for the previous implant, and some facilities have the ability to ultrasound the arm in the room to help in the identification for removal. Stitches or surgical tape may be used for closure.

Cultural/Religious Considerations

1. Views of foreign body implantation for medical use

Referrals

1. Other urologic provider if unable to extract implant
2. Medical oncology in setting of castrate resistance

Resources and References

Websites
1. Vantas® official website: http://www.vantasimplant.com
2. Vantas® website for video of placement: http://www.vantasimplant.com/hcp/administration/
3. Vantas® website for patient brochures: http://www.vantasimplant.com/hcp/resource-center/

Dose Efficacy
1. Djavan et al. (2010)
2. Altarac (2011)
3. Schlegel (2009)
4. Chertin et al. (2000)
5. Schlegel and Histrelin Study Group (2006)
6. Mariani et al. (2001)
7. Weckermann and Harzmann (2004)

Tolerability
1. Shore et al. (2012)

Patient Safety
1. Ricker et al. (2010)
2. Labrie et al. (1987)
3. Kuhn et al. (1989)

Book Chapter
1. Nelson (2013)

Other Suggested Readings
1. Messing et al. (1999)
2. Prostate Cancer Trialists' Collaborative Group (2000)

Seminars

1. Local national meetings for SUNA, UAPA, and AUA with search of "Hands on Course"

Penile Nerve Block

Define the Procedure

Many in-office urologic procedures require regional anesthesia. A penile nerve block involves local infiltration of an injectable anesthetic into the base of the penis prior to proceeding with other penile procedures (Yachia 2007a, b).

Indications

- Circumcision
- Paraphimosis
- Dorsal slit
- Priapism
- Penile laceration
- Meatotomy
- Optical urethrotomy

Pre-procedure Preparation

- Informed consent should be obtained from the patient or patient's guardian prior to proceeding.
- Aseptic precautions should be used when prepping the patient.
- Avoid the use of epinephrine due to risk of ischemia.

Post Dorsal Penile Block Complications

- Pain at the injection site.
- Hematoma.
- Edema.
- Compression or vasospasm is rare but can occur with large volumes of anesthetic.

Follow-up

- As directed, based on the indication for the nerve block

Insurance Coverage

- Issues of coverage may come into play for the procedure being conducted, i.e., circumcision.

Resources

Online Videos
- Several videos are available through www.youtube.com.

Guidelines
- No current guidelines exist for dorsal penile block.

Book Chapters
- Lewis and Stephan (1997)
- Yachia (2007a, b)

Journal Articles on Penile Nerve Block
- Choe (2000)
- Serour et al. (1995)
- Kirya and Werthmann (1978)
- Stav et al. (1995)
- Snellman and Stang (1995)

Online Resources
- Up to date: Management of Zipper Injuries

References
1. Choe (2000)
2. Serour et al. (1995)
3. Kirya and Werthmann (1978)
4. Stav et al. (1995)
5. Snellman and Stang (1995)
6. Lewis and Stephan (1997)
7. Yachia (2007a)
8. Bothner (2014)

Reduction of Paraphimosis

Define the Procedure

Paraphimosis is a condition where the foreskin of the penis is retracted for a prolonged period of time, preventing normal advancement of the foreskin. This urologic emergency causes engorgement of the glans that can eventually result in infection, ischemia, and gangrene of the glans (Wein 2012b; Vunda et al. 2013). The procedure redues the paraphimosis through replacement of the foreskin to its normal anatomical position.

Indications

Reduction should be performed immediately once paraphimosis has been identified (Vunda et al. 2013).

Procedure

Paraphimosis reduction requires reducing the edema in the glans, ultimately allowing placement of the foreskin to its normal anatomical position (Turner et al. 1999; Dubin and Davis 2011; Pohlman 2012). Paraphimosis and reduction techniques can be very painful and should be conducted with analgesics (Turner et al. 1999; Pohlman 2012). Noninvasive manual compression and reduction should be attempted first; this procedure requires steady compression of the distal penis with a gloved hand for several minutes followed by manual traction applied to the foreskin by the provider's fingers. Traction with Babcock or Adson forceps can also be used to aid in reduction (Turner et al. 1999; Chambers 2008). If no ischemia is present, adjunctive methods can aid in reducing swelling and include ice, compression bandages, and osmotic agents (Houghton 1973; Dubin and Davis 2011; Cahill and Rane 1999; Pohlman 2012; Kerwat et al. 1998; Anand and Kapoor 2013). Invasive techniques include puncture techniques, glans aspiration, and dorsal slit (Little and white 2005; Reynard and Barua 1999; Barone and Fleisher 1993; Hamdy and Hastie 1990; Raveenthiran 1996; Choe 2000).

Pre-procedure Preparation
- Careful examination of the penis should be done to rule out other causes of edema.
- Informed consent should be obtained from the patient or patient's guardian prior to proceeding.
- A topical or a local anesthetic is used to anesthetize the area (Vunda et al. 2013). Some patients may also need oral opioids or anxiolytics to help with pain and anxiety.

Post-procedure Instruction
- The foreskin should not be retracted for 1 week after procedure (Vunda et al. 2013).
- If minor tears occur during the procedure, topical antibiotics can be applied to prevent infection.

Follow-up

- Patients should have a follow-up appointment 1 week after reduction to reevaluate the penis. Patient education should be provided concerning proper hygiene of the penis and gentle retraction of the foreskin to avoid recurrence (Vunda et al. 2013).
- Patients are at risk of scarring and recurrence of paraphimosis. Circumcision may be needed.

Insurance Coverage

Since this is a medical emergency, prior authorization is not warranted.

Resources

Online Videos
- Vunda et al. (2013)

Guidelines
No current guidelines exist for paraphimosis reduction.

Book Chapters
- Chapter 36: Surgery of the Penis and Urethra
- Chambers (2008)
- Yachia (2007a, b)

Journal Articles on Paraphimosis Reduction
- Reynard and Barua (1999)
- Dubin and Davis (2011)
- Vunda et al. (2013)
- Cahill and Rane (1999)
- Choe (2000)
- Turner et al. (1999)
- Little and White (2005)
- Houghton (1973)
- Pohlman et al. (2013)
- Ganti et al. (1985)

- Kerwat et al. (1998)
- Anand and Kapoor (2013)
- Coutts (1991)
- Barone and Fleisher (1993)
- Hamdy and Hastie (1990)
- Kumar and Javle (2001)
- Raveenthiran (1996)

Online Resources
- Up to date: Paraphimosis Reduction

Paraphimosis References

1. Reynard and Barua (1999)
2. Dubin and Davis (2011)
3. Vunda et al. (2013)
4. Cahill and Rane (1999)
5. Choe (2000)
6. Turner et al. (1999)
7. Little and White (2005)
8. Houghton (1973)
9. Pohlman et al. (2013)
10. Ganti et al. (1985)
11. Kerwat et al. (1998)
12. Anand and Kapoor (2013)
13. Coutts (1991)
14. Barone and Fleisher (1993)
15. Hamdy and Hastie (1990)
16. Kumar and Javle (2001)
17. Raveenthiran (1996)
18. Vunda et al. (2013)
19. Wein (2012b)
20. Chambers (2008)
21. Yachia (2007b)
22. Tews (2013)

Penile Duplex Doppler Ultrasound

Description of Procedure

Penile duplex Doppler ultrasound uses high-resolution real-time ultrasound with color-pulsed Doppler to analyze the blood flow of the deep penile arteries. It can assess for arterial obstruction and venous leak (Wein 2012c).

Indications

- Evaluation of erectile dysfunction (ED)
- Evaluation of priapism
- Evaluation of penile trauma
- Evaluation of Peyronie's disease

Pre-procedure Preparation

- None unless indication requires injection or anesthetic prior to proceeding with study.
- Erectile dysfunction evaluation generally requires intracavernous injection with vasodilator(s). Informed consent should be obtained and risks of priapism should be discussed (Wein 2012d).

Post-procedure Instruction

- Dependent on indication.
- If patients are given intracavernous injection, the patient should not leave until the penis is flaccid (Wein 2012e).

Follow-up

- As directed based on the indication for the penile duplex Doppler ultrasound.

Insurance Coverage

- Prior authorization may be required for evaluation of ED and Peyronie's disease.
- Documentation of both the images and interpretation is vital for reimbursement. Images of all areas should be recorded, and variations from normal should be measured and documented. The images should have the patient's name, date, anatomical location, and right vs. left (Martino et al. 2014).
    - More information can be found on the AUA website at: http://www.auanet. org/resources/billing-for-ultrasound.cfm

Resources

National and Local Meeting Courses
- 2014 Doppler and Advances Techniques in Urologic Ultrasound Video (must purchase course)

Online Videos
- AUA Videos and CME Videos:
  - 2014 Doppler and Advanced Techniques in Urologic Ultrasound Video (requires purchase)
- Several videos are available for penile duplex Doppler ultrasound and intracavernous injections through www.youtube.com.

Book Chapters
- Chapter 24: Evaluation and Management of Erectile Dysfunction
- Chapter 25: Priapism

Journal Articles on Penile Duplex Doppler Ultrasound
- Martino et al. (2014)
- Wilkins et al. (2003)
- Chiou et al. (1998)
- Mihmanil and Faith (2007)
- Fitzgerald et al. (1992)
- Bhatt et al. (2005)
- Sadeghi-Nejad et al. (2004)

Online Resources
AUA Core Curriculum: Available at auanet.org with membership

- Uroradiology: Ultrasound
- Sexual Medicine: Peyronie's Disease Epidemiology, Pathophysiology, Evaluation
- Sexual Medicine: ED Patient Evaluation, Investigations

Guidelines
No current guidelines exist for penile duplex Doppler ultrasound but, there are AUA guidelines discussing the use of this procedure with priapism.

Penile Duplex Doppler Ultrasound References
1. Wein (2012c)
2. Wein (2012d)
3. Martino et al. (2014)
4. Wilkins et al. (2003)
5. Chiou et al. (1998)
6. Mihmanil and Faith (2007)
7. Fitzgerald et al. (1992)
8. Bhatt et al. (2005)
9. Sadeghi-Nejad et al. (2004)
10. Cunningham (2015)
11. O'Brant (2014)
12. Deveci (2014)

13. Figler
14. Muhlhall
15. Shindell

Xiaflex® (Collagenase Clostridium Histolyticum) Injections

Description of Procedure

Several injectable therapies have been used to manage Peyronie's disease, but collagenase clostridium histolyticum (Xiaflex) became the first FDA-approved agent in 2013. Penile plaques are infused with the medication followed by wrapping the penis with an elastic bandage for a few hours.

Indications

- Peyronie's disease

Pre-procedure Preparation

- Patient should be repeatedly reminded, and this should be documented, that sexual activity (both intercourse and masturbation) is prohibited from after the first injection to at least 14 days after the final injection of the series, depending on the degree of ecchymosis and swelling.
- Patients should be advised that the bruising that can occur is very deep purple, described as "eggplant".
- The medication must be stored according to manufacturer's instructions.
- Documentation prior to the procedure must include degree of curvature to ensure the patient meets the criteria for the medication.
- If the is no previous documentation, induce a penile erection with an intracavernous injection of a 10 to 20 µg of alprostadil. Anesthetic can be injected prior to intracavernous injection.
- Lyophilized Xiaflex powder must be reconstituted with the sterile diluent provided with the medication.

Post-procedure Instruction/Red Flags

- Sexual activity for 2 weeks after the second in the series of two injections is prohibited.
- Daily at-home penile modeling activities shown in the office for 6 weeks after the injection.
- Immediate follow-up is needed if penile facture or anaphylaxis occurs.
- Most common reactions include bruising/hematoma at the injection site.

Follow-up

- 1 to 3 days after the first injection, the provider performs in-office penile modeling and performs the second Xiaflex injection to complete one cycle. Up to four cycles can be completed for each patient.

Insurance Coverage

Treating with Xiaflex can be very costly. Prior authorization should be completed so that patients are informed about their out-of-pocket expenses. Some insurance companies consider the procedure experimental, and submission of the above journal articles and a letter of necessity may be required. Some insurance companies require documented failure of two non-FDA-approved treatments prior to accepting preauthorization paperwork. Auxilium Pharmaceuticals has information concerning CPT codes and financial assistance for patients at https://peyronies-disease.xiaflex.com/hcp/copay-program.php.

Resources

Online Videos
- Xiaflex website: https://peyronies-disease.xiaflex.com/hcp/

Book Chapters
- Campbell-Walsh Chapter 28: Peyronie's Disease

Journal Articles on Penile Duplex Doppler Ultrasound
- Jordan (2008)
- Gelbard et al. (1993)
- Gelbard et al. (2013)

Online Resources
- Up To Date Topics: Peyronie's Disease (diagnosis and medical management)
- AUA Core Curriculum: Available at auanet.org with membership
- Sexual Medicine: Peyronie's Disease Medical Treatment

Guidelines

- No current guidelines exist for Xiaflex.

Collagenase Clostridium Histolyticum (Xiaflex) Injections References
1. Treatment of Peyronie's Disease: Curved or Bent Penis
2. Wein (2012e)
3. Jordan (2008)

4. Gelbard et al. (1993)
5. Gelbard et al. (2013)
6. O'Brant (2013)

Transrectal Ultrasound (TRUS)-Guided Prostate Needle Biopsy

Description of Procedure

TRUS prostate biopsy remains the gold standard for diagnosing prostate cancer and uses ultrasound to aid in removing core samples of tissue from the prostate to be analyzed for cancer. An ultrasound probe is inserted into the rectum to visualize the prostate while a spring-driven biopsy gun is passed through the needle guide of the ultrasound probe into the prostate to obtain tissue core samples (Wein 2012a).

Indications

*   Elevated or rising PSA
*   Abnormal prostate exam
*   Inadequate initial sampling on prior prostate biopsy

Pre-procedure Preparation

*   Prophylactic antibiotics: To help lower the risk of post-biopsy infection, prophylactic antibiotics are recommended. Typically, a fluoroquinolone or first-, second-, or third-generation cephalosporin antibiotic has been the standard practice (Kapoor et al. 1998; Aron et al. 2000; Sabbagh et al. 2004; Shigemura et al. 2005). Studies have also shown that a single dose of antibiotics is as effective as 1- or 3-day regimens (Sabbagh et al. 2004; Shigemura et al. 2005). The AUA Best Practice Policy on antimicrobial prophylaxis was updated on 1/1/2014 to include trimethoprim-sulfamethoxazole as an alternative therapy, and when using an IM/IV aminoglycoside or aztreonam, clindamycin or metronidazole is no longer required. Bacterial resistance to fluoroquinolones contributes to infectious complications following prostate biopsy. One study showed that 22% of patients undergoing a rectal swab prior to a prostate biopsy harbored fluoroquinolone-resistant bacteria (Liss et al. 2011). However, at this time the AUA guidelines do not recommend rectal swabs prior to prostate biopsy.
*   Bowel prep: A standard bowel preparation has not been established due to limited research. One study found a decreased number of infectious complications with the use of a bisacodyl rectal suppository done the night prior to the biopsy (Jeon et al. 2003). However, two studies found no benefit with the use of sodium bisphosphonate enema or pre-procedural povidone-iodine (Otrock et al. 2004; Carey and Korman 2001). Mechanical enema in conjuncture with antimicrobial

prophylaxis decreases the risk of bacteremia according to the literature. However, it does not reduce the risk of fever (Zani et al. 2011).

- Anticoagulation medications: Per AUA best practice statement, 1 to 4% of patients experience signification post prostate biopsy bleeding. However, a significant number of patients experience some post-procedure bleeding whether it be hematuria, hematospermia, or rectal bleeding (Kariotis et al. 2010; Halliwell et al. 2006; Ihezue et al. 2005; Carmignani et al. 2011). Literature reviews are mixed on the use of anticoagulant/antiplatelet medication during biopsy, but given the high number of patients experiencing some bleeding, discontinuation of anticoagulation medication may be warranted.

Post-procedure Complications

- Infection: All patients should be instructed to call if they develop a fever.
- Bleeding: Patients should be counseled on the bleeding risk.
- Urinary retention: Although rare, occurring in 0.2 to 1.1% of men, patients should be instructed to call their urologist or proceed to the ER if they are in retention (Berger et al. 2004; Raaijmakers et al. 2002; Zaytoun et al. 2011; Kakehi et al. 2008).
- Hematospermia.

Follow-up

- Pending biopsy results or if post-procedure complications occur.

Insurance Coverage

- Prior authorization may be required for coverage.
- The AUA has information about CPT coding for TRUS prostate biopsy at: www.auanet.org/resources/biopsy-procedures.cfm

Resources

Online Videos
- AUA Videos and CME Videos:
  - 2008 Transrectal Ultrasound of the Prostate (must purchase)
  - Basic Urologic Ultrasound (must purchase)

National and Local Meeting Courses
- AUA National Meeting: Hands on Urologic Ultrasound
  - Check for course offerings on AUA website.

- SUNA National Meeting: Prostate Ultrasound Workshop
  - Check for course offerings on SUNA website.
- UAPA National Meeting: Ultrasound Breakout Session
  - Check for course offerings on UAPA website.

Book Chapters
- Chapter 97: Ultrasound and Biopsy of the Prostate
- Wieder

Journal Articles on TRUS and Prostate Biopsy
- Matlaga et al. (2003)
- El-Hakim and Moussa (2010)

Journal Articles on Ultrasound of the Prostate
- Martino et al. (2014)
- Boczko et al. (2006)

Online Resources
- Up To Date Topics: Prostate Biopsy
- AUA Core Curriculum: Available at auanet.org with membership
- Uroradiology: Ultrasound

Guidelines

AUA/SUNA White Papers
- Optimal Techniques of Prostate Biopsy and Specimen Handling
- AUA Quality Improvement Summit 2014: Conference Proceedings on Infectious Complications of Transrectal Prostate Needle Biopsy
- The Incidence, Prevention, and Treatment of Complications Related to Prostate Needle Biopsy

TRUS Prostate Biopsy Resources
1. Kapoor et al. (1998)
2. Aron et al. (2000)
3. Sabbagh et al. (2004)
4. Shigemura et al. (2005)
5. American Urological Association. Prostate-Specific Antigen Best Practice Statement. Revised (2014)
6. Roberts et al. (2014)
7. Liss et al. (2011)
8. Jeon et al. (2003)
9. Otrock et al. (2004)

10. Carey and Korman (2001)
11. Zani et al. (2011)
12. Halliwell et al. (2008)
13. Kariotis et al. (2010)
14. Halliwell et al. (2006)
15. Ihezue et al. (2005)
16. Carmignani et al. (2011)
17. Raheem et al. (2011)
18. Berger et al. (2004)
19. Raaijmakers et al. (2002)
20. Zaytoun et al. (2011)
21. Kakehi et al. (2008)
22. Biopsy Procedures: American Urological Association
23. https://www.auanet.org/university/product-detail-cme.cfm?typeID=1&produc tID=474
24. https://www.auanet.org/university/product-detail-cme.cfm?typeID=1&produc tID=476
25. Wein (2012a)
26. Weider (2010)
27. Matlaga et al. (2003)
28. El-Hakim and Moussa (2010)
29. Martino et al. (2014)
30. Boczko et al. (2006)
31. Benway (2014)
32. Gonzolez et al. (2012)
33. Averch et al. (2014)
34. Samir et al. (2015)

Clinical Pearls

- When anticipating expanding one's practice to include procedures, it is imperative that the APP confirm their state scope of practice, malpractice provider, and facility credentialing supports this expansion in practice.
- Always confirm patient allergies.
- Expansion into common procedures can improve patient access and satisfaction, decrease wait times, promote continuity of care, and improve patient adherence to surveillance guidelines.
- APPs performing procedures can represent a "hidden role" and hidden revenue generated by APPs if the procedures must be billed under an MD for insurance/ reimbursement requirements.

References

Altarac S (2011) [Histrelin acetate--the first once yearly LHRH agonist]. Lijec Vjesn 133(9–10):320–322. Croatian

American Urological Association (2014) Prostate-specific antigen best practice statement. Revised. Available at: http://www.auanet.org/common/pdf/education/clinical-guidance/Antimicrobial-Prophylaxis.pdf. Accessed 2 Jan 2015

Anand A, Kapoor S (2013) Mannitol for paraphimosis reduction. Urol Int 90:106

Aron M, Rajeev TP, Gupta NP (2000) Antimicrobial prophylaxis for transrectal needle biopsy of the prostate: a randomized controlled study. BJU Int 85:682

Athanassopoulos A, Liatsikos EN, Barbalias GA (2005) The difficult urethral catheterization: use of a hydrophilic guidewire. BJU Int 95:192

Averch T et al (2014) AUA quality improvement summit 2014: conference proceedings on infectious complications of transrectal prostate needle biopsy. AUA white paper. American Urological Association Education and Research, Inc, Linthicum, MD

Barone JG, Fleisher MH (1993) Treatment of paraphimosis using the "puncture" technique. Pediatr Emerg Care 9:298

Beaghler M, Grasso M 3rd, Loisides P (1994) Inability to pass a urethral catheter: the bedside role of the flexible cystoscope. Urology 44:268

Benway B (2014) Prostate biopsy. Available at: https://www.uptodate.com/contents/prostate-biopsy. Accessed 8 Feb 2015

Berger AP, Gozzi C, Steiner H et al (2004) Complication rate of transrectal ultrasound guided prostate biopsy: a comparison among 3 protocols with 6, 10 and 15 cores. J Urol 171:1478

Bhatt S, Kocakoc E, Rubens DJ, Seftel AD, Dogra VS (2005) Sonographic evaluation of penile trauma. J Ultrasound Med 24:993–1000

Blitz BF (1995) A simple method using hydrophilic guide wires for the difficult urethral catheterization. Urology 46:99

Boczko J, Messing E, Dogra V (2006) Transrectal sonography in prostate evaluation. Radiol Clin N Am 44:679

Bothner J (2014) Management of zipper injuries. Available at: https://www.uptodate.com/contents/management-of-zipper-injuries. Accessed 31 Jan 2015

Cahill D, Rane A (1999) Reduction of paraphimosis with granulated sugar. BJU Int 83:362

Carey JM, Korman HJ (2001) Transrectal ultrasound guided biopsy of the prostate. Do enemas decrease clinically significant complications? J Urol 166:82

Carmignani L, Picozzi S, Bozzini G et al (2011) Transrectal ultrasound-guided prostate biopsies in patients taking aspirin for cardiovascular disease: a meta-analysis. Transfus Apher 45:275–280

Chambers P (2008) Paraphimosis reduction. In: King C, Henretig FM (eds) Textbook of pediatric emergency procedures, 2nd edn. Lippincott, Williams & Wilkins, Philadelphia, PA, p 904

Chatterton K (2010) A bladder cancer nurse-led flexible cystoscopy service. Eur Urol Today 22(3). Available at: http://www.uro.web.org/news/?act=showfull&aid=104

Chelladurai AJ, Srirangam SJ, Blades RA (2008) A novel technique to aid urethral catheterization in patients presenting with acute urinary retention due to urethral stricture disease. Ann R Coll Surg Engl 90:77

Chertin B, Spitz IM, Lindenberg T, Algur N, Zer T, Kuzma P, Young AJ, Catane R, Farkas A (2000) An implant releasing the gonadotropin hormone-releasing hormone agonist histrelin maintains medical castration for up to 30 months in metastatic prostate cancer. J Urol 163(3):838–844

Chiou RK, Pomeroy BD, Chen WS, Anderson JC, Wobig RK, Taylor RJ (1998) Hemodynamic patterns of pharmacologically induced erection: evaluation by Color Doppler sonography. J Urol 159(1):109–112

Choe JM (2000) Paraphimosis: current treatment options. Am Fam Physician 62:2623

Coutts AG (1991) Treatment of paraphimosis. Br J Surg 78:252

Cunningham G (2015) Evaluation of male sexual dysfunction. Available at: https://www.uptodate.com/contents/evaluation-of-male-sexual-dysfunction. Accessed 31 Jan 2015

Deveci   S   (2014)   Priapism.   Available   at: http://www.uptodate.com/contents/
priapism?source=search_result&search=Priapism&selectedTitle=1~14. Accessed 31 Jan 2015

Djavan B, Schlegel P, Salomon G, Eckersberger E, Sadri H, Graefen M (2010) Analysis of testosterone suppression in men receiving histrelin, a novel GnRH agonist for the treatment of
prostate cancer. Can J Urol 17(4):5265–5271

Dubin J, Davis JE (2011) Penile emergencies. Emerg Med Clin North Am 29:485

El-Hakim A, Moussa S (2010) CUA guidelines on prostate biopsy methodology. Can Urol Assoc
J 4(2):89–94

Erickson B, Han Y, Meeks W, Gulig S, Fang R, Annam K, Nepple K (2017) Increasing use of
advanced practice providers for urological office procedural care in the United States. Urol
Pract 4(2):169–175

Fagerberg M, Nostell PO (2005) Follow up of urinary bladder cancer – a task for the urology
nurse? Lakartidningen 102:2149–2150

Fairman JA, Rowe JW, Hassmiller S, Shalala DE (2010) Broadening the scope of nursing practice.
N Engl J Med 364(3):193–196

Fitzgerald SW, Erickson SJ, Foley WD, Lipchik EO, Lawson TL (1992) Color Doppler sonography in the evaluation of erectile dysfunction. Radiographics 12:3–17

Freid RM, Smith AD (1996) The Glidewire technique for overcoming urethral obstruction. J
Urol 156:164

Ganti SU, Sayegh N, Addonizio JC (1985) Simple method for reduction of paraphimosis.
Urology 25:77

Gelbard MK, James K, Riach P et al (1993) Collagenase versus placebo in the treatment of
Peyronie's disease: a double-blind study. J Urol 149:56

Gelbard M, Goldstein I, Hellstrom WJ et al (2013) Clinical efficacy, safety and tolerability of collagenase clostridium histolyticum for the treatment of peyronie disease in 2 large double-blind,
randomized, placebo controlled phase 3 studies. J Urol 190:199

Gidlow AB, Laniado ME, Ellis BW (2000) The nurse cystoscopist: a feasible option? Br J Urol
Int 85:651–654

Gonzolez CM et al (2012) AUA/SUNA white paper on the incidence, prevention and treatment
of complications related to prostate needle biopsy. AUA white paper. American Urological
Association Education and Research, Inc, Linthicum, MD

Halliwell OT, Lane C, Dewbury KC (2006) Transrectal ultrasound-guided biopsy of the prostate:
should warfarin be stopped before the procedure? Incidence of bleeding in a further 50 patients.
Clin Radiol 61:1068–1069

Halliwell OT, Yadegafar G, Lane C, Dewbury KC (2008) Transrectal ultrasound-guided biopsy
of the prostate: aspirin increases the incidence of minor bleeding complications. Clin Radiol
63:557–561

Hamdy FC, Hastie KJ (1990) Treatment for paraphimosis: the 'puncture' technique. Br J
Surg 77:1186

Herr HW (2014) Should antibiotics be given prior to outpatient cystoscopy? A plea to urologists to
practice antibiotic stewardship. Eur Urol 65(4):839–842

Hess MJ, Zhan EH, Foo DK, Yalla SV (2003) Bladder cancer in patients with spinal cord injury. J
Spin Cord Med 26:335–338

Ho KJ, Thompson TJ, O'Brien A et al (2003) Lignocaine gel: does it cause urethral pain rather
than prevent it? Eur Urol 43:194–196

Houghton GR (1973) The "iced-glove" method of treatment of paraphimosis. Br J Surg 60:876

Ihezue CU, Smart J, Dewbury KC, Mehta R, Burgess L (2005) Biopsy of the prostate guided by
transrectal ultrasound: relation between warfarin use and incidence of bleeding complications.
Clin Radiol 60:459–463. Discussion 7–8

Institute of Medicine (2010) The future of nursing: leading change, advancing health. National
Academies Press, Washington, DC. Available at: http://www.iom.edu.libproxy.lib.unc.edu/
Reports/2010/The-Future-of-Nursing-Leading-Change-Advancing-Health.aspx

Jeon SS, Woo SH, Hyun JH, Choi HY, Chai SE (2003) Bisacodyl rectal preparation can
decrease infectious complications of transrectal ultrasound-guided prostate biopsy. Urology
62(3):461–466

Jiménez-Pacheco A, Lardelli Claret P, López Luque A, Lahoz-García C, Arrabal Polo MA, Nogueras Ocaña M (2012) Arch randomized clinic trial on antimicrobial prophylaxis for flexible urethrocystoscopy. Esp Urol 65(5):542–549

Jordan GH (2008) The use of intralesional clostridial collagenase injection therapy for Peyronie's disease: a prospective, single-center, non-placebo-controlled study. J Sex Med 5:180

Kakehi Y, Naito S, Japanese Urological Association (2008) Complication rates of ultrasound-guided prostate biopsy: a nation-wide survey in Japan. Int J Urol 15:319

Kapoor DA, Klimberg IW, Malek GH, Wegenke JD, Cox CE, Patterson AL et al (1998) Singledose ciprofloxacin versus placebo for prophylaxis during transrectal prostate biopsy. Urology 52:552

Kariotis I, Philippou P, Volanis D, Serafetinides E, Delakas D (2010) Safety of ultrasound-guided transrectal extended prostate biopsy in patients receiving low-dose aspirin. Int Braz J Urol 36:308–316

Kelleher S, Turner L, Howe C, Conway AJ, Handelsman DJ (1999) Extrusion of testosterone pellets: a randomized controlled clinical study. Clin Endocrinol 51(4):469–471

Kelleher S, Howe C, Conway AJ, Handelsman DJ (2004) Testosterone release rate and duration of action of testosterone pellet implants. Clin Endocrinol 60(4):420–428

Kerwat R, Shandall A, Stephenson B (1998) Reduction of paraphimosis with granulated sugar. Br J Urol 82:755

Kirya C, Werthmann M (1978) Neonatal circumcision and penile dorsal nerve block: a painless procedure. J Pediatr 92:998–1000

Kleier JA (2009) Procedure competencies and job functions of the urologic advanced practice nurse. Urol Nurs 29(2):112–117. Available at: https://auth.lib.unc.edu/ezproxy_auth.php?url=https://search.proquest.com/docview/220%20160997?accountid=14244

Kovac JR, Rajanahally S, Smith RP, Coward RM, Lamb DJ, Lipshultz LI (2014) Patient satisfaction with testosterone replacement therapies: the reasons behind the choices. J Sex Med 11(2):553–562. https://doi.org/10.1111/jsm.12369

Krikler SJ (1989) Flexible urethroscopy: use in difficult male catheterization. Ann R Coll Surg Engl 71:3

Kuhn JM, Billebaud T, Navratil H, Moulonguet A, Fiet J, Grise P, Louis JF, Costa P, Husson JM, Dahan R et al (1989) Prevention of the transient adverse effects of a gonadotropin-releasing hormone analogue (buserelin) in metastatic prostatic carcinoma by administration of an antiandrogen (nilutamide). Engl J Med 321(7):413–418

Kumar V, Javle P (2001) Modified puncture technique for reduction of paraphimosis. Ann R Coll Surg Engl 83:126

Labrie F, Dupont A, Belanger A, Lachance R (1987) Flutamide eliminates the risk of disease flare in prostatic cancer patients treated with a luteinizing hormone-releasing hormone agonist. J Urol 138(4):804–806

Langston JP, Orcutt VL, Smith AB, Schultz H, Hornberger B, Deal AB, Doran TJ, McKibben MJ, Kirby EW, Nielsen ME et al (2017a) Advanced practice providers in U.S. urology: a national survey of demographics and clinical roles. Urol Pract 4(5):418–424. https://doi.org/10.1016/j.urpr.2016.09.012. ISSN 2352-0779

Langston JP, Duszak R, Orcutt VL, Schultz H, Hornberger B, Jenkins LC, Hemingway J, Hughes DR, Pruthi RS, Nielsen ME (2017b) The expanding role of advanced practice providers in urologic procedural care. Urology 106:70–75. https://doi.org/10.1016/j.urology.2017.03.047. ISSN 0090-4295

Latthe PM, Foon R, Toozs-Hobson P (2008) Review – infections antibiotic prophylaxis in urologic procedures: a systematic review. Eur Urol 54:1270–1286

Lewis LS, Stephan M (1997) Local and regional anesthesia. In: Henretig FM, King C (eds) Textbook of pediatric emergency procedures. Williams & Wilkins, Baltimore, MD

Liss MA, Chang A, Santos R et al (2011) Prevalence and significance of fluoroquinolone resistant Escherichia coli in patients undergoing transrectal ultrasound guided prostate needle biopsy. J Urol 185:1283

Little B, White M (2005) Treatment options for paraphimosis. Int J Clin Pract 59:591

Mariani AJ, Glover M, Arita S (2001) Medical versus surgical androgen suppression therapy for prostate cancer: a 10-year longitudinal cost study. J Urol 165(1):104–107

Martino P, Galosi AB, Bitelli M, Imaging Working Group-Societa Italiana Urologia (SIU); Società Italiana Ecografia Urologica Andrologica Nefrologica (SIEUN) et al (2014) Practical recommendations for performing ultrasound scanning in the urological and andrological fields. Arch Ital Urol Androl 86(1):56–78

Matlaga BR, Eskew AL, McCullough DL (2003) Prostate biopsy: indications and technique. J Urol 169(1):12–19

McCullough A (2014) A review of testosterone pellets in the treatment of hypogonadism. Curr Sex Health Rep 6(4):265

McCullough AR, Khera M, Goldstein I, Hellstrom WJ, Morgentaler A, Levine LA (2012) A multi-institutional observational study of testosterone levels after testosterone pellet (Testopel®) insertion. J Sex Med 9(2):594–601. https://doi.org/10.1111/j.1743-6109.2011.02570.x

Mechlin CW, Frankel J, McCullough A (2014) Coadministration of anastrozole sustains therapeutic testosterone levels in hypogonadal men undergoing testosterone pellet insertion. J Sex Med 11(1):254–261

Mendez-Probst CE, Razvi H, Denstedt JD (2012) Management of the difficult-to-catheterize patient. In: Wein AL, Kavoussi LR, Partin AW, Peters CA (eds) Campbell-Walsh urology, 11th edn. Elsevier, Philadelphia, PA, pp 177–191.e4

Messing EM, Manola J, Sarosdy M et al (1999) Immediate hormonal therapy compared with observation after radical prostatectomy and pelvic lymphadenectomy in men with nodepositive prostate cancer. N Engl J Med 341:1781–1788

Mihmanil I, Faith K (2007) Erectile dysfunction. Seminars in ultrasound, CT and MRI. Semin Ultrasound CT MR 28(4):274–286

Nelson JB (2013) Chapter 109: Hormone therapy for prostate cancer. In: Wein AL, Kavoussi LR, Partin AW, Peters CA (eds) Campbell-Walsh urology, 11th edn. Elsevier, Philadelphia, PA, pp 2934–2953

O'Brant W (2013) Peyronie's disease: diagnosis and medical management. Available at: https://www.uptodate.com/contents/search?search=peyronies-disease-diagnosis-and-medical%2D%2Dmanagement&sp=0&searchType=PLAIN_TEXT&source=USER_INPUT&searchControl=TOP_PULLDOWN&searchOffset=1&autoComplete=false&languag e=&max=0&index=&autoCompleteTerm=. Accessed 6 Feb 2015

O'Brant W (2014) Surgical management of peyronie's disease. Available at: https://www.uptodate.com/contents/surgical-management-of-peyronies-disease. Accessed 31 Jan 2015

Otrock ZK, Oghlakian GO, Salamoun MM, Haddad M, Bizri AR (2004) Incidence of urinary tract infection following transrectal ultrasound guided prostate biopsy at a tertiary-care medical center in Lebanon. Infect Control Hosp Epidemiol 25:873

Pastuszak AW, Mittakanti H, Liu JS, Gomez L, Lipshultz LI, Khera M (2012) Pharmacokinetic evaluation and dosing of subcutaneous testosterone pellets. J Androl 33(5):927–937

Patel AR, Jones JS, Babineau D (2008) Lidocaine 2% gel versus plain lubricating gel for pain reduction during flexible cystoscopy: a meta-analysis of prospective, randomized, controlled trials. J Urol 179:86

Pohlman GD, Phillips JM, Wilcox DT (2013) Simple method of paraphimosis reduction revisited: point of technique and review of the literature. J Pediatr Urol 9:104

Prostate Cancer Trialists' Collaborative Group (2000) Maximum androgen blockade in advanced prostate cancer: an overview of randomized trials. Lancet 255:1491–1498

Quallick S, Lajiness S, Koviark J, Doran T, Shultz H, Langston JP (2020) Standardized Office Cystoscopy for Advanced Practice Providers in Urology. Urology Practice (7):228–233

Quallich SA (2011) A survey evaluating the current role of the nurse practitioner in urology. Urol Nurs 31(6):328–326. Available at: https://auth.lib.unc.edu/ezproxy_auth.php?url=https://search.proquest.com/docview/91143460%205?accountid=14244

Raaijmakers R, Kirkels WJ, Roobol MJ, Wildhagen MF, Schrder FH (2002) Complication rates and risk factors of 5802 transrectal ultrasound-guided sextant biopsies of the prostate within a population-based screening program. Urology 60:826

Radhakrishnan S, Dorkin TJ, Johnson P, Menezes P, Greene D (2006) Nurse-led flexible cystoscopy: experience from one UK center. Br J Urol Int 98(2):256–258

Raheem O, Casey RG, Lynch TH (2011) Does anticoagulant or antiplatelet therapy need to be discontinued for transrectal ultrasound-guided prostate biopsies? A systematic literature review. Curr Urol 5:121–124

Raveenthiran V (1996) Reduction of paraphimosis: a technique based on pathophysiology. Br J Surg 83:1247

Reynard JM, Barua JM (1999) Reduction of paraphimosis the simple way – the Dundee technique. BJU Int 83:859

Ricker JM, Foody WF, Shumway NM, Shaw JC (2010) Drug-induced liver injury caused by the histrelin (Vantas) subcutaneous implant. South Med J 103(1):84–86

Roberts MJ, Williamson DA, Hadway P, Doi SA, Gardiner RA, Paterson DL (2014) Baseline prevalence of antimicrobial resistance and subsequent infection following prostate biopsy using empiric or altered prophylaxis: a bias-adjusted meta-analysis. Int J Antimicrob Agents 43(4):301–309

Sabbagh R, McCormack M, Péloquin F, Faucher R, Perreault JP, Perrotte P et al (2004) A prospective randomized trial of 1-day versus 3-day antimicrobial prophylaxis for transrectal ultrasound guided prostate biopsy. Can J Urol 11:2216

Sadeghi-Nejad H, Dogra V, Seftel AD, Mohamed MA (2004) Priapism. Radiol Clin N Am 42:427–443

Samir ST et al (2015) Optimal techniques of prostate biopsy and specimen handling. AUA White paper. Available at: www.AUAnet.org

Schlegel P (2009) A review of the pharmacokinetic and pharmacological properties of a once-yearly administered histrelin acetate implant in the treatment of prostate cancer. BJU Int 103(Suppl 2):7–13

Schlegel PN, Histrelin Study Group (2006) Efficacy and safety of histrelin subdermal implant in patients with advanced prostate cancer. J Urol 175(4):1353–1358

Schultz H (2011) Practical and legal implications of nurse practitioners and physician assistants in cystoscopy. Urol Nurs 31(6):355–358. Available at: https://auth.lib.unc.edu/ezproxy_auth.php?url=https://search.proquest.com/docvie%20w/911434610?accountid=14244

Serour F, Reuben S, Ezra S (1995) Circumcision in children with penile block alone. J Urol 153(2):474–476

Shigemura K, Tanaka K, Yasuda M, Ishihar S, Muratani T, Deguchi T et al (2005) Efficacy of 1-day prophylaxis medication with fluoroquinolone for prostate biopsy. World J Urol 23:356

Shore N, Cookson MS, Gittelman MC (2012) Long-term efficacy and tolerability of once-yearly histrelin acetate subcutaneous implant in patients with advanced prostate cancer. BJU Int 109(2):226–232. https://doi.org/10.1111/j.1464-410X.2011.10370.x

Smith RP, Khanna A, Coward RM, Rajanahally S, Kovac JR, Gonzales MA, Lipshultz LI (2013) Factors influencing patient decisions to initiate and discontinue subcutaneous testosterone pellets (Testopel) for treatment of hypogonadism. J Sex Med 10(9):2326–2333

Snellman L, Stang H (1995) Prospective evaluation of complications of dorsal penile nerve block for neonatal circumcision. Pediatrics 95:705–708

Stav A, Gur L, Gorelik U, Ovadia L, Isaakovich B, Sternberg A (1995) Modification of the penile block. World J Urol 13:251–253

Subramonian K, Cartwright RA, Harnden P, Harrison SC (2004) Bladder cancer in patients with spinal cord injuries. BJU Int 93:739–743

Sung JC, Springhart WP, Marguet CG et al (2005) Location and etiology of flexible and semirigid ureteroscope damage. Urology 66:958–963

Taghizadeh AK, El Madani A, Gard PR et al (2006) When does it hurt? Pain during flexible cystoscopy in men. Urol Int 76:301–303

Tews M (2013) Paraphimosis reduction. Available at: https://www.uptodate.com/contents/search?search=paraphimosis-reduction&sp=0&searchType=PLAIN_TEXT&source=USER_INPUT&searchControl=TOP_PULLDOWN&searchOffset=1&autoComplete=false&language=&max=0&index=&autoCompleteTerm=. Accessed 3 Jan 2015

Turner CD, Kim HL, Cromie WJ (1999) Dorsal band traction for reduction of paraphimosis. Urology 54:917

Tzortzis V, Gravas S, Melekos MM, de la Rosette JJ (2009) Intraurethral lubricants: a critical literature review and recommendations. J Endourol 23:821–826

Villanueva C, Hemstreet G (2010) Experience with a difficult urethral catheterization algorithm at a university hospital. Curr Urol 4:152

Villanueva C, Hemstreet GP 3rd (2008) Difficult male urethral catheterization: a review of different approaches. Int Braz J Urol 34:401

Vunda A, Lacroix LE, Schneider F et al (2013) Videos in clinical medicine. Reduction of paraphimosis in boys. N Engl J Med 368:e16

Weckermann D, Harzmann R (2004) Hormone therapy in prostate cancer: LHRH antagonists versus LHRH analogues. Eur Urol 46(3):279–283

Weider A (2010) Prostate cancer, 4th edn. Griffith Publishing, Caldwell, ID, pp 113–117

Wein A (2012a) Ultrasound and biopsy of the prostate, vol 3, 10th edn. Saunders, an imprint of Elsevier, Philadelphia, PA

Wein A (2012b) Surgery of the penis and urethra. In: Campbell-Walsh urology, vol 3, 10th edn. Saunders, an imprint of Elsevier, Philadelphia, PA

Wein A (2012c) Evaluation and management of erectile dysfunction. In: Campbell-Walsh urology, vol 3, 10th edn. Saunders, an imprint of Elsevier, Philadelphia, PA

Wein A (2012d) Priapism. In: Campbell-Walsh urology, vol 3, 10th edn. Saunders, an imprint of Elsevier, Philadelphia, PA

Wein A (2012e) Peyronie's disease. In: Campbell-Walsh urology, vol 3, 10th edn. Saunders, an imprint of Elsevier, Philadelphia, PA

Wilkins CJ, Sriprasad S, Sihus PS (2003) Colour Doppler ultrasound of the penis. Clin Radiol 58(7):14–23

Wilson LR, Thelning C, Masters J, Tuckey J (2005) Is antibiotic prophylaxis required for flexible cystoscopy? A truncated randomized double-blind controlled trial. J Endourol 19(8):1006–1008

Wolf JS, Bennett CJ, Dmochowski RR et al (2008) Best practice policy statement on urologic surgery antimicrobial prophylaxis. J Urol 179:1379–1390

Yachia D (2007a) Chapter 2: Anesthesia for penile surgery. In: Text atlas of penile surgery. CRC Press, Boca Raton, FL, pp 9–11

Yachia D (2007b) Chapter 4: Paraphimosis. In: Text atlas of penile surgery. Informa Healthcare, London, pp 17–19

Zani EL, Clark OA, Rodrigues NN Jr (2011) Antibiotic prophylaxis for transrectal prostate biopsy. Cochrane Database Syst Rev 5:CD006576

Zaytoun OM, Anil T, Moussa AS, Jianbo L, Fareed K, Jones JS (2011) Morbidity of prostate biopsy after simplified versus complex preparation protocols: assessment of risk factors. Urology 77(4):910–914

Further Reading

Wieder JA (ed) (2014) Pocket guide to urology, 5th edn. J. Wieder Medical, Oakland, CA

Pain Management and the Urology Patient

23

Susanne A. Quallich

Contents

Objectives
1. Define the types of pain
2. Discuss the basics of pain assessment
3. Compare effective options for pain management in urology patients
4. Examine issues with postsurgical pain management

Introduction

"Pain is whatever the experiencing person says it is, existing whenever the experiencing person says it does" (McCaffery 1968)—and this highlights the challenges of addressing pain in any population of patients. Chronic pain is a very expensive

S. A. Quallich (✉)
Division of Andrology, General and Community Health, Department of Urology, Michigan Medicine, University of Michigan, Ann Arbor, MI, USA
e-mail: quallich@umich.edu

© Springer Nature Switzerland AG 2020
S. A. Quallich, M. J. Lajiness (eds.), *The Nurse Practitioner in Urology*,
https://doi.org/10.1007/978-3-030-45267-4_23

public health problem and affects millions of people each year. In 1994 The International Association for the Study of Pain (IASP) developed its taxonomy for pain. "Pain is an unpleasant sensory or emotional experience associated with actual or potential tissue damage, or described in terms of such damage" (Mersky and Bogduk 1994). IASP supports that pain is always subjective; its interpretation by an individual is heavily influenced by their previous experiences with pain, their previous experiences with pain management and their larger social and psychological context for that pain. Unfortunately, "pain" can also be a catchall phrase for when patients lack the vocabulary or experience to describe the sensations that they are feeling. "If they regard their experience as pain and if they report it in the same ways as pain caused by tissue damage, it should be accepted as pain" (IASP 1994, para. 5). Inherent in this IASP definition is the multifactorial nature of pain, and this definition implies that management of any chronic pain occurs within me an individual the larger social and healthcare context (which can include insurance coverage) and providers must acknowledge pain's effects on quality of life, and work to address psychosocial components that create and sustain pain (Rosenquist et al. 2010). Pain therefore, becomes a multidimensional construct that includes sensory components, emotional or interpretive components, and any identifiable physical changes to tissues and organs.

Within the realm of urology chronic pain patients can be particularly challenging, and providers who evaluate a large number of patients with kidney stones are well-versed with the contemporary challenges of pain management due to the identified opioid epidemic. Providers face a daily challenge in managing the multidimensional aspects of pain management that include compromises to patients functions, overall quality of life, quality of relationships and social roles, their emotional state (Duenas et al. 2016), and their general well-being within the expectations for treatment.

Incidence

Chronic pain patients have urology issues, and urology patients may have chronic pain issues. Identifying the level and amount of pain experienced by the general population is a difficult task. The United States 2012 National Health Interview Survey reported that 25.3 million adults (11.2%) reported suffering from daily (chronic) pain and 23.4 million (10.3%) are reported "a lot" of pain (Nahin 2015; Stanos et al. 2016). These authors also stated that females in the database had a higher incidence of category 3 and 4 pain (0–10 scale), particularly non-Hispanic, English preferred, African-American, and Caucasian females. The cost of chronic pain in the United States has been reported as being as high as $635 billion/year (Murphy et al. 2017) representing lost wages and lost productivity, in addition to healthcare costs.

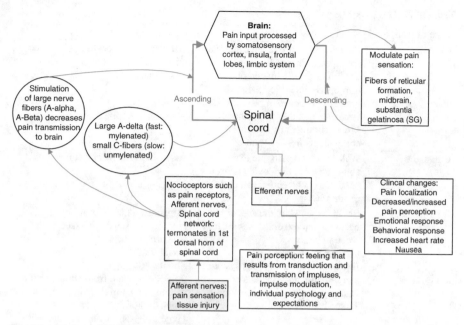

Fig. 23.1 Schematized pain conduction

Pathophysiology of Pain and Types of Pain

Pain is described in two ways: normal or nociceptive (e.g., incision pain) and abnormal or pathophysiologic (e.g., chronic pain conditions such as interstitial cystitis or chronic pelvic pain). Pain involves both the afferent pathway (nerves that receive information or stimuli) and the efferent pathway (nerves that carry sensation to muscles and stimulate responses). The afferent portion includes pain receptors (nociceptors), afferent nerve fibers, and the spinal cord network (Fig. 23.1).

Pain is classified as acute (again, such as incision pain) and chronic (such as chronic bladder or pelvic pain). Acute pain can be easily identified by its sudden onset, and usually easily identifiable cause; it is also of short duration (<1 month). Patients may be observed crying, moaning, crying, protecting, and holding the affected area or limb. Chronic pain may not have a cause that is remembered by the patient, as some point they became aware that their pain did not resolve, or the patient and provider recognize that surgical pain persists beyond the time of average healing post-procedure (Price et al. 2014). Table 23.1 offers a discussion of the various categories of pain.

There is no distinct or precise "pain center" of the brain (Jensen 2010; Jensen and Turk 2014) that can be considered analogous to the visual process center, for example. Both input and output related to pain are processed and evaluated in multiple

Table 23.1 Discussion of pain types[a]

Type of pain	Description	Descriptors and examples
Chronic	Pain that does not resolve after an anticipated time of healing; can be a result of poorly treated or improperly identified pain that gradually becomes more complex Persists beyond 3–6 months More prominent psychosocial components may be seen	Will depend on location, suspected origin of the pain (deep vs. superficial)
Cutaneous	Well-localized pain due to an abundance of nerve endings from cutaneous nociceptors just under the dermis	Also called superficial somatic pain
Inflammatory	Begins when skin, muscle, or bone becomes injured and inflammatory reaction begins Generally adaptive pain Interaction of the nervous system and inflammatory mediators causing peripheral sensitization Tissue heals, the pain resolves	Depends on nature of injury, e.g., burning and sensitivity seen with sunburn Usual triad: Spontaneous pain Allodynia—pain from stimuli that is usually not painful (pain from the touch of clothing) Hyperesthesia—Unusual sensitivity to stimuli; chronic burning type pain, increased sensitivity to touch
Neuropathic	Clinical description: can be pain that happens without distinct injury Damage to the system that *reports/interprets* pain Generated by nerves; due lesion or disease of somatosensory nervous system Can result after trauma or infection Central neuropathic pain: caused by a lesion or disease of the central somatosensory nervous system. CNS undergoes remodeling and sustains and, in many cases, amplifies pain	Burning, shooting, tingling, numb, radiating, stabbing, "electric" Hyperalgesia: Increased pain stimuli that normally provokes pain Indicators of central sensitization: sensitivity in areas without pathology, pain at the end of the stimulus, maintenance of pain by low-intensity stimuli that typically do not provoke pain
Referred	Pain perceived at a location other than the site of the painful stimulus	Depends on site Examples include referred pain from myocardial infarction, appendicitis, "brain freeze" pattern of referred pain from trigeminal nerve
Somatic (deep)	Arises from nerves in the skin, tendons, deep tissue and visceral, originating in internal organs or viscera fewer nociceptors, resulting in longer duration of a diffuse aching sensation	Squeezing, cramping, pressure, distention, deep pain/discomfort, dull aching Site of pain poorly localized

Table 23.1 (continued)

Type of pain	Description	Descriptors and examples
Superficial	Arising from skin and mucous membranes	Dull, achy, throbbing, sore
Visceral	Originates in organs or visceral cavities Fewer nociceptors, resulting in longer duration of a diffuse aching sensation Diffuse, poorly localized Due to changes in visceral hypersensitivity at peripheral or central level	Examples include kidney stone pain, gastric dysmotility pain, pancreatitis, organ ischemia, pain from cancer

Some definitions adapted from "Part III: Pain Terms, A Current List with Definitions and Notes on Usage" (pp. 209–214) Classification of Chronic Pain, Second Edition, IASP Task Force on Taxonomy, edited by H. Merskey and N. Bogduk, IASP Press, Seattle, 1994
[a]A full discussion of these conditions is beyond the scope of the chapter; this summary is simply to provide an introduction of relevant pain concepts

centers of the brain (Fig. 23.1), resulting in an evaluation of pain that happens due to synchronization of non-localized brain areas that are primarily involved in sensory, emotional, motivational, and cognitive processes (Tracey and Johns 2010). This provides evidence for the "pain matrix" first described by Melzack (1999) but also results in a multidimensional perception, followed by interpretation, of one's pain.

Assessment of Pain

It is critical that the provider obtain an accurate and careful assessment of the pain (Stanos et al. 2016), including whether or not a patient is currently experiencing pain. Within a surgical planning context, this is helpful to aid with assessment postoperatively, especially if the pain is the reason for surgery. For example, men undergoing epididymectomy for pain will report relief of that focal pain, with only incision pain after surgery, while patients undergoing bladder hydrodistension often note resolution of bladder pain after the procedure. Within the context of addiction or psychological concerns, a careful validation of any pain-related distress will encourage compliance with treatment.

Patient Pain History

Ask specific questions to elicit a full understanding of the patient's pain complaint, keeping in mind that their focus for pain management may be different from your assessment as the provider. Have patients detail the location, quality, and intensity of the pain, its characteristics, and any aggravating or alleviating factors. Explore

Table 23.2 Guide to pain assessment

Dimension	Considerations
Quality	Burning, aching, stabbing, nauseating, etc. (Table 23.1)
Impact	How often do they need OTC medications, prescription medications? Ability to maintain work/family/social roles Sleep quality Anxiety/depression
Site/radiation of pain	Helps determine potential mechanisms (Table 23.1)
Severity	Pain scale 0–10
Temporal characteristics	Does pain wax/wane, during the day or with activity; worse in am/pm, constant
Aggravating/alleviating factors	Position, activity; voiding/defecating Use of medication, positional changes
Past response to treatment	Success vs. intolerance due to medication side effects
Physical exam	As indicated based on complaint
Diagnostics	Imaging study indications, trigger point injections, spermatic cord block, cystoscopy, lab work
Previous evaluations outside urology	Pain clinic, Physical Medicine and Rehabilitation, physical therapy, occupational therapy, psychology, yoga, chiropractor, acupuncture
Expectations, goals for treatment	Allows provider insight into need for referrals Promotes patient engagement in self-care Interest in support groups

previous treatments and the success/failure of these attempts. If the pain is chronic, explore how the pain has impacted impacts the patient's lifestyle, relationships, work functions, and quality of life, and what their expectations for treatment are (Table 23.2).

Physical Exam

The physical examination should be system-driven, and can include a general physical examination. Within the context of urology-related pain, the exam will focus of GU-related structures as a way to establish the possible role of GU pathology. The general appearance of the patient, including apparent level of anxiety and affect, should be noted. Assessment should include sexual function, given the proximity of the sexual organs and GU system.

Laboratory and Imaging Studies

Additional investigations will be influenced by the examination and suspected causes for the pain. (See Chap. 21, and diagnosis specific chapters).

Comorbid Conditions that Impact Acute and Chronic Pain

Acute pain is far less subject to the effects of comorbid, or co-occurring conditions than chronic pain. Acute pain demands attention and is designed to be protective and prevent further injury. Chronic pain is associated with comorbid conditions that have a direct influence on the patient's pain experience, but also increases the risk for other health issues. These associated conditions contribute to psychological and often financial, strain (IOM 2011). A full description of this illness burden is complex, and beyond the scope of this chapter. However, clinicians should be aware that the following domains are impacted by chronic pain (Duenas et al. 2016):

- Quality of life;
- Functional capacity/limited activity;
- Fatigue;
- Sleep disturbance/sleep deprivation/poor sleep hygiene;
- Mood (depression/anxiety/anger);
- Dyscognition (memory/attention);
- Coping mechanisms;
- Gender-specific issues.

Pain behaviors (such as guarding, adjusting gait/posture) can contribute to and sustain pain, and in turn create disability that is not actually a function of the pain itself, such as a lack of movement leading to muscle weakness (Jensen and Turk 2014).

Anxiety, depression, and anger/frustration can create functional limitations, and affect one's judgments of control over pain. For example, anxiety has been implicated in maladaptive pain behaviors, because anxiety represents uncertainty about the future and uncertainty about the meaning of the pain (Gatchel et al. 2007; Serbic et al. 2016), which in turn can result in avoidance of activities that promote recovery. As a further example, anxiety has been evaluated prospectively to its role as a risk factor that may predict chronic postoperative pain. Anxiety preoperatively was the primary predictor of chronic postsurgical pain (Jackson et al. 2016; Powell et al. 2012), suggesting that patients with higher baseline anxiety may be more prone to develop chronic pain. Anxiety can also transition into hypervigilance or catastrophizing, both of which predict a low incidence of treatment success (Karoly and Ruehlman 2007; Sullivan et al. 2001).

Postsurgical Pain Management

Surgical expenditures in the US exceed $500 billion/year, and account for approximately 40% of the national healthcare spending (Muñoz et al. 2010). Many patients have their first exposure to opioids after surgery and the prescribing guidelines for postsurgical dosing and amounts are inconsistent across specialties even in regards to minor surgical procedures. This creates substantial geographic, institutional, and personal variation in postsurgical prescription of opioids.

Recently, there has been increased attention on postoperative pain management, across all specialties. There remains a lack of consensus about pain management strategies, although several authors have offered guidelines. Overton et al. (2018) aimed to create prescribing guidelines for the quantity of opioids after surgery, by using the Delphi method to include a variety of multidisciplinary stakeholders that included patients. Only one urology procedure was included in this process: robotic prostatectomy; these authors' recommendation included 0–10 oxycodone 5 mg tablets as an appropriate postoperative prescription. The authors concluded their study by acknowledging that time pressure is a significant influence on prescribing practices, as was continuity of care.

A 2017 systematic review reported that the incidence of unused opioids was high in all studies, and that for both inpatient and outpatient surgeries more than two-thirds of the patients surveyed reported unused opioids. The authors listed reasons for the unused opioids as patients felt their pain control is adequate (71–83%) and a concern for adverse effects seen with opioid medication (16–29%) (Bicket et al. 2017). These authors also reported that this review revealed that opioids were poorly stored as patients arrived home.

Another area of concern is persistent opioid use postoperatively. Brummett et al. (2017) examined nationwide insurance claims data from 2013 to 2014, including 13 common procedures, with adults aged 18–64. The only urologic procedure included in this review was TURP, but the review did include 31,177 patients with a mean age of 44.6. These authors reported that the primary risk factors for new, persistent opioid use among opioid-naïve patients included use of tobacco, alcohol and previously documented substance abuse. Preexisting diagnoses of anxiety, depression, and other preexisting pain disorders also increased the potential risk for persistent opioid use. Furthermore, these authors reported that for patients receiving opioid prescriptions in the 30 days before their procedure, there was a twofold higher risk of continued use postoperatively. Although this study did not include specific evaluation of patients being treated for stone disease, the finding of increased risk with prescriptions in the 30 days before their procedure is noteworthy.

The AUA has developed a statement regarding for opioid management postoperatively (2019), stating:

> Urologists should manage their patients' pain in a way that addresses the needs of the individual patient while also considering the impact of opioid use on the larger population and society. When opioids are necessary, the lowest dose and lowest potency to adequately control pain from surgery and other conditions should be used and discontinued as soon as possible … Through careful opioid prescribing, patient education, and awareness of risk, urologists can provide quality care for patients and positively impact a critical public health epidemic.

The AUA position statement also endorses the use of Prescription Drug Monitoring Programs (PDMP) while acknowledging that there may be additional improvements necessary in these systems. Furthermore, the AUA agrees with the

FDA and its position that patients must be counseled about the safe use of opioids and proper disposal.

Acebedo et al. (2020) investigated opioid prescribing specifically within the urologic surgery population, based on evidence in the literature that detailed overprescribing in the urologic surgery population. These authors developed guidelines (Fig. 23.2) based on the invasiveness of the procedure and calculating a morphine milligram equivalent (MME) that was then divided into daily dosing based on length of stay. This daily dosing then guided calculation of a discharge regimen for the opioid. The authors also included non-opioid medications into the discharge

1. Consult the Controlled Substance Utilization Review and Evaluation System (CURES) before prescribing opioid analgesics at discharge (State of California Department of Justice, n.d.).
2. In-patient providers should consider non-opioid discharge pain regimen for older adult patients and for patients who underwent minimally invasive urologic procedures (Large et al., 2018).
3. In-patient providers should communicate with out-patient opioid prescriber regarding discharge opioid analgesic plan for patients with prescribed opioid analgesics before admission.
4. In-patient providers should honor patients' pre-existing pain contract with outpatient opioid prescriber.
5. In-patient providers should consult acute pain management service for patients with more than usual postoperative pain response (Chen et al., 2016).
6. For patients with more than usual postoperative pain response, in-patient providers should consider discharge referral to pain specialist or advise patient to follow up with out-patient opioid prescriber for opioid dose adjustment and refill.
7. Unless contraindicated, in-patient providers should prescribe patients with acetaminophen and ibuprofen at discharge (Wick et al., 2017).
8. Unless contraindicated, patients who are post-cystourethroscopy ureteroscopy should be prescribed:
   a. Ibuprofen 400 mg orally every 8 hours around the clock for the first 48 hours, then every 8 hours as needed for pain thereafter.
   b. Tamsulosin (Flomax) orally once daily at bedtime for at least 30 days.
   c. Ditropan 5 mg every 8 hours orally as needed for bladder spasms until the scheduled clinic follow up.
9. Follow the recommended procedure-specific discharge opioid guideline below. The guideline is intended as a point-of-care clinical decision aid and is not intended to replace providers' prudent clinical judgment.

Procedure Type	Recommended Discharge Opioid Quantity
Cystourethroscopies a) Simple cystoscopy b) Ureteroscopy c) Ureteral stent placement	Either: • 10 tablets of hydrocodone 5/acetaminophen 325 mg • 7 tablets of oxycodone 5 mg
Laparoscopic Procedures a) Laparoscopic nephrectomy b) Laparoscopic decortication c) Laparoscopic pyeloplasty	Either: • 40 tablets of hydrocodone 5/325 mg • 25 tablets of oxycodone 5 mg
Male Implants a) Inflatable/malleable penile prosthesis b) Artificial urinary sphincter c) Sling	Either: • 30 tablets of hydrocodone 5/325 mg • 20 tablets of oxycodone 5 mg
Male Reconstruction a) Urethroplasty b) Scrotoplasty c) Phalloplasty	Either: • 15 tablets of hydrocodone 5/325 mg • 10 tablets of oxycodone 5 mg
Percutaneous Access Procedures	Either: • 15 tablets of hydrocodone 5/325 mg • 10 tablets of oxycodone 5 mg
Prostate Procedures a) Holmium laser enucleation of the prostate (HoLEP) b) Transurethral resection of the prostate (TURP)	Either: • 5 tablets of hydrocodone 5/325 mg • 4 tablets of oxycodone 5 mg • 5 tablets of tramadol 50 mg

Fig. 23.2 Urological surgery procedure-specific discharge prescription guideline. (Reprinted with permission. Acebedo, C., Hung, N., & Heshmati, C. (2020). Discharge opioid prescribing guideline for the urologic surgery patient population. *Urologic Nursing, 40*(1), 23–30, 33. https://doi.org/10.7257/1053-816X.2020.40.1.23) (Large et al. 2018; Chen et al. 2016; Wick et al. 2017)

regimen, being mindful of the use of NSAIDs in patients with elevated creatinine. The authors reported that after implementation of these guidelines, 90% of patients surveyed ($n = 158$) reported pain control that was "adequate" or "excellent."

Providers working with postoperative patients should keep in mind that even with guidelines, there is likely to be variation among patients in their use of opioid medications. Facilities may also have their own guidelines in place for determining appropriate opioid prescriptions at discharge. In those states where PDMPs are available, should be certain to check patient previous prescription and usage prior to initiating a new prescription. Providers also need to be aware of the requirements and restrictions that may be unique to their individual state regarding opioid prescription.

Chronic Postsurgical Pain (CPSP)

Describing and defining chronic postsurgical pain (CPSP) suffers from a variety of barriers. Across the literature, there are various terms that have been used: persistent postoperative pain (PPOP) acute or persistent postsurgical neuropathic pain (PPSNP), or chronic postsurgical neuropathic pain (CPSNP). This clearly creates issues with measurement and comparisons across studies. In addition, studies do not agree on a general definition for surgical pain that persists. A general definition is pain that lasts more than 3 months after surgery, with the acknowledgment that some studies define it as greater than 6 months after surgery, while others define it pain that persists for more than 2 months after surgery.

The lack of a standardized definition also creates issues with determining the true incidence of chronic postsurgical pain. There are reports in the literature that CPSP ranges from 10% to 50%, depending on the procedure, and postoperative pain that becomes chronic is independent of an individual's education, socioeconomic status, or insurance type (Niraj and Rowbotham 2011).

There are limited studies globally of CPSP specifically as it relates to urologic procedures. Althaus et al. (2012) reported that patients undergoing GU surgeries reported less chronic pain ($n = 150$ for the study). Alper and Yuksel (2016) compared open vs. laparoscopic nephrectomy, and reported that pain scores between the two sets of patients were very similar, with similar risk for developing CPSP.

Table 23.3 discusses factors that have been identified to be contributors to the risk of developing chronic postsurgical pain (Chapman and Vierck 2017; Schnabel 2018), with the acknowledgment that surgical time and surgical approach cannot always be adjusted.

Furthermore, there are distinct risk factors that place patients at a higher risk for development of CPSP, independent of gender. These include chronic pain in the same area as the planned surgery, chronic pain in general, abdominal pain syndromes, and visceral hyperalgesia syndromes.

Table 23.3 Contributors to chronic postsurgical pain

Preoperative risk	Intraoperative risk	Postoperative risk

• Pain >1 month prior to surgery
• At site or remote from site of planned procedure
• Hyperalgesia: increased response to painful stimuli
• Repeat surgery
• Anxiety; catastrophizing
• Age: younger = higher risk
• Genetics
• Social isolation/poor social support
• (Worker's compensation)
• Female gender/pelvic surgery specific (Butrick 2016)
  – Dyspareunia/vulvodynia
  – PTSD
  – LUTS
  – Recurrent UTIs
  – Defecation issues
  – Urologic chronic pelvic pain syndrome (UCPPS)
• Low sense of control
• Illness perception
• Poor coping mechanisms
• Comorbid symptoms
  – Poor sleep hygiene
  – Use of sleeping medication
  – Fatigue
  – Intrusive/fearful thoughts
	• Procedure in area of large nerves, nerve trunk
	• Procedure with risk of crushing nerves
	• Retraction/cutting fascia, joints, muscles, viscera
	• sensory nerves
	• Operative time: Increased risk with >3 h
	• Open procedures
		• Pain; pain severity post-op
		  – Complaints consistent with neuropathic pain
		• Inadequate pain control POD 1
		• Adjunct therapies
		• Radiation treatment to area
		• Neurotoxic chemotherapy after surgery
		• Depression
		• Psychological vulnerability
		• Anxiety
		• Neuroticism
		• Exaggerated stress response

Butrick, C. W. (2016). Persistent postoperative pain: pathophysiology, risk factors, and prevention. *Female pelvic medicine & reconstructive surgery, 22*(5), 390–396

Anticipating Chronic Postsurgical Pain

Providers can be aware of certain warning signs and help anticipate an individual's risk for development of chronic pain postoperatively. This includes taking steps to prevent new central sensitization that would promote the development of chronic pain (Chapman and Vierck 2017). Goals:

- Aim to resolve or manage any chronic pain that is in the same area as the plan surgery;
- Target close management, when possible, of any existing chronic pain syndromes;
- Consider surgical approaches that minimize tissue trauma when possible;
- Aim for the shortest intraoperative time;

- Consider regional anesthesia and or opioid use that decreases the overall anal-gesia use;
- Postoperatively monitor for a patient's passive response to pain (victim mentality);
- Monitor for a patient's delay in returning to their usual level of activity;
- and remember that the single best predictor of recovery is a patient's preopera-tive anxiety level (Schnabel 2018).

Many of these concerns can be addressed simply by managing patient expecta-tions both preoperatively and postoperatively, by individualizing treatment plans and preoperative education. This means involving patients in their pain manage-ment to encourage self-efficacy through means such as control over their medica-tion. It is also vital to engage partners and family members in the care and management of patients postoperatively.

Barriers to Effective Pain Management

The Institute of Medicine (IOM; 2011) acknowledged the lack of specific chronic pain management training in all healthcare provider curricula. Management of pain by nurse practitioners (NP) and physician assistants (PA) is directly impacted by the absence of urology and pain topics from their curricula, and opportunities for clini-cal training while in school. Prior to recognition of the country-wide the opioid epidemic, there had been little attention to pain management practices in primary care settings, and investigation of the pain management prescribing habits of NPs and PAs was also neglected. Graduate education should include a focus on potential psychosocial issues of the patients and their families, and move to address barriers and the challenges of clinicians for pain management. Current debate centers around the value of curriculum content versus competencies for pain management educa-tion (Gereau et al. 2014), but there is a need to define curricula in order to promote effective pain evaluation and management.

The Department of Health and Human Services (HHS) was tasked with develop-ment of a national curriculum and standards of care for opioid prescribers by the President's Commission on Combating Drug Addiction and the Opioid Crisis (Christie et al. 2017). This included the recommendation that there be guidelines for specialty practitioners, and that multiple specialties be stakeholders in future guide-line development. Additionally, this document recommends that agencies work with stakeholders to develop statutes and regulations and policies to ensure informed patient consent prior to opioid prescribing for chronic pain. The Commission report also recommends that Centers for Medicare and Medicaid Services (CMS) abolish pain assessment as a dimension of patient satisfaction surveys as a way to avoid improper use of these surveys as "savvy providers have figured out that opioids are a way to manipulate satisfaction" (Christie et al. 2017, p. 49). Furthermore, the document recommends removal of pay or barriers to reimbursement of multimodal and interdisciplinary treatments for chronic pain.

In 2015 enough prescription opioids were sold to medicate every US adult with 5 mg hydrocodone every 4 hours for 3 weeks (Jones et al. 2015). In early 2016, The Joint Commission began a project to revise its pain assessment and management standards and to develop standards related to safe and judicious prescribing of opioids. Three main areas were identified: assessment and management of acute pain; assessment and management of chronic pain; and recognition, management, and/or referral of patients addicted to opioids.

Undertreatment of pain, and chronic pain in particular, contributes to decreased quality of life, psychosocial decline, and potential for decreased functional status. This turn creates poorer outcomes, resulting in higher healthcare costs.

Clinical Pearls
- Pain is always subjective.
- Superficial pain is initiated by activation of nociceptors in the skin or other superficial tissue, and is sharp, well-defined, and clearly located.
- Chronic opioid use can cause endocrine abnormalities in both men and women.
- In June 2016, The American Medical Association removed pain as a vital sign.
- In 2018, CMS reimbursement was no longer tied to pain management scores.

Resources for Nurse Practitioners and Physician Assistants

The International Association for the Study of Pain (IASP): www.iasp-pain.org
The IASP Terminology: https://www.iasp-pain.org/Education/Content.
American Urological Association (AUA) Position Statement: Opioid Use (2018 and revised 2019): www.auanet.org/guidelines/opioid-use
Relieving Pain in America: A Blueprint for Transforming Prevention, Care, Education, and Research - summary: https://www.iprcc.nih.gov/sites/default/files/IOM_Pain_Report_508comp_0.pdf
National Pain Strategy: https://www.iprcc.nih.gov/sites/default/files/HHSNational_Pain_Strategy_508C.pdf
CDC Guideline for Prescribing Opioids for Chronic Pain: https://www.cdc.gov/drugoverdose/prescribing/guideline.html

Resources for Patients

American Chronic Pain Association: http://www.theacpa.org
Pain Connection-Chronic Pain Outreach Center: http://www.painconnection.org
Patient Advocate Foundation: http://www.patientadvocate.org
Pain Toolkit: http://www.paintoolkit.org

References

Alper I, Yuksel E (2016) Comparison of acute and chronic pain after open nephrectomy versus laparoscopic nephrectomy: a prospective clinical trial. Medicine 95(16)

Althaus A, Hinrichs-Rocker A, Chapman R, Becker OA, Lefering R, Simanski C, Weber F, Moser KH, Joppich R, Trojan S, Gutzeit N, Neugebauer E (2012) Development of a risk index for the prediction of chronic post-surgical pain. Eur J Pain 16(6):901–910

American Urological Association (AUA) (2018–2019) Position statement: opioid use. www.aua-net.org/guidelines/opioid-use

Bicket MC, Long JJ, Pronovost PJ, Alexander GC, Wu CL (2017) Prescription opioid analgesics commonly unused after surgery: a systematic review. JAMA Surg 152(11):1066–1071

Brummett CM, Waljee JF, Goesling J, Moser S, Lin P, Englesbe MJ, ASB B, Kheterpal S, Nallamothu BK (2017) New persistent opioid use after minor and major surgical procedures in US adults. JAMA Surg 152(6):e170504–e170504

Chapman CR, Vierck CJ (2017) The transition of acute postoperative pain to chronic pain: an integrative overview of research on mechanisms. J Pain 18(4):359–3e1

Chen JH, Hom J, Richman I, Asch SM, Podchiyska T, Johansen NA (2016) Effect of opioid prescribing guidelines in primary care. Medicine 95(35):e4760. https://doi.org/10.1097/MD.0000000000004760

Christie C, Baker C, Cooper R, Kennedy PJ, Madras B, Bondi P (2017) Final report of the president's commission on combating drug addiction and the opioid crisis. Available from https://www.whitehouse.gov/sites/whitehouse.gov/files/images/Meeting%20Draft%20of%20Final%20Report%20-%20November%201%2C%202017.pdf

Duenas M, Ojeda B, Salazar A, Mico JA, Failde I (2016) A review of chronic pain impact on patients, their social environment and the health care system. J Pain Res 9:457–467. https://doi.org/10.2147//JPR.S105892

Gatchel RJ, Peng YB, Peters ML, Fuchs PN, Turk DC (2007) The biopsychosocial approach to chronic pain: scientific advances and future directions. Psychol Bull 133(4):581–624. https://doi.org/10.1037/0033-2909.133.4.581

Gereau RW, Sluka KA, Maixner W, Savage SR, Price TJ, Murinson BB, Sullivan MD, Fillingim RB (2014) A pain research agenda for the 21st century. J Pain 15(12):1203–1214

Institute of Medicine (2011) Relieving pain in America: a blueprint for transforming prevention, care, education and research. The National Academies Press, Washington, DC

International Association for the Study of Pain (1994) Part III: Pain terms, a current list with definitions and notes on usage. In: IASP Task Force on Taxonomy, Merskey H, Bogduk N (eds) Classification of chronic pain, 2nd edn. IASP Press, Seattle, WA. Available from http://www.iasp-pain.org/AM/Template.cfm?Section=Pain_Definitions&Template=/CM/HTMLDisplay.cfm&ContentID=1728#Pain

Jackson T, Tian P, Wang Y, Iezzi T, Xie W (2016) Toward identifying moderators of associations between presurgery emotional distress and postoperative pain outcomes: a meta-analysis of longitudinal studies. J Pain 17(8):874–888. https://doi.org/10.1016/j.jpain.2016.04.003

Jensen MP (2010) A neuropsychological model of pain: research and clinical implications. J Pain 11(1):2–12

Jensen MP, Turk DC (2014) Contributions of psychology to the understanding and treatment of people with chronic pain: why it matters to ALL psychologists. Am Psychol 69(2):105

Jones CM, Logan J, Gladden RM, Bohm MK (2015) Vital signs: demographic and substance use trends among heroin users—United States, 2002–2013. MMWR Morb Mortal Wkly Rep 64(26):719

Karoly P, Ruehlman LS (2007) Psychosocial aspects of pain-related life task interference: an exploratory analysis in a general population sample. Pain Med 8(7):563–572

Large T, Heiman J, Ross A, Anderson B, Krambeck A (2018) Initial experience with narcotic-free ureteroscopy: a feasibility analysis. J Endourol 32:907. https://doi.org/10.1089/end.2018.0459

McCaffery M (1968) Nursing practice theories related t cognition, bodily pain, and man-environment interactions. UCLA Students' Store, Los Angeles, CA

Melzack R (1999) From the gate to the neuromatrix. Pain 82:S121–S126

Mersky H, Bogduk N (1994) Classification of chronic pain: descriptions of chronic pain syndromes and definitions of pain terms, 2nd edn. International Association for the Study of Pain (IASP) Press, Seattle, WA

Muñoz E, Muñoz W III, Wise L (2010) National and surgical health care expenditures, 2005–2025. Ann Surg 251(2):195–200

Murphy KR, Han JL, Yang S, Hussaini SMQ, Elsamadicy AA, Parente B, Xie J, Pagadala P, Lad SP (2017) Prevalence of specific types of pain diagnoses in a sample of United States adults. Pain Phys J 20:E257. Available from www.painphysicianjournal.com

Nahin R (2015) Estimates of pain prevalence and severity in adults: United States, 2012. J Pain 16(8):769–780. https://doi.org/10.1016/j.pain.2015.05.002

Niraj G, Rowbotham DJ (2011) Persistent postoperative pain: where are we now? Br J Anaesth 107(1):25–29

Overton HN, Hanna MN, Bruhn WE, Hutfless S, Bicket MC, Makary MA et al (2018) Opioid-prescribing guidelines for common surgical procedures: an expert panel consensus. J Am Coll Surg 227(4):411–418

Powell R, Johnston M, Smith WC, King PM, Chambers WA, Krukowski Z, McKee L, Bruce J (2012) Psychological risk factors for chronic post-surgical pain after inguinal hernia repair surgery: a prospective cohort study. Eur J Pain 16(4):600–610

Price C, Lee J, Taylor AM, Baranowski AP (2014) Initial assessment and management of pain: a pathway for care developed by the British pain society. Br J Anaesth 112(5):816–823. https://doi.org/10.1093/bja/aet589

Rosenquist RW et al (2010) Practice guidelines for pain management. Anesthesiology 112:810–833

Schnabel A (2018) Acute neuropathic pain and the transition to chronic postsurgical pain. Pain Manag 8(5):317–319

Serbic D, Pincus T, Fife-Schaw C, Dawson H (2016) Diagnostic uncertainty, guilt, mood, and disability in back pain. Health Psychol 35(1):50–59. https://doi.org/10.1037/hea0000272

Stanos S, Brodsky M, Argoff C, Clauw DJ, D'Arcy Y, Donevan S (2016) Rethinking chronic pain in a primary care setting. J Postgrad Med 128(5):502–515. https://doi.org/10.1080/0032548 1.2016.1188319

Sullivan MJ, Thorn B, Haythornthwaite J, Keefe F, Martin M, Bradley L, Lefebvre J (2001) Theoretical perspectives on the relation between catastrophizing and pain. Clin J Pain 17(1):52–64

Tracey I, Johns E (2010) The pain matrix: reloaded or reborn as we image tonic pain using arterial spin labelling. Pain 148:359–360

Wick EC, Grant MC, Wu CL (2017) Postoperative multimodal analgesia pain management with nonopioid analgesics and techniques: a review. JAMA Surg 152(7):691–697

LGBTQ Cultural Humility for the Urology Healthcare Provider

24

Elizabeth K. Kuzma ⓘ and Brooke C. Acarregui Lehmann

Contents

E. K. Kuzma (✉) · B. C. A. Lehmann
University of Michigan School of Nursing, Ann Arbor, MI, USA
e-mail: ekuzma@med.umich.edu

© Springer Nature Switzerland AG 2020
S. A. Quallich, M. J. Lajiness (eds.), *The Nurse Practitioner in Urology*,
https://doi.org/10.1007/978-3-030-45267-4_24

Objectives
1. Understand that LGBTQ people face health disparities for a variety of reasons.
2. Identify several ways the urologic healthcare provider can create safe, inclusive, and affirming spaces and care for LGBTQ patients with cultural humility to help reduce those health disparities.
3. Recognize a variety of unique urologic needs of LGBTQ people.
4. Locate references and resources for more in-depth evidence-based care guidelines for the urologic care of LGBTQ people.

Introduction

It is well documented in the literature that people who identify as lesbian, gay, bisexual, transgender, queer, or questioning (LGBTQ) face many health disparities, for both physical and mental health conditions, including urologic conditions. Some of the disparities are the result of limited access to high-quality, affirming, inclusive, and welcoming healthcare environments resulting from a combination of factors (Kuzma et al. 2019). An important factor is the limited LGBTQ health education that clinicians receive during their formal education. On top of that discriminatory practices of individual providers and health systems further exacerbate challenges that LGBTQ individuals face when trying to access care. Many healthcare providers, including physicians, physician assistants (PAs), nurse practitioners (NPs), and allied health professionals have not received adequate education and training on the unique general and specialty specific care needs of LGBTQI patients (Hollenbach et al. 2014; Kuzma et al. 2019; Lim et al. 2013).

Unfortunately, urology physicians, nurse practitioners, physician assistants in urology, and allied healthcare providers are no exception. One study surveyed Canadian medical residents in several different subspecialties to assess whether or not they felt that caring for transgender patients fell within their scope of practice and if they felt prepared to care for transgender patients (Coutin et al. 2018). Only 50% of the urology residents felt that transgender care fell under their scope of practice, and only 12% felt their medical training prepared them to care for transgender patients. As insurers are broadening coverage for gender affirming surgeries for surgical transition, it is likely that more transgender patients will be accessing urologic specialty care, making it imperative for urology healthcare providers to become more knowledgeable and experienced in caring for these patient populations (Dy et al. 2016).

Having a healthcare workforce that has received inadequate training in LGBTQ health issues contributes to health disparities, because many LGBTQ patients do not receive appropriate preventive services and often experience delays in treatment of common health conditions, which can result in late identification of problems, advanced progression at diagnosis, and unnecessary complications of care (Hickerson et al. 2018; James et al. 2016). Urologic NPs, PAs, and allied health providers can play an important role in reducing health disparities for LGBTQ patients by creating welcoming, inclusive, and affirming spaces and providing care with cultural humility.

About Terms and Language

Before diving further into details about LGBTQ health, it is essential to first provide a brief foundation about terms and language as they relate to the LGBTQ populations. While the common acronym, LGBTQ or another variation (i.e., LGBT, LGBT+, etc.), is used, each component represents diverse and unique populations of people (Hollenbach et al. 2014). Each group within the acronym, which represents a variety of sexual orientations and gender identities, all have diverse and unique social and healthcare needs as a whole as well as for individuals within each separate group (Hollenbach et al. 2014; Makadon et al. 2015). For the purpose of this chapter, LGBTQ will be used as a shorthand term, understanding that language evolves over time making it nearly impossible to list every identity on the gender identity and sexual orientation spectrum. Table 24.1 provides a list of terms and definitions that may be helpful to understand some of the most common terms currently used related to gender identity and sexuality.

Existing State of LGBTQ Healthcare

Health disparities faced by LGBTQ individuals and populations are staggering and will be briefly outlined below to provide important context for providing care to LGBTQ patients. It is also imperative to note that LGBTQ populations and individuals have many strengths, resilience, and powerful inner networks of support (Makadon et al. 2015). Understanding these strengths can help healthcare providers utilize, highlight, and capitalize on the resources to work with their LGBTQ patients to improve their health and well-being.

Healthcare Providers and Access to Care

Access to care can be limited for LGBTQ patients receiving routine care when providers inadvertently perpetuate stereotypes and make assumptions. This can make it more difficult for LGBTQ patients to *come out*, disclose their sexual orientation or gender identity, to their healthcare provider (Zestcott et al. 2016). When providers make assumptions about their patients, avoid discussions, or do not make an effort to intentionally ask about gender identity and sexual orientation, they can miss important information about their patients. Some providers make *heteronormative* and *cisnormative* assumptions, where they automatically assume a patient is heterosexual or cisgender, which are seen as the default/normal sexuality and gender identity (Merriam-Webster n.d.; TheGayUK 2019). Thus, making it difficult to

Table 24.1 Helpful terms and definitions

Terms	Definitions
Asexual	A person with little or no sexual attraction to any gender.
Biological sex	The sum of the biological (chromosomal, hormonal, and anatomical) factors that make an individual male, female, or intersex.
Cisgender	This term refers to someone whose gender identity is the same as the biological sex they were assigned at birth.
Gender diverse, expansive, neutral, queer, or variant, fluid, nonbinary	A person who views their gender identity as one of many possible genders beyond strictly woman/female or man/male
Gender identity	A person's self-identified sense of being male or female (or neither or both). This term refers to how people think about and express their gender.
Gender pronouns	Personal pronouns are used in place of nouns referring to people. Some examples include: • He/him/his • She/Her/Hers • They/Them/Theirs/Themself • Ze/Zie/Hir/Hirs/Hirself • Xe/Xem/Xyr/Xyrs/Xemself • Ey/Em/Eir/Eirs/Emself
Intersex	A person born with sex chromosomes, external genitalia, and/or an internal reproductive system that is not considered "standard" for either male or female.
Passing	This is a term that is used when a transgender person "passes" socially as their gender identity, typically in a binary way—as a man or a woman.
Transgender	This term refers to someone whose gender identity is different from the biological sex they were assigned to at birth.
Transition	The process a gender diverse person undergoes when changing their bodily appearance to be more congruent with the gender/sex they feel themselves to be. Transition can be social (how one dresses and presents oneself to the outside world), legal (changing legal name and gender markers), medical (use of medication, usually hormones and adjuvant medication), and/or surgical (there are a variety of options for gender affirming surgeries).
Sexual and gender minority (SGM)	These are terms that you may see in the literature as another way to describe LGBTQ populations and are used frequently in research.
Sexual orientation	This term refers to how a person identifies sexually—meaning the physical and emotional ways we are attracted to persons of the same gender, another gender, or all genders

Note. From Michigan Medicine, Adolescent Health Initiative, 2014; Oxford University Press, 2018; OK2BME, 2018; http://www.whatisasexuality.com/, nd

understand who their patients are and appreciate their unique health needs, which can lead to substandard care. To provide high-quality patient-centered care, patients must feel affirmed, included, and welcomed in healthcare spaces (Kuzma et al. 2019).

Disclosure of Sexual Orientation and Gender Identity to Healthcare Providers

In order for healthcare providers to offer the most comprehensive, evidence-based, individualized care to their patients, they must first seek to understand who their patients are and how they identify, including sexual orientation and gender identity. However, healthcare providers do not regularly ask about gender identity or sexual orientation, for a variety of reasons, including lack of comfort with such discussions (Rossman et al. 2017). Beyond that, avoidance may be unintentional when clinicians make heteronormative and cisnormative assumptions. In some extreme cases, LGBTQ patients have been outright refused care by providers due to homophobia and transphobia (Hollenbach et al. 2014).

If healthcare providers do not assess sexual orientation and gender identity routinely, it puts pressure on LGBTQ individuals to disclose this information. Yet, for LGBTQ individuals, disclosing this information, or *coming out* to their healthcare providers can be just as challenging as *coming out* to their loved ones because they fear or anticipate judgment or refusal of care (Law et al. 2015). LGBTQ patients who do not disclose their identity often experience worse mental health status when compared with those who do share their identity with their healthcare providers (Durso and Meyer 2013). Thus, highlighting the need for healthcare providers to create safe, inclusive, and affirming spaces where patients receive a positive and supportive response when they disclose their identity (Rossman et al. 2017).

To better understand the unique perspectives and needs of LGBTQ patients, providers need to also understand the societal issues many LGBTQ communities face and have faced historically, including systematic discrimination and oppression as well as interpersonal violence and trauma (Hollenbach et al. 2014; Makadon et al. 2015). Healthcare systems and providers share some responsibility in perpetuating the discrimination and oppression that LGBTQ individuals and communities have endured.

Health Disparities

LGBTQ people face staggering health disparities, such as higher rates of a variety of illnesses, poorer health outcomes, and increased morbidity and mortality when compared with their *cisgender* (sex assigned at birth is consistent with gender identity) and straight (heterosexual) peers (Mogul-Adlin 2015; Ward et al. 2014). Some examples of health disparities include (a) decreased rates of preventive care (i.e., lesbian women are screened less often for cervical cancer), (b) gay men have higher rates of sexually transmitted infections (STIs), including the human immunodeficiency virus (HIV), (c) two to three times higher rates of homelessness, (d) more likely to experience trauma and victimization, and (e) higher rates of depression and suicide (CDC 2019c). The LGBTQ populations with the greatest health disparities are LGBTQ youth, transgender people, and most significantly transgender people of color (CDC 2019c).

Minority Stress Theory

There are a number of theories why the health disparities of LGBTQ people are so significant, including the minority stress theory. Ihan Meyer's minority stress model posits that systemic and cultural stigma (i.e., transphobia, binary gender norms, homophobia, etc.) results in a series of proximal and distal stressors between the LGBTQ individual and interactions with the surrounding environment, the community, and oneself that may negatively affect the minority individual (2003). Minority stress is "to distinguish the excess stress to which individuals from stigmatized social categories are exposed as a result of their social, often a minority, position" (Meyer 2003, pp. 675). Consider an LGBTQ individual encountering a health system. The individual may incur distal stress through their interaction with the health system environment to include health system personnel. Next, proximal stressors affect the individual's perception of the environment. Proximal stressors include the individual's internalized minority status (i.e., societal stigma against LGBTQ people) and their interaction with the external environment (Meyer 2003). As a result of systemic and internalized stigma, the individual may anticipate prejudice to occur as they go about their encounters. The model further explains layers of minority status for individuals who are, for example, a racial minority and a sexual or gender minority, also known as intersectionality. In such case, the individual would incur additional layering of minority stressors related to their multiple identities (Meyer 2003).

Coping and resilience is, in part, fostered by the camaraderie that exists from the minority status itself. According to Meyer, individuals who identify as LGBTQ are able to find resilience through their social support from other LGBTQ members and allies (Meyer 2003). When social support is positive for the individual, it lends to positive coping and increased resilience combating the minority stressors.

Longstanding societal discrimination and oppression may increase the stress faced by LGBTQ people, leading to the initiation and progression of maladaptive and often unhealthy coping methods and self-care strategies which may worsen health status and disparities (Makadon et al. 2015). Additionally, seminal research, led by Drs. Felitti and Anda in 1998, identified the association between exposure to adverse childhood experiences (ACE), chronic stress, trauma, and disparities in chronic health problems, including early morbidity and mortality (Felitti et al. 1998). The results of the study found that even in the absence of unhealthy risk-behaviors, those with exposure to these adverse experiences and chronic stress still faced significant health disparities, likely due to physiologic changes in the brain and body in response to the chronic stress (Felitti et al. 1998).

When the minority stress model is applied to understand LGBTQ patients' encounters accessing healthcare, the importance of providing inclusive, welcoming environments and culturally competent care cannot be overstated. When there is inclusive, affirming and culturally competent care, the LGBTQ individual's minority stress experience decreases, their coping and resilience increase, and slowly trust is introduced. The goal is to support improved health status and outcomes by virtue of an increase in healthcare utilization on behalf of the individuals.

Oppression and Discrimination

LGBTQ individuals and communities have a long history of oppression and discrimination in healthcare and in society (Hollenbach et al. 2014). LGBTQ identities were criminalized socially and pathologized in healthcare, for example homosexuality was considered a mental illness until the 1970s when it was de-classified (Hollenbach et al. 2014). Transgender people were previously diagnosed with *gender identity disorder* if they identified as transgender, pathologizing the identity itself (APA 2013). That has since changed to *gender dysphoria*, where a person does not receive a diagnosis for being transgender, rather a diagnosis is made for transgender patients who experience distress or discomfort with the fact that their gender identity does not match their biologic sex (APA 2013). The history of pathologization of LGBTQ identities perpetuates stigma and magnifies the distrust LGBTQ people have with healthcare providers and systems (Hollenbach et al. 2014).

The reason for health disparities faced by LGBTQ individuals and communities are not fully understood, but many believe they are likely due to a combination of factors, including the health impact of chronic stress from persistent, systematic, societal discrimination, and oppression. Additionally, health disparities may be attributed to the negative health effects associated with the development of maladaptive coping strategies as well as the barriers LGBTQ patients face in accessing inclusive, affirming, and welcoming healthcare provided by knowledgeable clinicians and staff. When healthcare providers better understand the origin of health disparities faced by their LGBTQ patients, they are armed with knowledge to improve their ability to provide equitable care to mitigate the adverse health effects.

Cultural Humility

While many healthcare providers have been taught about cultural competence, the concept of cultural humility is fairly new. Although it is important to understand that cultural competence can present foundational information to understand norms within certain cultures and unique experiences or challenges faced, it is not enough (Chang et al. 2012). No one can become truly competent in understanding another person's or communities' culture. Individuals within cultures have unique experiences and beliefs that may or may not align with cultural norms.

Cultural humility is a novel way of striving to understand the culture of others that is particularly helpful for healthcare providers. Approaching patients with cultural humility, means the healthcare provider may have learned information about cultural norms, but they understand that all people are unique, with their own individual beliefs, and may express their culture and heritage differently (Chang et al. 2012; Moncho 2013). Thus, requiring the healthcare provider to truly provide patient-centered care by using self-reflection, improving self-awareness, avoiding assumptions, accepting limitations, and partnering with patients to better understand their needs (Kuzma et al. 2019). In partnering or collaborating with patients, healthcare providers understand that patients are experts about themselves, and therefore they can learn from their patients as much as their patients can learn from them (Hohman 2013). The practice of caring with cultural humility requires lifelong learning and self-reflection (Hohman 2013; Kuzma et al. 2019).

Providing Inclusive and Affirming Care

All patients deserve to be able to access healthcare settings that are inclusive and affirming of their identity. Being inclusive is when all patients are welcomed and affirmed regardless of their race, socioeconomic status, level of education, culture, gender identity, and sexual orientation (Kuzma et al. 2019). To be affirming, one must be nonjudgmental, accepting of others as they are and respecting them as people (Makadon et al. 2015). Healthcare providers can practice with cultural humility to foster inclusive and affirming care in welcoming, safe spaces (Makadon et al. 2015).

Cultural Humility: Self-reflection

Self-reflection is the first step in caring for patients with cultural humility. All people have biases about various aspects of the world around them, both conscious and unconscious or implicit (Staats et al. 2017). Conscious biases are those that the conscious mind is aware of (Hannah and Carpenter-Song 2013). Implicit or unconscious biases are deeper in the brain, develop over time as the brain categorizes things in the world based on socialization and past experiences, and are more automatic (Staats et al. 2017). Implicit biases often come out in times of stress or when quick decisions need to be made (Hannah and Carpenter-Song 2013). Unconscious biases can conflict with a person's conscious beliefs and values (Staats et al. 2017).

However, healthcare providers' implicit biases can impact the care they provide and outcomes for the patients they serve. Therefore, healthcare providers must first self-reflect to become aware of their own beliefs and intentionally work to overcome or resist their biases to improve their relationships with patients, the quality of care they provide, and outcomes of care (Kuzma et al. 2019).

Education

The Institute of Medicine (2011) emphasized the need for an adequately educated healthcare workforce on the unique needs of LGBTQ communities as a key component to reducing the staggering health disparities these communities face, by improving access to appropriate, evidence-based care. As noted earlier, healthcare providers receive inadequate formal education about LGBTQ patient care. Medical and nursing schools offer a range from no content to up to 5 hours throughout their programs and nursing schools have a median of 2.13 hours on LGBTQ health (Lim

Table 24.2 Communication best practices

Best practice	Example
When addressing new patients, avoid pronouns or gendered words like "sir" or "ma'am."	"How may I help you today?"
When talking to coworkers about new patients, also avoid pronouns and gender terms. Or, use gender-neutral words such as "they." Never refer to someone as "it."	"Your patient is here in the waiting room." "They are here for their 3 o'clock appointment."
Politely and privately ask if you are unsure about a patient's preferred name or pronouns.	"What name and pronouns would you like us to use?" "I would like to be respectful—how would you like to be addressed?"
Ask respectfully about names if they do not match in your records.	"Could your chart be under another name?" "What is the name on your insurance?"
Avoid assuming the gender of patient's partners.	"Are you in a relationship?"
Use the terms people use to describe themselves.	If someone calls himself "gay," do not use the term "homosexual." If a woman refers to her "wife," then say "your wife" when referring to her; do not say "your friend."
Only ask for information that is required.	Ask yourself: What do I know? What do I need to know? How can I ask in a sensitive way?
Did you make a mistake? Apologize.	"I apologize for using the wrong pronoun. I did not mean to disrespect you."

National LGBT Health Center. (2016). *Providing inclusive services and care for LGBTQ people: A guide for healthcare staff*

et al. 2013). Urologic residents have reported specifically feeling inadequately prepared to care for transgender patients (Coutin et al. 2018).

Therefore, practicing healthcare providers must take initiative themselves to learn more about the unique needs of these patient populations to better provide care by seeking out educational opportunities at conferences, reading articles, and books (like this one). Table 24.2 lists a variety of resources and references for healthcare providers to learn more about evidence-based LGBTQ healthcare. When equipped with the knowledge about best practices and evidence-based care for LGBTQ patients, healthcare providers could improve health promotion, disease prevention, early identification of diseases, and improve morbidity and mortality.

Creating Safe Spaces

The physical environment and space in which care is provided in healthcare is often cold, sterile, and provider or system-centric. An important step to improve LGBTQ patient access to care is creating physical spaces and environments that is welcoming to all patients (Makadon et al. 2015). By altering the physical environment to be more inclusive, safe spaces can be created. There are a number of ways this can be achieved, including adding visual cues in common spaces, such as: (a) posters and pamphlets with photos and information LGBTQ patients can identify with in common areas, (b) having rainbow stickers visible, and (c) having gender-neutral or gender-inclusive bathrooms available (National LGBT Health Center, no date). Beyond adding visual cues, all providers and staff must be trained in providing inclusive, affirming care with cultural humility, beginning with the use of appropriate terms and language.

Healthcare providers can decrease the pressure for LGBTQ patients to disclose their identity by consistently asking all of their patients direct, respectful, and clear questions about sexual orientation or gender identity. Tables 24.2 and 24.3 provides

Table 24.3 Provider and patient resources for LGBTQ health

Highlights	Website
CDC: Lesbian, Gay, Bisexual, and Transgender Health: Health statistics reports and resources	https://www.cdc.gov/lgbthealth/
Fenway Health's National LGBT Health Education Center: Provider resources, online modules, training sessions, conferences, patient resources	https://www.lgbthealtheducation.org/
InterAct is an organization that advocates for intersex youth. Information on intersex advocacy, policy, and education for the public.	https://interactadvocates.org/
Lambda Legal serves to achieve full civil rights for LGBTQ people and provides legal references and learning	https://www.lambdalegal.org/
Project Implicit: Offers a variety of tests to assess your own implicit biases	https://implicit.harvard.edu/implicit/
Trans Guys Supply Blog Post: Helpful information for educating transmasculine patients on the care of their packing devices	https://transguysupply.com/blogs/news/how-to-care-for-your-packer
UCSF Center for Excellence in Transgender Health: Online resources, guidelines for primary care of transgender individuals	http://transhealth.ucsf.edu/
What Is Asexuality: Definitions, information, and resources to learn more about asexuality	http://whatisasexuality.com
World Professional Association for Transgender Health: International guidelines for transgender healthcare, online resources for providers and patients	http://www.wpath.org/
Highlights	Book
This is a comprehensive book that covers broad-ranging healthcare information and guidelines for caring for LGBTQ patients	Fenway Guide to Lesbian, Gay, Bisexual, and Transgender Health, Second edition Harvey J. Makadon, Kenneth H. Mayer, Jennifer Potter, and Hilary Goldhammer, MS
This is a comprehensive book that covers broad-ranging healthcare guidelines for primary and specialty care of LGBTQ patients	Lesbian, Gay, Bisexual, and Transgender Healthcare: A Clinical Guide to Preventive, Primary, and Specialty Healthcare Kristen Eckstrand and Jessie M. Ehrenfield, *Editors*

examples of best practices for communication from Fenway Health. Once this information is collected, healthcare providers should respect the patients' identity and use their pronouns and preferred name (Rossman et al. 2017).

Urology-Specific Considerations for LGBTQ Patients

The purpose of this section is not to outline the management of specific urologic conditions as those are outlined elsewhere in the book. Rather the point is to focus on how these common urologic conditions might impact LGBTQ patients and to outline unique considerations.

Health Promotion and Disease Prevention

Obesity

Obesity has an impact on bladder health (Mobley and Baum 2015b). When compared to heterosexual women, lesbian and bisexual women have higher rates of being overweight or obese (Fallin-Bennett et al. 2016). While gay men tend to have lower, more healthy body mass index (BMI), some gay men are part of a "bear" subculture, where they tend to be stockier, have hairy bodies, and appear rugged (Fallin-Bennett et al. 2016; Flores 2015). Within this subculture it may be considered normal or celebrated to have a larger body and high body mass index (BMI) (Fallin-Bennett et al. 2016). Obesity has been tied to higher rates of prostate cancer, hypogonadism, erectile dysfunction, lower urinary tract infections, lower urinary tract symptoms (i.e., bladder leaking, urinary frequency, etc.), and natal male infertility (Mobley and Baum 2015b).

Tobacco Use

LGBTQ people have higher rates of tobacco use than their heterosexual peers, nearly twice as high (Fallin-Bennett et al. 2016). This disparity is due to a number of factors, including minority stress. Tobacco use is of particular concern for the urology provider due to the negative impact smoking has on urologic health. For instance, the main risk factor for developing bladder cancer is cigarette smoking (Mobley and Baum 2015a). As LGBTQ people have higher rates of smoking, there is also an associated increased risk of developing bladder cancer (Fallin-Bennett et al. 2016). Tobacco use has also been linked to an increased risk of prostate cancer and associated increased mortality (over 40% higher in smokers) from the disease (Mobley and Baum 2015a). Additionally, tobacco use has been associated with higher rates of erectile dysfunction, incontinence, infertility, benign prostatic hyperplasia, and interstitial cystitis. Thus highlighting why screening LGBTQ patients for tobacco use and providing tobacco cessation counseling is necessary.

Prostate Cancer Screening

The U.S. Preventive Services Task Force (USPSTF) advises against routine screening for prostate cancer using prostate-specific antigen (PSA) screening test (USPSTF 2019). Gay and bisexual men and transgender women age 55–69 with an intact prostate should be counseled by a clinician about the risks and benefits of the use of PSA screening for prostate cancer and offered the opportunity to be screened (Fallin-Bennett et al. 2016). Lastly, when providing care to transgender women after gender confirmation vaginoplasty, it is important to note that the prostate is retained during the surgery and the possibility of prostate cancer remains (Wesp 2016). Estrogen hormone therapy for transgender women may reduce the risk of prostate cancer; however, should the provider need to examine the prostate this should be done via the neovagina by palpating along the ventral aspect of the neo-vaginal wall or through transvaginal ultrasound (Wesp 2016).

Sexual History

The importance of performing a sensitive discussion inclusive of sexual issues cannot be overstated. Discussing sexuality and sexual or urinary issues can be challenging for any patient, but it can be particularly stressful for LGBTQ people (Truesdale et al. 2015). Patients should be able to access care where they feel comfortable sharing sensitive information about their history, gender identity, and sexuality without having to worry about experiencing discrimination or judgment. LGBTQ patients who do not disclose their gender identity and/or sexual orientation experience poorer health outcomes and face increased health disparities (Hollenbach et al. 2014). Therefore it is essential for urologic providers to create open and inclusive healthcare environments, to be able to obtain essential details of their patients' histories, including LGBTQ identities, and provide individualized, evidence-based care.

When collecting a sexual history, one must suspend judgment, avoid assumptions, and use inclusive language. Try to avoid any assumptions about an individual's sexual practices based on their stated sexual orientation or relationship status. People's sexual behaviors do not always align with their reported sexual orientation (Truesdale et al. 2015). For example, approximately 7% of adult women under the age of 60 in the United States (U.S) have reported having sexual experiences with other women, of which more than half identified as heterosexual (Truesdale et al. 2015). Over two-thirds of lesbian women have had a sexual relationship with a man in the past and about 6% did in the past year (Truesdale et al. 2015). There are also a number of men who identify as heterosexual, but have sex with other men and those who identify as gay, but also have sex with women. Some clinicians and researchers use the terms men who have sex with men (MSM) or women who have sex with women (WSW) instead of lesbian, gay, or bisexual to differentiate identity from behavior.

Specific to the transgender patient population, it is important to recognize that gender identity does not indicate sexual orientation. Moreover, a transgender person who elects to have gender affirmation surgery, specifically genitoplasty (i.e., phalloplasty, vaginoplasty, etc.), does not correlate with their sexual preference nor does it imply a specific sexual function preference. Completing an "organ inventory" is a helpful tool the urology provider can use to identify which organs the transgender person has retained during their transition (Makadon et al. 2015). It is up to the urology provider to assess for specific sexual history and preference should the clinical scenario indicate the need to know.

When asking sexual health questions during a clinical encounter it is helpful to preface the questions with a statement about the nature of the questions you will be asking and why you are going to ask them. For example, "I am going to ask you some sensitive questions about your sexual health and sexual practices, which may seem intrusive. However, this information is important for me to understand as a clinician so I can better understand you, your health needs, and how we can work together to help you be as healthy as possible." Below are some examples of questions that could be included on patient history forms or during the patient encounter:

- "Do you have any questions or concerns regarding your sexual health?"
- "What are the genders of your partners (i.e., cisgender men, cisgender women, trans men, trans women)?"
- "What type of sex do you engage in—anal, oral, vaginal?"
  - "If you are a man who has anal sex with other men do you have insertive (top), receptive (bottom), or both?"
- "What type of practices do you use to prevent/reduce the risk of sexually transmitted infections (i.e., pulling out, condoms, oral versus anal/vaginal penetrative sex, dental dam)?"
- "Do you have a history of a sexually transmitted infection (i.e., gonorrhea, chlamydia, trichomonas, syphilis, Hepatitis C, etc.)?"
- "Have you ever been tested for HIV?"
- "Do you have questions about family planning for yourself or your partner (i.e., preventing pregnancy)?"
- "Do you have questions about fertility preservation?"

Sexual Function and Satisfaction
Assessing sexual function and satisfaction is important for providing holistic, patient-centered care to all patients, and is particularly important for LGBTQ patients, because of the potential impact on their relationship dynamics and mental health.

Anal Intercourse
When cisgender men and transgender women engage in sexual activity, an area in the center of the brain, the mesodiencephalic transition zone, is activated (Truesdale et al. 2015). Of particular interest, this area of the brain has dopaminergic nerve cells and is controlled by the neurotransmitter dopamine, which is connected to pleasure and reward behaviors. The spinal cord carries sensory information from the rectum, anus, and genitals to the mesodiencephalic region of the brain during ejaculation, which is likely the reason that stimulation of the anus and genitals cause such great pleasure and are rewarding. Beyond that, the prostate itself also produces sexual stimulation and pleasure. Many gay or bisexual men, some transgender

women, and other men who have sex with men, engage in anal intercourse, therefore it is important to understand the role of the anus, prostate, and rectum in providing pleasure during anal receptive intercourse or stimulation.

Screening for STIs, Including HIV

Gay and bisexual men are known to experience STIs at a much higher rate than their heterosexual peers, with a prevalence of 11.2% for Chlamydia and 14.9% for gonorrhea (CDC 2015). Most notably, men who have sex with men represent 62% of all syphilis cases (both primary and secondary) and 70% of new HIV cases in the U.S. (CDC 2016; CDC 2019a). Transgender women, particularly transgender women of color have disproportionate rates of STIs, most notably for HIV (account for more than half of the cases for transgender men and women) (CDC 2019b). While the risk for STIs is somewhat lower for women who have sex with women due to less efficient transmission, they remain at risk for contracting STIs (CDC 2015). HIV transmission in women who have sex with women is possible, though extremely rare.

Performing a comprehensive sexual history for LGBTQ patients is important to identify sexual practices, partners, and methods used to protect from STIs to help identify individualized risks (Fallin-Bennett et al. 2016). STI screening for LGBTQ patients should align with the type of sex they engage in and which body parts they and their partners have (Fallin-Bennett et al. 2016). For example, if a cisgender man or transwoman has oral or anal sex (receptive and insertive) with cisgender men or transgender women, they should be screened for STIs (i.e., gonorrhea and chlamydia) from oral, urine or genital, and anal samples (CDC 2015).

Family Planning

Family planning is a topic to address with any patient, regardless of sexual orientation or gender identity. The literature supports that LGBTQ patients are interested in becoming parents through surrogacy, adoption, and pregnancy (Fallin-Bennett et al. 2016). However, likely due to existing prejudice toward the LGBT community related to childbearing and childrearing, these individuals often are discriminated against by providers when seeking care for family planning and fertility (Klein et al. 2018). Thus, it is paramount that the urologic provider intentionally addresses family planning with LGBTQ patients so as not to make assumptions about the patient's preferences. To address family planning with cultural humility, it is important that the urologic provider consider the possibility of their own heteronormative and cisnormative implicit bias. When discussing options with patients, it is important to also suggest legal counsel to navigate state-specific laws related to custody and LGBTQ families (Eyler et al. 2014).

Options for biological offspring and family planning continue to evolve. It is important that the urologic provider strive to address each couple with the same respect they would be addressing a heterosexual couple. According to expert review, lesbian and bisexual female couples have the following options for family planning: donor sperm insemination, including home self-insemination, and also in-vitro fertilization (IVF) and donor sperm (Eyler et al. 2014). A new trend emerging called "reciprocal" IVF female couples allows one female partner to serve as the egg donor and the other female partner to carry the pregnancy via IVF and sperm donation to allow both partners a biological attachment to the pregnancy (Eyler et al. 2014). Gay male couples may parent offspring via egg donor and gestational surrogacy (Eyler et al. 2014). In some cases, surrogates may even be family members (sisters or cousins) of the gay couple, or good friends.

Family planning should also be addressed with transgender individuals. Transgender individuals who retain natal sex organs, specifically transgender males, have been able to achieve pregnancy and carry a pregnancy to term (Fallin-Bennett et al. 2016). Of note, testosterone is a teratogen to the fetus, and testosterone is not a reliable form of birth control for the transgender man. Even if he stops menstruation as a result of hormone therapy, he may still become pregnant if having vaginal sexual intercourse with a cisgender male (Fallin-Bennett et al. 2016). Transgender women who have already been on estrogen therapy may have a return of spermatogenesis when going off of estrogen therapy, but the sperm counts drop often requiring infertility intervention (Eyler et al. 2014).

Sexual Functioning

Adult men and women in the U.S. rate satisfaction with their sex life and sexual health highly important for their quality of life (Flynn et al. 2016). Clinicians should incorporate an assessment of sexual health, including sexual functioning, desire, and pleasure as part of routine care for their patients. Performing a thorough, inclusive, and sensitive sexual health assessment can help identify important sexual health concerns for all patients, including those who identify as LGBTQ.

Erectile Dysfunction

Research has found that approximately 58% of gay and bisexual men have experienced at least one episode of erectile dysfunction, which is higher than their heterosexual peers of which 46% have (Fallin-Bennett et al. 2016). Men who have sex with men have higher rates of tobacco use, which also increases their risk for erectile dysfunction. Other contributing factors for erectile dysfunction include: decreased libido, single relationship status, increased age, and passive or versatile sexual role. Acquired immunodeficiency syndrome (AIDS) and a history of lower urinary tract symptoms (LUTS) were also associated with erectile dysfunction.

Erectile dysfunction is a particularly important issue for men who engage in anal intercourse, including men who have sex with men (Fallin-Bennett et al. 2016). A very firm erection is needed for anal sex in order to penetrate through the muscle tone of the anal sphincter. Therefore, small changes in the ability to obtain a firm erection can have a significant effect on sexual performance and satisfaction for gay and bisexual men who have insertive anal sex (top) (Fallin-Bennett et al. 2016).

Premature Ejaculation

Clinical premature ejaculation is the ejaculation that occurs in under 1 min following penetration that is associated with distress and loss of the sense of control (Porst and Burri 2019). The definition for premature ejaculation has a heterosexist lens as the most recognized definition is specifically related to vaginal penetration with no mention of anal penetration. While the definition is not inclusive for men who engage in anal sex, premature ejaculation has similar prevalence (about 5%) for heterosexual men and men who have sex with men (Fallin-Bennett et al. 2016; Porst and Burri 2019).

Decline in Sexual Desire

Low sexual desire, also defined as hypoactive sexual desire disorder, occurs in a number of men and women. It has been found that between 17% and 35% of women and 15–25% of men experience low sexual desire, though both are understudied (McCabe et al. 2016). There is limited to no evidence in the literature regarding the prevalence of low sexual desire for LGBTQ individuals; however, one could presume that if it is a problem for heterosexual individuals, it is also a problem for a subset of LGBTQ people as well and can significantly impact one's sexual satisfaction and quality of life. Having low sexual desire can be impacted by a number of factors, including poor mental health, which has high prevalence in LGBTQ populations (Fallin-Bennett et al. 2016).

Sexual Dysfunction, HIV, and AIDS

Men who have sex with men with AIDS are at risk for developing problems with sexual function, including premature ejaculation and/or erectile dysfunction (Fallin-Bennett et al. 2016). This is possibly due to low CD4 levels, long-term use of antiretroviral medications, and exposure to opportunistic infections (Fallin-Bennett et al. 2016). Other possible contributing factors are: long-term antidepressant therapy, chronic need for antihypertensive medications, and testosterone deficiency which can be common among HIV positive men. Another hypothesis is the effect of psychological stressors associated with HIV status may impact sexual functioning.

Treating erectile dysfunction in men with HIV takes some special considerations, particularly the risk or concern of transmission of HIV to their sexual partners (Fallin-Bennett et al. 2016). Condom use is an important method to prevent or reduce the risk of HIV transmission from one sexual partner to another. Yet, condom use may lead to additional erectile challenges for men with erectile dysfunction, making it more likely that an HIV positive man may not use a condom during sex. Treatment of erectile dysfunction in HIV positive men when paired with counseling on safe sex practices could facilitate condom use and safer sex practices.

Lower Urinary Tract Symptoms (LUTS)

Lower urinary tract symptoms are common complaints that present to urology. Cisgender men and transgender women with a history of STIs or urinary tract infections, increasing prostate size, and those who are HIV positive are more likely to develop LUTS (Truesdale et al. 2015). As gay and bisexual cisgender men and transgender women have higher rates of STIs and HIV, they may also have higher rates of LUTS. LGBTQ individuals experience significantly higher rates of depression. Major depression has also been found to contribute to the development of LUTS, potentially due to an increase in inflammatory markers associated with depression. As mentioned above, bisexual and lesbian women have higher incidence of obesity, which is also another key risk factor for the development of LUTS (Truesdale et al. 2015).

Prostate Cancer Care: Special Considerations

In general, sexual and gender minority cancer survivors report experiencing discrimination during their care, experience gaps in care, have less social support during their treatment, and experience greater social isolation (Wheldon et al. 2018). Commonly used tools to evaluate treatment effects after prostate cancer are not inclusive of non-heterosexual sexual behaviors (Fallin-Bennett et al. 2016). For example, some questions focus on whether or not an erection is vigorous enough for vaginal penetration. Regardless, gay men with prostate cancer report more severe scores on health-related quality of life scales, compared with their heterosexual peers (Hart et al. 2014). Men who have sex with men experience similar side effects related to prostate cancer treatment (i.e., urinary incontinence, painful anal receptive intercourse, erectile dysfunction, and loss of ejaculation) and the associated impact on quality of life (Fallin-Bennett et al. 2016). Yet, the side effects may have a unique impact for men who have sex with men relative to their sexual behaviors, and are associated with increased distress, more dissatisfaction with care, and fear of recurrence (Hart et al. 2014).

Gay men who engage in receptive anal sex (bottom) may be disproportionately impacted by prostate cancer treatment (Fallin-Bennett et al. 2016). For instance, radiation-induced rectal wall fibrosis, surgical removal of the prostate, or other changes in the pelvic anatomy that can cause chronic pelvic pain have a particular impact on men who enjoy anal receptive sex. Prostate cancer treatment has also been associated with decreased penile size, which can be distressing to any man, but is extremely distressing to gay and bisexual men (Fallin-Bennett et al. 2016). As noted earlier, it is important for clinicians to perform a comprehensive sexual health history; this is also true for patients diagnosed with prostate cancer. Gathering this information would be helpful to evaluate what elements of their patients' sexual expression are important to them. For gay men in particular, this means assessing the importance of penis size, and their ability to engage in receptive or insertive anal sex.

Counseling patients on the potential side effects of treatment and discussing how treatment may also impact relationship dynamics is important for same sex couples. The dynamics in an established relationship for a same sex couple can change following prostate cancer treatment. For example, consider this scenario: a man with prostate cancer treated with a radical prostatectomy who previously enjoyed having receptive anal sex (bottom) and their partner who enjoyed having insertive anal sex (top). Following surgery, the couple would likely need to renegotiate their sexual roles and practices, which would inherently change their relationship dynamics. It would be helpful to discuss this possibility prior to treatment to help the patient and their partner prepare for their role change.

Urology and Transgender Men and Women

Access to Bathrooms

All transgender individuals are likely to experience challenges in accessing a bathroom that they would be welcome to use (James et al. 2016). Often bathrooms are gendered, for "men" or "women." This is particularly challenging for transgender youth in the school setting. Schools may not have many, if any, gender-neutral, gender-inclusive, or unisex bathrooms, and those that are available may be in locations that are far away, difficult to get to, or associated with school personnel (i.e., Principal's Office). While different schools may have different rules on which bathrooms transgender youth are able to use, they may not be safe using the bathroom that aligns with their sex assigned at birth. For example, transgender women face victimization and trauma at alarming rates, and requiring them to use the "men's" bathroom, could put them at risk for experiencing violence (Herman 2013). Transgender people's access to bathrooms is becoming more of an issue as some states are working on legislation that would restrict their access to bathrooms, and require them to use a bathroom that aligns with their sex assigned at birth (Herman 2013). Challenges in accessing bathrooms in a timely manner can have an impact on urologic health, requiring transgender individuals to restrict their fluid intake, or hold their urine for excessive periods of time, potentially leading to impaired bladder function.

According to one study where transgender women and transgender men were surveyed, 70% reported experiencing at least one of the following problems related to bathroom use: denied access, verbal harassment, or physical assault because of their gender identity (Herman 2013). Among those surveyed, 54% reported a health problem as a result of avoiding public bathroom use including dehydration, urinary tract infections (UTI), pyelonephritis, and other kidney-related problems (Herman 2013). The 2015 United States Transgender Survey ($n = 27,715$) reflects similar numbers (James et al. 2016). Fifty-five percent indicated they avoided using public restrooms out of fear of discrimination, harassment, or physical violence (James et al. 2016). Almost one-third of respondents indicated they had avoided eating or drinking to prevent needing to use the public restroom which, in some cases, resulted in health problems including UTI, pyelonephritis, and incontinence among other urologic health conditions (James et al. 2016).

Tucking

Many transgender individuals use different practices to change their physical appearance during their social transition to affirm their gender and *pass* (see Table 24.1 for definition), including *tucking* and *packing*. *Tucking* is a practice that some transgender women use to present a smooth contour to their crotch by moving the scrotum and penis back and between the legs in the perineal region and moving testicles (if still present) into the inguinal canal (Deutsch 2016). The position of the genitals is held in place by either adhesive tape, tight fitting underwear, or a special garment called a gaffe. As this practice helps transgender women affirm their gender, the position of the tucking may even be maintained during sleep (Zevin 2016). This practice, while important for transgender women to affirm their gender, is dangerous and has risks of complications, including scrotal pain from neuropathic, traumatic, or mechanical sources (Deutsch 2016). If the practice of tucking is longstanding it may cause the anus to be a source of urinary tract infections or more seriously, lead to the compression of the urethral meatus.

Packing

Packing is a practice that some transgender men use to present a bulge in their crotch for social transition, to affirm their gender, to *pass*, and reduce gender dysphoria (Deutsch 2016). Packing can be done with various items that give the outward appearance of "male" genitals, such as penis and scrotum, including penile prosthesis (Underwood 2016). Additionally, some transgender men use stand-to-pee devices to allow them to urinate standing up, which may or may not be the same device used for packing. When used for urination, they often are made out of rubber or silicone. The device forms a seal around the user's urethra, has a hollow tube in the center, and urine comes out of a hole at the tip of the device that appears like a urethra (Underwood 2016). Some devices used for packing can also double as sex toys and come with silicone shafts so they can be used for penetration. Underwear made specifically for packing can also be purchased to be used with a packer.

While there is no information in the literature regarding the use of genital packers and risk for infection, it is likely that when a device is used in the genital area that gets moist from sweat and vaginal secretions, used for urination and possibly sexual use, that it could transmit infections, urinary or sexually transmitted. Therefore, it is important for healthcare providers to educate their transmasculine patients who are packing about the care and cleaning of the device to prevent the risk of infection. Each device will likely have their own care instructions. However, in general the packer should be washed with warm water and gentle soap before and after each use and disinfected with an antibacterial toy cleanser, making sure to use a brush or tool to clean the inside and small opening when applicable (Underwood 2016). Devices made out of silicone can also be boiled in water for 5–10 min or washed in the dishwasher on the top rack (Brown University 2015).

Fertility Preservation for Transgender Individuals

Transgender men and women, like any others, should be provided accurate information about oocyte and spermatozoa preservation regardless of their sexual orientation or gender identity. Being that multiple avenues exist for individuals to have biological children, it is incumbent upon the healthcare provider to ensure that the patient receives all information when faced with prescribed therapies or disease that is threatening to one's fertility (Johnson and Finlayson 2016). Fertility preservation becomes especially important to address with transgender individuals preparing to start hormone therapy as the literature still remains unclear about population-wide effects of transgender hormone replacement therapy on natal gonads (Johnson and Finlayson 2016). For both transgender men and women, the option of cryopreservation should be addressed. Moreover, as younger transgender individuals begin hormone replacement therapy sometimes in their late teens after puberty blocking medications, addressing the issue of fertility preservation early in treatment is important and may require the assistance of an endocrinologist who is familiar with transgender care and specializes in fertility.

Gender Affirming Surgeries and Urologic Complications

Surgical transition is the process where a transgender person will elect surgical procedures to affirm their gender identity. Gender affirmation surgery (also known as gender reassignment surgery or gender confirmation surgery) is one of many options available to transgender people used to treat gender dysphoria (Keatly et al. 2015). According to the 2015 United States Transgender Survey ($n = 27,715$), 25% of participants reported having had a transition-related surgery (James et al. 2016). This is illustrative of the importance that a provider not assumes all transgender individuals opt for surgical transition. Lastly, it is unknown how these rates would change if all transgender people had access to surgical transition through both insurance coverage and surgical providers who accepted the varying insurance types.

There are a variety of surgical options for transgender people seeking gender affirming surgery (i.e., facial feminization and masculinization, breast augmentation, chest reconstruction, etc.) (Keatly et al. 2015). However, this section of chapter will only present information that is pertinent to urologic care; further discussion is presented in Chap. 26. Genital reconstructive surgical procedures have urologic implications and fall under the umbrella of gender confirmation surgery. Genital reconstructive procedures are often referred to as "bottom surgery" within the transgender community. It is important to note that these surgeries are multidisciplinary and surgical techniques are still being standardized (Berli et al. 2017). Because these surgeries are only offered at a few institutions nationally whereby transgender individuals may travel across states for surgery, urology providers local to these patients may encounter individuals requiring follow-up with complications (Dreher et al. 2018). Thus, when providing care to a patient, if the clinical scenario warrants, it may be beneficial to the urology provider to elicit patient records and notes from the original surgeon(s) who completed the surgery to understand the urologic implications for the patient. The World Professional Association for Transgender Health (WPATH) currently sets the standard of care for transgender healthcare including genital surgery (Coleman et al. 2012). The following section will summarize both masculinizing and feminizing genital reconstructive surgeries.

Transgender Women (Male to Female Surgeries): Feminizing Genitoplasty

The surgeries offered to transgender women are orchiectomy, vaginoplasty (penile inversion or intestinal conduit), clitoroplasty, labiaplasty (Berli et al. 2017). Penile inversion vaginoplasty (PIV) is the most commonly performed (Berli et al. 2017; Coleman et al. 2012). While the specific techniques for PIV vary among surgeons, the procedure includes orchiectomy, removal of phallus tissues, creation of a neovagina and labia (Dreher et al. 2018; Bryson and Honig 2019). The prostate and seminal vesicles are not removed during surgery and remain (Bryson and Honig 2019). PIV typically involves the following steps: orchiectomy, dissection and removal of phallus tissue including corpora spongiosum and neurovascular bundles, neovaginal cavity creation between the bladder and rectum within the rectoprostatic fascia (Denonvilliers' fascia), inversion of penile skin and often scrotal skin (with or without graft) creating the neovagina, the native urethra is reduced in length to the anatomical female position, a miniaturized and neurologically intact glans penis forms the neoclitoris, and remaining scrotal skin forms the labia minora and majora (Bryson and Honig 2019; Dreher et al. 2018; Berli et al. 2017).

Common Urologic Complications with Penile Inversion Vaginoplasty There are a number of complications noted in the literature for penile inversion vaginoplasty. Those most relevant to the urology provider are listed here. Stenosis or stricture of the neomeatus and neourethral structures are the most common complications with reported frequencies of 10% (Bryson and Honig 2019) to 14.4% (Dreher et al. 2018) and is also one of the most common reasons for surgical revision. Urethral injuries occur and are rare (Bryson and Honig 2019; Dreher et al. 2018); urinary retention (noting that sometimes the prostate can be the source of urinary retention especially in elderly transgender patients) (Bryson and Honig 2019); urinary incontinence, which may complicate the patient's healing and quality of life; atypical urine stream (especially up to 6 weeks postoperatively), and urinary tract infections as a result of the shortened neourethra (Bryson and Honig 2019). Neovaginal stenosis is reported at rates of 9.8% (Dreher et al. 2018) especially if the patient is not vaginally dilating as prescribed by the surgeon—vaginal dilation is required indefinitely in most cases (Bryson and Honig 2019).

Of note, if the transgender woman engages in receptive vaginal intercourse, neovaginal stenosis may have significant impact on the individual's sexual health, satisfaction, and mood. Wound infection with an incidence of 3.2% (Dreher et al. 2018) has the potential to complicate healing of the labia, neovagina, and neomeatus. The following are rare but have significant impact on healing, and may impact the patient's quality of life and sexual health: rectal injury 2%, hematoma 1.7%, prolapse of neovagina 1.6%, tissue necrosis including necrosis of neoclitoris 1.4%, and rectovaginal fistula 1.0% (Dreher et al. 2018).

Transgender Men (Female to Male Surgeries): Masculinizing Genitoplasty

Surgical transition for transgender men is complex, and requires interdisciplinary care management involving multiple surgical disciplines including urologic, plastic, and gynecologic surgeons. Current gender affirmation surgeries offered to transgender men include hysterectomy and salpingo-oopherectomy, colpectomy, metoidioplasty, phalloplasty (includes phallus, glansplasty, urethroplasty, and erectile prosthesis), and scrotoplasty with testicular implants (Berli et al. 2017). While there are exceptions, most often a transgender man who is seeking metoidioplasty or phalloplasty will first have a hysterectomy and salpingo-oopherectomy (Berli et al. 2017). If the patient opts for phalloplasty, the patient typically will have a colpectomy after phalloplasty is completed, as some of the natal vaginal tissues may be used to complete an urethroplasty (Bryson and Honig 2019).

Metoidioplasty Androgen hormonal replacement therapy for medical transition hypertrophies the clitoris. Techniques vary among surgeons for metoidioplasty, but generally the surgeon will complete the following and may or may not include urethral lengthening per patient goals (Hadj-Moussa et al. 2019): release the suspensory ligaments of the clitoris. Buccal grafts and genital flaps (typically labia minora) are most commonly used for urethral lengthening to provide a pendulous urethra to allow micturition while standing. The clitoral glans is also reconstructed and skin flaps cover the neophallus. The urethra heals with the support of a catheter and urine is diverted suprapubically through a catheter until healing has completed.

Common Urologic Complications from Metoidioplasty Metoidioplasty is less complex and has lower rates of complications than phalloplasty. According to a recent review, metoidioplasty has an overall complication rate of 10–37% (Hadj-Moussa et al. 2019). The most common complication is urinary dribbling or spraying stream that affects almost a third of patients and often resolves 3–6 months (Hadj-Moussa et al. 2019). Reportedly, urethrocutaneous fistulas occur in 5–23% depending on the literature (Hadj-Moussa et al. 2019). Rare complications include flap necrosis and wound infection (Hadj-Moussa et al. 2019).

Phalloplasty Phalloplasty is most commonly completed in multiple stages over a series of months to a year to optimize healing and reduce complications. The phalloplasty allows for a neophallus resembling that of a natal male, micturition while standing, and may allow for penetrative intercourse with an erectile implant device—staged at least 9–12 months after initial surgery (Berli et al. 2017; Hadj-Moussa et al. 2019). There are many surgical techniques for phalloplasty. Currently, the most commonly used is a radial forearm free flap (RFP) phalloplasty; the second most common is the anterolateral thigh (ALT) phalloplasty. The radial forearm free flap phalloplasty is briefly summarized here. This phalloplasty approach allows for the construction of the neophallus and urethra during a single operation using a "tube-within-a-tube" technique (Berli et al. 2017; Hadj-Moussa et al. 2019).

A full thickness, skin flap from the nondominant forearm provides the tissue for the neophallus. The native urethra, or "pars fixa," is attached using natal genital tissue in combination with the ulnar aspect of the flap that becomes the neourethra as it is constructed and rolled around a catheter (this skin must be hairless). Microscopic surgical techniques ensue to provide the anastomosed blood supply and neurologic sensation to the neophallus. The clitoris is de-epithelialized and buried in the neophallus. Once healed, the glans is often tattooed. Once sensation returns, an erectile prosthesis can be implanted (Hadj-Moussa et al. 2019).

Common Urologic Complications from Phalloplasty A multi-institutional retrospective review that included 55 patients, 40 of whom had phalloplasty (surgical type nondescript), indicated that urethral fistula, stricture, and vaginal tissue remnants were among the most common complications (Dy et al. 2019). Additional complications included pars fixa urethrocutaneous fistula and meatal stenosis ($n = 25$) (Dy et al. 2019) and often require surgical attention (Bryson and Honig 2019). Bryson and Honig (2019) also note that post-void dribbling or spraying is also a problem that affects almost one-third of patients; urinary stasis and infection secondary to hair growing in urethra may pose complications; urinary retention, which should only be addressed by a urologist familiar with phalloplasty anatomy; and flap failure or necrosis is rare, but a severe complication that can be devastating for the patient. If the patient has had an implanted penile prosthesis, reported rates of infection and erosion in phalloplasty are 30–70% and often require surgical attention (Bryson and Honig 2019).

Urological Physical Examination

The urologic physical exam is a very sensitive exam and cause anxiety for any patient because it requires an examination of the genitals and/or prostate. Transgender patients may find the urologic exam extremely distressing and particularly traumatic, especially those with gender dysphoria (Feldman and Spencer 2015). Therefore the urologic physical examination must be approached with sensitivity and patience. A particularly useful approach to this type of exam is the trauma-informed approach. Trauma-informed care is an approach to patients with the understanding that traumatic experiences (i.e., interpersonal violence, sexual assault, neglect, abuse, household dysfunction, chronic stress from minority status or discrimination, etc.) are fairly common, and any patient could have experienced trauma in the past (Li et al. 2019). With that understanding, the healthcare provider can then create a universal approach to patient care, where the focus is on developing a strong patient–provider relationship built upon mutual respect and trust (Feldman and Spencer 2015).

Also central to this approach is the need to balance the power differential between the patient and provider. This can be done by explaining the reason for certain exams or procedures and giving the patient choices where possible, including simple choices such as would you like to sit or stand, and ultimately allowing the patient to say when they are ready for their examination, and how they would prefer it be performed (Feldman and Spencer 2015). Before proceeding with the examination, the clinician should give clear, direct instructions about what to expect, including how it will feel, where they can expect to be touched, and when it will be performed (Feldman and Spencer 2015). When describing the exam use anatomical terms (i.e., penis, testicles, prostate, urethra), noting the organs that will be examined and try to refrain from describing anatomy based on gender (i.e., male or female anatomy) (Feldman and Spencer 2015). As is the case with any other patient, it is generally helpful in establishing a trusting environment between provider and patient to mimic the language the patient uses to refer to their genitalia and other body parts.

Gender Affirmation Surgery Summary

Gender affirmation surgery is a means of surgical transition and is one of many treatments available for gender dysphoria. The penile inversion vaginoplasty is among the most common genitoplasty procedures for transgender women. Genitoplasty procedures available to transgender men are phalloplasty, metoidioplasty, and scrotoplasty. WPATH currently sets the standards of care in the seventh edition for the comprehensive healthcare and surgical care for transgender people (Coleman et al. 2012), and an updated eighth version is forthcoming. It is important to note and consider that genitoplasty procedures are still evolving in technique, best practices, and standards. Additionally, there is a lack of standardization of reporting complications and rates thereof in the literature. Moreover, many transgender individuals may not have local access to a surgical team performing genitoplasty. Thus, the urology provider should anticipate there may be patient encounters where transgender individuals with complications may seek care in their local geographic area that is far removed from the institution providing the gender affirmation surgery.

Urology for Intersex Individuals

Disorders of sexual development, also defined as intersex, are extremely rare and have a wide range of presentations (AUA 2019). Intersex individuals' families often seek medical treatment for their children from a pediatric urologist to determine how to best work with the patient and family to determine if any treatment is recommended and discuss potential treatment options (AUA 2019). The discussion about urologic concerns for intersex individuals is beyond the scope of the chapter, so will not be discussed further.

Summary and Clinical Pearls

This chapter presented foundational information on how the urology healthcare provider can care for LGBTQ patients with cultural humility. Cultural humility is a unique perspective to help clinicians provide safe, affirming, and inclusive environments for all patients, especially LGBTQ patients. LGBTQ individuals may seek care from a urology healthcare provider for a variety of urologic health issues.

Urologic-specific considerations for LGBTQ patients include health promotion and disease prevention for obesity, tobacco use, and prostate cancer screening. Providing comprehensive, high-quality, and affirming care to LGBTQ patients includes completing a nonjudgmental, candid, and affirming sexual health history. Providers may consider practicing this skill outside of clinic to improve their comfort prior to assessing the patient's sexual health history.

Understanding unique considerations for LGBTQ patients regarding sexual function further illustrates the importance of a comprehensive sexual health history. Urologic-specific considerations for LGBTQ patients include erectile dysfunction, premature ejaculation, HIV/AIDS, lower urinary tract infections, and prostate cancer care. Urology for the transgender patient includes the following issues: accessing public bathrooms, practices of tucking and packing, fertility preservation, gender affirmation surgery, and sensitive exam considerations. In conclusion, while urologic treatment options often do not differ for LGBTQ patients, there are some unique considerations that the urology healthcare provider should include in the assessment and plan of care for these individuals.

Clinical Pearls
- LGBTQ patients experience health disparities, including those related to urologic health.
- The urology healthcare provider can create safe spaces and care for patients with cultural humility to improve LGBTQ patients access to high-quality, evidence-based care for urological conditions.
- LGBTQ patients experience common concerns managed in urology, but may have some unique considerations for care.
- The use of an inclusive, affirming health history, specifically sexual health history can help the urology provider gather essential information that impacts LGBTQ patients' health.
- When performing a physical exam that requires an assessment of sensitive body parts, such as the genitals and/or p0rostate, it is important to create a strong patient relationship built on mutual respect and trust, clearly explain what needs to be done, when, and how, and to allow patients choice wherever possible.

References

American Psychiatric Association (2013) Gender dysphoria. Available from APA_DSM-5-Gender-Dysphoria.pdf

American Urological Association (2019) Pediatric decision making and differences of sex development: a societies for pediatric urology and American Urological Association joint position statement. Available from https://www.auanet.org/guidelines/joint-statement-on-dsd

Berli JU, Knudson G, Fraser L, Tangpricha V, Ettner R, Ettner FM, Safer JD, Graham J, Monstrey S, Schechter LJ (2017) What surgeons need to know about gender confirmation surgery when providing care for transgender individuals: a review. JAMA Surgery 152(4):394–400. https://doi.org/10.1001/jamasurg.2016.5549

Brown University (2015) What is the best way to clean sex toys? BWell Health Promotion. Available from https://www.brown.edu/campus-life/health/services/promotion/content/whats-best-way-clean-sex-toys

Bryson C, Honig SC (2019) Genitourinary complications of gender-affirming surgery. Current Urology Reports 20(6):31. https://doi.org/10.1007/s11934-019-0894-4

Centers for Disease Control and Prevention [CDC] (2015) Gay, bisexual and other men who have sex with men (MSM). Available from https://www.cdc.gov/std/life-stages-populations/msm.htm

Centers for Disease Control and Prevention [CDC] (2016) Syphilis statistics. Available from https://www.cdc.gov/std/syphilis/stats.htm

Centers for Disease Control and Prevention [CDC] (2019a) HIV and gay and bisexual men. Available from https://www.cdc.gov/hiv/group/msm/index.html

Centers for Disease Control and Prevention [CDC] (2019b) HIV and transgender people. Available from https://www.cdc.gov/hiv/group/gender/transgender/index.html

Centers for Disease Control and Prevention [CDC] (2019c) Risks among sexual minority youth. Available from https://www.cdc.gov/healthyyouth/disparities/health-considerations-lgbtqouth.htm?CDC_AA_refVal=https%3A%2F%2Fwww.cdc.gov%2Fhealthyyouth%2Fdisparities%2Fsmy.htm

Chang E, Simon M, Dong X (2012) Integrating cultural humility into healthcare professional education and training. Advances in Health Sciences Education 17(2):269–278. https://doi.org/10.1007/s10459-010-9264-1

Coleman E, Bockting W, Botzer M, Cohen-Kettenis P, DeCuypere G, Feldman J, Fraser L, Green J, Knudson G, Meyer WJ, Monstrey S, Adler RK, Brown GR, Devor AH, Ehrbar R, Ettner R, Eyler E, Garofalo R, Karasic DH, Monstrey S (2012) [WPATH] Standards of care for the health of transsexual, transgender, and gender-nonconforming people, version 7. International Journal of Transgenderism 13(4):165–232. https://doi.org/10.1080/15532739.2011.700873

Coutin A, Wright S, Li C, Fung R (2018) Missed opportunities: are residents prepared to care for transgender patients? A study of family medicine, psychiatry, endocrinology, and urology residents. Canadian Medical Education Journal 9(3):e41–e55

Deutsch MB (2016) Binding, packing, and tucking. Available from https://transcare.ucsf.edu/guidelines/binding-packing-and-tucking

Dreher PC, Edwards D, Hager S, Dennis M, Belkoff A, Mora J, Tarry S, Rumer KL (2018) Complications of the neovagina in male-to-female transgender surgery: a systematic review and meta-analysis with discussion of management. Clinical Anatomy 31(2):191–199

Durso LE, Meyer IH (2013) Patterns and predictors of disclosure of sexual orientation to healthcare providers among lesbians, gay men, and bisexuals. Sexuality Research and Social Policy 10(1):35–42. https://doi.org/10.1007/s13178-012-0105-2

Dy GW, Osbun NC, Morrison SD, Grant DW, Merguerian PA (2016) Exposure to and attitudes regarding transgender education among urology residents. The Journal of Sexual Medicine 2016(13):1466–1472

Dy GW, Granieri MA, Fu BC, Vanni AJ, Voelzke B, Rourke KF, Elliott SP, Nikolavsky D, Zhao LC (2019) Presenting complications to a reconstructive urologist after masculinizing genital reconstructive surgery. Urology 132:202–206. https://doi.org/10.1016/j.urology.2019.04.051

Eyler AE, Pang SC, Clark A (2014) LGBT assisted reproduction: current practice and future possibilities. LGBT health 1(3):151–156

Fallin-Bennett K, Henderson SL, Nguyen GT, Hyderi A (2016) Primary care, prevention, and coordination of care. In: Eckstrand KL, Ehrenfeld JM (eds) Lesbian, gay, bisexual, and transgender healthcare: a clinical guide to preventive, primary, and specialist care. Springer International Publishing, New York, NY. https://doi.org/10.1007/978-3-319-19752-4

Feldman J, Spencer K (2015) Medical and surgical management of the transgender patient: what the primary clinician needs to know. In: Makadon H, Mayer K, Potter J, Goldhammer H (eds) The Fenway guide to lesbian, gay, bisexual, and transgender health. American College of Physicians, Philadelphia, PA. Available from https://store.acponline.org

Felitti VJ, Anda RF, Nordenberg D, Williamson DF, Spitz AM, Edwards V, Koss MP, Marks JS (1998) Relationship of childhood abuse and household dysfunction to many of the leading causes of death in adults - the adverse childhood experiences (ACE) study. American Journal of Preventive Medicine 14:245–258

Flores JZ (2015) A reference guide to the gay bear culture. Available from http://www.jacobz-flores.com/2011/09/18/a-reference-guide-to-the-gay-bear-culture/

Flynn KE, Lin L, Watkins Bruner D, Cyranowski JM, Hahn EA, Jeffrey DD, Barsky Reese J, Reeve BB, Shelby RA, Weinfurt KP (2016) Sexual satisfaction and the importance of sexual health to quality of life throughout the life course of U.S. adults. The Journal of Sexual Medicine 13(11):1642–1650

Hadj-Moussa M, Agarwal S, Ohl DA, Kuzon WM Jr (2019) Masculinizing genital gender confirmation surgery. Sexual medicine reviews 7(1):141–155. https://doi.org/10.1016/j.sxmr.2018.06.004

Hannah S, Carpenter-Song E (2013) Patrolling your blind spots: introspection and public catharsis in a medical school faculty development course to reduce unconscious bias in medicine. Culture, Medicine, and Psychiatry 37(2):314–339. https://doi.org/10.1007/s11013-013-9320-4

Hart TL, Coon DW, Kowalkowski MA, Zhang K, Hersom JI, Goltz HH, Wittmann DA, Latini DM (2014) Changes in roles and quality of life for gay men after prostate cancer: challenges for sexual health providers. Journal of Sexual Medicine 2014(11):2308–2317. https://doi.org/10.1111/jsm.12598

Herman JL (2013) Gendered restrooms and minority stress: the public regulation of gender and its impact on transgender people's lives. Journal of Public Management & Social Policy 19(1):65

Hickerson K, Hawkins LA, Hoyt-Brennan AM (2018) Sexual orientation/gender identity cultural competence: a simulation pilot study. Nursing 16:2–5. https://doi.org/10.1016/j.ecns.2017.10.011

Hohman M (2013) Cultural humility: a lifelong practice. "IN SITU" - the Blog of the SDSU School of Social Work. Available from https://socialwork.sdsu.edu/insitu/diversity/cultural-humility-a-lifelong-practice/

Hollenbach A, Eckstrand K, Dreger A (2014) Implementing curricular and institutional climate changes to improve healthcare for individuals who are LGBTQ, gender nonconforming, or born with DSD: a resource for medical educator. Available from https://members.org/eweb/upload/Executive%20LGBT%20FINAL.pdf

Institute of Medicine (IOM) (2011) The health of lesbian, gay, bisexual, and transgender people: building a foundation for better understanding. Available from http://www.nationalacademies.org/hmd/Reports/2011/The-Health-of-Lesbian-Gay-Bisexual-and-Transgender-People.aspx

James SE, Herman JL, Rankin S, Keisling M, Mottet L, Anafi M (2016) The report of the 2015 U.S. transgender survey. National Center for Transgender Equality, Washington, DC. Available from https://www.transequality.org/sites/default/files/docs/USTS-Full-Report-FINAL.PDF

Johnson EK, Finlayson C (2016) Preservation of fertility potential for gender and sex diverse individuals. Transgender Health 1 1(2016):41 44

Keatly JG, Deutsch MB, Sevelius JM, Gutierrez-Mock L (2015) Creating a foundation for improving trans health: understanding trans identities and health care needs. In: Makadon H, Mayer K, Potter J, Goldhammer H (eds) The Fenway guide to lesbian, gay, bisexual, and transgender health. American College of Physicians, Philadelphia, PA. Available from https://store.acponline.org

Klein DA, Berry-Bibee EN, Baker KK, Malcolm NM, Rollison JM, Frederiksen BN (2018) Providing quality family planning services to LGBTQIA individuals: a systematic review. Contraception 97(5):378–391. https://doi.org/10.1016/j.contraception.2017.12.016

Kuzma EK, Pardee M, Darling-Fisher CS (2019) LGBT health: creating safe spaces and caring for patients with cultural humility. Journal of the American Association of Nurse Practitioners. 31(3):167–174. https://doi.org/10.1097/JXX.0000000000000131

Law M, Mathai A, Veinot P, Webster F, Mylopoulos M (2015) Exploring lesbian, gay, bisexual, and queer (LGBQ) people's experiences with disclosure of sexual identity to primary care physicians: a qualitative study. BMC Family Practice 16(175):1–8. https://doi.org/10.1186/s12875-015-0389-4

Li Y, Cannon LM, Coolidge EM, Darling-Fisher CS, Pardee M, Kuzma EK (2019) Current state of trauma-informed education in the health sciences: lessons for nursing. Journal of Nursing Education 58(2):93–101. https://doi.org/10.3928/01484834-20190122-06

Lim FA, Brown DV, Jones H (2013) Lesbian, gay, bisexual, and transgender health: fundamentals for nursing education. Journal of Nursing Education 52(4):198. https://doi.org/10.3928/01484834-20130311-02

Makadon H, Goldhammer H, Davis JA (2015) Providing optimal health care for LGBT people: changing the clinical environment and educating professionals. In: Makadon H, Mayer K, Potter J, Goldhammer H (eds) The Fenway guide to lesbian, gay, bisexual, and transgender health. American College of Physicians, Philadelphia, PA. Available from https://store.acponline.org

McCabe MP, Sharlip ID, Lewis R, Atalla E, Balon R, Fisher AD, Laumann E, Lee SW, Segraves RT (2016) Incidence and prevalence of sexual dysfunction in women and men: a consensus statement from the fourth international consultation on sexual medicine 2015. The Journal of Sexual Medicine 13(2):144–152. https://doi.org/10.1016/j.jsxm.2015.12.034

Merriam-Webster (n.d.) Heteronormative. Available from https://www.merriam-webster.com/dictionary/heteronormative. Accessed 20 Jan 2020

Meyer IH (2003) Prejudice, social stress, and mental health in lesbian, gay, and bisexual populations: conceptual issues and research evidence. Psychological Bulletin 129:674–697. https://doi.org/10.1037/0033-2909.129.5.674

Mobley D, Baum N (2015a) Smoking: its impact on urologic health. Reviews in Urology 17(4):220–225. Available from https://www.ncbi.nlm.nih.gov/pmc/articles/PMC4735668/

Mobley D, Baum N (2015b) The obesity epidemic its impact on urologic care. Reviews in Urology 17(3):165–170

Mogul-Adlin H (2015) Unanticipated: healthcare experiences of gender nonbinary patients and suggestions for inclusive care. Available from ProQuest Dissertations & Theses: Open. http://pqdtopen.proquest.com/doc/1680223938.html?FMT=AI

Moncho C (2013) Cultural humility, part I — what is 'cultural humility'? The Social Work Practitioner. Available from https://thesocialworkpractitioner.com/2013/08/19/cultural-humility-part-i-what-is-cultural-humility/

National LGBT Health Center (2016) Providing inclusive services and care for LGBTQ people: a guide for healthcare staff. National LGBT Health Center: A Program of the Fenway Health Institute, Boston, MA. Available from http://www.lgbthealtheducation.org/wp-content/uploads/Providing-Inclusive-Services-and-Care-for-LGBT-People.pdf

Porst H, Burri A (2019) Novel treatment for premature ejaculation in the light of currently used therapies: A review. Sexual Medicine Reviews 7(1):129–40. https://doi.org/10.1016/j.sxmr.2018.05.001. Epub 2018 Jul 26

Rossman K, Salamanca P, Macapagal K (2017) A qualitative study examining young adults' experiences of disclosure and nondisclosure of LBGTQ identity to health care providers. Journal of Homosexuality 64(10):1390–1410. https://doi.org/10.1080/00918369.2017.1321379

Staats C, Capastosto K, Tenney L, Mamo S (2017) Implicit Bias Review. Available from http://kirwaninstitute.osu.edu/wp-content/uploads/2017/11/2017-SOTS-final-draft-02.pdf

TheGayUK (2019) What does cisnormative mean? Available from https://www.thegayuk.com/what-does-cisnormative-mean/

Truesdale MD, Breyer BN, Shindel AW (2015) Urologic issues in LGBT health. In: Eckstrand KL, Ehrenfeld JM (eds) Lesbian, gay, bisexual, and transgender healthcare: a clinical guide to preventive, primary, and specialist care. Springer International Publishing, New York, NY. https://doi.org/10.1007/978-3-319-19752-4

U. S. Preventive Services Task Force [USPSTF] (2019) Final recommendation statement: prostate cancer screening. Available from https://www.uspreventiveservicestaskforce.org/Page/Document/RecommendationStatementFinal/prostate-cancer-screening1

Underwood T (2016) A guide to packers for transmen. Available from https://ftm-guide.com/guide-to-packers-for-transmen/

Ward BW, Dahlhamer JM, Galinsky AM, Joestl SS (2014) Sexual orientation and health among U.S. adults: National health interview survey, 2013. National Health Statistic Report 15(77):1–10. PMID: 25025690

Wesp L (2016) Prostate and testicular cancer considerations in transgender women. Available from https://transcare.ucsf.edu/guidelines/prostate-testicular-cancer

Wheldon CW, Schabath MB, Hudson J, Bowman Curci M, Kanetsky PA, Vadaparampil ST, Simmons VN, Sanchez JA, Sutton SK, Quinn GP (2018) Culturally competent care for sexual and gender minority patients at national cancer institute-designated comprehensive cancer centers. LGBT Health 5(3):203–211. https://doi.org/10.1089/lgbt.2017.0217

Zestcott CA, Blair IV, Stone J (2016) Examining the presence, consequences, and reduction of implicit bias in health care: a narrative review. Group Processes & Intergroup Relations 19(4):528–542. https://doi.org/10.1177/1368430216642029

Zevin B (2016) Testicular and scrotal pain and related complaints. Available from https://transcare.ucsf.edu/guidelines/testicular-pain

The Medical/Nursing Expert Witness: A Primer and Considerations for the Practitioner and the Profession

25

Patrick J. Quallich

Contents

Objectives
1. Discuss legal requirements of an expert witness.
2. Define terms that are relevant to functioning as an expert witness.
3. Describe challenges to functioning as an expert witness.
4. Review tips for medical documentation.

Disclaimer: Not legal advice
The views depicted or expressed in this chapter do not constitute legal advice; do not create any warranties; do not form or create an attorney–client relationship; should not serve as a basis for legal decision-making. Any participants/viewers should obtain qualified legal counsel from a qualified legal professional specific to their own unique circumstances/needs.

P. J. Quallich (✉)
Managing Trial Attorney, Nationwide Trial Division Mediator, and United States Equal Employment Opportunity Commission, Cleveland, OH, USA

© Springer Nature Switzerland AG 2020
S. A. Quallich, M. J. Lajiness (eds.), *The Nurse Practitioner in Urology*,
https://doi.org/10.1007/978-3-030-45267-4_25

Disclaimer: Not purport to be opinions/views of any affiliated institution/company

The views expressed in this chapter are those solely of the author and do not necessarily reflect the positions, policies, or views of others.

Introduction

Serving as a medical expert witness can be an enriching and rewarding professional experience. Medical expert witnesses can have a powerful and enduring impact on their profession, particularly in a specialized area of medicine, such as urologic nursing and urologic care. When serving as an expert witness, a nurse practitioner (NP) or physician assistant (PA) is acting in a professional capacity (though not necessarily engaging in the practice of medicine). As such, conduct as an expert can be viewed as a reflection of one's profession. Most malpractice lawsuits name physicians, surgeons, or hospitals.

For the individual practitioner, there are many potential reasons why an NP/PA may consider serving as a medical expert: satisfy intellectual curiosity; confront a new professional challenge; or experience the excitement of serving as a courtroom expert. From the perspective of the healthcare profession, having its practitioners serve as experts presents potentially another area for further professional oversight, as well as an opportunity to provide clear, consistent guidance to its members.

The decision to serve as an expert witness should be an informed and deliberative process. There are quite a number of important issues and considerations that should be part of the decision-making process.

The Nurse Practitioner or Physician Assistant Expert Witness: Considerations and Discussion

I. The Expert Witness

1. Helps the jury understand the medical aspects of cases or claims
   (a) Historically, should practice is same area as defendant, but this no longer true
      • Limited pool of experts
      • Some subspecialties are restricted to large cities/academic medical centers
   (b) "Expert" more likely to be established by a national standard
      • Relevant experience
      • Relevant education
      • Relevant skill(s)
      • Relevant Knowledge
   (c) Experts usually
      • have advanced degrees in their fields
      • have published in the literature in their field
      • have spoken at professional conferences
      • belong to professional societies

    (d) Able to present an opinion without having been a witness to the issue/occurrence that generated the lawsuit
- Opinion based on evidence and information
- Opinion not based on speculation

    (e) Must be familiar with the type of care at the heart of the suit (Pollin, 2017) and is often trained in the discipline

    (f) Plaintiff and defendant use expert testimony to define the standard of care differently

    (g) Provide an impartial opinion on the liability implicated and on the damages that warrant compensation to the judge, who is not a medical professional

2. Why? What interests you about serving as a medical expert?
    (a) Challenge
    (b) Excitement
    (c) Justice
    (d) Compensation
    (e) Professionalism

3. Measure your motivation versus that of the civil justice system
    (a) Achieve balance or rectify imbalance
- Actual
- Perceived

4. How did we get here?—Lawsuits
    (a) Abdication of responsibility
    (b) Failure to appreciate true cause of an adverse event
- Injury/death/wrong not necessarily redressable
- Suspected agent/reason unfounded
- Plaintiff must show evidence of inadequate care
- Help establish that the minimally competent care was not met
- Harm was done to plaintiff
- Harm was due to a failure of competent care

5. Keep things in perspective
    (a) Reality—99% of lawsuits settle
    (b) Cases—range of defensibility

6. Who does a medical expert "work" for—Pick a side?
    (a) Not a battle of **good** vs. **evil**
    (b) Both sides fulfill an essential role

7. How do you win in court—civil matters
    (a) Preponderance of evidence—greater weight of the evidence required in a civil (noncriminal) lawsuit for the trier of fact (jury or judge without a jury) to decide in favor of one side or the other
    (b) Arena in which an expert witness can demonstrate authority or truth and accuracy
    (c) Ultimately a subjective determination
    (d) Contrasted with "beyond a reasonable doubt" needed for criminal case

8. When may an expert get consulted?
    (a) Pre-suit/claims process for review of chart and care process
    (b) Following commencement of suit

9. The typical life process of a lawsuit
   (a) Claim/pre-suit: making of a demand (asserting a claim) for money due from damages
   (b) Discovery: obtaining information before trial; can include documents, depositions, potential witnesses, written depositions
   (c) Disclosures
   (d) Deposition: testimony under oath that is not in the courtroom and can happen prior to the trial
   (e) Trial: examination of facts and law presided over by a judge (or other magistrate); will include various motion by both attorneys; can include a jury
10. Where may a medical practitioner serve as an expert witness?
   (a) Dependent upon the jurisdiction

II. What Are the Relevant Rules and Regulations for Medical Experts

1. The Law—state vs. federal law
   (a) Federal Rules of Evidence—apply to any proceedings in US courts, civil, or criminal proceeding
2. Two types of legal witnesses
   (a) Fact witness: person with knowledge of what is purported to have happened in a case. This can be a professional such as forensic psychologist.
   (b) Expert witness
3. Fact witness—testimony as to perception
   (a) *Federal Rules Of Evidence 602 Need for Personal Knowledge*:
      • A witness may testify to a matter only if evidence is introduced sufficient to support a finding that the witness has personal knowledge of the matter.
4. Fact witness—opinion testimony
   (a) First-hand knowledge about the events and/or facts in a case
   (b) *Federal Rules of Evidence 701:* Opinion testimony of fact witness limited to that which is:
      • based on the witness's perception; what they saw, heard, smelled, tasted, felt.
      • testify as to what happened during a situation or event, e.g., events things noted during direct patient contact
      • helpful to clearly understand the testimony or to determine a fact in issue
      • NOT based on scientific, technical, or other specialized knowledge.
5. An expert witness (see above)
   (a) Must be qualified as an expert
   (b) May provide competent, qualified opinions
   (c) Deemed "expert" based on state definitions
   (d) Simplifies complex issues and provides clear explanations
   (e) Demonstrate "medical certainty": opinion grounded in evidence
   (f) Understands the jury's right to a solid opinion established on evidence-based medicine
   (g) Effective communication skills are paramount when addressing the court and jury

III. How to Qualify as a Medical Expert

1. Expert—qualifications: *Federal Rules Of Evidence 702*—A witness who is qualified as an expert by knowledge, skill, experience, training, or education may testify
2. How to qualify as an expert—requirements: *Federal Rules Of Evidence 702* provides the requirements for an expert to testify
   (a) the expert's scientific/technical knowledge will help the jury understand the evidence;
   (b) based on sufficient facts or data;
   (c) reliable principles/methods; and
   (d) reliably applied the principles/methods to the case.
3. Two different tests to qualify as an expert witness (*Frye* test vs. *Daubert* test)
   (a) *Frye*—embraced by a minority of states rule (California, Illinois, Maryland, Minnesota, New Jersey, New York, Pennsylvania, Washington)
   (b) Qualifying as an expert under *Frye* test (1923)
   - General acceptance test
   - Focus is on the methodology
   - Expert opinion admissible only if the technique is generally accepted as reliable in the relevant scientific community
4. Qualifying as an expert witness—What is the role of the court
   (a) *Daubert* (1993): rule of evidence regarding the admissibility of expert witness testimony.
   (b) Components
   - Judge is gatekeeper—determine whether an expert is qualified
   - Is expert testimony relevant/reliable?
   - Scientific knowledge = scientific method
   - Illustrative factors that support scientific method
5. Qualifying as an expert witness—What is the role of the court?
   (a) Considerable leeway and discretion
   (b) Liberal introduction of expert evidence
   (c) Experts can be powerful and misleading
6. How does a court fulfill its role as gatekeeper?
   (a) Preliminary assessment whether the methodology underlying the expert witness' testimony is valid
   (b) Keep the scientific standard with the practitioners
7. Judicial determination of the validity of an expert opinion
   (a) Reliability
   (b) Relevance (aid fact finder in the task at hand)
8. Judicial determination if an expert's opinion is reliable (*Daubert* factors)
   (a) Technique/theory tested
   (b) Technique/theory subject to peer review/publication
   (c) Known/potential rate of error of the technique/theory
   (d) Existence of standards
   (e) Technique/theory generally accepted in the scientific community

9. Judicial determination whether an expert's opinion is reliable (*Daubert* factors)
    (a) Court's inquiry must be specific to the particular issues in each case
    (b) Sufficient specialized knowledge to assist the jury in deciding the issues
    (c) Expert's conclusions must have a basis in established fact
10. *Federal Rules Of Evidence 703*—Foundation of an expert's opinions/testimony
    (a) An expert may base an opinion on:
        • Facts/data the expert has been made aware of or personally observed
        • Sufficient reliable principles and methods
        • Expert must be able to identify their methodology and its underlying assumptions
        • May disclose opinion if the probative value in helping the jury evaluate the opinion substantially outweighs the prejudicial effect
11. Expert Opinions—reliability threshold
    (a) Reasonable degree of medical certainty
    (b) Probability
    (c) Likelihood

IV. What Is Expected of a Medical Expert?

1. What is the role of the expert
    (a) Fully evaluate
    (b) Fairly evaluate
2. What is the role of the expert—fully evaluate
    (a) Strengths
    (b) Weaknesses
3. What is the role of the expert—fairly evaluate
    (a) Be candid!
    (b) Do NOT overstate/embellish
    (c) Do NOT placate
4. What is expected—the expert's opinions
    (a) Provide opinion
    (b) Maintain that opinion
    (c) Supplement opinion
    (d) Will not change that opinion (absent new information)
5. What is expected—Timely provision of opinions
    (a) Significant consequences for untimely disclosure
6. What is the role of the expert
    (a) Treating Practitioner
    (b) Consultant
    (c) Expert
7. What is the expert's role—educate or persuade?
    (a) Observational reporter
    (b) Impassioned advocate

8. What is the expert's role—review or examine?
   (a) Record review
   (b) Independent Medical Examination
9. What is the expert's role—Independent medical examination
   (a) FRCP 35—Physical examination of a party by court order
   (b) No medical/patient privilege is established
   (c) Findings memorialized
10. Independent medical examination
   (a) Recording
   (b) Video
   (c) Interference by counsel
   (d) Interference by examinee
11. How will the expert's opinions be made known—Expert disclosures
12. What are the different forms of expert disclosures
   (a) Identification only
   (b) Attorney Disclosures
      • Whose opinions are these?
   (c) Report
13. Expert Disclosures—Witnesses who do not provide a written report: FRCP Rule 26(a)(2)(C)
   (a) must provide:
      • subject matter on which the witness is expected to present evidence
      • summary of facts/opinions to which the witness is expected to testify
14. Expert Disclosures—Attorney Disclosures (various state courts)
   (a) subject matter on which each expert is expected to testify
   (b) substance of facts/opinions on which each expert is expected to testify
   (c) qualifications of each expert witness
   (d) summary of the grounds for each expert's opinion.
15. Expert Disclosures—Witnesses Who Must Provide a Written Report: Federal Rules of Civil Procedure (FRCP) Rule 26(a)(2)(B)
   (a) Unless otherwise stipulated or ordered by the court, this disclosure must be accompanied by a written report—prepared and signed by the witness—if the witness is one retained or specially employed to provide expert testimony in the case or one whose duties as the party's employee regularly involve giving expert testimony.
16. Expert Disclosures—Required Contents of the Expert's Report
   (a) FRCP 26 provides what must the report contain:
      • all opinions and their basis
      • facts/data considered
      • exhibits used to support them
      • qualifications, listing of publications (past 10 years)
      • prior testimonial history (4 years)
      • statement of compensation

IV. What Standard Is Used by the Expert in Evaluating the Medical Care

1. The legal elements/standard for medical negligence/malpractice
   In order to establish medical malpractice:
   (a) the standard of care recognized by the medical community;
   (b) breach of the standard of care; and
   (c) direct causal connection between the medically negligent act and the injury.
2. What is the Standard of Care
   (a) Largely determined from the testimony of experts
   (b) Technical literature/periodicals
   (c) Standards
3. What constitutes medical malpractice/breach of the standard of care?
   (a) Act or omission that a medical practitioner of ordinary skill/care would not have done under similar circumstances
4. Standard of Care—Generalist vs. Specialist
   (a) Specialist is held to the standard of care "of a reasonable specialist practicing in that same specialty"
5. Standard of Care—timing
   (a) SOC assessed in the light of the then present day scientific knowledge in the specialty field
   (b) SOC not assessed with benefit of hindsight
6. Causation
   (a) Connection between breach and injury
   (b) Breach can exist without malpractice
   (c) Probable non-causes
   (d) Potential vs. probable causes
7. The determination whether malpractice has occurred
   (a) Jury weighs evidence
   (b) Jury decides who to believe
   (c) Jury determines whether malpractice has been proven

V. WHAT ARE the Challenges and Potential Perils of Being a Medical Expert?

1. Understand your case and the issues
   (a) Be prepared
   (b) Mock examination/deposition
   (c) Review/refresh
   (d) Get what you need to fully/fairly evaluate
   (e) Stay in your lane/backyard
2. Two fundamental approaches of attacking/challenging an expert
   (a) Attack the person (expert)
   (b) Attack the testimony

3. Challenges to the expert—qualifications
   (a) Educational/Experiential deficiency
       • Timing
       • Length
       • Teaching
       • Practice
       • Subject matter
4. Challenges to the expert—jurisdictional/procedural deficiency
   (a) Timing of submission
   (b) Jurisdictional specific requirements
5. Challenges to the expert—financial motivation
   (a) Avarice/remuneration
   (b) Fees/income derived from expert work
   (c) Percentage of income due to litigation
6. Challenges to the expert—objectivity
   (a) Pattern of testimony—plaintiff/defense oriented
   (b) Not review all necessary materials
   (c) Not request/provided all pertinent materials
   (d) Stay current in specialty area
   (e) Maintain accurate perspective
   (f) Have a clear understanding of what they know and what they do not know
   (g) Admit when they cannot answer a question or subject/topic is outside their
       scope of practice
   (h) Avoid overstating opinions
   (i) Be consistent from case-to-case
7. Challenges to the expert testimony
   (a) Expert's manner of practice
   (b) Expert's institution's manner of practice
   (c) Variance from established standards
   (d) Variance with peer reviewed literature
   (e) Divergence of opinion among defense experts
8. Challenges to the expert testimony
   (a) Inconsistency—logic, reason, common sense
   (b) Care by providers
   (c) *Daubert*-based challenges

VI. How to Substantially Mitigate Professional Risk as an Expert

1. Agreement/understanding of the expert's role
   (a) Memorialized—agreement between counsel and expert
   (b) What specifically is the expert being asked to do?
   (c) Should there be a written agreement?

2. What should the agreement address or consist of?
   (a) Rate of pay
   (b) Fees
   (c) Timing
   (d) Billing
   (e) Documentation
   (f) Forum for disputes
   (g) Arbitration clause: arbitration is a mini-trial, which may be for a lawsuit ready to go to trial, held in an attempt to avoid a court trial and conducted by a person or a panel of people who are not judges
   (h) Mutual obligation to cooperate
   (i) Cancellation timing/requirements
   (j) Notice and challenges to the expert/testimony
   (k) Disclaimer for responsibility
   (l) Advance, sufficient notice of deadlines
3. Payment considerations
   (a) Customary/prevailing rates of remuneration
   (b) Retainer for review
   (c) IME fees
   (d) Pre-payment (deposition/trial)
4. Corporate entity vs. individual witness
5. Practical considerations/impact of expert work on your practice
   (a) Centralization/coordination of litigation-related tasks
   (b) Office Manager
   (c) Agreement of partners/employers
   (d) Agreement as to fees/funds
   (e) Agreement as to time
      • during vs. outside office hours

VII. What Are the Opportunities/Challenges for the Profession?

1. Opportunities and challenges for the profession
   (a) How can the profession oversee its practitioners as experts
   (b) To what extent should the profession oversee its practitioners as experts
   (c) Consensus statement on expert witnesses within the specialty
2. How have other medical specialties addressed the serving as a medical expert?
   (a) American College of Vascular Surgery—Guidelines
   (b) American Academy of Pediatrics—Policy Statement—Guidelines for Expert Witness Testimony in Medical Malpractice Litigation
   (c) American College of Emergency Medicine Physicians
   (d) American College of Physicians
   (e) American College of Radiology Practice Parameter on the physician expert
   (f) The Journal of Legal Nurse Consulting: Standards for Nurse Expert Witnesses: A Recommendation

    (g) American Association of Legal Nurse Consultants
    (h) American Medical Association Code of Ethics
  3. Opportunities and challenges for the practitioner in serving as an expert
    (a) Different professional challenge
    (b) Play a role in policing your own profession
    (c) Defend fellow practitioners
    (d) Remunerative
    (e) More conscientious, self-aware practitioner

Clinical Pearls

- Nurse practitioners and physician assistant are held to the same standard of care as physicians. There is no separate standard for the NP or PA; this may be especially relevant as NPs and PAs begin to perform and bill independently for procedures in urology.
  - Despite the fact that this standard must be equal, a PA may not offer expert testimony concerning the standard of care of a physician.
  - Unclear with respect to NPs, as in 26 states NP have full practice authority.
- Documentation is vital. If is not documented, it did not happen, was not ordered or discussed.
  - Charts must be completed in a timely fashion.
  - Records that are complete and well-kept are easy to evaluate and defend.
  - Documentation should permit an accurate reconstruction of patient assessments/contact/education/direction, e.g., direction to go to ER.
  - Avoid scenarios that create an absence of proof of consent or traceability of information given to patients.
  - Copies of letters to referring provider, primary care providers.
  - Oral and written communication deficits are often a source of litigation.
- Consider adding a phrase to your note (inpatient or outpatient) similar to "all questions were addressed to his/her/their satisfaction, and he/she/they/guardian verbally agree with plan of care."
- Every time a lab or imaging study is ordered, it is the provider's obligation to retrieve it, interpret it and act on it accordingly—and document.
- Adhere to policies and procedures; work-arounds create liability.
  - This also avoids relieving employers of responsibility.
- Beware of the "autofill" function of electronic medical records—do not let the EMR document an examination or care that did not happen.
- Charting by exception— documenting only findings that vary from the norm, or variance charting, *does not* provide sufficient evidence of compliance with the standards of care.
- Be cautious when leaving messages on answering machines, particularly sensitive information—it can create a HIPPA violation and can result in liability.
- Be mindful of professional boundaries; personal relationships with patients/families can be red flags for juries.

- Any request for medical records, especially with a case or patient that was difficult, should prompt the provider to notify the employer and insurer of a potential suit.
- Some states only accept nurses as expert witnesses in nursing malpractice lawsuits involving nursing standards of practice and breach of duty; some states permit non-nurses (e.g., physicians) to testify as experts in *nursing* care.

Listing of Sources

1. *Daubert v. Merrell Dow Pharmaceuticals, Inc.*, 509 U.S. 579, 113 S.Ct. 2786, 125 L.Ed.2d 469 (1993)
2. *Frye v. United States*, 293 F. 1013 (D.C. Cir. 1923)
3. Federal Rule of Evidence 601 (2019)
4. Federal Rule of Evidence 701 (2019)
5. Federal Rule of Evidence 702 (2019)
6. Federal Rule of Evidence 703 (2019)
7. Federal Rule of Evidence 705 (2019)
8. Federal Rule of Civil Procedure 26 (2019)
9. Federal Rule of Civil Procedure 35 (2019)
10. Ohio Rule of Evidence 601 (2019)
11. New York CPLR 3101
12. Michigan Compiled Law Service 600.2169 (2018)
13. *Barnette v. Grizzly Processing, LLC*, 2012 WL 293305 (E.D.Ky., 2012)
14. *Hamilton v. Pike County, Ky.*, 2012 WL 6570508 (E.D.Ky., 2012)
15. *U.S. v. Beverly*, 369 F.3d 516 (2004)
16. *Early v. Toyota Motor Corp.*, 277 Fed.Appx. 581, 2008 WL 2001727 (6th Cir. 2008)
17. *Early v. Toyota Motor Corp.*, 486 F.Supp.2d 633 (E.D.Ky. 2007)
18. *Kumho Tire Co., Ltd. v. Carmichael*, 526 U.S. 137, 119 S.Ct. 1167, 143 L.Ed.2d 238 (1999).
19. *McLean v. 988011 Ontario, Ltd.*, 224 F.3d 797 (6th Cir. 2000)
20. *Smelser v. Norfolk Southern Ry. Co.*, 105 F.3d 299 (6th Cir.1997)
21. *Tamraz v. Lincoln Elec. Co.*, 620 F.3d 665(2010)
22. *Yurkowski v. Univ. of Cincinnati*, 2017-Ohio-7681
23. *Stanley v. Ohio State Univ. Med. Ctr.*, 10th Dist. No. 12AP-999, 2013-Ohio-5140
24. *Westberry v. Gislaved Gummi AB*, 178 F.3d 257 (4th Cir. 1999)
25. *Mathias v. Shoemaker*, 2017 U.S. Dist. LEXIS 132999
26. *Bresler v. Wilmington Trust Co.*, 855 F.3d 178 (4th Cir. 2017)
27. *Cooper v. Smith & Nephew, Inc.*, 259 F.3d 194 (4th Cir. 2001)
28. *Westberry v. Gislaved Gummi AB*, 178 F.3d 257 (4th Cir. 1999)
29. *United States v. McLean*, No. 16-4673, 695 Fed.App'x 681, 2017 U.S. App. LEXIS 10380, 2017 WL 2533381 (4th Cir. June 12, 2017)
30. *United States v. Wilson*, 484 F.3d 267 (4th Cir. 2007)

31. *Rockman v. Union Carbide Corp.*, RDB-16-1169, 266 F. Supp. 3d 839, 2017 U.S. Dist. LEXIS 110181, 2017 WL 3022969 (D. Md. July 17, 2017)
32. Medical Association and Society's Professional and Ethical Requirements/ Guidelines for expert witness testimony
    (a) American Medical Association
    (b) American College of Vascular Surgery
    (c) American College of Emergency Medicine Physicians
    (d) American College of Physicians
    (e) American College of Radiology and Radiation Oncology
    (f) American Academy of Pediatrics
    (g) American Association of Legal Nurse Consultants
    (h) American College of Obstetricians & Gynecologists
    (i) American College of Orthopedic Surgery
33. Pollin D. Requisites of Expert Witness, 33 AM. JUR. PROOF OF FACTS 2D 179 § 5 (Feb. 2017 Update).

Special Topics for the Advanced Practice Provider in Urology

26

Roberto Navarrete, Miriam Hadj-Moussa, Susanne A. Quallich, Michelle J. Lajiness, Kenneth A. Mitchell, and Katherine Marchese

Contents

R. Navarrete · M. Hadj-Moussa
Department of Urology/Michigan Medicine, University of Michigan, Ann Arbor, MI, USA

S. A. Quallich (✉)
Division of Andrology, General and Community Health, Department of Urology, Michigan Medicine, University of Michigan, Ann Arbor, MI, USA
e-mail: quallich@umich.edu

M. J. Lajiness
Department of Urology, University of Toledo, Toledo, OH, USA
e-mail: Michelle.Lajiness@utoledo.edu

K. A. Mitchell
Meharry Medical College Physician Assistant Sciences Program, Nashville, TN, USA
e-mail: kmitchell@mmc.edu

K. Marchese
Department of Urology, RUSH University Medical Center, Chicago, IL, USA

© Springer Nature Switzerland AG 2020
S. A. Quallich, M. J. Lajiness (eds.), *The Nurse Practitioner in Urology*,
https://doi.org/10.1007/978-3-030-45267-4_26

Objectives

1. Recognize potential short- and long-term complications of gender-affirming surgery.
2. Summarize "Competencies for the nurse practitioner working with adult urology patients."
3. Discuss the basics of the male infertility evaluation.
4. Identify the issues inherent in Men's Health for urology providers.
5. Describe the process of vasectomy and potential for non-surgical male contraception.
6. Review inflammatory conditions of the penis and urgent urology conditions.

Urologic Complications of Genital Gender Confirmation Surgery

Roberto Navarrete and Miriam Hadj-Moussa

Introduction

Gender dysphoria is distress caused by an incongruence between gender identity and biologically determined sex. Multidisciplinary treatment of gender dysphoria seeks to affirm a patient's gender identity and is individualized based on each patient's goals for gender expression. Interventions may include social gender transition, psychotherapy, cross-sex hormone therapy, permanent hair removal, vocal coaching, and/or gender confirmation surgery (GCS). GCS can include any number of procedures that alter the face, chest, genitals, etc. and is performed by a combination of Plastic Surgeons, Urologists, and Gynecologists.

For appropriately selected patients, GCS is effective and medically necessary treatment for gender dysphoria because it enhances the physical characteristics corresponding with their gender identity (WPATH 2012). The benefits of GCS to treat gender dysphoria have been well established, despite the overall lack of high-quality studies in transgender care (WPATH 2012). Surgery has been shown to enhance the benefits of psychotherapy, social gender transition, and hormone therapy to alleviate gender dysphoria (Hadj-Moussa et al. 2018a, b).

The number of patients seeking all forms of GCS has increased dramatically in recent years (Ridgeway et al. 2018). Although only an estimated 10% of transgender patients undergo gender-affirming surgery, the incidence of genital surgery in this cohort has increased from 72.0% to 83.9% (Canner et al. 2018).

Surgeons performing GCS follow guidelines published by the World Professional Association for Transgender Health (WPATH 2012) to determine surgical eligibility. Criteria for genital procedures includes two letters of referral from mental health providers with experience in transgender care, 12 months of cross-sex hormone therapy, and a 12-month social gender transition (WPATH 2012). Obtaining the patient's informed consent preoperatively is of paramount importance given the irreversibility, complex nature, and high risk of complications for genital GCS procedures.

Evaluation and management of a transgender patient who may be suffering a complication of genital GCS begins with a thorough review of the patient's history—specifically surgical history and any available operative notes or clinic notes from their GCS surgeon. Address the patient by their preferred name and pronoun as documented in their clinical chart. It may be necessary to modify medical history forms and interview questions to build rapport and avoid miscommunication (Puechl et al. 2019; Hadj-Moussa et al. 2018a, b). In most cases, the patient's GCS surgeon(s) will have supported them through any immediate postoperative complications like bleeding or wound dehiscence. Long-term complications are more likely to be encountered in the urology office.

Evaluation and Management of Complications Following Feminizing Genitoplasty

Feminizing genitoplasty can include bilateral orchiectomy alone, performed to eliminate endogenous testosterone and reduce anti-androgen medication requirements, or full genital reconstruction with vaginoplasty to create an esthetic and functional neovagina. During vaginoplasty, the penis and testicles are removed and a space for the neovagina is created anterior to the rectum and posterior to the bladder and prostate, which is left in situ. The neovagina is created either using an inverted penile skin tube (penile inversion vaginoplasty) or a segment of intestine (intestinal transposition vaginoplasty) (Hadj-Moussa et al. 2018a, b). Penile inversion vaginoplasty (PIV) does not require intraabdominal surgery or bowel resection, hence its preferential use (Pan and Honig 2018).

Vaginoplasty is associated with a diverse side effect profile; however, major systemic adverse events are very rare (Hadj-Moussa et al. 2018a, b). The most common complications are related to delayed wound healing and localized infections. These are underreported in the literature and most often managed with local wound care and/or antibiotics.

Evaluation of potential complications should include a thorough history and physical exam. Query patients regarding specific urinary symptoms, including a spraying or split urinary stream, obstructive voiding symptoms, incontinence, and recurrent urinary tract infections. The use of validated questionnaires (American Urological Association Symptom Score and Incontinence Symptom Index) are helpful. An adequate physical exam will require visual examination of the neovagina with a speculum. Post-void residual testing is important when there is concern for urinary retention. A urinalysis and urine culture is used to evaluate for urinary tract infection. Additional workup with cystoscopy, voiding cystourethrogram, cross-sectional imaging, etc. may be required.

Urinary Complications

Urinary symptoms are common following vaginoplasty. A spraying stream affects up to 33% of patients and a smaller percentage are affected by urgency, frequency, urinary incontinence (stress, urge, or mixed), urinary tract infections, and/or weak stream (WPATH 2012; Hadj-Moussa et al. 2018a, b). The etiology of incontinence after vaginoplasty is not well understood since neither the internal or external sphincters are directly manipulated during the procedure, however, one theory is that the external urinary sphincter complex may be damaged during dissection of the neovaginal space. Unmasking of detrusor overactivity by shortening the urethra and the development of periurethral fibrosis may also play a role in the development of incontinence following vaginoplasty (Hadj-Moussa et al. 2018a, b). Transwomen who have been on anti-androgen medications rarely have obstructive urinary symptoms related to benign prostatic hyperplasia (BPH). Patients who started anti-androgenic hormones later in life are the exception. Consider pelvic floor physical therapy (PFPT) for bothersome urinary complaints, as they may improve or resolve with therapy (Ridgeway et al. 2018). Lower urinary tract symptoms may require pharmacologic intervention with anticholinergics or alpha blockers. Symptoms refractory to medical management should be referred to a Urologist for surgical intervention.

A spraying and/or weak stream may be due to meatal stenosis, which affects less than 10% of patients, and can be associated with an elevated post-void residual (PVR). More proximal urethral strictures are very rare (Hadj-Moussa et al. 2018a, b). Patients presenting with urinary retention due to meatal stenosis should have their bladders decompressed with a urethral catheter or a suprapubic tube. Rarely, dilation of the meatus is effective treatment, surgical intervention with meatoplasty is usually necessary.

Neovaginal Stenosis

Without regular postoperative dilation or penetrative intercourse to maintain the width and depth of their neovagina, patients can develop neovaginal stenosis (<10%)

or introital stenosis (<15%) following vaginoplasty (WPATH 2012). The patient may report a feeling of loss of depth or inadequate depth that prevents penetrative intercourse or difficulty performing neovaginal dilation. Physical exam may demonstrate a short neovaginal cavity on speculum exam. In some cases sequential dilation can restore length and width to the neovagina (Nolan et al. 2019). Severe cases should be referred back to the patient's urologist or plastic surgeon for surgical reconstruction.

Rectovaginal Fistula

Rectovaginal fistulas only affect approximately 1% of vaginoplasties, but the morbidity is extensive (Levy et al. 2019; Ferrando 2018). Rectal injury during dissection of the neovaginal space, revision vaginoplasty, and postoperative hematoma or abscess have been shown to increase the risk of rectovaginal fistula (Van Der Sluis et al. 2016). Rarely, the presence of a fistula may signal the presence of malignancy (Van Der Sluis et al. 2016). Presenting symptoms include passage of flatus or foul-smelling discharge from the neovagina. Small fistulas may be managed conservatively with a low residual diet. Formal fistula repair with advancement flaps is usually required and may be augmented by bowel diversion with assistance from a General or Colorectal Surgeon (Vogel et al. 2016).

Evaluation and Management of Complications Following Masculinizing Genitoplasty

Surgical creation of a neophallus can be performed via metoidioplasty or flap-based phalloplasty. During metoidioplasty, the hormonally hypertrophied clitoris is mobilized to create a small neophallus (its embryologic equivalent) capable of standing micturition when combined with urethral lengthening using tubularized labia majora flaps and buccal grafts, sexual sensation, and erection but that is too short for penetrative intercourse (Vogel et al. 2016). Flap-based phalloplasty uses nongenital tissue, most commonly from the radial forearm (RFP), to construct an anatomically sized neophallus that can be used for standing micturition but that does not have any inherent sexual sensation or the ability to become erect without placement of a penile prosthesis (Morrison et al. 2017). Metoidioplasty and flap-based phalloplasty are associated with a reported a 10–37% and up to 50% risk of complications, respectively (Hadj Moussa et al. 2019). Complication rates are likely underreported since patients often travel long distances for surgery, staged procedures are common, and these procedures remain extremely technically challenging (Hadj-Moussa et al. 2019). The most common complications following masculinizing genitoplasty are urologic, owing to the difficulty in creating a urethra long enough to allow the patient to stand to void, while using non-urethral tissue for the procedure. Urologic complications following these procedures can present at any time.

Along with obtaining a thorough history and physical exam, a review of prior reconstructive procedures is important. Questions regarding specific urinary symptoms, including post-void dribbling, urinary leakage, weak stream, frequency, dysuria, or poor local wound healing should be asked as these may signal presence of a urethral stricture, persistence of the vaginal cavity, urinary tract infection, or urethrocutaneous fistula formation (Santucci 2018). The use of validated question-naires (American Urological Association Symptom Score and Incontinence Symptom Index) can be helpful and determine degree of patient bother. A post-void residual should be obtained when there is concern for urinary retention. A urinalysis and urine culture should be performed to rule out urinary tract infection. Physical examination may reveal meatal stenosis or a urethrocutaneous fistula. Additional workup with cystoscopy, retrograde urethrogram, voiding cystourethrogram, cross-sectional imaging, or other imaging may be required.

Urethrocutaneous Fistula

Patients with urethrocutaneous fistulae can describe leakage of urine from a site other than the neomeatus. Local tissue changes such as induration, erythema, or visible mucosa at the fistula site may also be detected and the fistula site can often be visual-ized (Dy et al. 2019). Fistulae after metoidioplasty usually occur at the anastomosis between the native urinary meatus and the labia majora flap, and complicate 5–23% of cases. Approximately half resolve with conservative management and prolonged catheter drainage (Djordjevic and Bizic 2013; Frey et al. 2016). The risk of urethrocu-taneous fistulae following phalloplasty is higher, complicating a reported 22–75% of cases (Nikolavsky et al. 2018). They usually occur at the anastomosis between the labia majora flap (pars fixa) and the nongenital tissue flap (pars pendulans) or between the native meatus and the labia majora flap (pars fixa). Some fistulae that form in the first few months after phalloplasty resolve with catheter drainage, though most will require surgical intervention, especially if they form after months or years.

Urethral Stricture

Urethral strictures lead to weak or spraying urinary stream, recurrent urinary tract infections, and/or urinary retention. Measurement of a post-void residual is important when there is suspicion of a urethral stricture. Bladder decompression with a Foley catheter or suprapubic tube is necessary for patients presenting with severe urinary retention from a stricture. Urethral strictures complicate 2–9% of metoidioplasties and occur at the anastomosis between the native meatus and the labia minora flap (Hadj-Moussa et al. 2019). Up to 60% of phalloplasties are complicated by urethral strictures which most commonly form at the anastomosis of the labia majora flap (pars fixa) and nongenital tissue flap (pars pendulans), but can occur at any point along the reconstructed urethra. Surgical intervention is typically necessary for ure-thral strictures. Less-invasive management with endoscopic urethral dilation or inci-sion may be indicated for short strictures. Unfortunately, the stricture is likely to recur, necessitating excision and reanastomosis, staged urethral reconstruction, or formation of a perineal urethrostomy depending on the patient (Jun and Santucci 2019).

Remnant Vaginal Cavity

Most transgender men who undergo metoidioplasty or phalloplasty also undergo hysterectomy and oophorectomy to eliminate the need for future gynecologic can-cer screenings and vaginectomy to remove the vaginal canal. Patients who develop strictures following phalloplasty can develop a urethrovaginal fistula because high voiding pressure created by the stricture forces urine into the obliterated vaginal space, especially if the vaginal mucosa was not completely excised at the time of their vaginectomy (Nikolavsky et al. 2018). These patients may present with obstructive urinary symptoms, urinary tract infections, or pelvic fullness. Cross-sectional imaging with CT or MRI may be used to diagnose the persistent vaginal cavity. Treatment includes surgical excision of the entire remnant vaginal cavity.

Clinical Pearls
- Long-term complications from these procedures are to be encountered in the urology office.
- Time since the procedure was completed is key when evaluating complications.
- Validated questionnaires can help with the assessment of symptoms.

Executive Summary: Competencies for the Nurse Practitioner Working with Adult Urology Patients

Susanne A. Quallich and Shelley Lajiness

Original Reference

Quallich, S.A., Bumpus, S.M., & Lajiness, S. (2015). Competencies for the nurse practitioner working with adult urology patients. Urologic Nursing, 35(5), 221–230. https://doi.org/10.7257/1053-816X.2015.35.5.221

Full text is also available in the first edition of this book.

Introduction

This paper highlights identified needs and gaps in knowledge for the role of the specialty urology Nurse Practitioner and works to fill these gaps by offering a template for providers who wish to document and evaluate their advancing skills in caring for adult urology patients. The paper describes a method for training and evaluating an NP in urology, using a stepwise approach grounded in theory and drawing from existing metrics, including the NP generalist curricula and the Urology Milestones used to evaluate residents.

Background

The need for urologic care is rapidly outpacing the number of available urologists. In this context, we are seeing increasing numbers of nurse practitioners moving into role that involve the care of urology patients. The AUA (2014) published a consensus statement endorsed both nurse practitioners and physician assistants in the current and future care of urology patients. However, there is rare specialty preparation for nurse practitioners specific to urology* that happens on the graduate or post certificate environment. This has created a gap in the preparation and knowledge base of nurse practitioners relative to care of patients with urologic issues. This results in a lack of standardization in the preparation of, and the knowledge base of, nurse practitioners who may already be working in urology environments.

The Certification Board for Urology Nurses and Associates (CBUNA) offers a certification exam for nurse practitioners to become a *Certified Urology Nurse Practitioner* (CUNP) after having worked a minimum of 800 direct patient care hours as a nurse practitioner providing care for urology patients (www.CUBUNA. org). Presently, there are less than 200 nurse practitioners who hold the certification.

Role and Scope of the Advance Practice Urology Nurse

A subspecialty focus allows nurse practitioners to focus on specific quality and access to that specialty service. Practice as a *urology nurse practitioner* does not have a concise definition at this time. This collection of competencies is a beginning step to establishing what a nurse practitioner can offer and achieve within the arena of urology.

These 24 urology NP competencies were created by synthesizing the core competencies for adult-gerontology nurse practitioner 2010 core competencies, family nurse practitioner 2013 core competencies, and the Society of Urologic Nurses and Associates (SUNA 2013) "Urologic Nursing: Scope and Standards of Practice" (2nd edition)**. These urologic care in these competencies influenced by the AUA consensus statement on Advanced Practice Providers (2014) and *The Urology Milestone Project* (Accreditation Council for Graduate Medical Education [ACGME]/AUA 2012).

Theoretical Framework

These 24 competencies are grounded in the work of Benner (1982) and her discussion of a progression from novice to expert. Benner's theory provides for distinction between theoretical and practical knowledge, and progression that is consistent with *advanced beginner*, *proficient*, and *expert* levels that are described in Benner's work. Automatic progression among the three levels described in these competencies is not guaranteed for every NP working in urology; some NPs may progress to Level I or "Expert Urology NP" for some domains but not others.

Overview of and Limitations of the Competencies

The competencies (Table 26.1) cover three general content areas: patient care, professional issues, and health system role for the nurse practitioner working in

Table 26.1 Selected competency examples

Competency (NONPF Competency)	Level 3 Newly graduated, and/or new to urology	Level 2 Experienced NP new to urology	Level 1 Expert Urology NP
Patient care activities			
1. **Obtains relevant health history, focused to genitourinary complaints, as comprehensive as needed to evaluate present issue** (*scientific foundation, independent practice*)	Incorporates knowledge of pediatric urologic issues and their impact on the care of adult urology patients. Evaluates signs and symptoms within context of a GU complaint to formulate plan of care. Developing skill with male and female GU examination	Prioritizes history and physical findings within context of GU complaint. Recognizes relevant history to prioritize evaluation of complaint. Developing skill in recognizing specifics of male and female GU examination, appropriately targeted to a patient's genitourinary complaints and medical condition. Developing skill with recognition of subtle GU physical exam findings	Distinguishes GU complaints that are a symptom of other health concerns from GU complaints that represents a specific GU health issue. Able to routinely identify subtle or unusual physical findings within context of GU complaints. Highly efficient at gathering pertinent information necessary to formulate specific GU plan of care
2. **Strives for patient-centered care based on respect and collaboration among team members** (*health delivery system, leadership*)	Responsive to patient needs and consistent follow-up based on results of evaluation. Communicates and coordinates plan of care with appropriate team members	Consistently prompt and responsive to patient care issues. Completes tasks and charting on time, and communicates with patient and family, and other team members as needed	Consistent in maintaining obligations to patient care. Always accepts feedback willingly. Plan of care issues completed in a careful and thorough manner, and communicated to patient and family
3. **Incorporates compassion, integrity, and respect for spiritual and cultural beliefs into genitourinary care** (*ethics, independent practice*)	Assists diverse panel of patients to obtain GU care. Honors requests for same gender provider when possible. Sensitive to psychological factors in GU conditions. Identifies need for background information (e.g., SES, sexual orientation) as issues emerge in GU patient care	Demonstrates sensitivity to cultural, ethnic and spiritual context when faced with patient or family emotions, within context of providing GU care	Willingness to express concerns regarding team behaviors that are inconsistent with culturally—and spiritually sensitive care

(continued)

Table 26.1 (continued)

Competency (NONPF Competency)	Level 3 Newly graduated, and/or new to urology	Level 2 Experienced NP new to urology	Level 1 Expert Urology NP
Patient care activities			
4. Provides genitourinary care in cost-aware fashion while accommodating risk-benefit issues (independent practice, health delivery system)	Understands coding issues that are specific to GU care Acknowledges socioeconomic barriers that influence patient-centered GU care Minimizes unnecessary care by adhering to established guidelines	Understands and follows established guidelines for GU management Focuses on patient-centered care by assessing economic impact of commonly performed GU procedures Able to envision long-term goals of GU care, and plan for patients and their support systems	Well-versed in coding issues specific to NP role within urology Leads and explores mechanism for cost containment, such as utilization of urologic supplies Practices within GU environment in a cost-effective fashion, including minimizing inappropriate medical resource use
5. Demonstrates leadership in the clinical environment (leadership, practice inquiry)	Participates in development of own orientation to urologic clinical environment Takes responsibility for actions and behavior and admits mistakes Seeks mentorship from GU providers with a complementary skill set	Seeks feedback on clinical role and emerging expertise Recognizes conflicts of interest Consistent in timely completion of medical records and patient communications	Willingness to function in an oversight capacity of the care team in the clinical environment Provides leadership for quality improvement initiatives
6. Continuously strives for evidence-based practice (practice inquiry, quality, scientific foundation)	Able to identify and utilize resources that promote evidence-based practice Identifies and refers patients as appropriate	Demonstrates ability to perform searches of the literature for evidence-based information Collaborates for GU research Aware of appropriate clinical trials or research studies, recruiting patients as appropriate	Synthesizes information by effectively and efficiently performing relevant reviews of literature Incorporates evidence based into helping patients to make informed decisions about GU care Promotes translational research to benefit GU patients

urology. The urology-specific competencies build on the population-based skills and knowledge of the nurse practitioner's generalist certification. The competencies also build on the emerging interdisciplinary model of care. Furthermore, the competencies offer a clear framework for progression, and a gauge for knowledge and skill acquisition as nurse practitioners remain in a urology clinical role.

The competencies are limited by the restrictions inherent in individual state scope of practice. The competencies support a broad in its scope of practice but are not a legal description of practice. For example, office-based cystoscopy is clearly implied within these competencies but whether or not an individual nurse practitioner can be privileged for this procedure will be determined based on the state scope of practice for nurse practitioners. These competencies also do not mandate specific didactic contents for the nurse practitioner in urology role; additional learning would be based on the specific role for an NP and the population that role serves.

Summary

This competency document can serve to standardize urology education and improve evaluation for nurse practitioners working in urology. Furthermore, it can offer a roadmap for nurse practitioners moving into urology to gauge their knowledge and skills as they progress from one level to the next. This is especially vital as increasing numbers of nurse practitioners are moving into specialty environments due to both need and attrition of physician numbers.

*At the time this paper was originally published, there were only 2 post-graduate fellowships in Urology for NPs.

** At the writing of this book the SUNA Scope and Standards of Practice were being updated.

Male Fertility Overview

Susanne A. Quallich

The World Health Organization describes "infertility is a disease of the reproductive system defined by the failure to achieve a clinical pregnancy after 12 months or more of regular unprotected intercourse" (Zegers-Hochschild et al. 2009). Infertility is disease of the reproductive system that affects about 6.1 million people in the United States, or about 15% of the reproductive age population globally (Agarwal et al. 2015). It affects men and women, and most cases are treated with conventional therapies such as medical management or surgery. Babies born by in vitro fertilization represent 1.5% of the children born in the US, as 2015.

Male factor infertility contributes to between 35% and 60% of the total cases of couples seeking fertility treatment and as many as 2% of men will have poor semen parameters (Kumar and Singh 2015), but the majority of male infertility is idiopathic. Male infertility is constructed as a medical condition with psychological consequences, and many disciplines have contributed to the study of the nonmedical aspects of infertility. Masculine norms (such as control, stoicism, or strength) impact the emotional well-being of men who do not live up to either reproductive or sexual cultural ideals. Little attention has been directed toward men's experience of infertility in differing social, cultural, and political contexts. Infertility challenges one's life expectations, and couples report disruptions in both their personal life, and emotional and sexual relationships,

There is a substantial amount of published literature that focuses on the impact of infertility on sexual and marital relationships, and women's reproductive lives have been extensively explored by social science research in the last 25 years. However, little research has been directed toward examination of the male infertility experience; available research is compounded by small sample sizes, uncontrolled study designs, and a lack of validated instruments. This limited body of social research marginalizes the experience of men and has left providers with little knowledge of the emotional repercussions of a diagnosis of male infertility. The few studies that have been completed confirm that infertility is experienced as a threat to masculinity.

Barriers to Care

Male infertility remains a hidden issue within the context of overall fertility care. Outcomes of fertility treatments are tracked only at conception or live birth, making a clear picture of the epidemiology of male fertility unclear. Study of male fertility issues is further hindered by the fact that male fertility is not a reportable disease, is almost exclusively treated outpatient, and is almost always paid for out-of-pocket. For *in vitro* fertilization cases, the Centers for Disease Control tracks only whether or not there was a male fertility factor present. This creates a scenario that results in an unclear public health burden for male sub- and in-fertility; there is evidence that it has been increasing over the past several decades (Winters and Walsh 2014). Authors have suggested that men with male factor infertility many have other health issues that contribute to decreased lifespan (Jensen et al. 2009). Furthermore, data related to male infertility and race is sparse, although Eisenberg et al. (2013) reported that Caucasian men are more likely to undergo evaluation.

The Affordable Care Act (2010) does not mention any mandate for infertility evaluation and treatment, leaving the issue to the individual states. Currently, only 16 states address coverage for infertility, and only six of these mandate male factor evaluation and treatment. This creates a disparity in coverage for identifying risks contributing to male health issues; it means that men are denied the opportunity to consider treatment for reversible causes; it means that men are denied the opportunity for interventions that may decrease the sophistication (and cost) of any assisted reproductive technology required.

Many urology practices may not have a provider that specializes in medical and/or surgical management of male infertility, and men may need to be referred. There are many areas of the US that do not have easy access to a male or female fertility specialist; in addition, there are clear knowledge gaps among providers and patients about what a male evaluation can yield or its utility (Mehta et al. 2016). These policy, socioeconomic, epidemiologic, and financial barriers contribute to access to care and a limited understanding of the true problem of male factor infertility.

When to Refer

Ideally, both partners should undergo evaluation at the same time, in order to coordinate care. While IVF can be a solution for many couples, it can be possible to address male factor diagnoses in a less invasive, and possible more cost-effective, manner. Consider referral to a male fertility specialist for:

- A patient or partner request;
- An abnormal semen analysis;
- Azoospermia (no sperm in ejaculate);
- A male with a spinal cord injury or other neurologic issue (including previous surgery) that compromises ejaculation;
- Male fertility evaluation before and after chemotherapy and/or treatment for any malignancy;
- A couple who has failed IVF cycles;
- A couple with a female partner age 40 or older;
- A male partner who has had a vasectomy;
- And a couple that has timed intercourse, and without a positive pregnancy test for >12 months.

History and Physical Examination

An infertility evaluation should be considered when there is a history of unprotected intercourse for at least 12 months without a positive pregnancy test, or if intercourse has been timed with ovulation. This length of time can be shortened if the female partner is age 35 or older, or if the couple is simply worried about their fertility status. There are other reasons to consider an evaluation, such as female infertility issues or a history of male risk factors for infertility, such as cryptorchidism or a history of cancer treatment.

A targeted history for potential fertility issues in the male includes general reproductive history including a history of previous paternity, any past medical history or surgical history that could affect the structure or function of the male genitalia, occupational exposure to temperature extremes and environmental toxins. Relevant surgical history includes any procedure that can alter the structure or function of the male genitalia, including retroperitoneal surgery or hernia repair. The sexual history and a history of female fertility evaluation are also necessary components.

Physical examination includes a general assessment special focus on the genitalia, the presence and consistency of the vas deferens. Men should be examined for unilateral or bilateral varicoceles (have patients Valsalva to reverse flow into the pampiniform plexus while standing to provoke palpable distention of the vessels; Table 26.2) and evidence of appropriate virilization including hair distribution. Varicoceles are associated with up to 40% of primary infertility cases and up to 80% of secondary infertility cases (difficulty establishing a pregnancy after minimal difficulty with first child).

Obesity by itself may be a risk factor for subfertility and/or infertility. This is in part due to its association with a body habitus that creates cloistered testes that are kept at a higher temperature, potential hormone derangements such as decreased free testosterone and increased estradiol, and associated conditions such as erectile dysfunction.

Laboratory evaluation is targeted at the hormones involved, and the actual quality of an ejaculated semen analysis (Table 26.2). Evaluation should be targeted at three semen analyses done at least 3 weeks apart, with 3 days' abstinence before sample is collected, to firmly establish a production pattern; the exception would be azoospermia (no sperm) that was analyzed at an andrology lab.

Table 26.2 Evaluation for male factor infertility

Test	Discussion
Semen analysis WHO parameters [Cooper et al. (2010)] Volume: 1.5 mL Sperm concentration: 15 million spermatozoa/mL Total sperm number: 39 million spermatozoa per ejaculate Morphology: 4% normal forms Progressive motility: 32% Total (progressive + nonprogressive motility): 40%	Men will be asked to provide a semen sample after a period of abstinence of 2–5 days. This can include a urine sample in the case of suspected retrograde ejaculation. Values that are evaluated are the volume of the ejaculate, sperm motility, total sperm count, and sperm morphology (shape)
Hormone studies	Total testosterone, luteinizing hormone (LH), follicle stimulating hormone (FSH), prolactin levels Estradiol may be included if the patient has a high body mass index (BMI)
Genetic testing	Karyotype analysis and Y-chromosome microdeletion testing may be included if the sperm counts are very low or zero Screening for cystic fibrosis may also be included if the vas deferens is not noted on physical examination
Other	Other tests, such as a scrotal ultrasound, can be included based on an individual's presentation and history
Exam: Estimation of testicular size/volume	Aid in establishing testicular function
Exam: Valsalva maneuver to evaluate for varicocele	Performed with patient standing, ideally in warm room; Valsalva reverses flow into pampiniform plexus and results in palpable distention of vessels
Exam: Presence/absence of vas deferens and spermatic cord	Absence bilaterally or unilaterally—cystic fibrosis or a variant

Table 26.3 Selected contributors to male factor infertility

Pre-testicular	Testicular	Post-testicular
• Anabolic steroid use • Diabetes with anejaculation • Idiopathic hypogonadotropic hypogonadism • Kallmann syndrome • Obesity • Pituitary or hypothalamic dysfunction Spinal cord injury Medications (antihypertensives psychotherapeutic agents, hormonal agents, antibiotics, cimetidine, cyclosporine, colchicine, allopurinol, sulfasalazine)	• Cryptorchidism Mumps orchitis • Klinefelter's syndrome • Previous chemotherapy or radiation treatment • Varicocele	• Antisperm antibodies • Congenital bilateral absence of the vas deferens (cystic fibrosis and its variants) • Erectile dysfunction • Failed vasectomy reversal • Inguinal hernia repair • Retrograde ejaculation • Vasectomy Pediatric hernia repair

Management

The goal of the male fertility evaluation is to identify any potentially reversible, treatable causes (Table 26.3). The goal is also to provide a treatment that may raise the overall semen quality into a range where less sophisticated assisted reproductive technologies may be appropriate. Referral to a male infertility specialist is recommended, but some tests can be ordered in advance: semen analysis, morning testosterone level, LH, FSH, and prolactin.

Behavioral and Conservative Management

Because obesity is associated with male factor infertility, weight loss and exercise is one of the primary recommendations for men who are overweight and obese. This is in part due to decreased serum testosterone levels seen with obese men, although the precise mechanism by which obesity influences male fertility is unknown.

Men should also be instructed to limit their exposure to known environmental toxins that affect semen quality such as pesticides, radiation, heavy metals, biopersistent chemicals, smoking, marijuana, and other drugs of abuse. Smoking, in particular, is a modifiable factor. Smokers have lower sperm concentrations, increased DNA damage and toxic metabolites in smoke impede successful spermatogenesis. In addition, smoking alone can lead to male subfertility or infertility by acting via hormones—suppressing FSH production.

Medical Management

Medical management for male infertility can be successful if a specific contributing factor is identified (Table 26.3). This can include removing environmental toxins, such as recommending smoking cessation, cessation of recreational drug use such as marijuana, and cessation of alcohol intake. Medical management can address endocrine abnormalities, and restore the patient to normal hormone levels. Medical management can include such options as selective estrogen receptor modulators (e.g., clomiphene citrate), aromatase inhibitors, antibiotics, FSH, human chorionic gonadotropin (hCG), or pseudoephedrine (Dabaja and Schlegel 2014) some of which are used "off label" in this context.

Oxidative stress can damage sperm, resulting in decreased motility, increased DNA damage, decreased fusion with the oocyte. Men with a history of cryptorchidsim, testicular torsion and repair, GU infections, and exposure to environmental toxins may be particularly as risk; aging itself may be a risk. Oxidative stress can also impair morphology and motility. Intake of antioxidant foods may improve sperm DNA integrity and overall semen quality. Antioxidants supplements may also be recommended, as these can work to combat the potential for sperm dysfunction or DNA damage (Dabaja and Schlegel 2014) that can be seen in some infertile men. A Cochrane review (2019) reported that 30–80% of male subfertility is suspected to be due to effects of reactive oxygen species on sperm; although there was only low-quality evidence from 4 studies, men who took antioxidants seemed to have a higher birth rate (Smits et al. 2019). However, no over-the-counter supplement is been conclusively proven to prove male fertility.

Men and their partners should be advised that it may take a few weeks to obtain prior authorization from their insurance for some of these medications. After a period of time, often 6 months or more (owing to the fact that sperm production takes 74–90 days), there can be improvements in overall semen parameters.

Surgical Management
Surgical management options include varicocele repair (Chap. 3) testicular or epididymal biopsy, microsurgical testicular sperm extraction (microTESE), vasectomy reversal, epididymal or testicular aspiration for IVF, transurethral resection (TUR) of the ejaculatory duct in cases of blockage.

Long-Term Follow-Up
Because sperm takes approximately 90 days to grow and mature, follow-up for male fertility treatment usually occurs every 3 months. At this point man can be expected to need a semen sample for analysis and to undergo repeat physical examination. Management of additional comorbid conditions should be encouraged, such as obesity, erectile dysfunction, ejaculatory dysfunction, and any depression or anxiety issues that may be impacting fertility management.

Clinical Pearls
- Male factor infertility is an under-acknowledged contributor couples' infertility, and some male infertility/subfertility responds to medical management.
- Male infertility is a hidden issue within the context of overall fertility care, and evaluation can be initiated if the male or couple is concerned about their fertility status.
- Most medical therapies for men are empiric.
- Elimination of known environmental spermatotoxins can preserve male fertility.
- Male infertility may be linked with higher risk for certain malignancies, decreased longevity.

Resources for the Nurse Practitioner or Physician Assistant

American Urological Association: The Optimal Evaluation of the Infertile Male: AUA Best Practice Statement http://www.auanet.org/common/pdf/education/clinical-guidance/Male-Infertility-d.pdf
> RESOLVE: The National Infertility Association: www.resolve.org
> American Society for Reproductive Medicine: http://www.reproductivefacts.org

Resources for the Patient

The Urology Care Foundation: www.urologyhealth.org
> RESOLVE: The National Infertility Association: www.resolve.org
> American Society for Reproductive Medicine: www.reproductivefacts.org

What Is Men's Health?

Kenneth A. Mitchell

When performing an internet search of men's health, the top 10 results yield an array of answers, ranging from *Men's Health* magazine, regional men's health clinics, Wikipedia definition of Men's Health magazine, to women's Health. Asking "What is Men's Health?", is a question which has multiple answers. Like religion and politics, its definition is directly related to whoever the question is being asked. Clinicians, scholars, and the public have defined and redefined men's health for almost a century.

In the 1940s the World Health Organization (WHO) defined men's health as a state of complete physical, mental, and social well-being, as experienced by men, and not merely the absence of disease or infirmity. These often relate to structure such as male genitalia or to conditions caused by hormones specific to, or most notable in, males (WHO 1948). Health experts at the time acknowledged the definition and attempted to educate men and boys about the importance of incorporating healthy lifestyle habits to establish and maintain good health throughout the lifespan. However, efforts by healthcare professionals since that time have been ineffective at reducing the morbidity and mortality of men versus that of women. Various reasons have been suggested to explain the disparity in lifespan between men and women including men's attitudes toward healthcare, clinician's attitudes regarding delivery of care to men, and social determinants of health.

Interestingly, men's healthcare disparity is truly a global issue as shown in a study conducted in 2010 by the Institute for Health Metrics and Evaluation. The study entitled the "Global Burden of Disease" showed that throughout the period from 1970 to 2010, women had a longer life expectancy than men. Furthermore, it was observed that over that 40-year period, female life expectancy at birth increased from 61.2 to 73.3 years, whereas male life expectancy rose from 56.4 to 67.5 years. This data indicates that the gap in life expectancy at birth widened between the sexes to men's disadvantage over that span of 40 years (Wang et al. 2012).

The past several decades have seen an increased interest in men's health by health-care providers largely related to advertising and the availability for both FDA-approved and over-the-counter supplements designed to improve or enhance sexual performance or restoring a youthful physical appearance. The public interest in has been further accentuated by a constant barrage of conventional and online media advertising that has redefined the public's perceived definition of men's health. Considering the WHO definition of men's health, this redefinition of men's health being related to a condition of failure to maintain sexual function, sexual prowess, vitality, and manhood has greatly contributed to a decrease in health literacy among men (Oliffe et al. 2019). Critics, including medical experts, have challenged this redefined perception of men's health as unethical and propagating an unwarranted anti-aging movement leading to medical treatments that yield no clinical benefit and/or may be harmful (Guardian 2008). This new definition of the healthy male feeds into the societal perception that good health in a man at any age is measured by the ability to achieve unrealistic, if not mythical, sexual prowess and physical appearance while ignoring the health issues that impact men's morbidity and mortality worldwide. Consequently, the promise of "turning back the clock" and increasing masculinity has perpetuated, if not worsened, the lack of engagement by men with the healthcare system.

Health Disparity and Social Determinants of Health

The disparity in Men's Health is believed to be attributed to several factors including economic, social, ethnic, accessibility, and men's perceived attitudes toward healthcare. Studies in the United States have pointed toward social determinants as being a major contributing factor for men's health disparities.

In 2015, Bruce et al., published an article highlighting the *Social Determinants of Men's Health Disparities* issue of *Family and Community Health* which included a collection of peer-reviewed articles designed to extend and stimulate discourse about social determinants, their interaction, and subsequent impact on the health outcomes of and among men. The collection of articles addressed various issues and arrived at several key considerations related to addressing men's health disparities. Topics included how African American men define manhood and health, the nature of disparities associated with increased morbidity and mortality–physical inactivity, current smoking, and current drinking–among Black and White men living in similar social and environmental conditions. Participants in one of the highlighted studies noted that these concepts were distinct, however, the authors found that manhood and health were interrelated. Both constructs were defined by constructs men embody, the behaviors men engage in and the goals and values men had to positively influence their families and communities. The authors concluded that these findings have important implications for understanding gender as a social determinant of men's health and how we approach health promotion among African American men.

Furthermore, the diversity of patterns of social determinants suggest that it may be useful to examine the additive effects of determinants of health but that it also will be important to consider the myriad ways that these factors may combine to affect specific populations of men differently and how these patterns of men's health may vary by health outcome (Bruce et al. 2015).

Gender and Men's Health Behaviors

Recognizing common phrases attributed to the attitudes of men and their health including "tough it out," "man up," and simply "be a man!" led experts to conduct studies that identified how masculinity has a profound impact on health behaviors. Although several factors mentioned previously contribute to male health behaviors, the male ideal of masculinity greatly contributes to the lack of engagement with the healthcare system. The design of the healthcare system in the United States, it can be argued, contributes to the lack of healthcare engagement by men. Consider that children from birth engage in the health system mandated by standards of health required by childcare, education, and athletic participation (e.g., immunizations and athletic physicals). However, girls reaching the age of menarche expect to remain engaged with the healthcare system and commonly remain engaged through adulthood primarily for fertility reasons.

In contrast, boys typically disengage once education or athletics no longer mandate healthcare requirements and thus are directed to only seek medical care when something is wrong rather than make efforts to prevent illness or injury. Male socialization, social connectedness, and work-life balance have also been shown to significantly impact overall health. The perception of masculinity begins early in boyhood and is perpetuated throughout the psychological and physical developmental stages, and has been identified as a *key factor* leading both men and boys to engage in risk taking and self-harming behavior.

Combined with societal expectations of male emotional responses, self-denial of access to the healing effects of emotional release, and valuing physical, emotional, and mental healthcare, men are further conditioned to engage in healthcare services much later when faced with illness, which may contribute to disease progression due to presenting with later-stage illness. Healthcare providers must consider and understand the variability of masculine identity and behavior over the course of a man's life as well as the cultural and ethnic background, sexual identity, socioeconomic, and geographical locations as factors.

Healthcare Providers Attitudes Toward Men's Health

On March 27, 1998, Viagra™ (sildenafil), became the first FDA-approved, oral, on-demand treatment for erectile dysfunction. The launch of this medication marked the beginning of a cultural and media revolution regarding male sexual dysfunction and represents one of the most successful launches of an FDA-approved medication in the history of the pharmaceutical industry (IMS Health 1998). In 2002, topical testosterone gels were approved by the FDA, with sales eventually following a similar trajectory as sildenafil. In that first year, there was an 87% increase in sales and a continued increase that ranged from 8% to 32% from year to year from 2002 to 2008 (IMS Health 2002).

Consequently, specialty healthcare providers (e.g., urology and endocrinology) faced increasing demands for evaluation and management of erectile dysfunction and testosterone deficiency. Moreover, general practitioners faced greater demands to provide this service combined with increasing demands from all other provided services. Additionally, increasing administrative workload, a shrinking physician workforce, media pressure, and resulting patient demand, all greatly contributed to a negative clinical bias toward testosterone deficiency and male-specific healthcare issues by many healthcare providers. This is further complicated by the lack of male-specific curricula content in healthcare providers' curricula. Generally, few healthcare providers receive specific training on how to effectively engage men regarding their health, or health issues that are unique to men, with the possible exception of STIs and their treatment. Carroll et al. reported that many healthcare providers view men as being "hard to reach" and are unclear about the type of services that might appeal to or engage men (Carroll et al. 2014).

Men's Health Reports

In 2016, the *Men's Health: Perceptions from Around the Globe* survey was commissioned by Sanofi Consumer Health Care in cooperation with Global Action on Men's Health (GAMH), the Men's Health Network (MHN), Men's Health Forum (MHF) UK, Australian Men's Health Forum (AMHF), and Men's Health Education Council (MHEC). The survey was conducted among 2000 demographically representative adults in 8 countries (Australia, France, Germany, Italy, Poland, Sweden, the United Kingdom, and the United States) examining attitudes toward men's health. The survey was carried out from August 31st to September 10th, 2016 by Opinium Research (Europe and Australia) and Harris (USA). Findings from the study revealed that majority of men wanted to take greater control of their health and wellness. Furthermore, participants reported they were as confident as women that they could do so.

This survey results challenged several well-established norms of healthcare seeking behavior of men. The survey reported that 87% of men wanted to take charge of their health, and 83% of the men were confident in managing their own health and felt like they knew what to do when they had a health problem. Interestingly, 55% of men agree there is plentiful information online to help them choose the right medication, while almost half of all men cited visiting a doctor as their first response when faced with a health problem and 80% of men believe that pharmacists can deal with nonserious and non-chronic health conditions. The findings clearly identified significant changes in men's attitudes and approaches to their health care. Furthermore, these findings further indicated significant opportunities for policymakers around the world who are looking for ways to improve men's health and well-being as part of more efficient and effective healthcare services.

In the United States, Tennessee (TN), is the only state that regularly published data on Men's Health. The Tennessee Men's Health Report Card monitors the health and well-being of men in Tennessee. Published in 2010, 2012, 2014 and 2017, the goal is to use the data to develop strategies to improve the health and well-being of men in the state. Remarkably, the TN Men's Health Report Card continues to distinguish Tennessee as the only state in the U.S. that has regularly published a report card to guide the planning, implementation, and evaluation of programs and policies to improve men's health (Tennessee Men's Health Report Card 2017).

Changing Attitudes and Perceptions of Men's Health

Healthcare providers and the public are becoming increasingly aware of the health disparity that exists between men and women. Academic and private practice groups are offering more Men's Health services than ever before. In 2017, Cleveland Clinic conducted a survey as part of an initiative to promote Men's Health. The results reported indicated younger generations of fathers are significantly more likely to have a father/father figure that has/does talk to them about their health (Millennials: 84% vs. Baby Boomers: 48%). However, 32% of fathers currently don't talk to their family about their health issues and concerns because they don't want to worry people. Eighty-five percent of fathers who talk to their son(s) about health, started the conversation when their son(s) were under 16 years old.

Racial differences in responses indicated that 50% of African American fathers whose family didn't openly talk about health issues and concerns wanted to break the pattern of silence with their families. Whereas about two-thirds (62%) of Hispanic fathers said that their family hid family health issues from them as a kid but talked to them more about it as an adult. Meanwhile, 31% of Hispanic fathers reported they wanted to talk to their sons about health topics but struggled to find the right words. The survey also indicated that more than 500 U.S. males over the age of 18, who are currently fathers or father figures to a boy, and who had a father and/or father figure growing up approximately 62% responded wishing that their own father/father figure had talked to them more about health topics. Forty-seven percent of participants reported that they didn't know about their family health history until they started to go to the doctor as an adult (Cleveland Clinic 2017). These responses demonstrate that men are beginning to understand the importance of maintaining their health and communicating to their sons at a younger age to do the same.

The Scope and Challenge of Men's Health

Men's Healthcare continues to be a controversial area of medicine. The initial emphasis on sexual health has clouded the original definition of men's health and has contributed to the increasing disparity in this area of medicine. The CDC reports that the top three leading causes of death in men have remained consistent (heart disease, cancer, and accidents). Despite the efforts by healthcare providers to address men's health issues, minimal progress has occurred toward reducing the morbidity and mortality of men versus women. Heidelbaugh (2018) reported that the well-male examination should consist of adherence to the recommended screening guidelines from the United States Preventive Services Task Force (USPSTF) and American Academy of Family Practice (AAFP) to best address the leading risks and causes of disease.

However, relentless marketing of sexual dysfunction, testosterone deficiency, and anti-aging solutions have skewed both the public and healthcare provider's perception of the true threats to health and wellness of men. Controversial and misinformation surrounding the effects of treatment for erectile dysfunction and testosterone deficiency have further compounded the public misconception of men's health. The overwhelming desire by men to treat sexual dysfunction has created an industry of Men's Health centers appearing in cities throughout the U.S., offering treatments for erectile dysfunction and "Low-T" and guaranteeing results. Men are lured into these centers with the promise of alleviating the embarrassment and worry of erectile and sexual dysfunction equating improved sexual prowess with wellness and vitality. Oftentimes, these centers are staffed with non-healthcare trained individuals or inadequately trained healthcare providers performing evaluations and treating men suffering from these ailments.

Typically, the style of patient engagement validates the masculine traits of stoicism and anonymity and further perpetuates men's lack of engagement with the healthcare system. Qualified healthcare providers continue to feel the increasing demand for treatments with expectations of restoring youthful appearances and sexual prowess without addressing the underlying causes that threaten the health and well-being of men. Yielding to such pressure, and not addressing the underlying or comorbid conditions related to sexual dysfunction can arguably contribute to disease progression.

Advanced Practice Providers in Men's Health

Healthcare providers in the twenty-first century have many more considerations regarding the care of men. Increasing numbers of aging men requiring services ranging from routine screening to specialized services put a significant demand on the healthcare system. As mentioned previously, continuing health disparities and the wide discrepancy in the life expectancy of men versus women continue to remain inadequately addressed both by men and healthcare providers. It is widely understood that patients and the medical community generally regard male sexual dysfunction to be best addressed by urology practices. However, the many comorbidities associated with erectile dysfunction and testosterone deficiency require a collaboration between primary care and other medical specialties to appropriately address men's health issues.

The emergence of Advanced Practice Providers (APP) in the discipline of Men's Health has already made a significant impact in the delivery of Men's Health care. Legitimate practices providing Men's Health care services staffed with well-trained APPs are increasing in number throughout the US, ensuring delivery of quality, evidence-based care to men. Urology practices in the United States predominately utilize APPs to deliver non-surgical care of male sexual dysfunction, and this trend will likely continue due to the shrinking urologist workforce.

The Future of Men's Health

The challenge of Men's Health will require that the medical community remain actively engaged with creating more increased public awareness of men's health issues. Healthcare providers must be committed to seizing opportunities to inform men and their significant others about the true threats to men's health and wellness and recognize the need to improve engagement of men with the healthcare system.

In Ireland, the ENGAGE training program was developed tailoring to the needs of health and allied health professionals delivering care to men. Participants' self-reported level of knowledge, skill and capacity in identifying priorities, engaging men and influencing practice beyond their own organization. Participants in the program (93.4%) reported improvements in delivering care to men were sustained 5-months post training. Researchers concluded that ENGAGE had succeeded in improving service providers' capacity to engage and work with men thus improving gender competency in the delivery of health and health-related services (Osborne et al. 2018). This study supports the incorporation of focused education in Men's Health in the curriculum of healthcare provider training as an essential component to meeting the healthcare needs of men.

Population health studies that continue to investigate and identify the specific variables that impact the disparity of men's health will be paramount to developing healthcare policy that ensures access to Men's Health services. Lastly, the combination of increased public awareness and improved training of healthcare professionals, will lead to a globally more accurate understanding of male health leading to earlier and continued engagement with healthcare throughout the lifespan resulting in improved health outcomes for men.

Clinical Pearls
- No single specialty "owns" the area of men's health.
- Men's health is influenced by social determinants of health and other factors can be corrected and positively influenced.
- Healthcare providers toward men can disadvantage them further, and have historically contributed to men disengaging with the healthcare system.

Vasectomy and Male Birth Control

Susanne A. Quallich and Kathy Marchese

Vasectomies are the most common nondiagnostic operation performed by urologists in the United States (AUA 2012): up to 500,000 vasectomies are performed in the United States each year. Although other providers will also perform this procedure, approximately 75% are done by trained urologists. It is an outpatient or clinic procedure, is covered to varying degrees by insurance, and involves far less cost and mortality than tubal ligation (the closest equivalent for female sterilization). It is usually performed under a local anesthetic, and sedation can be an option. Men or couples must understand that although a vasectomy is very effective, it is not 100% reliable in preventing pregnancy. The risk of pregnancy after vasectomy is approximately 1 in 2000 for men who have post-vasectomy azoospermia (AUA 2012).

Consultation and Evaluation

As with any invasive procedure, there should be a formal consultation, either with the patient himself or with the couple together. Minimal age for a vasectomy is the legal age of consent in the location where the procedure will be performed. Emphasis should be placed on the intended permanent nature of this procedure, and the discussion will help ensure appropriate expectations regarding the preoperative, operative, and postoperative consequences of this choice are understood. This consultation allows the provider to assess for any anxiety that may suggest sedation as an option for the procedure, and allows for an examination that ensures the procedure can be safely and effectively performed in the outpatient setting.

Vasectomy does not increase one's risk for prostate cancer, coronary heart disease, stroke, hypertension, dementia, hypogonadism, or testicular cancer. Physical examination findings such as varicoceles do not prevent a vasectomy form being an outpatient procedure.

Post-procedure instructions should be reviewed (Box 26.1) and men should be informed that there is a risk of developing chronic post-vasectomy pain. Short-term discomfort may also be associated with formation of a sperm granuloma. Antibiotics are not usually necessary after this procedure.

Follow-Up

A post-vasectomy semen analysis (PVSA) is key to establishing the success of the procedure. While there is some controversy regarding the timing of PVSA, the most current guidelines recommend examination of the first sample 8–16 weeks after the procedure (AUA 2012). Specific guidelines will be provider-dependent, and there may be a higher rate of first-sample compliance when men are given a specific appointment.

Male Birth Control

In the United States, almost 45% of pregnancies are unplanned; options for female contraception are varied and have been available for years. These include the contraceptive pill, hormonal injections, copper and hormonal intrauterine device (IUD), diaphragms, cervical caps, sponges, spermicidal agents and tubal ligations. Historically, the priority has always been given to developing options for female contraception; male were offered the options of condoms, withdrawal, and vasectomy. Condoms have a failure rate of 3–14%; withdrawal as a form of birth control is a game of chance with a failure rate of 19%; vasectomies have a failure rate of about 1% (AUA 2012).

About 15% of couples in the United States indicate that their primary form of birth control is condom use. Efficacy of this method is tempered by their knowledge of correct use and consistency of use. Annual sales for condoms are between six and

Box 26.1 Sample Vasectomy Post-procedure Instructions
1. You must have a companion to drive you home after your procedure.
2. Avoid strenuous exercise or activity for at least 7–10 days after your pro-cedure, as long as there is no pain. This includes any heavy lifting and vigorous exercise. You may return to work the next day, as long as no strenuous activity is required.
3. You may shower after 24 h. Do not take a bath or use a hot tub for five (5) days.
4. You may apply ice or a cold pack to the scrotum as needed, for 10 min of every hour. (A bag of frozen peas will mold to the area). This may help reduce any pain or swelling. It may also be helpful to wear supportive underwear, such as briefs.
5. Expect some mild pain, mild swelling of the scrotum and possible slight fluid leak from the site of the puncture. A gauze pad may be applied to the scrotum if there is any leakage from the puncture site. Drainage may continue for several days and is normal.
6. Take extra-strength acetaminophen or ibuprofen as needed for any pain or discomfort; follow the package directions regarding dose. Stronger pre-scription pain medication is provided, but most men do not find that it is necessary.
7. Continue your normal diet.
8. Avoid sexual activity *for at least 7 days* after your procedure. You may resume having sex after a week, if comfortable enough.
9. Until you are told that you are sterile, it is essential that you use another form of birth control. No method is 100% successful, and post-vasectomy pregnancies have been documented, but are rare. After two (2) zero sperm counts, you may stop other methods of birth control. If any sperm are seen on the first two counts, additional checks will be necessary.
10. If you experience unusual or severe pain that is not relieved by pain medi-cation, excessive bleeding or drainage, excessive swelling or redness, foul odor or a fever over 101 °F, please contact the clinic.

You will usually receive a phone call within 7–10 days after a specimen is dropped off, explaining the results. Please make sure that you provide an up-to-date phone number. If we *cannot* leave a message at that number, please let us know. **If you prefer to receive a message via the EMR portal, this will result in sooner access to your results.**

nine billion. In a survey regarding male birth control options, the majority of men and women responded that are interested in alternative male contraceptive choices. Science and research is catching up and new options for men are currently in trials here in the United States.

Dimethandrolone undecanoate (DMAU; 7a, 11bmethyl-19-nortestosterone undecanoate) is currently in clinical trials by the National Institute of Child Health and Human Development as an oral male contraceptive pill. This Phase 1b, double-blinded, randomized, placebo-controlled study of daily dosing of DMAU met their primary outcomes of safety and tolerability parameters with no significant adverse events as well as meeting their secondary outcomes of drug PK profiles and PD effects (serum FSH, LH and sex hormones). Eighty-two subjects completed the trial. This is obviously an early stage in the development of male birth control pills for men. Ongoing trials are expected to begin soon and will hopefully result in an oral birth control pill for men in the future (Thirumalai et al. 2019).

Another drug in research trials is a male contraceptive gel form which combines testosterone with a progestin compound called Nestorone. This gel is applied daily to the shoulders and back for 4–12 weeks. If the treatment is tolerated, they may continue on it for up to 16 weeks. Men will remain in the study for observation for 24 weeks after they discontinue use of the gel. The gel will decrease spermatogenesis by blocking the naturally produced testosterone but still maintain other testosterone functions through the addition of exogenous testosterone. This Phase IIb open label, single arm, multicenter trial will be conducted at 9 sites and enroll 450 men and will last up to 24 months. The endpoint of this trial will be assessed by the pregnancy prevention statistics.

One nonhormonal male contraceptive device which has completed Phase III clinical trials in India but not currently available in the United States is a polymer gel that is injected into the vas deferens blocking the passage of sperm. This polymer will allow fluid to pass thru but not the larger molecules like sperm. The product termed a RISUG (reversible inhibition of sperm under guidance) is marketed as Vasalgel. When the men decide they are ready to start a family, another fluid is used to dissolve and flush out the Vasalgel.

Although there is ongoing research in developing new pathways for male contraception, the traditional options are still the mainstay.

Clinical Pearls
- Guidelines for vasectomy counseling do not *require* the female partner's presence.
- Vasectomy does not increase risk for other diseases, such as prostate cancer or dementia.
- Forms of male contraception similar to those available for women remain elusive.

Inflammatory Conditions of the Penis and Urgent Urology Conditions (Tables 26.4 and 26.5)

Susanne A. Quallich

Table 26.4 Inflammatory conditions of the penis

Condition	History	Signs and symptoms	Evaluation	Therapeutic interventions
Phimosis	• Seen only in males who are uncircumcised • History of progressive difficulty at retracting the foreskin • History of poor personal hygiene and/or a recent groin skin infection • Creates risk for chronic inflammation and squamous cell cancer of the penis	• Foreskin may show signs of chronic irritation: erythema, fissuring, tightening of opening of foreskin • Possible urinary obstruction or "ballooning" of the foreskin when voiding as it traps urine • Pain • Balanitis or balanoposthitis	• History and presentation sufficient to confirm diagnosis	• Consider circumcision or dorsal slit • May require catheter if urinary function has been compromised
Balanitis	• Greatest risk: uncontrolled and poorly controlled diabetes mellitus • Seen in uncircumcised males and obese males with buried penis • Inflammation of the glans • Commonly caused by *Candida albicans*	• Symptoms can include edema, erythema, and pain of the glans • Dysuria • Urethral discharge • Scaling of skin • Possible history of discharge from between the foreskin and glans • Phimosis • Meatal stenosis • Rash to genitals	• Consider screening for diabetes, especially with higher BMI • Culture for STDs, and for other viral and fungal organisms • KOH (potassium hydroxide) and Tzanck preparations can be included • If ulcers are present, screen for herpes and syphilis • Biopsy may be indicated in refractory cases (no response to treatment after 6 weeks)	• Empiric treatment without cultures is common • NSAIDs may improve comfort level • If patient is diabetic, his diabetes must be controlled in order to help eradicate any infection and prevent recurrence • Retract foreskin and clean daily with warm saline and hypoallergenic soap • Depending on severity, can treat with oral antifungal ± topical antifungal alone or combined topical antifungal and low-strength steroid • Topical antibiotics may have a role in suspected anaerobic infection • Consider circumcision or dorsal slit in refractory cases

(continued)

Table 26.4 (continued)

Condition	History	Signs and symptoms	Evaluation	Therapeutic interventions
Balanoposthitis	• Greatest risk: uncontrolled and poorly controlled diabetes mellitus • Seen in uncircumcised males and obese males with buried penis • Inflammation of both the glans and foreskin	• Similar to balanitis • Can include an edematous and painful foreskin that may not retract	Same as for balanitis	Same as for balanitis
Balanitis Xerotica Obliterans (BXO) or Lichen Sclerosis	• Common in middle-aged men • Result of chronic infection or inflammation, or trauma • Uncircumcised and diabetic males have an increased risk • A personal history of long-standing BXO creates higher risk for squamous cell carcinoma of the penis • Can also been seen to external genitalia of females	• Painful condition associated with flat patches of white, thinned skin (mosaic pattern) • Localized penile discomfort • Painful erections • Urinary obstruction • Meatus may become edematous, indurated • Possible erosions, fissures • Often results in meatal stenosis and urethral strictures • Foreskin may adhere to the glans	Diagnosis can be made only via tissue biopsy	• If asymptomatic—no treatment • Manage associated symptoms • Low-strength steroid can improve comfort level • Yearly follow-up due to risk for malignancy

Table 26.5 Urgent urologic conditions

Condition	Clinical history	Signs/symptoms	Recommended evaluation	Therapeutic interventions
Priapism	• 38–42% of adult patients with sickle cell disease reported at least one episode of priapism • Overall incidence is 1.5 cases per 100,000 person years • Erection that has lasted >4 h beyond cessation of sexual activity • Common for men to delay seeking evaluation and treatment for several hours • Direct penile trauma may result in priapism (cycling) • Recent illicit drug use (cocaine, ecstasy, marijuana)	• Persistent, painful erection (low-flow or veno-occlusive priapism) • Present for hours or days • Erect but nontender penis (high-flow or nonischemic priapism)	• Penile Doppler • Penile blood gases • Arteriography • CBC if malignancy suspected	• Provide analgesia and sedation as needed • Manage any underlying conditions • Epinephrine, phenylephrine, pseudoephedrine, or terbutaline can be injected into the penis to help reverse engorgement • The corpora may also be irrigated with normal saline. Urgent urologic consultation: • The patient may need a needle aspiration to remove trapped blood • if this does not improve the condition, a shunt may be attempted • If this is unsuccessful, the patient may be taken to the operative room for a more aggressive shunt procedure
Acute Retention	• Recent GU instrumentation • Use of over-the-counter cold medicines (men on α-blockers for cold or allergy symptoms) • Recent back injury that may have compromised lumbosacral spine • In men, symptoms consistent with acute prostatitis • In the elderly, recent general anesthesia	• Lower abdominal discomfort/increasing size • Bladder distention (palpable just above symphysis pubis)	• Bladder ultrasound • Catheterization • Eventual spine imaging as indicated	• Insert an indwelling urinary catheter for immediate relief • Rapid drainage avoids stretch injury to the bladder • Investigate the cause and treat as indicated • Consider consultation with urologist to further investigate functional status of the bladder • Establish why this occurred

(continued)

Table 26.5 (continued)

Condition	Clinical history	Signs/symptoms	Recommended evaluation	Therapeutic interventions
Fournier's gangrene	• Progressive necrotizing infection of the external genitalia or perineum • 1.6/100,000 males • Peaks in males 50–79 years old (3.3/100,000) • Highest rate in the South (1.9/100,000) • Overall case fatality rate 7.5% • Also happens in women, incidence is much less • Obesity • Possible history of some break in the skin within the preceding 48 h • Recent poor blood sugar control, with recent rising levels/difficulty managing levels	• Painful swelling, erythema, and induration of the genitalia • Cellulitis, odor, tissue necrosis • Fever/chills and other systemic complaints, such as anxiety • Pain that seems in excess of the visible skin changes Essential to appreciate that the degree of internal necrosis is much greater than suggested by the external signs; adequate (repeated) surgical debridement is necessary to save patient's life	• Typically a type 1 necrotizing fasciitis that is polymicrobial in origin, including *Staphylococcus aureus, Streptococcus* sp., *Klebsiella* sp., *Escherichia coli,* and anaerobic bacteria • Plain films or computed tomography may demonstrate gas in the subcutaneous tissue • Elevated WBC • Serum blood sugar or finger stick	• Broad spectrum antibiotics—antibiotic treatment should be given that covers all causative organisms and can penetrate inflammatory tissue • Provide analgesia and sedation • Admission to hospital • Plan for extensive debridement • Surgical consultations: urology, general surgery, plastics
Paraphimosis	• Phimosis, with increasing difficulty advancing the foreskin • History of recent increased phimosis • History of frequent catheterizations, poor hygiene and/or chronic balanoposthitis leading to phimosis	• Swollen, painful edematous glans • Tight ring of skin apparent behind glans on examination • Discolored, necrotic areas may be noted to the glans	**True urologic emergency:** Necrosis of glans may occur secondary to arterial occlusion	• Provide nonsteroidal antinflammatory drugs for pain management • Initiate antibiotic therapy as indicated • Manual reduction can be attempted, by applying pressure with the thumbs to reduce the edema and advance the foreskin • If this is unsuccessful, local anesthetic may be given in order that a small incision be made in order to correct the restriction Advise patient to consider a circumcision or dorsal slit to prevent further episodes

References

Agarwal A, Mulgund A, Hamada A, Chyatte MR (2015) A unique view on male infertility around the globe. Reprod Biol Endocrinol 13(1):37

American Urological Association (2012) Vasectomy: AUA guideline. AUA Board of Directors. http://www.auanet.org/common/pdf/education/clinical-guidance/Vasectomy.pdf

American Urological Association (2014) AUA Consensus statement on advanced practice providers. Available from http://www.auanet.org/common/pdf/advocacy/advocacy-by-topic/AUA-Consensus-Statement-Advanced-Practice-Providers-Full.pdf

Benner P (1982) From novice to expert. Am J Nurs 82(3):402–407

Bruce MA, Griffith DM, Thorpe RJ Jr (2015) Social determinants of men's health disparities. Fam Commun Health 38(4):281–283

Canner JK et al (2018) Temporal trends in gender-affirming surgery among transgender patients in the United States. JAMA Surg 153:609

Carroll P, Kirwan L, Lambe B (2014) Engaging 'hard to reach' men in community based health promotion. Int J Health Promot Educ 52:120–130

Cleveland Clinic (2017) MENtion It. https://health.clevelandclinic.org/2017/09/american-dads-sons-keep-health-themselves-infographic/

Cooper TG, Noonan E, von Eckardstein S, Auger J, Baker HW, Behre HM et al (2010) World Health Organization reference values for human semen characteristics. Hum Reprod Update 16(3):231–245

Dabaja AA, Schlegel PN (2014) Medical treatment of male infertility. Transl Androl Urol 3(1):9

Djordjevic ML, Bizic MR (2013) Comparison of two different methods for urethral lengthening in female to male (metoidioplasty) surgery. J Sex Med 10(5):1431–1438. https://doi.org/10.1111/jsm.12108

Dy GW et al (2019) Presenting complications to a reconstructive urologist after masculinizing genital reconstructive surgery. Urology 132:202–206

Eisenberg ML, Lathi RB, Baker VL et al (2013) Frequency of the male infertility evaluation: data from the national survey of family growth. J Urol 189(3):1030–1034

Ferrando CA (2018) Vaginoplasty complications. Clin Plast Surg 45:361–368

Frey JD, Poudrier G, Chiodo MV, Hazen A (2016) A systematic review of metoidioplasty and radial forearm flap phalloplasty in female-to-male transgender genital reconstruction: is the "ideal" neophallus an achievable goal? Plast Reconstruct Surg Global Open 4(12):e1131

Hadj-Moussa M, Ohl DA, Kuzon WM (2018a) Evaluation and treatment of gender dysphoria to prepare for gender confirmation surgery. Sex Med Rev 6:607–617

Hadj-Moussa M, Ohl DA, Kuzon WM Jr (2018b) Feminizing genital gender-confirmation surgery. Sex Med Rev 6(3):457–468

Hadj-Moussa M, Agarwal S, Ohl DA, Kuzon WM (2019) Masculinizing genital gender confirmation surgery. Sex Med Rev 7:141–155

Heidelbaugh JJ (2018) The adult well- male examination. Am Fam Physician 98(12):729–737

IMS Health, Retail and Provider Perspective (1998) National Prescription Audit 1998

IMS Health, Retail and Provider Perspective (2002) National Prescription Audit 2002

Jensen TK, Jacobsen R, Christensen K et al (2009) Good semen quality and life expectancy: a cohort study of 43,277 men. Am J Epidemiol 170(5):559–565

Jun MS, Santucci RA (2019) Urethral stricture after phalloplasty. Transl Androl Urol 8:266–272

Kumar N, Singh AK (2015) Trends of male factor infertility, an important cause of infertility: a review of literature. J Hum Reprod Sci 8(4):191

Levy JA et al (2019) Male-to-female gender reassignment surgery: an institutional analysis of outcomes, short-term complications, and risk factors for 240 patients undergoing penile-inversion vaginoplasty. Urology 131:228–233

Mehta A, Nangia AK, Dupree JM, Smith JF (2016) Limitations and barriers in access to care for male factor infertility. Fertil Steril 105(5):1128–1137

Morrison SD, Chen ML, Crane CN (2017) An overview of female-to-male gender-confirming surgery. Nat Rev Urol 14:486–500

Nikolavsky D, Hughes M, Zhao LC (2018) Urologic complications after phalloplasty or metoidioplasty. Clin Plast Surg 45:425–435

Nolan IT, Dy GW, Levitt N (2019) Considerations in gender-affirming surgery: demographic trends. Urol Clin North Am 46:459–465

Oliffe JL, Rossnagel E, Kelly MT, Bottorff JL, Seaton C, Darroch F (2019) Men's health literacy: a review and recommendations. Health Promot Int:daz077. https://doi.org/10.1093/heapro/daz077

Osborne A, Carroll P, Richardson N, Doheny M, Brennan L, Lambe B (2018) From training to practice: the impact of ENGAGE, Ireland's national men's health training programme. Health Promot Int 33:458–467. https://doi.org/10.1093/heapro/daw100

Pan S, Honig SC (2018) Gender-affirming surgery: current concepts. Curr Urol Rep 19:62

Puechl AM, Russell K, Gray BA (2019) Care and cancer screening of the transgender population. J Women's Health 28:761–768

Ridgeway BM, Weintein M, Tunitsky-Bitton E (2018) AUGS best practice statement on evaluation of obstructed defecation. Fem Pelvic Med Reconstr Surg 24:383–391

Santucci RA (2018) Urethral complications after transgender phalloplasty: strategies to treat them and minimize their occurrence. Clin Anat 31(2):187–190. https://doi.org/10.1002/ca.23021

Smits RM, Mackenzie-Proctor R, Yazdani A, Stankiewicz MT, Jordan V, Showell MG (2019) Antioxidants for male subfertility. Cochrane Database Syst Rev 3

Society of Urologic Nurses and Associates (2013) Urologic nursing: scope and standards of practice, 2nd edn. Society of Urologic Nurses and Associates, Pitman, NJ

The Guardian (2008) Ten years on: it's time to count the cost of the Viagra revolution. https://www.theguardian.com/theobserver/2008/feb/24/controversiesinscience

Thirumalai A, Ceponis J, Amory JK, Swerdloff R, Surampudi V, Liu PY, Bremner WJ, Harvey E, Blithe DL, Lee MS, Hull L, Wang C, Page ST (2019) Effects of 28 days of oral dimethandrolone undecanoate in healthy men: a prototype pale pill. J Clin Endocrinol Metab 104(2):423–432

Van Der Sluis WB et al (2016) Clinical characteristics and management of neovaginal fistulas after vaginoplasty in transgender women. Obstet Gynecol 127:1118–1126

Vanderbilt (2017) Tennessee men's health report card. https://www.vanderbilt.edu/crmh/2017TNMensHealthReportCard.pdf

Vogel JD et al (2016) Clinical practice guideline for the management of anorectal abscess, fistula-in-ano, and rectovaginal fistula. Dis Colon Rectum 59:1117–1133

Wang H, Dwyer-Lindgren L, Lofgren KT, Rajaratnam JK, Marcus JR, Levin-Rector A et al (2012) Age-specific and sex-specific mortality in 187 countries, 1970–2010: a systematic analysis for the Global Burden of Disease Study 2010. Lancet 380:2071–2094

WHO (1948) Definition of Health.html. Preamble to the Constitution of the World Health Organization as adopted by the International Health Conference, New York, 19–22 June 1946; signed on 22 July 1946 by the representatives of 61 States (Official Records of the World Health Organization, no. 2, p. 100) and entered into force on 7 April 1948. http://www.who.int/about/definition/en/print

Winters BR, Walsh TJ (2014) The epidemiology of male infertility. Urol Clin 41(1):195–204

World Professional Association for Transgender Health (WPATH) (2012) WPATH standards of care. Int J Transgender 13:165–232

Zegers-Hochschild F, Adamson GD, de Mouzon J, Ishihara O, Mansour R, Nygren K et al (2009) (2009). International Committee for Monitoring Assisted Reproductive Technology (ICMART) and the World Health Organization (WHO) revised glossary of ART terminology, 2009. Fertil Steril 92:1520–1524

Printed in the United States
By Bookmasters